D0221462

PREVENTIVE CARDIOLOGY

NOTICE

Medicine is an ever-changing science. As new research and clinical experience broaden our knowledge, changes in treatment and drug therapy are required. The editors and the publisher of this work have checked with sources believed to be reliable in their efforts to provide information that is complete and generally in accord with the standards accepted at the time of publication. However, in view of the possibility of human error or changes in medical sciences, neither the editors nor the publisher nor any other party who has been involved in the preparation or publication of this work warrants that the information contained herein is in every respect accurate or complete, and they are not responsible for any errors or omissions or for the results obtained from use of such information. Readers are encouraged to confirm the information contained herein with other sources. For example and in particular, readers are advised to check the product information sheet included in the package of each drug they plan to administer to be certain that the information contained in this book is accurate and that changes have not been made in the recommended dose or in the contraindications for administration. This recommendation is of particular importance in connection with new or infrequently used drugs.

PREVENTIVE CARDIOLOGY

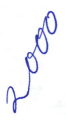

Editor-in-Chief

NATHAN D. WONG, Ph.D., F.A.C.C.

Associate Professor
Director, Heart Disease Prevention Program
Division of Cardiology, College of Medicine, University of California,
Irvine, California, and
Department of Epidemiology, School of Public Health, University of California,
Los Angeles, California

Associate Editors

HENRY R. BLACK, M.D., F.A.C.P.

Charles J. and Margaret Roberts Professor and Chair
Department of Preventive Medicine
Rush University College of Medicine
Chicago, Illinois

JULIUS M. GARDIN, M.D., F.A.C.C., F.A.C.P.

Professor of Medicine, Division of Cardiology, College of Medicine, and
Professor of Electrical and Computer Engineering
University of California, Irvine, California
Past President, American Society of Echocardiography

McGraw-Hill
Health Professions Division
New York   St. Louis   San Francisco   Auckland   Bogotá   Caracas   Lisbon
London   Madrid   Mexico City   Milan   Montreal   New Delhi   San Juan
Singapore   Sydney   Tokyo   Toronto

McGraw-Hill

A Division of The **McGraw·Hill** *Companies*

PREVENTIVE CARDIOLOGY

Copyright © 2000 by The McGraw-Hill Companies, Inc. All
rights reserved. Printed in the United States of America.
Except as permitted under the United States Copyright Act of
1976, no part of this publication may be reproduced or
distributed in any form or by any means, or stored in a data
base or retrieval system, without the prior written permission
of the publisher.

1 2 3 4 5 6 7 8 9 0 DOCDOC 9 9

ISBN 0-07-071856-3

This book was set in Times Roman by York Graphic
Services, Inc.
The editors were Darlene B. Cooke, Susan R. Noujaim,
and Lester A. Sheinis.
The production supervisor was Catherine H. Saggese.
The cover designer was Patrice Fodero Sheridan.
The indexer was Barbara Littlewood.
R.R. Donnelley and Sons Company was printer and
binder.

This book is printed on acid-free paper.

Library of Congress Cataloging-in-Publication Data

Preventive Cardiology / editors, Nathan D.
  Wong, Henry R. Black, Julius M. Gardin.
      p.   cm.
  Includes bibliographical references and index.
    ISBN 0-07-071856-3
    1. Heart—Diseases—Prevention.   2. Heart—Diseases—Epidemiology.
  3. Heart—Diseases—Risk Factors.   I. Wong, Nathan D.   II. Black.
  Henry R. (Henry Richard), date.   III. Gardin, Julius M.
    [DNLM: 1. Heart Diseases—prevention & control.   2. Preventive
  Medicine—methods.   3. Risk Factors.   WG 210 P8955 2000]
  RC682.P69   2000
  616.1′205—dc21
  DNLM/DLC
  for Library of Congress   99-34769
                                                  CIP

WG
210
P9441
2000

TO

Mia, my loving wife, and Don and Lunny, my devoted parents

NDW

Hallie, Matthew, and Dana for all their support these many years

HRB

My beloved wife, Susan, a woman of valor, and our three jewels—Adam, Tova, and Margot

JMG

AND

To all those who have in this century dedicated and will in the next millennium dedicate themselves to understanding the causes of and the mission to prevent and reduce the burden of cardiovascular diseases throughout the world

Contents

Contributors

Wilbert S. Aronow, M.D. [17]*
Medical Director
Hebrew Hospital Home
Adjunct Professor of Medicine
Mount Sinai School of Medicine
New York, New York

David R. Baines, M.D. [21]
Medical Director
Kamiah Health Center
Kamiah, Idaho

Stanley L. Bassin, Ed.D. [12, 19]
Professor
Department of Physical Education
California Polytechnic University
Pomona, California, and
Clinical Professor of Medicine
Division of Cardiology
College of Medicine
University of California
Irvine, California

Ronny A. Bell, Ph.D., M.S. [2]
Assistant Professor of Public Health Sciences
Department of Public Health Sciences
Wake Forest University School of Medicine
Wake Forest, North Carolina

Henry R. Black, M.D. [24]
Charles J. and Margaret Roberts Professor and Chair
Department of Preventive Medicine
Rush Medical College
Chicago, Illinois

George L. Blackburn, M.D., Ph.D. [10]
Associate Professor of Surgery
Beth Israel Deaconess Medical Center
Harvard Medical School
Boston, Massachusetts

Robert D. Brook, M.D. [23]
Fellow, Hypertension Division

*Numbers in brackets refer to chapters written or cowritten by the contributors.

University of Michigan School of Medicine
Ann Arbor, Michigan

Gregory L. Burke, M.D., M.S. [2]
Professor and Interim Chair
Department of Public Health Sciences
Wake Forest University School of Medicine
Wake Forest, North Carolina

Michael H. Criqui, M.D., M.P.H. [3]
Professor
Department of Family and Community Medicine and
Department of Medicine
University of California
San Diego School of Medicine
San Diego, California

Dennis M. Davidson, M.D. [16]
Clinical Professor of Medicine
Division of Cardiology
College of Medicine
University of California
Irvine, California

Prakash C. Deedwania, M.D. [20]
Chief, Division of Cardiology
VAMC/UCSF Program at Fresno
Fresno, California
Professor of Medicine
University of California
San Francisco, California

Robert C. Detrano, M.D., Ph.D. [3]
Professor of Medicine
Division of Cardiology
Harbor-UCLA Medical Center
UCLA School of Medicine
Torrance, California

Terence M. Doherty, B.A. [3]
Cardiovascular Technician
Division of Cardiology
Harbor-UCLA Medical Center
UCLA School of Medicine
Torrance, California

Charles K. Francis, M.D. [18]
President
Charles Drew University of Medicine and Science
University of California
Los Angeles, California

Gail C. Frank, Dr.P.H., R.D., C.H.E.S. [13]
Professor of Nutrition
Department of Family and Consumer Sciences
California State University
Long Beach, California
Adjunct Professor of Pediatrics
Department of Pediatrics
College of Medicine
University of California
Irvine, California

Julius M. Gardin, M.D. [4, 24]
Professor of Medicine
Division of Cardiology
College of Medicine, and
Professor of Electrical and Computer Engineering
University of California
Irvine, California

Philip Greenland, M.D. [23]
Harry W. Dingman Professor
Chair, Department of Preventive Medicine
Professor of Medicine (Cardiology)
Northwestern University Medical School
Chicago, Illinois

Rajeev Gupta, M.D. [20]
Head, Department of Medicine
Director of Research
Monilek Hospital and Research Centre
Jaipur, India

Victoria C. Hammonds, M.D. [6]
Fellow, Division of Geriatrics
Case Western Reserve University School of Medicine
Cleveland, Ohio

Paul N. Hopkins, M.D. [5]
Associate Professor of Medicine
Cardiovascular Genetics Research Clinic
University of Utah School of Medicine
Salt Lake City, Utah

Steven C. Hunt, Ph.D. [5]
Professor of Medicine
Cardiovascular Genetics Research Clinic
University of Utah School of Medicine
Salt Lake City, Utah

William B. Kannel, M.D., M.P.H. [1]
Professor of Medicine and Public Health
Boston University School of Medicine
Head, Visiting Scientist Program
Framingham Heart Study
Framingham, Massachusetts

Jennifer Kaseta, M.D. [8]
Fellow, Division of Endocrinology and Hypertension
Wayne State University
School of Medicine
Detroit, Michigan
(Currently Clinical Instructor, Department of Medicine
University of Michigan School of Medicine, Ann
Arbor, Michigan)

Moti L. Kashyap, M.D. [7]
Director
Cholesterol Clinic
Veterans Affairs Medical Center
Long Beach, California
Professor of Medicine
College of Medicine
University of California
Irvine, California

Penny M. Kris-Etherton, Ph.D., R.D. [13]
Distinguished Professor of Nutrition
Nutrition Department
The Pennsylvania State University
University Park, Pennsylvania

Harry A. Lando, Ph.D. [9]
Professor of Epidemiology
Division of Epidemiology
University of Minnesota School of Public Health
Minneapolis, Minnesota

Marian C. Limacher, M.D. [15]
Professor of Medicine
Division of Cardiovascular Medicine
University of Florida College of Medicine
Gainesville, Florida

Russell V. Luepker, M.D. [9]
Professor of Epidemiology and Medicine
Division of Epidemiology
University of Minnesota School of Public Health
Minneapolis, Minnesota

Alice G. Luten, Ph.D. [14]
Assistant Professor, Section of Epidemiology
Department of Preventive Medicine
Rush–Presbyterian–St. Luke's Medical Center
Rush Medical College
Chicago, Illinois

Karen C. McCowen, M.B., M.R.C.P.I. [10]
Instructor in Medicine
Beth Israel Deaconess Medical Center
Harvard Medical School
Boston, Massachusetts

Keith C. Norris, M.D. [18]
Professor of Medicine
Division of Nephrology
Department of Medicine
Charles Drew University of Medicine and Science
University of California
Los Angeles, California

Thomas A. Pearson, M.D., M.P.H., Ph.D. [22]
Albert D. Kaiser Professor and Chair
Department of Community and Preventive Medicine
University of Rochester School of Medicine
Rochester, New York

Lynda H. Powell, Ph.D. [14]
Director, Section of Epidemiology
Associate Professor of Preventive Medicine and
    Psychology
Rush–Presbyterian–St. Luke's Medical Center
Rush Medical College
Chicago, Illinois

Paul M. Ridker, M.D. [11]
Associate Professor of Medicine
Division of Cardiology, Department of Medicine
Brigham and Women's Hospital
Harvard Medical School
Boston, Massachusetts

Geeta Sikand, M.S., R.D. [13]
Assistant Clinical Professor of Medicine
Division of Cardiology,
College of Medicine
University of California
Irvine, California

James R. Sowers, M.D. [8]
Professor of Medicine
Division of Endocrinology and Hypertension
Wayne State University School of Medicine
Detroit, Michigan

Elaine J. Stone, Ph.D. [16]
Health Scientist Administrator
Division of Epidemiology and Clinical Applications
National Heart, Lung and Blood Institute
National Institutes of Health
Bethesda, Maryland

Cynthia Iftner Traum, M.S., R.D. [16]
Project Manager
Kaiser Permanente
Oakland, California

Roger R. Williams, M.D. [5]*
Professor of Medicine
Cardiovascular Genetics Research Clinic
University of Utah School of Medicine
Salt Lake City, Utah

Nathan D. Wong, Ph.D. [3, 4, 7, 11, 12, 16, 24]
Director, Heart Disease Prevention Program
Associate Professor
Division of Cardiology
College of Medicine, University of California, and
Department of Epidemiology, School of Public Health
University of California
Los Angeles, California

Jackson T. Wright, M.D., Ph.D. [6]
Professor of Medicine
Director, Clinical Hypertension Program
Department of Medicine
Case Western Reserve University School of Medicine
Cleveland, Ohio

Lily L. Wu, Ph.D. [5]
Associate Professor of Medicine
Cardiovascular Genetics Research Clinic
University of Utah School of Medicine
Salt Lake City, Utah

*Deceased.

Foreword

This comprehensive text, *Preventive Cardiology,* is indeed timely. It can help meet an important challenge, fundamentally strategic in nature:

The decades-long effort to control the epidemic of coronary heart disease (CHD) in the United States has apparently stalled after years of progress. It seems we are at a watershed, and the outcome for the next phase remains to be determined.

From the mid-1960s through the 1980s, CHD (and stroke) mortality rates declined steadily and substantially. This advance involved all adult age strata, men and women, all regions of the country, and all ethnic and socioeconomic groups (although it was smaller among the less educated and affluent). Correspondingly, since the major cardiovascular diseases (CVD) have been responsible for a majority of all adult deaths, the CVD downtrend produced a decline in all causes of mortality and an increase in life expectancy.

But in the 1990s the favorable CHD mortality trend slowed, and the decline in stroke mortality ceased. Will this adverse pattern of the 1990s persist? Even get worse? Will the CHD-CVD death rates increase again, as they did earlier in the century? Or can the interruption in the downtrend be halted and the declines be made to resume and accelerate? This is the strategic challenge as we enter the new century—to get this trend back on track, and keep it there.

This is vital for the decade ahead, both to achieve national health goals for the year 2010 and to position us to tackle the "bottom line" objective of not only curbing but also *ending the CHD-CVD epidemic* well before midcentury. Population-wide practical and effective CHD-CVD prevention, particularly primary prevention, and most particularly *primordial prevention*—the primary prevention of the major risk factors responsible for the epidemic—is of the essence in regard to these goals. Hence the relevance and potential importance of this text.

The unfavorable CHD-CVD mortality trend of the 1990s developed despite multiple advances in clinical treatment for patients with acute CHD or with major CHD risk factors (e.g., high blood pressure, hypercholesterolemia)—coronary artery bypass surgery, coronary angioplasty, antithrombotic and thrombolytic drugs, antihypertensives, statins, etc. Trials have demonstrated that these interventions improve prognosis for CHD patients and for the coronary-prone, and the results have been widely applied by practitioners. Interventional cardiology has become a new subspecialty. And it has been implied that in this high-tech era, further development and application of these secondary preventive, high-risk strategies are all that is needed to curb the CHD epidemic, i.e., the basic concept of the 1960s and 1970s—population-wide primary prevention is an essential strategic thrust to control epidemic CHD—may now be "old hat."

But critical scrutiny of recent data compels a different conclusion: First of all, despite all the progress, sudden death (usually out-of-hospital and unattended) with first heart attack remains a common problem resistant to high-tech approaches. And acute death (30-day mortality) with first heart attacks in persons not dying suddenly has proven to be only partially amenable to modern treatment. In fact, review of data from treatment trials in patients at high risk or with CHD reveals a downside generally left unmentioned amidst the emphasis on favorable effects of the newer interventions: Invariably, despite the benefits from the newer treatments, morbidity and mortality risks for these patients remain greater, and years of life expectancy remain fewer, than for people at low risk thanks to favorable status for all major CHD-CVD risk factors. This is the case, for example, for long-term prognosis of myocardial infarction (MI) patients treated in-hospital with thrombolytics, for patients with high blood pressure treated with antihypertensives, and for patients with above-optimal serum cholesterol treated with statins. The problem is not with the interventions, all of them important advances. The problem is the pathobiology of the underlying disease, severe atherosclerosis. Once the heart is damaged, there is no cure, no return to *status quo ante*; there is only palliation, amelioration, and slowing and avoidance of further progression. Even for higher-risk persons without clinical evidence yet of CHD-CVD, it is not possible fully to overcome the decades-long adverse effects of exposure to above-optimal blood pressure, above-optimal serum cholesterol, the adverse lifestyles—especially dietary patterns—playing a major causative role in the epidemic occurrence of these established major risk factors. And, correspondingly, long-term adverse effects of smoking, sedentary habits, diabetes, and obesity are also reversible only in part by the interventions for high-risk and already-afflicted adults. Valuable though they are, these interventions—given the pathobiology of the disease—are at that point little and late, however high tech.

Thus, the fundamental strategy—set down 30 years ago—remains valid and critically important:

> . . . a strategy of primary prevention of premature atherosclerotic diseases be adopted as long-term national policy for the United States and to implement this strategy adequate resources of money and manpower be committed to accomplish:
>
> a. Changes in diet to prevent or control hyperlipidemia, obesity, hypertension and diabetes.
> b. Elimination of cigarette smoking.
> c. Pharmacologic control of elevated blood pressure.

(Recommendations for the Primary Prevention of the Atherosclerotic Diseases, Inter-Society Commission for Heart Disease Resources, *Circulation* 1970.[1])

That strategy has been U.S. policy for many years. Three comments are in order here, by way of update, based on experiences in the effort to implement this strategy, and relevant research data accrued since 1970:

1. Epidemic CHD-CVD is absent among the small proportion (<10 percent) of young adult and middle-aged Americans with favorable levels for *all* quickly measurable major risk factors, i.e., men and women with serum cholesterol <200 mg/dL and systolic/diastolic blood pressure (SBP/DBP) ≤120/≤80 mmHg, who are also nonsmokers, not diabetic, and free of prior MI history.[2] Their long-term CHD-CVD mortality rates are a small proportion of mortality from all causes; all causes of death rates are low, i.e., about half those of all other persons of corresponding age and gender; their life expectancy is greater by several years.

   These facts underscore and refine the foregoing strategy: The need is not only to prevent and control high levels of the major risk factors, but it is also to achieve *favorable levels of all these traits* concurrently for more and more people, so that low-risk status becomes commonplace throughout the population. That is, the need is for primordial prevention of all the adverse lifestyles and lifestyle-related risk factors producing the CHD-CVD epidemic—primordial prevention from conception and weaning on, by mass improvement in lifestyles.

   While the national policy is population-wide primary prevention, there is as yet no commitment to population-wide primordial prevention—by the federal government, the American Heart Association, the American College of Cardiology, or other professional organizations. This policy matter—on the key component of strategy for ending the CHD-CVD epidemic—needs attention and action.

2. Scientifically, all the essential knowledge is in hand to enable adoption and implementation of this policy. Thus, for decades, it has been known that population serum cholesterol-lipid levels can be favorably influenced by nutritional-hygienic means, i.e., lower intake of saturated fats and cholesterol; higher intake of unsaturated fats (mono-and poly-) and water-soluble fiber; favorable calorie balance (to prevent and correct obesity). Public and professional education, particularly on dietary lipid composition, has led to favorable population-wide trends in this area, and average serum cholesterol of adults has declined from 1950 to 1960 levels of about 235 to 240 mg/dL to 200 to 205 mg/dL nowadays, i.e., within hailing distance of the national goal of no more than

200 mg/dL, showing what can be done. (All this, despite a steady increase in population body mass—a challenge for preventive cardiology.)

Research advances of the late 1980s and 1990s on nutrition and blood pressure make clear that multiple improvements in dietary pattern can favorably influence this major risk factor as well. These encompass lower salt intake, avoidance of high alcohol consumption, increased potassium ingestion, favorable calorie balance, and the several components of the Dietary Approaches to Stop Hypertension (DASH) clinical trial combination diet, i.e., increased intake of fruits, vegetables, fat-free and low-fat dairy products, and reduced consumption of total fat, saturated fat, and cholesterol. Note the concordance between the dietary recommendations for favorable plasma cholesterol-lipid and blood pressure levels.

With effective implementation and adoption of these recommendations, it is reasonable to expect lower population-wide average levels of serum cholesterol and SBP/DBP in youth and young adulthood, and little or no rise with age (contrary to the present situation). That is, with improved norms of human behavior, favorable levels—low-risk levels—can become the rule throughout adulthood, for all strata of the population, rather than the exception. The same holds for the other traits contributing to the epidemic—obesity, sedentary habits, and smoking.

3. To achieve these goals, both the long-term policy commitment and mobilization of resources are needed, as the 1970 statement noted.[1] To date, "resources of money and manpower" for population-wide CHD-CVD primary prevention, particularly primordial prevention, have been modest. This is so when the reckoning includes the total commitment of all agencies (official, voluntary, professional). Given the present-day challenge, the opportunities, and the potential benefits for all population strata, it is reasonable to say at this juncture that they are insufficient, by several orders of magnitude. This is a key aspect of policy also requiring attention.

This is being written on the eve of an NHLBI-sponsored "National Conference on CVD Prevention: Meeting the Healthy People Objectives for Cardiovascular Health"—a Conference mandated by the U.S. Congress—aiming to address these matters, overall, and in regard to the socioeconomic and ethnic strata of the population with more adverse lifestyles, risk factor patterns, and CHD-CVD rates. So this is indeed a "right" moment for *Preventive Cardiology*.

References

1. Inter-Society Commission for Heart Disease Resources, Atherosclerosis Study Group and Epidemiology Study Group: Primary prevention of the atherosclerotic diseases. *Circulation* 1970;42:A55–A95.
2. Stamler J, Stamler R, Neaton JD, et al: Relationship of baseline low risk factor profile to long-term cardiovascular and non-cardiovascular mortality and to life expectancy: findings for five large cohorts of young adult and middle-aged men and women. *JAMA* 1999, in press.

Jeremiah Stamler, M.D.
Professor Emeritus
Northwestern University Medical School
Chicago, Illinois

Preface

In *Preventive Cardiology,* we seek to provide the reader with a practical approach toward understanding the etiology of coronary artery disease, as well as novel and standard approaches to its identification and prevention. Unique to this text are the significant materials for the health care provider relating to the identification and management of key risk factors, dietary, physical activity, and behavioral strategies, and to the development of a preventive cardiology clinic. Distinctive aspects of the book include its detailed discussion of screening for risk factors for cardiovascular disease, the most current clinical guidelines for the management of these risk factors, and noninvasive techniques for measuring subclinical disease—a modifiable state beyond the presence of risk factors, but prior to clinical manifestations. Other chapters provide detailed discussion on nutritional approaches and counseling, physical activity recommendations, evaluation and management of psychosocial factors, and screening for genetic factors that may predispose to cardiovascular risk. The book also provides separate chapters regarding the prevention of heart disease in special populations—

women, the elderly, children and adolescents, and specific ethnic groups, including African Americans, Hispanic Americans, Asians (including South Asians) and Pacific Islanders, and Native Americans. The last section of the book concentrates on practical strategies for the primary and secondary prevention of cardiovascular diseases and approaches to setting up a preventive cardiology clinic.

We give special thanks to our contributors for their devoted efforts, without which this text would not be possible. We also thank our students and colleagues for their inspiration, among which will emerge tomorrow's leaders of the field.

This text would not have been possible without the efforts and dedication of Susan Noujaim, Catherine Saggese, Lester Sheinis, Darlene B. Cooke, and Martin Wonsiewicz of McGraw-Hill.

Finally, we wish to acknowledge the support of our families and the many sacrifices they have made to make this text possible. Our wives remain our greatest support and strength: Mia K. Wong, Hallie Black, and Dr. Susan Gardin.

Part I

Epidemiology

Epidemiologic Contributions to Preventive Cardiology and Challenges for the Twenty-First Century

William B. Kannel

Epidemiologic research conducted over the past five decades has contributed to an explosive expansion of knowledge regarding the natural history of cardiovascular disease (CVD). This research has provided significant information that has helped public health workers, scientists, physicians, and researchers increase their understanding of the factors predisposing to the occurrence of cardiovascular disease. These have come to be known as *risk factors*, a term coined by the Framingham Heart Study.[1] Identification of these modifiable risk factors helped stimulate an interest in preventive cardiology worldwide and has made cardiovascular epidemiology the basic science of preventive cardiology. The increased awareness of the major cardiovascular risk factors promulgated by the Framingham Heart Study and corroborated by other investigators encouraged public health initiatives against smoking in the 1960s, hypertension in the 1970s, and hypercholesterolemia in the 1980s.[2]

The initiation of epidemiologic research exploring the evolution of CVD was stimulated by a mounting epidemic of CVD in the 1930s through the 1950s, such that it became the leading cause of death in 1949, accounting for half of all deaths. The U.S. Public Health Service decided to explore the problem, seeking out modifiable predisposing conditions using an epidemiologic approach, which, at the time, was a novel concept.[3] This entailed long-term prospective observational investigation of suspected host and environmental factors that might be expected to promote cardiovascular disease in a representative general population sample.

The population approach used provided a less distorted appraisal of the evolution of cardiovascular disease than was obtained from clinical studies subject to selection bias. It soon became apparent that coronary heart disease (CHD) is an extremely common and highly lethal disease that attacks one in five persons before they attain 60 years of age, that women lag men in incidence by 20 years, and that sudden death is a prominent feature of CHD. One in every six coronary attacks was found to present with sudden death as the first, last, and only symptom.[4] It also became evident that the disease can be asymptomatic in its most severe form, with one in three myocardial infarctions going unrecognized because it is either silent or atypical.[5] Because of this clinical profile, a preventive approach seemed essential. Fortunately, epidemiologic research was able to identify a number of modifiable predisposing factors, making it possible to identify high-risk candidates for preventive measures long in advance of the appearance of symptoms.

Misconceptions Corrected

Before epidemiologic research examined the relationship of hypertension to CVD, it was believed that the common variety of hypertension was a benign condition and that it was essential that the blood pressure rise with age to ensure adequate perfusion of the tissues as the arterioles narrowed.[6,7] All of the cardiovascular sequelae were thought to derive from the diastolic blood pressure and it was held that the disproportionate rise in systolic blood pressure as age advanced was an innocuous accompaniment of arterial stiffening.[6,7] Further, it was believed that treatment of isolated systolic hypertension would not only be fruitless but also produce intolerable and dangerous side effects. Women were thought to tolerate hypertension well, and it was believed that normal blood pressures in both sexes were substantially higher in the elderly than in the middle-aged.

It took epidemiologic research to convince the skeptical that serum cholesterol was a true risk factor for CHD, that the lipoprotein-cholesterol fractions were fundamental to atherogenesis, and that diets rich in saturated fat and cholesterol—presumed to be healthy—promoted dyslipidemia and its cardiovascular sequelae.[8] Population research established that HDL cholesterol was actually a strong independent risk factor inversely related to the development of CHD.[9,10] Epidemiologic research was required to demonstrate that cigarette smoking was not only a carcinogen for lung cancer but also a substantial risk factor for atherosclerotic CVD. Population research has established that smoking is a major risk factor for CHD, precipitating coronary attacks and sudden deaths, especially in high-risk coronary candidates. Epidemiologic research has shown that the risk of coronary attacks could be promptly halved in smokers who quit, regardless of how long or how much they previously smoked.[11,12] Before epidemiologic investigation, physical exercise was considered dangerous for CHD candidates. Population research has established that physical activity is actually protective. There was skepticism about the importance of obesity as a risk factor for CVD, but this has been dispelled by epidemiologic research demonstrating that it promotes all the major cardiovascular risk factors. Left ventricular hypertrophy was shown to be an ominous harbinger of CVD rather than an incidental compensatory response to hypertension, CHD, and valve deformity.[13]

Before prospective epidemiologic investigation was performed to determine how those who devel-

oped atherosclerotic CVD differed from those who escaped it, it was held that a single etiology would be found to be essential and, in most instances, sufficient to produce the pathology. However, five decades of epidemiologic research have indicated that atherosclerotic disease is distinctly multifactorial, giving rise to the risk-factor concept. Certain living habits promote atherogenic traits in genetically susceptible persons. After prolonged exposure, these result in a compromised circulation, leading to clinical events. Thus, atherosclerotic cardiovascular disease is now regarded as a multifactorial process involving a variety of predisposing risk factors, each of which is best considered as an ingredient of a cardiovascular risk profile.[14–18]

Cardiovascular Risk Profiles

A preventive approach to atherosclerotic CVD is feasible and justified, because once clinically manifest, the disease is apt to be progressive and often lethal, and the patient can seldom be cured or restored to full function. Prevention is now feasible because epidemiologic research has identified a number of modifiable predisposing lifestyles and personal attributes that, when corrected, have been shown to reduce the likelihood of the development of clinical atherosclerotic CVD.[19–21] To cost-effectively evaluate candidates for the major cardiovascular events, multivariate risk profiles have been formulated; these facilitate targeting those at high risk for preventive measures.[14–18] The American Heart Association (AHA) Task Force on Risk Reduction[22] recently emphasized the importance of these risk profiles for motivating as well as reassuring patients and in assisting in selection of therapy. They concluded that these scores direct health care professionals to look at the whole patient and to recognize the cumulative nature of risk factors.

A half century of epidemiologic research at the Framingham Heart Study and elsewhere have identified a number of major cardiovascular risks that have a strong independent impact on the rate of development of the major atherosclerotic CVD.[20] These risk factors can be readily ascertained from ordinary office procedures and formulated into a predictive risk profile.[14-18] The Framingham Heart Study and others have identified and quantified several classes of cardiovascular risk factors—including atherosclerotic personal attributes, lifestyles that promote risk, signs of organ damage, and innate susceptibility. Those easy to ascertain during an office visit are a cigarette smoking history, blood lipids, glucose intolerance, blood pressure, and left ventricular hypertrophy as seen on the electrocardiogram.[20,21]

All the major established risk factors were shown to contribute powerfully and significantly to CHD risk (Table 1–1). For atherothrombotic brain infarction, the relevant factors are hypertension, left ventricular hypertrophy, and diabetes, but dyslipidemia appears to play a minor role (Table 1–2). For peripheral artery disease, glucose intolerance, cigarette smoking, and left ventricular hypertrophy are the most influential factors (Table 1–3). For heart failure, important factors are hypertension, diabetes, and reduced vital capacity, whereas total cholesterol appears unrelated (Table 1–4).

The standard risk factors were shown to influence CVD rates with different strengths in men and women. Diabetes was shown to operate more powerfully in women, eliminating their advantage over men for most atherosclerotic cardiovascular events.[23,24] Cigarette smoking was found to be more influential in men.

Some of the standard risk factors—including glucose intolerance, smoking, dyslipidemia, and hypertension—tend to have lower risk ratios in advanced age, causing some to question the relevance of risk factors in later life. However, this reduced relative risk has been shown to be offset by a higher absolute incidence of disease and a large excess risk in advanced age. Thus, the standard risk factors continue to be important in the elderly. Atherosclerotic cardiovascular events in the heart, brain, and limbs can now be predicted from epidemiologic data.[14-18]

Clinical categorical risk assessments according to the number of arbitrarily defined abnormalities present can identify high-risk persons, but epidemiologic research has pointed out that this approach tends to overlook persons at high risk because of multiple marginal abnormalities. Identification for treatment of persons with several borderline risk-factor values is important because such persons have a high risk and produce most of the cardiovascular events in the general population.

TABLE 1–1 Risk of Coronary Heart Disease According to Standard Risk Factors: Framingham Heart Study—36-Year Follow-up

	Age 35–64 Years				Age 65–94 Years			
	Age-Adjusted Biennial Rate per 1000		Age-Adjusted Relative Risk		Age-Adjusted Biennial Rate per 1000		Age-Adjusted Relative Risk	
Factors	Men	Women	Men	Women	Men	Women	Men	Women
Cholesterol ≥240 mg/dL	34	15	1.9*	1.8†	59	39	1.2‡	2.0*
Hypertension ≥140/90 mmHg	45	21	2.0*	2.2*	73	44	1.6†	1.9*
Diabetes	39	42	1.5*	3.7*	79	62	1.6†	2.1*
ECG-LVH	79	55	3.0*	4.6*	134	94	2.7*	3.0*
Smoking	33	13	1.5†	1.1	53	38	1.0	1.2

*$p < .001$.
†$p < .01$.
‡$p < .05$.

Source: From Kannel WB, Wilson PWF: Comparison of risk profiles for cardiovascular events: implications for prevention. *Adv Intern Med* 1997; 42:39–66, with permission.

TABLE 1–2 Risk of Atherosclerotic Brain Infarction According to Standard Risk Factors: Framingham Heart Study—36-Year Follow-up

	Age 35–64 Years				Age 65–94 Years			
	Age-Adjusted Biennial Rate per 1000		Age-Adjusted Relative Risk		Age-Adjusted Biennial Rate per 1000		Age-Adjusted Relative Risk	
Factors	Men	Women	Men	Women	Men	Women	Men	Women
Cholesterol ≥240 mg/dL	3	2	1.0	1.1	10	12	1.0	1.0
Hypertension ≥140/90 mmHg	7	4	5.7*	4.0*	20	17	2.0*	2.6*
Diabetes	7	4	3.0†	2.4‡	20	28	1.6	2.9*
ECG-LVH	13	13	5.1*	8.1*	44	51	3.6*	5.0*
Smoking	4	1	2.5†	1.0	17	20	1.4	1.9*

*$p < .001$.
†$p < .01$.
‡$p < .05$.

Source: From Kannel WB, Wilson PWF: Comparison of risk profiles for cardiovascular events: implications for prevention. *Adv Intern Med* 1997; 42:39–66, with permission.

TABLE 1–3 Risk of Peripheral Artery Disease by Standard Risk Factors: Framingham Heart Study—36-Year Follow-up

	Age 35–64 Years				Age 65–94 Years			
	Age-Adjusted Biennial Rate per 1000		Age-Adjusted Relative Risk		Age-Adjusted Biennial Rate per 1000		Age-Adjusted Relative Risk	
Factors	Men	Women	Men	Women	Men	Women	Men	Women
Cholesterol ≥240 mg/dL	3	2	1.0	1.1	10	12	1.0	1.0
Hypertension ≥140/90 mmHg	7	4	5.7*	4.0*	20	17	2.0*	2.6*
Diabetes	7	4	3.0†	2.4‡	20	28	1.6	2.9*
ECG-LVH	13	13	5.1*	8.1*	44	51	3.6*	5.0*
Smoking	4	1	2.5†	1.0	17	20	1.4	1.9*

*$p < .001$.
†$p < .01$.
‡$p < .05$.

Source: From Kannel WB, Wilson PWF: Comparison of risk profiles for cardiovascular events: implications for prevention. *Adv Intern Med* 1997; 42:39–66, with permission.

TABLE 1–4 **Risk of Cardiac Failure by Standard Risk Factors: Framingham Heart Study—36 Year Follow-up**

	Age 35–64 Years				Age 65–94 Years			
	Age-Adjusted Biennial Rate per 1000		Age-Adjusted Relative Risk		Age-Adjusted Biennial Rate per 1000		Age-Adjusted Relative Risk	
Factors	Men	Women	Men	Women	Men	Women	Men	Women
Cholesterol ≥240 mg/dL	7	4	1.2	1.1	21	18	1.0	1.0
Hypertension ≥140/90 mmHg	14	6	4.0*	3.0*	33	24	1.9*	1.9*
Diabetes	23	21	4.4†	8.0*	40	51	2.0*	3.6*
ECG-LVH	71	36	15.0*	13.0*	99	84	4.9*	5.4*
Smoking	7	3	1.5*	1.1	23	22	1.0	1.3‡

*$p < .001$.
†$p < .01$.
‡$p < .05$.

Source: From Kannel WB, Wilson PWF: Comparison of risk profiles for cardiovascular events: implications for prevention. *Adv Intern Med* 1997; 42:39–66, with permission.

Epidemiologic research has shown that prevention based on individual risk-factor assessment and treatment is inefficient and misleading. This approach often falsely reassures or needlessly alarms potential candidates for cardiovascular disease because the risk of such events for any particular risk factor varies widely depending on the burden of associated risk factors (Fig. 1–1). Another reason for quantitative multivariate risk assessment is the epidemiologically established fact that all the standard risk factors tend to cluster together because they are metabolically linked (Table 1–5). Clusters of three or more risk factors have been shown to occur at four to five times the expected rate.

pendent risk factors (Figs. 1–2 and 1–3).[14–18] A simplified version of the Framingham Heart Study profile for CHD risk allows for classification based on Joint National Committee (JNC)-V blood pressure and National Cholesterol Education Program (NCEP) cholesterol categories in addition to age, HDL cholesterol, diabetes, and smoking.[18] The risk of developing CHD increases with the burden of these risk factors, depending on the intensity of exposure to them. The risk-factor score corresponds to the probability of a coronary event over a specified interval of time. These estimated event rates can be compared with the average risk for persons of the same age, providing absolute and relative risk estimates.

Coronary Risk Profile

Prevention of CHD by risk-factor control deserves a high priority because the incidence of CHD equals that of all the other atherosclerotic cardiovascular sequelae combined (Table 1–6). Multivariate formulations for quantifying risk of developing CHD have been developed from Framingham Heart Study data that enable physicians to estimate their patients' probability of an event from a set of established inde-

Stroke Profile

Epidemiologic research has also yielded a risk profile for estimating the risk of developing an atherothrombotic brain infarction, the most common variety of stroke and the most feared of the atherosclerotic sequelae of identified risk factors. The predisposing risk factors and cardiac conditions include the standard risk factors plus atrial fibrillation, CHD, and heart failure (Table 1–7). These independent risk

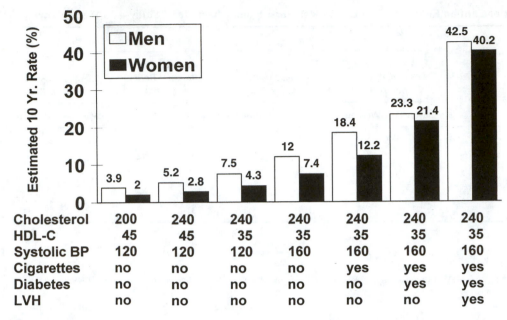

FIGURE 1–1 Incidence of CHD in 42-year-old adults; Framingham Heart Study 1972–1984. *Key:* HDL-C, high-density lipoprotein cholesterol; BP, blood pressure; LVH, left ventricular hypertrophy.

TABLE 1–5   Risk-Factor Clustering of Framingham Offspring, Exam 1—Age 18–74 Years

Index Quintile Variable (sex-specific)	Sex	Number	Distribution of RF Scores (presence in top quintile) [entries in percent]					
			$n = 0$	$n = 1$	$n = 2$	$n = 3$	$n = 4$	$n = 5$
High cholesterol	Men	$n = 505$	29	28	23	15	4	1
	Women	$n = 519$	26	26	23	17	5	2
Low HDL-cholesterol	Men	$n = 501$	27	27	26	14	4	1
	Women	$n = 544$	38	26	18	11	5	2
High BMI	Men	$n = 497$	23	29	27	15	5	1
	Women	$n = 533$	15	31	27	18	7	2
High systolic BP	Men	$n = 530$	25	29	24	16	5	1
	Women	$n = 545$	19	28	26	18	7	2
High triglycerides	Men	$n = 491$	11	28	33	21	6	1
	Women	$n = 522$	20	29	23	18	7	2
High glucose	Men	$n = 477$	23	31	22	17	5	1
	Women	$n = 608$	29	26	21	15	6	2
Expected			33	41	20	5	0.6	0.03

Key: HDL, high-density lipoprotein; BMI, body mass index; BP, blood pressure; RF, risk factor.

TABLE 1-6 Incidence of Major Cardiovascular Events: Framingham Heart Study 40-Year Follow-up*

Age	Cardiovascular Disease (all types)		Coronary Heart Disease		Stroke and Transient Ischemic Attack		Congestive Heart Failure		Peripheral Arterial Disease	
	Men	Women	Men	Women	Men	Women	Men	Women	Men	Women
36–44	5	2	6	1	+	+	+	+	+	+
45–54	15	7	11	4	2	1	2	1	2	1
55–64	28	16	21	11	5	3	6	3	6	3
65–74	39	24	26	14	10	8	9	6	7	4
75–84	59	40	33	19	21	14	19	13	6	4
85–94	73	58	31	22	9	26	28	26	4	1

*Average annual incidence per 1000 persons free of specified disease.
†Results are omitted when fewer than five individuals experience an event.
‡Age-adjusted rates.

factors have been formulated into a stroke risk profile based on Framingham Heart Study data and made available by the AHA.[16] Risk of stroke in persons with any of these risk factors varies widely depending on the number of accompanying risk factors (Fig. 1–4). The risk profile tables that have been developed enable estimates of the joint effect of any combination of the predisposing factors, providing estimates of absolute and relative risks of developing a stroke (Table 1–8).

Peripheral Artery Disease Profile

Population research at the Framingham Heart Study has also produced multivariate risk profiles for the estimation of occurrence of intermittent claudication, the cardinal clinical manifestation of peripheral artery disease.[17] The major cardiovascular risk factors have been shown to predict intermittent claudication better than they predict CHD.[25] Modification of these independent risk factors may reduce the probability of developing peripheral artery disease, and, in turn, improve cardiovascular morbidity and mortality. Using this risk formulation, an individual's probability of developing intermittent claudication can be readily assessed on routine examination and laboratory analysis performed in a physician's office. The risk factors needed, aside from age and sex, are a blood pressure and cholesterol determination, a blood glu-

cose and history of cigarette smoking, and determination of the presence of CHD. As for other atherosclerotic cardiovascular disease outcomes, the risk of intermittent claudication varies over a wide range depending on the burden of the aforementioned risk factors (Fig. 1–5). Cigarette smoking substantially escalates the risk at any level of other risk factors. The multivariate risk formulation enables physicians easily to estimate the probability of developing peripheral artery disease based on data collected as part of a routine examination (Tables 1–9 and 1–10). The risk profile can be used to motivate patients to modify risk factors to avoid not only intermittent claudication but also CHD and stroke.

Heart Failure Profile

Epidemiologic research has pointed out that cardiac failure is a terminal condition with a survival experience little better than that of cancer. Once CHD is clinically overt, the median survival in the Framingham Heart Study subjects with heart failure was only 1.7 years in men and 3.2 years in women; sudden death was a common feature of this mortality.[26] Major independent contributors to the occurrence of heart failure have been identified and quantified by population research; from these, multivariate risk profiles have been formulated that efficiently predict these lethal events and provide estimates of the

STEP 1

Age		
Years	LDL Pts	Chol Pts
30–34	−1	[−1]
35–39	0	[0]
40–44	1	[1]
45–49	2	[2]
50–54	3	[3]
55–59	4	[4]
60–64	5	[5]
65–69	6	[6]
70–74	7	[7]

STEP 2

LDL-C		
(mg/dL)	(mmol/L)	LDL Pts
<100	<2.59	−3
100–129	2.60–3.36	0
130–159	3.37–4.14	0
160–190	4.15–4.92	1
≥190	≥4.92	2

Cholesterol		
(mg/dL)	(mmol/L)	Chol Pts
<160	<4.14	[−3]
160–199	4.15–5.17	[0]
200–239	5.18–6.21	[1]
240–279	6.22–7.24	[2]
≥280	≥7.25	[3]

STEP 3

HDL-C			
(mg/dL)	(mmol/L)	LDL Pts	Chol Pts
<35	<0.90	2	[2]
35–44	0.91–1.16	1	[1]
45–49	1.17–1.29	0	[0]
50–59	1.30–1.55	0	[0]
≥60	≥1.56	−1	[−2]

STEP 4

Blood Pressure					
Systolic (mmHg)	Diastolic (mmHg)				
	<80	80–84	85–89	90–99	≥100
<120	0 [0] pts				
120–129		0 [0] pts			
130–139			1 [1] pts		
140–159				2 [2] pts	
≥160					3 [3] pts

Note: When systolic and diastolic pressures provide different estimates for point scores, use the higher number

STEP 5

Diabetes		
	LDL Pts	Chol Pts
No	0	[0]
Yes	2	[2]

STEP 7 (sum from steps 1–6)

Adding up the Points	
Age	_____
LDL-C or Chol	_____
HDL-C	_____
Blood Pressure	_____
Diabetes	_____
Smoker	_____
Point Total	_____

* Hard CHD events exclude angina pectoris.
+ Low risk was calculated for a person the same age, optimal blood pressure, LDL-C 100–129 mg/dL or cholesterol 160–199 mg/dL, HDL-C 45 mg/dL for men or 55 mg/dL for women, nonsmoker, no diabetes.
  Risk estimates were derived from the experience of the Framingham Heart Study, a predominantly Caucasian population in Massachusetts, USA.

STEP 6

Smoker		
	LDL Pts	Chol Pts
No	0	[0]
Yes	2	[2]

STEP 8 (determine CHD risk from point total)

CHD Risk			
LDL Pts Total	10 Yr CHD Risk	Chol Pts Total	10 Yr CHD Risk
<−3	1%		
−2	2%		
−1	2%	[<−1]	[2%]
0	3%	[0]	[3%]
1	4%	[1]	[3%]
2	4%	[2]	[4%]
3	6%	[3]	[5%]
4	7%	[4]	[7%]
5	9%	[5]	[8%]
6	11%	[6]	[10%]
7	14%	[7]	[13%]
8	18%	[8]	[16%]
9	22%	[9]	[20%]
10	27%	[10]	[25%]
11	33%	[11]	[31%]
12	40%	[12]	[37%]
13	47%	[13]	[45%]
≥14	≥56%	[≥14]	[≥53%]

STEP 9 (compare to average person your age)

Comparative Risk			
Age (years)	Average 10 Yr CHD Risk	Average 10 Yr Hard* CHD Risk	Low+ 10 Yr CHD Risk
30–34	3%	1%	2%
35–39	5%	4%	3%
40–44	7%	4%	4%
45–49	11%	8%	4%
50–54	14%	10%	6%
55–59	16%	13%	7%
60–64	21%	20%	9%
65–69	25%	22%	11%
70–74	30%	25%	14%

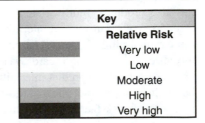

Key	
Relative Risk	
	Very low
	Low
	Moderate
	High
	Very high

FIGURE 1–2 CHD score sheet for men using TC or LDL-C categories. Uses age, TC (or LDL-C), HDL-C, blood pressure, diabetes, and smoking. Estimates risk for CHD over a period of 10 years based on Framingham experience in men 30 to 74 years old at baseline. Average risk estimates are based on typical Framingham subjects and estimates of idealized risk are based on optimal blood pressure, TC 160 to 199 mg/dL (or LDL 100 to 129 mg/dL), HDL-C of 45 mg/dL in men, no diabetes, and no smoking. Use of the LDL-C categories is appropriate when fasting LDL-C measurements are available. Pts indicates points. (From Wilson et al.,[18] with permission.)

STEP 1

Age		
Years	LDL Pts	Chol Pts
30–34	−9	[−9]
35–39	−4	[−4]
40–44	0	[0]
45–49	3	[3]
50–54	6	[6]
55–59	7	[7]
60–64	8	[8]
65–69	8	[8]
70–74	8	[8]

STEP 2

LDL-C		
(mg/dL)	(mmol/L)	LDL Pts
<100	<2.59	−2
100–129	2.60–3.36	0
130–159	3.37–4.14	0
160–190	4.15–4.92	2
≥190	≥4.92	2

Cholesterol		
(mg/dL)	(mmol/L)	Chol Pts
<160	<4.14	[−2]
160–199	4.15–5.17	[0]
200–239	5.18–6.21	[1]
240–279	6.22–7.24	[1]
≥280	≥7.25	[3]

STEP 3

HDL-C			
(mg/dL)	(mmol/L)	LDL Pts	Chol Pts
<35	<0.90	5	[5]
35–44	0.91–1.16	2	[2]
45–49	1.17–1.29	1	[1]
50–59	1.30–1.55	0	[0]
≥60	≥1.56	−2	[−3]

STEP 4

Blood Pressure					
Systolic (mmHg)	Diastolic (mmHg)				
	<80	80–84	85–89	90–99	≥100
<120	−3 [−3] pts				
120–129	0 [0] pts				
130–139		0 [0] pts			
140–159			2 [2] pts		
≥160					3 [3] pts

Note: When systolic and diastolic pressures provide different estimates for point scores, use the higher number

STEP 5

Diabetes		
	LDL Pts	Chol Pts
No	0	[0]
Yes	4	[4]

STEP 7 (sum from steps 1–6)

Adding up the Points	
Age	_____
LDL-C or Chol	_____
HDL-C	_____
Blood Pressure	_____
Diabetes	_____
Smoker	_____
Point Total	_____

* Hard CHD events exclude angina pectoris.
+ Low risk was calculated for a person the same age, optimal blood pressure, LDL-C 100–129 mg/dL or cholesterol 160–199 mg/dL, HDL-C 45 mg/dL for men or 55 mg/dL for women, nonsmoker, no diabetes.

Risk estimates were derived from the experience of the Framingham Heart Study, a predominantly Caucasian population in Massachusetts, USA.

STEP 6

Smoker		
	LDL Pts	Chol Pts
No	0	[0]
Yes	2	[2]

STEP 8 (determine CHD risk from point total)

CHD Risk			
LDL Pts Total	10 Yr CHD Risk	Chol Pts Total	10 Yr CHD Risk
≤−2	1%	[<−2]	[1%]
−1	2%	[−1]	[2%]
0	2%	[0]	[2%]
1	2%	[1]	[2%]
2	3%	[2]	[3%]
3	3%	[3]	[3%]
4	4%	[4]	[4%]
5	5%	[5]	[4%]
6	6%	[6]	[5%]
7	7%	[7]	[6%]
8	8%	[8]	[7%]
9	9%	[9]	[8%]
10	11%	[10]	[10%]
11	13%	[11]	[11%]
12	15%	[12]	[13%]
13	17%	[13]	[15%]
14	20%	[14]	[18%]
15	24%	[15]	[20%]
16	27%	[16]	[24%]
≥17	≥32%	[≥17]	[≥27%]

STEP 9 (compare to average person your age)

Comparative Risk			
Age (years)	Average 10 Yr CHD Risk	Average 10 Yr Hard* CHD Risk	Low+ 10 Yr CHD Risk
30–34	<1%	<1%	<1%
35–39	<1%	<1%	1%
40–44	2%	1%	2%
45–49	5%	2%	3%
50–54	8%	3%	5%
55–59	12%	7%	7%
60–64	12%	8%	8%
65–69	13%	8%	8%
70–74	14%	11%	8%

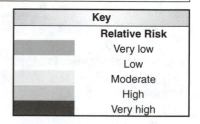

Key	
Relative Risk	
	Very low
	Low
	Moderate
	High
	Very high

FIGURE 1–3 CHD score sheet for women using TC or LDL-C categories. Uses age, TC (or LDL-C), HDL-C, blood pressure, diabetes, and smoking. Estimates risk for CHD over a period of 10 years based on Framingham experience in women 30 to 74 years old at baseline. Average risk estimates are based on typical Framingham subjects and estimates of idealized risk are based on optimal blood pressure, TC 160 to 199 mg/dL (or LDL 100 to 129 mg/dL), HDL-C of 55 mg/dL in men, no diabetes, and no smoking. Use of the LDL-C categories is appropriate when fasting LDL-C measurements are available. Pts indicates points. (From Wilson et al.,[18] with permission.)

TABLE 1–7 Multivariate Risk Factors for Stroke from the Framingham Heart Study—Subjects Aged 55 to 84 Years

Factor	Multivariate Risk Ratio	
	Men	Women
Age (10 years)	1.66	1.93
Systolic blood pressure (10 mmHg)	1.91	1.68
Antihypertensive medication	1.39	—
Diabetes	1.40	1.72
Cigarette smoking	1.67	1.70
Cardiovascular disease	1.68	1.54
Atrial fibrillation	1.83	3.16
Left ventricular hypertrophy	2.32	2.34

Note: Each relative risk is adjusted for the effects of the other risk factors.

Source: Adaped from Wolf et al.,[16] with permission.

risk.[27] The risk relevant factors include electrocardiographic left ventricular hypertrophy, cardiac enlargement on chest x-ray, rapid heart rate, reduced vital capacity, presence of significant heart murmurs, CHD, and systolic blood pressure. Multivariate risk formulations for estimating the probability of developing heart failure from the burden of these risk factors are being devised, based on Framingham Heart Study data.[27] Using such multivariate risk assessments, it will be possible to identify high-risk candidates for heart failure among those with either normal or impaired left ventricular function.

Refinements in Risk Assessment

Further refinements in risk-factor assessment for predicting and controlling atherosclerotic cardiovascu-

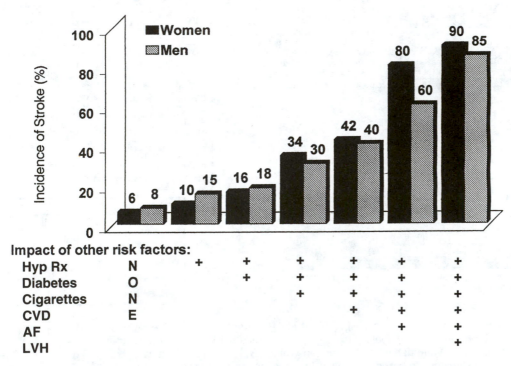

FIGURE 1–4 Probability of stroke (percent) during 10 years in men and women aged 70 years, systolic blood pressure, 160 mmHg. *Key:* Hyp Rx, under antihypertensive therapy; CVD, cardiovascular disease; AF, atrial fibrillation; LVH, left ventricular hypertrophy by electrocardiogram. (From Kannel WB: Blood pressure as a contributor to stroke. *Fed Pract* 1995; Nov suppl:14–20, with permission.)

TABLE 1–8 Stroke Risk Factor Prediction Chart

1. Find Points for Each Risk Factor

Men

Age	SBP	HYP RX	Diabetes	Cigs	CVD	AF	LVH
54 – 56 = 0	95 – 105 = 0	No = 0	No = 0	No = 0	No = 0	No = 0	No = 0
57 – 59 = 1	106 – 116 = 1	Yes = 2	Yes = 2	Yes = 3	Yes = 3	Yes = 4	Yes = 6
60 – 62 = 2	117 – 126 = 2						
63 – 65 = 3	127 – 137 = 3						
66 – 68 = 4	138 – 148 = 4						
69 – 71 = 5	149 – 159 = 5						
72 – 74 = 6	160 – 170 = 6						
75 – 77 = 7	171 – 181 = 7						
78 – 80 = 8	182 – 191 = 8						
81 – 83 = 9	192 – 202 = 9						
84 – 85 = 10	203 – 213 = 10						

Women

Age	SBP	HYP RX	Diabetes	Cigs	CVD	AF	LVH
54 – 56 = 0	95 – 104 = 0	No = 0	No = 0	No = 0	No = 0	No = 0	No = 0
57 – 59 = 1	105 – 114 = 1	If Yes see below	Yes = 3	Yes = 3	Yes = 2	Yes = 6	Yes = 4
60 – 62 = 2	115 – 124 = 2						
63 – 65 = 3	125 – 134 = 3						
66 – 68 = 4	135 – 144 = 4						
69 – 71 = 5	145 – 154 = 5						
72 – 74 = 6	155 – 164 = 6						
75 – 77 = 7	165 – 174 = 7						
78 – 80 = 8	175 – 184 = 8						
81 – 83 = 9	185 – 194 = 9						
84 – 86 = 10	196 – 204 = 10						

If Currently Under Antihypertensive Therapy Add the Following Points Depending on SBP Level

SBP	95–104	105–114	115–124	125–134	135–144	145–154
Points	6	5	5	4	3	3

SBP	155–164	165–174	175–184	185–194	195–204
Points	2	1	1	0	0

2. Sum Points For All Risk Factors:

Age ___ + SBP ___ + HYP RX ___ + Diabetes ___ + CIGS ___ + CVD ___ + AF ___ + LVH ___ = ___ Point Total

3. Look Up Risk Corresponding to Point Total

Men 10 Yr.

Pts.	Prob.	Pts.	Prob.	Pts.	Prob.
1	2.6%	11	11.2%	21	41.7%
2	3.0%	12	12.9%	22	46.6%
3	3.5%	13	14.8%	23	51.8%
4	4.0%	14	17.0%	24	57.3%
5	4.7%	15	19.5%	25	62.8%
6	5.4%	16	22.4%	26	68.4%
7	6.3%	17	25.5%	27	73.8%
8	7.3%	18	29.0%	28	79.0%
9	8.4%	19	32.9%	29	83.7%
10	9.7%	20	37.1%	30	87.9%

Women 10 Yr.

Pts.	Prob.	Pts.	Prob.	Pts.	Prob.
1	1.1%	11	7.6%	21	43.4%
2	1.3%	12	9.2%	22	50.0%
3	1.6%	13	11.1%	23	57.0%
4	2.0%	14	13.3%	24	64.2%
5	2.4%	15	16.0%	25	71.4%
6	2.9%	16	19.1%	26	78.2%
7	3.5%	17	22.8%	27	84.4%
8	4.3%	18	27.0%		
9	5.2%	19	31.9%		
10	6.3%	20	37.3%		

4. Compare to Average 10-Year Risk

Avg. 10 Yr. Prob. by Age

	Men	Women
55 – 59	5.9%	3.0%
60 – 64	7.8%	4.7%
65 – 69	11.0%	7.2%
70 – 74	13.7%	10.9%
75 – 79	18.0%	15.5%
80 – 84	22.3%	23.9%

Key: SBP, systolic blood pressure; HYP RX, under antihypertensive therapy; Diabetes, Diabetes, history of diabetes; Cigs, Smokes cigarettes; CVD, History of myocardial infarction, angina pectoris, coronary insufficiency, intermittent claudication or congestive heart failure; AF, History of atrial fibrillation; LVH, Left ventricular hypertrophy on ECG.

Source: From the Framingham Heart Study and the American Heart Association, with permission.

FIGURE 1–5 Estimated 4-year probability of intermittent claudication in 70-year-old men; Framingham Heart Study. *Key:* BP indicates blood pressure; NL, normal; Stg 1, stage 1 hypertension; Stg 2+, stage 2 or greater hypertension; CHD, coronary heart disease; cigs, cigarettes. (From Murabito J: Intermittent claudication: a risk profile from the Framingham Heart Study. *Circulation* 1997; 96:44–49, with permission.)

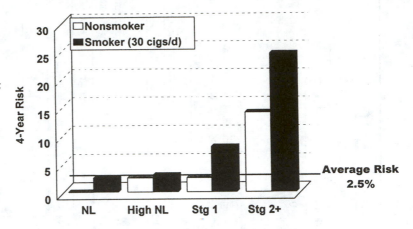

lar disease have evolved, often stimulated by epidemiologic research. The atherogenic aspect of the serum total cholesterol is now known to be its low-density lipoprotein (LDL) component; furthermore, a high-density lipoprotein (HDL) involved in the removal of cholesterol from the tissues and inversely related to the incidence of CHD is now an established protective factor. [28–30] The strength of the association between total cholesterol (TC) and CHD was found to decline with advancing age in men, but the TC:HDL-C ratio has been demonstrated to be a reliable predictor of CHD at all ages in both sexes (Table 1–11). [28,31]

Assessment of hypertension now places greater emphasis on the systolic blood pressure and isolated systolic hypertension as a hazard for all cardiovascular sequelae of hypertension. [32] The additional potential significance of pulse pressure, [33] ambulatory blood pressure monitoring, and circadian blood pressure variation are currently under investigation.

Interest in diabetes now focuses on lesser degrees of glucose intolerance and the influence of this condition as an ingredient of an insulin-resistance syndrome. [34] Epidemiologic research has shifted the attention of obesity investigation from the body mass index (BMI) to patterns of obesity, and abdominal

TABLE 1–9 Four-Year Probability of Intermittent Claudication for Persons Aged 45 to 84 Years: Framingham Heart Study

Risk Factor	0	1	2	3	4	5	6	7	Line Score
Age, years	45–49	50–54	55–59	60–64	65–69	70–74	75–79	80–84	5
Sex	Female			Male					3
Cholesterol, mg/dL	<170	170–209	210–249	250–289	>289				3
Blood pressure	Normal	High Normal	Stage 1		Stage 2+				2
Cigarettes per day	0	1–5	6–10	11–20	>20				3
Diabetes	No					Yes			5
CHD	No					Yes			
								Point Total	21

Source: From Murabito et al.,[17] with permission.

TABLE 1–10 Four-Year Probability of Intermittent Claudication for Persons Aged 45 to 84 Years: Framingham Heart Study

Points	4-Year Probability	Points	4-Year Probability
<10	<1%	22	8%
10–12	1%	23	10%
13–15	2%	24	11%
16–17	3%	25	13%
18	4%	26	16%
19	5%	27	18%
20	6%	28	21%
21	7%	29	24%
		30	28%

Source: From Murabito et al.,[17] with permission.

TABLE 1–12 Established Cardiovascular Disease Risk Factors

Nonmodifiable factors
  Age
  Sex
  Family history
Modifiable factors
  Cigarette smoking
  Obesity
  Hypertension
  Physical inactivity
  Diabetes mellitus
  Cholesterol
  Elevated low-density lipoprotein cholesterol
  Reduced high-density lipoprotein cholesterol

Reproduced, with permission, from Hoeg.[36]

obesity in particular.[35] It too is now regarded as a component of the insulin-resistance syndrome comprising dyslipidemia, hypertension, abnormal lipoprotein lipase, hyperinsulinemia, and abdominal obesity.

Newer Risk Factors

Although there is general agreement on the established cardiovascular risk factors (Table 1–12), epidemiologic research continues to identify or evaluate additional risk factors that contribute to the occurrence of atherosclerotic CVD and warrant fur-

ther clarification (Table 1–13).[36] A variety of lipid measurements now available to researchers await long-term evaluation to determine whether they should be included in vascular disease risk formulations. Subgroups of HDL and LDL have been shown to be associated with CHD, but the utility of these refinements over the standard lipoprotein determinations is not established.[37–39] Similarly, increased lipoprotein(a) has been shown to be associated with greater risk of CHD and stroke in some but not all studies.[40–43]

The antioxidant vitamins E and C and beta-carotene have been found in observational studies to

TABLE 1–11 Risk Ratio for Development of CHD by Total/HDL Cholesterol Ratio According to Age: Framingham Heart Study 16-Year Follow-up

Age (years)	Total/HDL-C Ratio Quintile 5/Quintile 1			Total Cholesterol (≥240 vs. <200 mg/dL)	
	49–59	60–69	70–81	35–64	64–94
Men	3.4*	2.9*	2.3*	1.9†	1.2
Women	3.7*	6.7*	3.3*	1.8‡	2.0†

*0.01 < p < 0.05.
†p < .001.
‡0.001 < p < 0.01.

TABLE 1–13 Proposed Cardiovascular Disease Risk Factors

Proatherogenic
  Homocysteine
  Lipoprotein particle oxidation
  Hyperinsulinemia
  Lipoprotein particle subspecies
  Apolipoprotein E isoforms
  Cholesteryl ester transferase protein

Prothrombogenic
  Plasminogen
  Fibrinogen
  Factor VII
  Plasminogen activator inhibitor 1
  Lipoprotein(a)

Antiatherogenic
  Apolipoprotein A-I
  Lecithin-cholesterol acyl transferase
  Hepatic lipase
  Low-density lipoprotein receptor
  Very low-density lipoprotein receptor
  Apolipoprotein E

Reproduced, with permission, from Hoeg.[36]

be associated with reduced risk of CHD.[44–46] However, clinical trials have not always confirmed the observational data.[47] Homocysteine, an amino acid regulated by vitamins B_{12}, B_6, and folate, is another factor that has been associated with CHD and atherosclerosis. Higher concentrations of homocysteine were found in 29 percent of Framingham Heart Study participants and in 5 percent of subjects in the Physicians' Health Study.[47–49] Although elevated homocysteine has been found to be associated with an increased risk of cardiovascular disease, no clinical trials have thus far tested whether reducing homocysteine by supplementation of these vitamins would decrease the risk of atherosclerotic events.

Challenges for the Twenty-First Century

Whereas CHD and stroke mortality have declined in the past several decades, the incidence of initial occurrence of these diseases and of heart failure has not shown a similar decrease. The result of these trends is an increasing pool of persons with established CHD, strokes, and heart failure. The long-term outlook of persons with any one of these conditions is guarded because they are at high risk of atherosclerotic disease in other vascular territories.[50] Persons with intermittent claudication are at a two- to fourfold increased risk of CHD, stroke, or heart failure. Following initial myocardial infarction, there is a three- to sixfold increased risk of heart failure and stroke. After a stroke, the risk of heart failure and CHD is increased twofold.[50] A better understanding of the reason for the difference in the impact of the major risk factors on the various clinical atherosclerotic disease outcomes is needed. It seems evident, however, that the measures taken to prevent one cardiovascular disease outcome should carry a bonus in preventing the others.

A major challenge for the future is to cost-effectively implement comprehensive preventive programs for initial CVD and their sequelae using multivariate risk assessment to target high-risk candidates so that fewer have to be treated to prevent one event. Because indiscriminate therapy focused on single risk factors requires that hundreds must be treated to prevent one event, we must find ways to better promote multifactorial risk assessment to target hypertensive, dyslipidemic and glucose-intolerant persons for long-term drug therapy. Only in this way will it be possible to avoid needlessly alarming or falsely reassuring possible candidates for atherosclerotic cardiovascular disease. Such an approach is needed to maintain the rate of decline in coronary and stroke mortality that has been observed since 1968 but which seems to be slackening lately. There is a need to reverse the upward trend in CHD mortality in eastern Europe and the former Soviet Union and to prevent the almost inevitable rise in CHD mortality in Asia as Asian nations westernize their diet and lifestyle.

Second, while multivariate risk assessment is vital, its effectiveness may also be enhanced with better screening modalities, particularly for subclinical atherosclerosis. The potential use of measurements from echocardiography and carotid ultrasound to further stratify risk needs to be reviewed, as do emerging technologies such as electron-beam computed tomography and magnetic resonance imaging,[36] although the initial investment, procedural costs, and practical application of all these vary substantially.

Also, improved campaigns focusing on improving awareness and treatment of major risk factors are needed. An investigation of population awareness and control of hypercholesterolemia in 1995 found that only 42 percent of hypercholesterolemic subjects were aware of their condition and only 4 percent were both treated and controlled.[51] Regarding high blood pressure, most recent data indicate that 68 percent are aware of their condition, 53 percent are on treatment, but only 27 percent are adequately controlled.[52] After the recent implementation of the National Cholesterol Education Program, the levels of treatment and control of hyperlipidemia have improved, but they are substantially lower than those for hypertension. Further improvement in the detection and control of these and other major risk factors—such as diabetes, and cigarette smoking especially in younger persons—is clearly needed, particularly in populations where cardiovascular risk is high or in those whose access to preventive services and health care is inadequate.

Enough information is available about major correctable risk factors for CVD to implement effective public health and physician-administered preventive measures designed to continue the decline in cardiovascular mortality. Reorganization of the health care delivery system is needed to put more emphasis on prevention, with reward structures in place for providers who are successful in identifying and controlling their patients at risk. More effort is needed to alter the ecology to one more favorable to cardiovascular health, so that the average blood pressures, lipid values, body weights, and glucose values are at more optimal levels. To achieve this, it will be necessary to alter the national diet, engineer physical activity back into daily life, curb unrestrained weight gain, and get rid of the cigarette. The less affluent segment of the public needs to be better educated about risk factors so that they can take measures to protect their own health.

As we begin the twenty-first century, we also face an emerging epidemic of diabetes. Although improved medications for controlling glucose levels, dyslipidemia, and proteinuria are becoming rapidly available, we must find a way to control the epidemic of obesity, which substantially contributes to the risk of diabetes and CVD. Methods to prevent unwanted weight gain and to safely achieve sustained weight reduction in those who have become obese need to be more widely understood. Abdominal obesity seems to be an important feature of the insulin-resistance syndrome that appears to be an important determinant of the tendency for atherogenic risk factors to cluster. We need an operational definition of this syndrome so that its prevalence, determinants and cardiovascular hazards can be better understood. There is a need to determine whether drug-specific correction of insulin resistance improves the cardiovascular risk profile and, in turn, the atherosclerotic CVD outlook.

With an aging population of increased size, it will be necessary to keep the elderly healthy enough to remain in the work force. More attention needs to be focused on the efficacy and cost-effectiveness of risk-factor control in the older segment of the population. More information is needed on the benefits of exercise in the old so as to determine the optimal frequency and duration of exercise and the minimal threshold for cardiovascular benefit in this age group.

Epidemiologic data have established that women undergoing menopause promptly face a threefold escalation in their risk of CHD over that of women who remain premenopausal at the same age. Hormonal replacement therapy with low-dose estrogen has been shown to be protective, but it is not clear how long this therapy should be continued and whether the protection extends into advanced age. Although results from observational studies suggest a strong protective role for estrogen replacement therapy in CVD, studies such as the Women's Health Initiative will document whether this hypothesis holds up in the primary prevention setting. The role of hormone replacement therapy in the very old needs further investigation because of conflicting effects on hormone-dependent cancers that may offset benefits for CVD and osteoporosis.

Clinical trials have demonstrated the efficacy of correcting dyslipidemia in persons with CHD and those at high risk of developing it. Aggressive lowering of LDL-C levels in high-risk individuals holds promise in reducing morbidity and mortality from CHD in the first third of the twenty-first century. But adequate control of other lipid abnormalities, cigarette smoking, hypertension, diabetes, and other risk factors must be obtained to realize the potential benefit of lipid lowering.[53] The reduction in clinical events has far exceeded expectations from the amount of regression of lesions induced, suggesting that lipid-lowering drugs may be stabilizing lesions that would otherwise be likely to undergo thrombotic occlusion. More research is needed to gain insight into the ways to stabilize lesions. There is also a need to further clarify the role of small, dense LDL, lipoprotein(a), oxidized LDL, and triglycerides in atherogenesis and the value of correcting these lipid abnormalities.

The need continues to identify additional risk factors that could explain the approximately one-fourth of patients with premature CVD who do not have one of the standard risk factors.[36] More investigation is needed to establish the role of newly discovered risk factors, such as homocysteine, lipoprotein oxidation, antioxidant vitamins, infectious agents such as *Chlamydia*, acute-phase reactants, lipoprotein(a), apoprotein E isoforms, and insulin resistance in accelerating atherogenesis and to determine the preventive efficacy of correcting them. Clotting factors, acute-phase reactants, indicators of inflammation, and infectious agents also deserve more attention. The importance of genetic determinants of risk factors and susceptibility to their influence need further investigation. Further research is needed to determine whether left ventricular hypertrophy, an ominous harbinger of cardiovascular events, can be better reversed by specific antihypertensive agents or by correction of ischemia and valve deformity and to determine the clinical benefit of this reversal.

An understanding of the multifactorial approach to risk reduction will offer the best opportunity both for primary and secondary prevention of cardiovascular disease. Risk-factor modification in the public and among those at highest risk offers the best chance for reducing the prevalence of CHD.[22] Although the concept of cardiovascular risk factors is well established in clinical practice, the emergence of more sensitive and specific screening methods for atherosclerosis as well as newer risk factors will further refine our ability to accurately identify and manage those at increased risk for CHD. Although there is clearly more to be learned about the evolution of atherosclerotic disease, we must press on in applying more vigorously the valuable information we already have which should enable us to further curb the epidemic of atherosclerotic CVD. We must come to regard the occurrence of an overt atherosclerotic event as a *medical failure* rather than the first indication for treatment.

References

1. Kannel WB, Dawber TR, Kagan A, et al: Factors of risk in development of coronary heart disease—six year follow-up experience: the Framingham Study. *Ann Intern Med* 1961; 55:33–50.
2. Report of Intersociety Commission for Heart Disease: Resources for primary prevention of atherosclerotic disease. *Circulation* 1984; 70(suppl A):155A–205A.
3. Dawber TR: *The Framingham Study: the Epidemiology of Atherosclerotic Disease.* Cambridge, MA: Harvard University Press, 1980:14–29.
4. Gordon T, Kannel WB: Premature mortality from coronary heart disease: the Framingham Study. *JAMA* 1971; 215:1617–1625.
5. Kannel WB, Abbott RD: Incidence and prognosis of unrecognized myocardial infarction: an update on the Framingham Study. *N Engl J Med* 1984; 311:1144–1147.
6. Wilking SVB, Belanger AJ, Kannel WB, et al: Determinants of isolated systolic hypertension. *JAMA* 1988; 260:3451–3455.
7. Kannel WB, Gordon T, Schwartz MJ: Systolic versus diastolic blood pressure and risk of coronary heart disease: the Framingham Study. *Am J Cardiol* 1971; 27:335–345.
8. Gotto AM Jr, LaRosa JC, Hunninghake D, et al: The cholesterol facts: a summary of the evidence relating dietary fats, serum cholesterol and coronary heart disease. A joint statement by the American Heart Association and the National Heart, Lung and Blood Institute. *Circulation* 1990; 81:1721–1733.
9. Grundy SM, Goodman DS, Rifkind BM, et al: The place of HDL in cholesterol management: a perspective from the National Cholesterol Education Program. *Arch Intern Med* 1989; 149:505–510.
10. Castelli WP, Garrison RJ, Wilson PWF, et al: Coronary heart disease incidence and lipoprotein levels: the Framingham study. *JAMA* 1986; 256:2835–2838.
11. Rosenberg L, Kaufman DW, Helmrich SP, et al: The risk of myocardial infarction after quitting smoking in men under 55 years of age. *N Engl J Med* 1985; 313:1511–1514.

12. Kannel WB, McGee DL, Castelli WP: Latest perspectives on cigarette smoking and cardiovascular disease: the Framingham Study. *J Cardiac Rehab* 1984; 4:267–277.

13. Kannel WB, Dannenberg AL, Levy D: Population implications of left ventricular hypertrophy. *Am J Cardiol* 1987; 60:851–931.

14. Kannel WB, McGee DL, Gordon T: A general cardiovascular risk profile: the Framingham Study. *Am J Cardiol* 1976; 38:46–51.

15. Anderson KM, Wilson PWF, Odell PM, et al: An updated coronary risk profile: a statement for health professionals. *Circulation* 1991; 83:357–363.

16. Wolf PA, D'Agostino RB, Belanger AJ, et al: Probability of stroke: a risk profile from the Framingham study. *Stroke* 1991; 3:312–318.

17. Murabito JM, D'Agostino RB, Silberschatz H, Wilson PWF: Intermittent claudication: a risk profile from the Framingham Heart Study. *Circulation* 1997; 96:44–49.

18. Wilson, PWF, D'Agostino RB, Levy D, et al: Prediction of coronary heart disease using risk factor categories. *Circulation* 1998; 97:1837–1847.

19. Manson JE, Tosteson H, Ridker PM, et al: The primary prevention of myocardial infarction. *N Engl J Med* 1992; 326:1406–1416.

20. Kannel WB: Contribution of the Framingham study to preventive cardiology. *J Am Coll Cardiol* 1990; 15: 206–211.

21. Kannel WB, Sytkowski PA: Atherosclerosis risk factors. *Pharmacol Ther* 1987; 32:207–235.

22. Grundy SM, Galady GJ, Criqui MH, et al: AHA Scientific Statement: primary prevention of coronary heart disease: guidance from Framingham. *Circulation* 1998; 97:1876–1887.

23. Kannel WB, McGee DL: Diabetes and glucose tolerance as risk factors for cardiovascular disease: the Framingham Study. *Diabetes Care* 1979; 2:120–126.

24. Manson JE, Colditz GA, Stampfer MJ, et al: A prospective study of maturity-onset diabetes and risk of coronary heart disease and stroke in women. *Arch Intern Med* 1991; 151:1141–1147.

25. Kannel WB, McGee DL: Update on some epidemiologic features of intermittent claudication: the Framingham Study. *J Am Geriatr Soc* 1985; 33:13–18.

26. Ho KK, Anderson KM, Kannel WB, et al: Survival after the onset of congestive heart failure in Framingham Heart Study subjects. *Circulation* 1993; 88:107–115.

27. Kannel WB, Belanger AJ: Epidemiology of heart failure. *Am Heart J* 1991; 121:951–957.

28. Kannel WB: High-density lipoproteins: epidemiologic profile and risks of coronary artery disease. *Am J Cardiol* 1983; 52:9B–12B.

29. Expert Panel on Detection, Evaluation and Treatment of High Blood Cholesterol in Adults: summary of the second report of the NCEP Expert Panel (Adult Treatment Panel II). *JAMA* 1993; 269:3015–3023.

30. NIH Consensus Development Panel: Triglyceride, high-density lipoprotein and coronary heart disease. *JAMA* 1993; 269:505–510.

31. Wilson PWF, Kannel WB: Hypercholesterolemia and coronary risk in the elderly: the Framingham Study. *Am J Geriatr Cardiol* 1993; 2:52–56.

32. Kannel WB, Dawber TR, McGee DL, et al: Perspectives on systolic hypertension: the Framingham Study. *Circulation* 1980; 61:1179–1182.

33. Franklin SS, Gustin W, Wong ND, et al: Hemodynamic patterns of age-related change in blood pressure: the Framingham Heart Study. *Circulation* 1997; 96:308–315.

34. Reaven GM: Banting Lecture 1988: role of insulin resistance in human disease. *Diabetes* 1988; 37:1595–1607.

35. Bjorntorp P: Regional patterns of fat distribution. *Ann Intern Med* 1985; 103:994–995.

36. Hoeg JM: Evaluating coronary heart disease risk: tiles in the mosaic. *JAMA* 1997; 277:1387–1390.

37. Buring JE, O'Conner GT, Goldhaber SZ, et al: Decreased HDL_2 and HDL_3 cholesterol, Apo A-I and Apo A-II and increased risk of myocardial infarction. *Circulation* 1992; 85:22–29.

38. Wilson PWF: Relation of high-density lipoprotein subfractions and apolipoprotein isoforms to coronary disease. *Clin Chem* 1995; 41:165–169.

39. Austin MA, Hokanson JE, Brunzell JD: Characterization of low-density lipoprotein subclasses: methodologic approaches and clinical relevance. *Curr Opin Lipid* 1994; 5:395–403.

40. Campos H, Genest JJ Jr, Blijlevens E, et al: Low-density lipoprotein particle size and coronary artery disease. *Arterioscler Thromb* 1992; 12;187–195.

41. Ridker PM, Stampfer MJ, Hennekens CH: Plasma concentration of plasma lipoprotein (a) and the risk of future stroke. *JAMA* 1995; 273:1269–1273.

42. Ridker PM, Hennekens CH. Lipoprotein (a) and risks of cardiovascular disease. *Ann Epidemiol* 1994; 4:360–362.

43. Schaefer EJ, Lamon-Fava S, Jenner JL, et al: Lipoprotein (a) levels and risk of coronary heart disease in men: the Lipid Research Clinics Coronary Primary Prevention Trial. *JAMA* 1994; 272:999–1003.

44. Hennekens CH, Buring JE, Peto R: Antioxidant vitamins: benefits not yet proved (editorial). *N Engl J Med* 1994; 330:1080–1081.

45. Stampfer MJ, Hennekens CH, Manson JE, et al: Vitamin E consumption and risk of coronary heart disease in women. *N Engl J Med* 1993; 328:1444–1449.

46. Rimm EB, Stampfer MJ, Aschero A: Vitamin E consumption and risk of coronary heart disease in men. *N Engl J Med* 1993; 328:1450–1456.

47. Genest JJ Jr, McNamara JR, Salem DN, et al: Plasma homocysteine levels in men with premature coronary artery disease. *J Am Coll Cardiol* 1990; 16;1114–1119.

48. Selhub J, Jacques PF, Boston AG, et al: Association between plasma homocysteine and extracranial carotid stenosis. *N Engl. J Med* 1995; 332:286–291.

49. Stampfer MJ, Malinow MR, Willett WC, et al: A prospective study of plasma homocysteine and risk of myocardial infarction in US physicians. *JAMA* 1992; 268:877–881.

50. Cupples LA, D'Agostino RB, Kiely D: The Framingham Heart Study. Section 35. *An Epidemiological Investigation of Cardiovascular Disease. Survival Following Cardiovascular Events: 30-Year Follow-Up.* Bethesda MD: National Heart Lung and Blood Institute, 1988.

51. Nieto FJ, Alonso J, Chambliss LE, et al: Population awareness and control of hypertension and hypercholes-terolemia: the Atherosclerosis in Communities Study. *Arch Intern Med* 1995; 155:677–684.

52. The Joint National Committee on Prevention, Detection, Evaluation, and Treatment of High Blood Pressure and the National High Blood Pressure Education Program Coordinating Committee: The Sixth Report of the Joint National Committee on Prevention, Detection, Evaluation, and Treatment of High Blood Pressure. *Arch Intern Med* 1997; 157:2413–2446.

53. Grundy SM. Cholesterol and coronary heart disease: the 21st century. *Arch Intern Med* 1997; 157:1177–1784.

CHAPTER 2

Trends in Cardiovascular Disease: Incidence and Risk Factors

Gregory L. Burke
Ronny A. Bell

Cardiovascular disease (CVD) has been and continues to be the leading cause of death in the United States and other developed countries. More recently, evidence points toward an increasing burden from CVD in developing countries. Current projections suggest that overall CVD rates will continue to increase in the twenty-first century and will be the leading cause of death in both the developed and developing world. The global increased burden of CVD is unfortunate, and although a substantial number of proven preventive strategies have become available for primary and secondary prevention efforts, these have not been effectively disseminated on a global basis. Prior to implementing a large-scale CVD prevention program, however, it is imperative that key decision makers be aware of the scope of the problem. The purpose of this chapter is to provide an overview of the data on differences between populations and secular trends in CVD risk factors, morbidity, and mortality. Specifically, data are presented across age, gender, and geographic entities; in addition, a brief overview of recent time trends in CVD incidence and risk factors is presented.

Cardiovascular Disease Morbidity and Mortality: Rates and Trends in the United States and Other Countries

In the following section, we review existing national and international data on CVD mortality and mor-

bidity. The focus of this section is to describe the current burden from CVD and recent trends in CVD events. The bulk of the U.S. data were obtained from published reports of the National Center for Health Statistics, the American Heart Association, and region-specific surveillance studies. International data were extracted primarily from World Health Organization (WHO) reports as well as the WHO Multinational Monitoring of Trends and Determinants in Cardiovascular Disease (WHO MONICA) Project.[1]

International Comparisons of Cardiovascular Disease Morbidity and Mortality

Cardiovascular disease (ICD-9 codes 390–450) is the leading cause of death in most countries, particularly in those that are economically developed. Significant international variation in CVD mortality and morbidity has been documented from nation-specific data and in WHO MONICA communities. Figure 2–1 shows 1995 mortality rates for CVD in 36 countries.[2] CVD accounts for about 25 to 45 percent of all deaths in these countries. CVD death rates (per 100,000 population) among men ages 35 to 74 in these select populations range from 1310 (Russian Federation) to 201 (Japan), a 6.5-fold variation. Among women ages 35 to 74, CVD death rates range from 581 (Russian Federation) to 84 (France), a nearly sevenfold difference. Among these countries, the U.S. rates rank sixteenth for both men (413) and women (201).

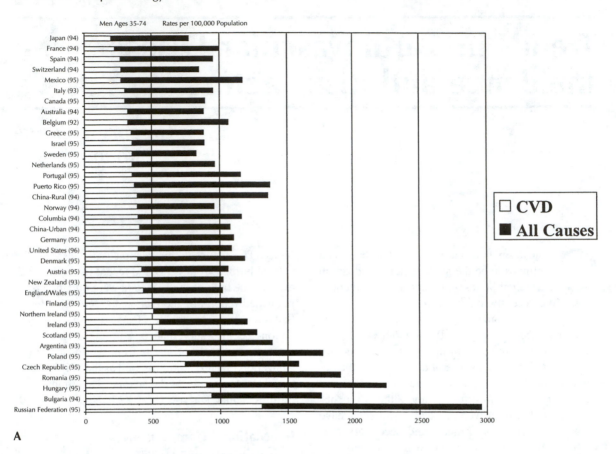

Men Ages 35-74   Rates per 100,000 Population

FIGURE 2-1 *A.* Death rates in men for cardiovascular diseases and all causes in selected countries (most recent year available). ICD-9 codes 390–459 for cardiovascular disease. Rates adjusted to the European standard population. (Data from the World Health Organization and the American Heart Association, with permission.)

Data from 35 participating WHO MONICA sites (population age 35 to 64 years) indicate similar international variation in CVD mortality. For men, the highest rates in these populations were 631 and 493 per 100,000 for CVD and ischemic heart disease (IHD), respectively, in North Karelia, Finland, and 122 per 100,000 for stroke in Pecs, Hungary. For women, overall CVD mortality rates ranged from 237 per 100,000 in Pecs, Hungary, to 42 per 100,000 in Catalonia, Spain; for IHD, rates ranged from 86 per 100,000 in Budapest, Hungary, to 11 per 100,000 in Catalonia, Spain; for stroke, rates varied from 65 per 100,000 in Pecs, Hungary, to 12 per 100,000 in Vaud/Fribourg, Switzerland.[3]

Data including CVD morbidity from 36 WHO MONICA population sites in 1985 to 1987[4] are presented in Fig. 2–2 to describe the geographic variation of CVD events (defined as "definite" fatal, "probable" fatal, "unclassified," and "definite" nonfatal). For all sites combined, a CVD event rate of 456 per 100,000 for men and 101 per 100,000 for women was observed. Population-specific event rates ranged from 915 per 100,000 in North Karelia, Finland, to 76 per 100,000 in Beijing, China, for men, and from 256 in

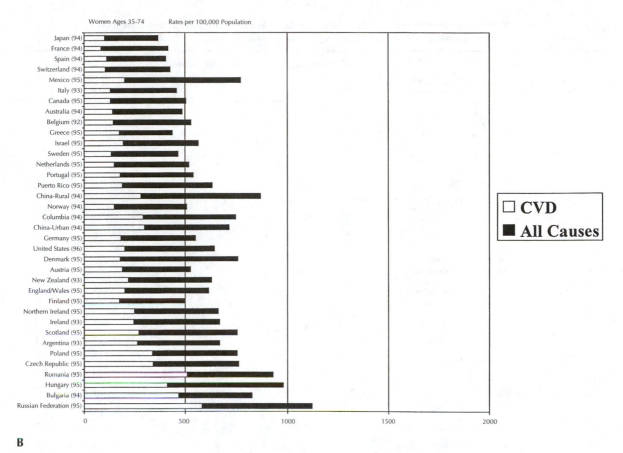

Women Ages 35-74   Rates per 100,000 Population

B

FIGURE 2–1 *B.* Death rates in women for cardiovascular diseases and all causes in selected countries (most recent year available). ICD-9 codes 390–459 for cardiovascular disease. Rates adjusted to the European standard population. (Data from the World Health Organization and the American Heart Association, with permission.)

Glasgow, United Kingdom, to 30 in Catalonia, Spain, for women. Importantly, these data indicate an even greater heterogeneity in CVD burden across populations when nonfatal events are included.

Cardiovascular Disease Mortality in the United States

In the United States, about 960,000 people died from CVD in 1995 (413 deaths per 100,000 people), representing approximately 42 percent of all deaths. CVD is the United States' overall leading cause of

death and is the leading cause of death in men greater than 45 years of age and in women greater than 65 years of age. In addition, CVD is the leading cause of death for all race/gender groups in the United States. Approximately 58 million Americans, or about 20 percent of the population, have some form of CVD. CVD accounted for about 5.8 million hospital discharges in 1995. About half of CVD deaths are due to coronary heart disease (CHD) and 16 percent to stroke. The economic costs of CVD in the United States are enormous, estimated to be $274 billion dollars in 1998.[2]

TABLE 2–1 Total Cardiovascular, Ischemic Heart Disease, and Stroke Mortality Rates (per 100,000 Population) across WHO MONICA Sites for Men and Women Ages 35 to 64

Population	Country	CVD Mortality		IHD Mortality		Stroke Mortality	
		Men	Women	Men	Women	Men	Women
Newcastle	Australia	309	136	231	81	41	37
Perth	Australia	215	75	161	42	25	19
Beijing	China	163	145	47	27	73	70
Czechoslovakia	Czechoslovakia	467	163	273	63	90	46
Glostrup	Denmark	285	95	195	44	30	17
Kuopio Province	Finland	514	134	382	55	71	50
North Karelia	Finland	631	132	493	63	75	37
Turku/Loimaa	Finland	382	97	296	57	50	28
Bas-Rhin	France	174	58	86	18	26	16
Lille	France	190	58	88	18	35	17
Augsburg (rural)	Germany	224	12	135	14	27	6
Augsburg (urban)	Germany	248	18	151	15	26	6
Bremen	Germany	302	92	158	31	45	26
DDR MONICA	Germany	305	124	150	45	29	15
Halle County	Germany	315	129	158	41	43	25
Karl-Marx-Stadt County	Germany	303	123	155	36	31	21
Rhien-Necker Region	Germany	218	71	134	28	28	15
Budapest	Hungary	555	227	294	86	108	55
Pecs	Hungary	530	237	260	80	122	65
Iceland	Iceland	260	59	202	26	29	18
Area Latina	Italy	200	77	92	20	47	28
Brianza Area	Italy	176	57	105	23	34	15
Fruili	Italy	190	70	99	23	38	23
Kaunas	Lithuania	469	139	326	66	74	34
Malta	Malta	330	111	209	60	77	24
Auckland	New Zealand	324	124	241	59	38	35
Tarnobrzeg Voivodship	Poland	399	166	172	31	44	35
Warsaw	Poland	421	164	184	47	77	45
Moscow (control)	Russia	487	168	321	72	90	52
Moscow (intervention)	Russia	492	164	316	75	109	53
Catalonia	Spain	135	42	66	11	29	13
Goteborg	Sweden	232	76	169	39	24	18
Northern Sweden	Sweden	275	73	215	37	23	20
Ticino	Switzerland	162	48	100	17	15	15
Vaud/Fribourg	Switzerland	172	51	94	16	16	12

Source: Adapted from the WHO MONICA Project.[3]

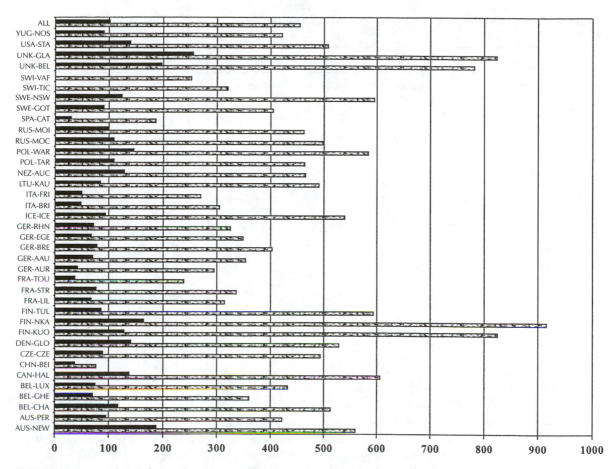

FIGURE 2–2 Coronary heart disease event rate (per 100,000 population) for 36 WHO MONICA communities. (Adapted from the WHO MONICA Project.[4])
Key: ■, women; ▨, men. AUS-NEW, AUS-PER, Australia; BEL-CHA, BEL-GHE, BEL-LUX, Belgium; CAN-HAL, Canada; CHN-BEI, China; CZE-CZE, Czech Republic; DEN-GLO, Denmark; FIN-KUO, FIN-NKA, FIN-TUL, Finland; FRA-LIL, FRA-STR, FRA-TOU, France; GER-AUR, GER-AUU, GER-BRE, GER-EGE, GER-RHN, Germany; HUN-BUD, HUN-PEC, Hungary; ICE-ICE, Iceland; ITA-BRI, ITA-FRI, Italy; LTU-KAU, Lithuania; NEZ-AUC, New Zealand; POL-TAR, POL-WAR, Poland; RUS-MOC, RUS-MOI, RUS-NOC, RUS-NOI, Russia; SPA-CAT, Spain; SWE-GOT, SWE-NSW, Sweden; SWI-TIC, SWI-VAF, Switzerland; UNK-BEL, UNK-GLA, UK; USA-STA, USA; YUG-NOS, Yugoslavia.

Table 2–2 presents 1996 U.S. data for all-cause and CVD mortality rates and years of potential life lost (YPLL) before the age of 75 by gender and race/ethnicity group.[5] Overall, heart disease contributed to 135 deaths and 1223 years of life lost prior to age 75 per 100,000 people, while stroke was associated with 26 deaths and 210 years of life lost per 100,000 people. The greatest CVD burden in the United States is found in the African-American population, with rates of heart disease mortality approximately 37 percent higher for African-American men than for non-Hispanic white men and approximately

TABLE 2–2   U.S. Mortality Rate and Years of Potential Life Lost before Age 75 for Heart Disease and Stroke, 1996

Race/Gender Group	All Causes		Diseases of the Heart		Cerebrovascular Disease	
	Mortality Rate*	YPLL†	Mortality Rate	YPLL	Mortality Rate	YPLL
All persons	491.6	7748	134.5	1,223	26.4	210
American Indian/Alaska Native						
Men	555.9	11,608	131.6	1,565	21.4	234
Women	367.7	6,797	74.9	739	20.6	195
Asian/Pacific islander						
Men	355.8	5,102	98.1	874	26.9	219
Women	214.4	2,950	50.9	319	21.5	159
Black						
Men	967.0	18,995	242.6	2,970	51.8	583
Women	561.0	10,013	153.4	1,636	39.2	423
Hispanic						
Men	474.8	8,861	117.6	1,125	22.3	234
Women	268.0	4,211	64.7	459	17.1	155
Non-Hispanic white						
Men	589.5	8,744	176.2	1,643	26.1	186
Women	364.1	4,875	93.6	644	23.0	156

*Age-adjusted mortality rate per 100,000 population.
†Years of potential life lost before age 75 per 100,000 population under 75 years of age.
Source: Adapted from National Center for Health Statistics.[5]

63 percent higher for African-American women than for non-Hispanic white women. This gap was even greater for stroke; mortality rates for African-American men were nearly twice as high as those for non-Hispanic white men (51.8 versus 26.1, respectively), and rates for African-American women were 70 percent higher than for non-Hispanic white women (39.2 versus 23.0, respectively). Heart disease rates for men and women were lowest for Asian/Pacific islanders (98 and 51 per 100,000, respectively). Stroke mortality rates in men were lowest for American Indian/Alaska Natives (21.4 per 100,000) while stroke mortality rates in women were lowest for Hispanics (17.1 per 100,000).[5] Thus, substantial ethnic differences in CVD burden in the United States were observed across race and gender groups.

There are also substantial differences in ischemic heart disease and stroke mortality within the United States. Table 2–3 presents 1995 death rates due to ischemic heart disease ranked by state from the highest to lowest incidence.[6] New York had the highest rate (179.7 per 100,000), more than double the rate of the lowest-ranked state, New Mexico (82.0 per 100,000). Table 2–4 presents 1995 death rates due to stroke.[6] South Carolina ranked the highest in stroke deaths (63.3 per 100,000), more than double the rate of New York (30.6 per 100,000), the lowest-ranking state for stroke deaths. Although the factors responsible for the great variation in ischemic heart disease and stroke rates are unclear, these data may suggest where statewide prevention programs are most needed.

Secular Trends in Cardiovascular Disease Mortality

Most industrialized nations have observed substantial reductions in CVD mortality since the 1960s, congruent with changes in major CVD risk factors (discussed below). Among 28 countries (Fig. 2–3), mortality rates for CHD in men aged 35 to 74 declined by approximately 3 to 7 percent per year for

TABLE 2–3 Rates of Death Due to Ischemic Heart Disease,* 1995†

Rank	State	Deaths per 100,000	Rank	State	Deaths per 100,000
1	New York	179.7	27	Wisconsin	125.6
2	Oklahoma	157.6	28	California	124.6
3	Missouri	156.1	28	Vermont	124.6
4	West Virginia	154.9	30	Virginia	122.3
5	Tennessee	154.1	31	Kansas	120.9
6	Ohio	153.7	32	Arizona	120.8
7	South Carolina	153.2	33	Delaware	117.7
8	Rhode Island	153.0	34	Massachusetts	117.1
9	Kentucky	152.7	35	Alabama	116.8
10	Indiana	148.3	36	Alaska	115.3
11	Arkansas	147.1	37	Nevada	115.0
12	Michigan	146.7	38	Connecticut	114.8
13	New Jersey	144.3	39	Maryland	114.4
14	Illinois	142.6	40	Wyoming	113.6
15	North Carolina	142.2	41	Nebraska	112.2
16	Pennsylvania	140.2	42	Idaho	109.8
17	Louisiana	137.0	43	Oregon	109.6
18	New Hampshire	133.9	44	Minnesota	107.4
19	South Dakota	132.7	45	District of Columbia	100.5
20	Florida	132.0	46	Montana	96.4
21	Mississippi	131.5	47	Washington	96.2
22	Texas	131.1	48	Colorado	94.0
23	Maine	130.5	49	Utah	88.7
24	North Dakota	128.1	50	Hawaii	85.5
25	Iowa	127.7	51	New Mexico	82.0
26	Georgia	126.2			

*ICD-9 codes: 410–414.

†All data are age-adjusted, 1970 total U.S. population.

Source: Centers for Disease Control and Prevention: *Chronic Diseases and Their Risk Factors: The Nation's Leading Causes of Death.* Bethesda, MD, U.S Department of Health and Human Services, 1998.

21 countries from 1985 to 1992, including an approximately 4 percent reduction per year for the United States.[7] Virtually all of these 21 countries saw changes in excess of 25 percent during this 7-year period. Two eastern European countries, Poland and Romania, observed substantial *increases* in CHD mortality, by approximately 12 to 20 percent. A similar pattern was observed for women; however, an even greater number of countries (25) observed reductions in CHD mortality.[7]

Stroke mortality rates have also steadily declined in recent years. Across 28 countries, 27 had average annual reductions in stroke mortality among men aged 35 to 74 from 1985 to 1992 of 0.5 to 8.0 percent, while only one country (Poland) had an increase in average annual stroke mortality during this

TABLE 2–4 Rates of Death Due to Stroke,* 1995†

Rank	State	Deaths per 100,000	Rank	State	Deaths per 100,000
1	South Carolina	63.3	27	California	42.9
2	Tennessee	56.0	28	Wisconsin	42.7
3	Arkansas	54.7	29	Minnesota	42.6
4	North Carolina	54.6	30	West Virginia	41.3
5	Mississippi	51.7	31	Kansas	41.0
6	Georgia	51.1	31	Ohio	41.0
7	Alaska	51.0	33	Pennsylvania	40.6
8	District of Columbia	50.5	34	Iowa	39.7
9	Oregon	48.7	34	Nebraska	39.7
10	Virginia	48.6	36	New Hampshire	39.6
11	Louisiana	48.2	37	Vermont	39.0
12	Indiana	47.3	38	Idaho	38.9
13	Alabama	46.6	39	South Dakota	38.6
14	Oklahoma	46.1	40	Utah	38.5
15	Michigan	45.6	41	Arizona	37.1
15	Wyoming	45.6	42	New Jersey	36.8
17	Texas	45.0	43	Rhode Island	36.8
18	Missouri	44.6	44	Delaware	36.6
19	Maryland	44.5	44	Florida	36.6
20	Montana	44.3	44	Maine	36.6
20	Nevada	44.3	47	Colorado	36.2
22	Illinois	44.0	48	Connecticut	36.1
22	Kentucky	44.0	49	New Mexico	35.5
24	Hawaii	43.9	50	Massachusetts	34.4
25	Washington	43.8	51	New York	30.6
26	North Dakota	43.1			

*ICD-9 codes 430–438.

†All data are age-adjusted, 1970 total U.S. population.

Source: Centers for Disease Control and Prevention: *Chronic Diseases and Their Risk Factors: The Nation's Leading Causes of Death.* Bethesda, MD, U.S. Department of Health and Human Services, 1998.

period (approximately 1.0 percent) (Fig. 2–4). Reductions during this time period were greatest in Australia, France, and Italy. Among women in this age group, all 28 countries observed reductions in average annual stroke mortality ranging from an approximately 9.0 percent decline in Australia to an approximately 0.8 percent decline in Denmark. Annual reductions of greater than 7.0 percent for women during this time period were observed in Australia, Italy, France, Spain, Germany, Austria, and Japan. In the United States, average annual reductions in stroke mortality during this period were approximately 3 percent for both men and women.[7]

Change in stroke attack rates for the 17 WHO MONICA sites are presented in Fig. 2–5. Among men aged 35 to 64, thirteen sites observed reductions in average annual stroke attack rates (fatal and nonfatal) over 5- or 6-year periods from 1982 to 1990.[8]

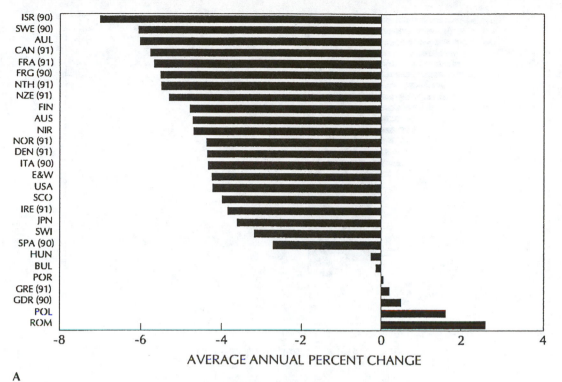

A

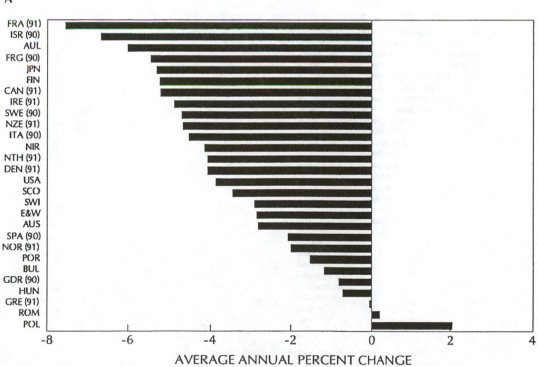

B

FIGURE 2–3   *A*. Percent change in death rates for CHD in men age 35–74 by country, 1985–1992. *B*. Percent change in death rates for CHD in women age 35–74 by country, 1985–1992. (From National Heart, Lung, and Blood Institute.[7])

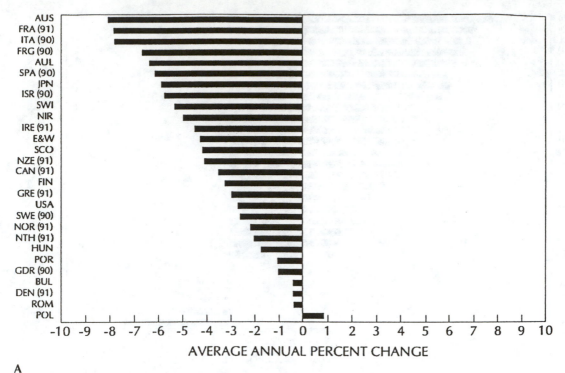

A

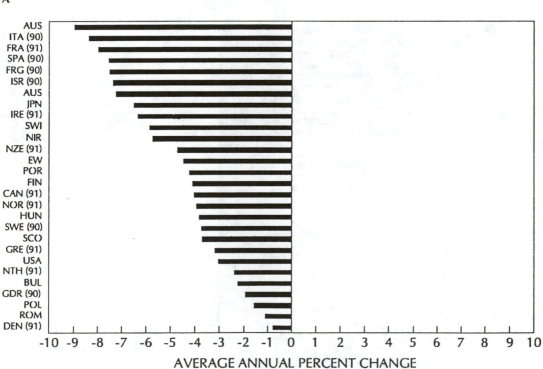

B

FIGURE 2–4 *A.* Percent change in death rates for stroke in men age 35–74 by country, 1985–1992. *B.* Percent change in death rates for stroke in women age 35–74 by country, 1985–1992. (From National Heart, Lung, and Blood Institute.[7])

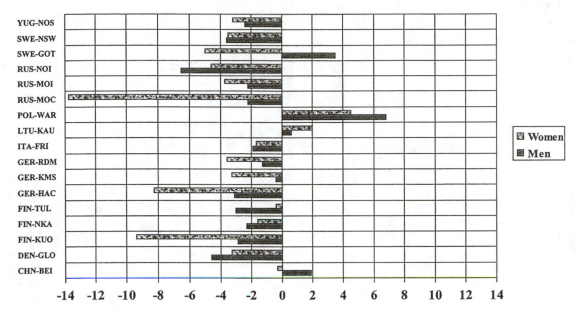

FIGURE 2–5 Relative change in stroke attack rates per year (per 100,000) for 17 selected WHO MONICA communities. YUG-NOS, Yugoslavia Novi Sad; SWE-NSW, Northern Sweden; SWE-GOT, Sweden Gothenburg; RUS-NOI, Russia Novosibirsk (intervention); RUS-MOI, Russia Moscow (intervention); RUS-MOC, Russia Moscow (control); POL-WAR, Poland Warsaw; LTU-KAU, Lithuania Kaunas; ITA-FRI, Italy Friuli; GER-RDM, Germany rest of DDR-MONICA; GER-KMS, Germany Karl-Marx-Stadt County; HRT-HAC, Germany Halle County; FIN-TUL, Finlad Turku/Loimaa; FINN-NKA, Finland North Karelia; FIN-KUO, Finland Kuopio Province; DEN-GLO, Denmark Glostrup; CHN-BEI, China Beijing. (Adapted from The WHO MONICA Project.[8])

Of 17 sites, 15 reported average annual reductions in stroke attack rates for women. For men, the greatest decrease in stroke rates were observed in Novosibirsk, Russia (6.5 percent) and Glostrup, Denmark (4.6 percent), while for women even larger reductions were observed in some sites (Moscow, Russia, 13.8 percent; Kuopio Province, Finland, 9.4 percent; and Halle County, Germany, 8.3 percent). Of the 15 sites, 5 with reductions in annual stroke attack rates for women observed reductions of 4.0 percent or greater, while only two sites observed similar reductions for men.[8]

Data reported by Kesteloot and Joossens[9] provide an opportunity to assess international variation in CVD mortality for men and women of different age groups over a 20-year period (1968 to 1988) (Table 2–5). Among men age 45 to 59, mean CVD mortality rates declined by 13.7 percent across 34 countries during this time period; for women of the same age

group, total CVD rates decreased by 34.2 percent. Rates declined for 27 of 34 countries for men and 31 of 34 countries for women. The largest reductions during this time period were observed in Australia (55.6 percent for men and 61.2 percent for women) and Japan (49.3 percent for men and 61.5 percent for women). Reductions of 50 percent or more during this time period were observed in nine countries for women (Japan, Australia, Spain, Iceland, Finland, Italy, Switzerland, France, and Canada), but only one country for men (Australia). For men, three countries (Hungary, Poland, and Bulgaria) had *increases* in CVD mortality of greater than 50 percent. The country with the highest increase in CVD mortality for women during this period was Poland (14.1 percent).

The age group with the greatest decline in CVD mortality in men was the 60- to 74-year group, while

TABLE 2–5 Percent Change in Cardiovascular Disease Mortality from 1968 to 1988 Across 34 Countries, by Gender and Age Group

Country	Age 45–59 Years		Age 60–74 Years		Age 75–84 Years		Age 85+ Years	
	Men	Women	Men	Women	Men	Women	Men	Women
Argentina	−12.6	−12.0	−11.0	−19.4	2.6	2.0	−11.2	13.4
Australia	−55.6	−61.2	−48.4	−53.7	−40.7	−42.7	−34.3	−31.6
Austria	−20.6	−43.2	−26.1	−39.3	−19.8	−27.0	−8.9	−11.5
Belgium	−46.4	49.1	−40.6	−47.0	−34.6	−39.3	−33.9	−33.6
Bulgaria	85.7	4.1	46.3	2.9	43.2	13.8	56.5	50.5
Canada	−49.3	−50.5	−38.5	−46.8	−34.1	−43.1	−30.8	−34.4
Czechoslovakia	22.8	−4.6	14.9	−1.7	8.2	−3.3	−5.9	−6.6
Denmark	−13.7	−18.2	−19.9	−37.1	−18.9	−35.9	−21.1	−22.2
England & Wales	−27.3	−36.9	−24.6	−30.7	−27.0	−33.7	−38.0	−33.5
Fed. Rep. Germany	−26.6	−40.6	−27.1	−40.2	−17.4	−31.9	−8.7	−9.0
Finland	−43.1	−56.8	−30.3	−47.2	−30.8	−44.7	−34.8	−37.4
France	−43.1	−51.5	−40.6	−51.4	−35.3	−39.6	−27.8	−19.4
Greece	16.1	−27.8	14.9	−8.8	29.1	16.0	31.5	44.7
Hong Kong	−48.5	−47.6	−46.0	−30.3	−37.5	−26.8	−6.1	−19.4
Hungary	58.3	8.1	10.8	−12.1	−11.5	−20.9	−19.3	−17.5
Iceland	−18.8	−58.3	−27.3	−32.4	−7.8	−34.5	−25.4	−22.0
Ireland	−11.7	−41.4	−8.5	−33.9	−7.9	−26.0	−8.4	−11.2
Italy	−36.0	−56.5	−39.7	−52.9	−29.4	−40.1	−19.6	−16.6
Japan	−49.3	−61.5	−60.6	−63.6	−49.0	−50.0	−20.1	−13.9
Netherlands	−27.0	−32.4	−18.2	−40.7	−17.9	−38.3	−23.4	−29.7
New Zealand	−35.0	−42.2	−30.5	−34.2	−26.6	−31.0	−32.7	−26.6
Northern Ireland	−24.4	−29.7	−14.7	−30.4	−23.0	−33.3	−22.0	−29.5
Norway	−11.0	−29.2	−11.6	−39.2	−11.4	−33.3	−8.1	−17.0
Poland	67.0	14.1	26.3	4.6	33.8	17.5	63.8	58.5
Portugal	−27.6	−43.3	−33.2	−43.0	−19.5	−29.1	20.9	28.5
Romania	45.9	−0.3	1.4	−12.5	2.1	−6.8	31.0	53.5
Scotland	−24.8	−36.2	−19.2	−26.5	−23.1	−30.9	−33.1	−35.0
Singapore	−17.1	−19.9	−20.7	−5.8	−26.1	4.9	23.8	50.0
Spain	−21.5	−58.3	−32.9	−49.9	−24.2	−32.1	4.4	1.0
Sweden	−12.1	−39.4	−16.2	−41.6	−19.8	−38.2	−22.3	−29.4
Switzerland	−33.4	−55.9	−33.6	−53.1	−32.6	−47.0	−21.7	−29.3
United Kingdom	−24.6	−35.0	−23.7	−30.3	−26.4	−33.6	−37.0	−34.3
USA	−46.1	−42.4	−44.2	−44.3	−34.6	−41.3	−29.3	−36.6
Yugoslavia	34.0	−7.1	19.0	−0.4	30.6	22.4	68.3	75.8
Mean ± SD	−13.7 ± 35.3	−34.2 ± 21.3	−19.2 ± 23.6	−32.1 ± 18.3	−15.8 ± 22.4	−25.2 ± 20.4	−8.3 ± 29.3	−6.8 ± 32.8

Source: Adapted from Kesteloot H, Joossens JV: Worldwide mortality changes from all-causes and from cardiovascular diseases between 1968 and 1988. *Acta Cardiolog* 1993;48:421–439.

in women, the 45- to 59-year group showed the greatest decline. In both men and women, the percent of decline in CVD mortality was greatest in younger age groups and changed the least in the oldest old (aged 85+ years).

The gap in percent CVD mortality reduction over these 20 years between men and women narrowed in older age groups. Specifically, the gender differences in rates in 75- to 84-year-olds were 15.8 percent in men versus 25.2 percent in women while among ≥85-year-olds, men had slightly higher rates in CVD mortality reduction between 1968 and 1988 (8.3 percent versus 6.8 percent, respectively). No countries had rate reductions of greater than 50 percent for men or women in either of the oldest age groups, while women aged 75 to 84 in Japan had a rate reduction of 50 percent. Among ≥85-year-olds, three countries had rate *increases* of greater than 50 percent (Bulgaria, Poland, and Yugoslavia for men; Romania, Poland, and Yugoslavia for women). It should be noted that some of the large differences observed in older age groups might be attributable to instability of the estimates because of the relatively small sample sizes.

In the United States, there was a 57 percent overall reduction in IHD mortality from 1950 (307.2 per 100,000) to 1996 (134.5 per 100,000) and a 10 percent reduction since 1980 (149.8 per 100,000).[5] Even more dramatic reductions were observed for stroke mortality during these time periods (70 percent reduction since 1950; 35 percent reduction since 1980). Table 2–6 shows age-adjusted mortality rates for heart disease, IHD, and stroke for 1980 and 1996 overall by gender and by race/ethnicity.[5] The reductions in mortality during this time period have been slightly greater for men than for women (36.2 versus 30 percent for diseases of the heart; 44.5 versus 38.9 percent for IHD; 36.5 versus 34.6 percent for stroke; and 19.8 versus 11.9 percent for total mortality).[5] Among racial/ethnic groups, although all groups showed reductions in CVD mortality, the greatest reductions during this time period were observed for non-Hispanic whites for diseases of the heart (34.3 percent), IHD (42.6 percent), and stroke (35.5 percent). Reductions in CVD mortality were a substantial contributor to the approximately 10 to 20

percent reduction in all-cause mortality across all five racial/ethnic groups.[5]

Rosemond and colleagues[10] examined trends in heart disease incidence and mortality across four racial/gender groups (white men and women, black men and women) in four U.S. communities (Forsyth County, NC; Jackson, MS; Minneapolis suburbs; Washington County, MD) from 1987 to 1994. While all four groups had reductions in CHD mortality, the largest decreases in CHD mortality were observed among white males (average annual rate change of 4.7 percent), while the smallest decline in CHD mortality was observed for black men (average annual rate change of 2.5 percent). Average annual rates of hospitalization for first myocardial infarction actually increased during this time period for black women (7.4 percent) and black men (2.9 percent) while remaining essentially unchanged for white men (0.3 percent) or lower for white women (2.5 percent). There was also evidence for a decrease in rates of recurrent myocardial infarction and improvement in survival after myocardial infarction.[10]

To summarize the CVD morbidity and mortality data, while most economically developed nations have had major reductions in CVD mortality and morbidity in the latter part of this century, there was still substantial heterogeneity in CVD rates and in the rates of reduction of CVD mortality between nations. A small number of eastern European nations have had increases in CVD mortality. In the United States, rates of CVD mortality and morbidity continue to decline, although there is still significant variation between regions (states) and among race/ethnic groups in the burden of CVD, with African Americans bearing the greatest burden from CVD. These data may suggest where preventive efforts and programs may be most needed or best targeted to high-risk groups or regions.

Cardiovascular Disease Risk Factors: National and International Rates and Trends

In this section, we present data on the prevalence and trends in "traditional" CVD risk factors (i.e.,

TABLE 2–6 U.S. Age-Adjusted All-Cause and CVD Mortality Rates (per 100,000 Population) and Percent Change from 1980 to 1996 for Selected Race/Gender Groups

Race/Gender Group	All Causes			Diseases of the Heart			Ischemic Heart Disease			Cerebrovascular Disease		
	1980	1996	% Change	1980	1996	% Change	1980	1996	% Change	1980	1996	% Change
All persons	585.5	491.6	−16.0%	202.0	134.5	−33.4%	149.8	86.7	−42.1%	40.8	26.4	−35.3%
Males	777.2	623.7	−19.8%	280.4	178.8	−36.2%	214.8	119.3	−44.5%	44.9	28.5	−36.5%
Females	432.6	381.0	−11.9%	140.3	98.2	−30.0%	98.8	60.4	−38.9%	37.6	24.6	−34.6%
American Indian/ Alaska Native	564.1	456.7	−19.0%	131.2	100.8	−23.2%	87.4	63.8	−27.0%	26.6	21.1	−20.7%
Asian/Pacific islander	315.6	277.4	−12.1%	93.9	71.7	−23.6%	67.5	44.8	−33.6%	29.0	23.9	−17.6%
Black	842.5	738.3	−12.4%	255.7	191.5	−25.1%	150.5	99.4	−34.0%	68.5	44.2	−35.5%
Hispanic*	397.4	365.9	−7.9%	116.0	88.6	−23.6%	77.8	58.2	−25.2%	23.8	19.5	−18.1%
Non-Hispanic white	559.4	466.8	−16.6%	197.6	129.8	−34.3%	150.6	86.4	−42.6%	38.0	24.5	−35.5%

* Baseline Data for 1985 presented for Hispanics.

Source: Adapted from National Center for Health Statistics.[5]

cigarette smoking, obesity, high blood pressure, and serum cholesterol). These data are presented both for the United States and other countries as potential mediating factors for the previously presented trends on CVD morbidity and mortality.

High Blood Pressure

Elevated systolic ($\geq$140 mmHg) and diastolic blood pressure ($\geq$90 mmHg) or hypertension greatly increases the risk of heart disease and stroke. International data indicate a great deal of geographic variation in the presence of hypertension.[11] Table 2–7 shows that among adults age 35 to 64 from WHO MONICA communities, the prevalence of hypertension (in men and women, respectively) varies from 6.3 and 3.6 percent (Catalonia, Spain) to 42.4 percent (Kuopio Province, Finland) and 34.5 percent (Novosibirsk intervention). Twelve of these communities had hypertension prevalence rates of greater than 30 percent for men, while, for women, only four communities had prevalence rates greater than 30 percent, documenting the substantial worldwide need for more intensive hypertension detection treatment and control programs.

Among 16 WHO MONICA sites, mean systolic blood pressure declined among 14 communities between 1982 and 1985 and 1987 and 1990, ranging from a decrease of 1.2 to 9.1 mmHg. In the two communities where increases in systolic blood pressure were observed, these increases were very modest (0.56 and 1.19 mmHg per year).[12]

In the United States, approximately 23 percent of the adult population aged 20 to 74 have high blood pressure (Table 2–8). Substantial reductions in hypertension have been observed from 1976 to 1994; prevalence rates among all persons have declined from 39 percent in 1976 to 1980 to 23 percent in 1988 to 1994.[5] Percent reductions have been greatest during this time period for non-Hispanic white men (45 percent), and lowest for African-American men and women (28 percent for both). Slight increases in the prevalence of hypertension among Mexican-American men and women have been observed during this time period, although the prevalence of hypertension in this population remains

lower than other racial groups. Across states, there is significant variation in the prevalence of self-reported hypertension, ranging from 16.3 percent in Arizona to 34.4 percent in Mississippi (Table 2–9).[6]

Cholesterol

Elevated serum cholesterol is an established risk factor for CVD among middle-aged adults. International data on median levels of serum cholesterol and the prevalence of hypercholesterolemia presented in this chapter were obtained from WHO MONICA study data.[10] The median total cholesterol value for the 30 WHO MONICA sites ranged from 4.1 mmol/L (158 mg/dL) (Beijing, China) to 6.4 mmol/L (246 mg/dL) (Luxembourg Province) in men and from 4.2 mmol/L (162 mg/dL) (Beijing, China) to 6.4 mmol/L (246 mg/dL) (Glasgow, United Kingdom) in women. This represents a difference between the highest and lowest centers of approximately 50 percent (Table 2–7). Substantial regional variability was observed in the prevalence of hypercholesterolemia in these populations (defined as total serum cholesterol $\geq$6.5 mmol/L, or 250 mg/dL) ranging from approximately 2 percent in Beijing, China, to approximately 50 percent in Lille, France.[11]

There have been modest declines in population cholesterol levels in recent years. In the 16 WHO MONICA populations observed over 5- to 6-year periods, 10 sites observed average annual reductions in mean serum total cholesterol ranging from 0.01 mmol/L (0.4 mg/dL) to 0.07 mmol/L (3 mg/dL), while six sites observed increased mean serum total cholesterol ranging from 0.02 mmol/L (0.8 mg/dL) to 0.07 mmol/L (3 mg/dL).[12]

In the United States, approximately 19 percent of persons aged 20 to 74 have high serum cholesterol.[5] The mean serum cholesterol value in the United States is approximately 203 mg/dL. The prevalence of elevated serum cholesterol is slightly higher among women (20.0 percent) than men (17.5 percent), with very little variation across race/ethnic groups. In the United States the overall prevalence of elevated serum cholesterol has declined by 28 to 29 percent from 1976 to 1994 (Table 2–8). In the United States, self-reported hypercholesterolemia in the adult population

TABLE 2–7 Prevalence of Major Cardiovascular Risk Factors for Men and Women Ages 35–64 Years across WHO MONICA Communities

Country	Regular Smokers (%)		Hypertension (%)*		Median Total Cholesterol (mmol/L)		Median BMI (kg/m²)	
	Men	Women	Men	Women	Men	Women	Men	Women
Auckland	28.7	24.9	15.8	8.7	5.7	5.7	25.4	23.7
Augsburg (rural)	29.6	12.0	18.9	14.3	6.1	5.9	27.3	25.8
Augsburg (urban)	36.2	18.4	24.7	15.4	6.2	6.0	26.8	25.1
Bas-Rhin	34.3	14.5	40.0	26.1	5.5	5.4	27.3	25.6
Beijing	58.2	17.5	22.9	16.3	4.1	4.2	23.4	23.9
Belfast	34.0	33.4	21.0	15.6	5.9	6.0	25.5	24.8
Berlin-Lichtenberg	32.3	22.8	30.8	22.5	N/A	N/A	25.9	24.7
Bremen	44.8	29.3	23.0	20.0	6.0	6.0	26.3	25.5
Brianza Area	43.5	18.4	29.1	20.2	5.6	5.5	25.5	24.3
Budapest	51.9	35.7	N/A†	N/A	5.7	5.8	25.8	25.5
Catalonia	47.3	5.5	6.3	3.6	N/A	N/A	26.5	26.3
Charleroi	50.2	23.7	12.9	5.4	6.1	5.8	26.3	26.0
Czechoslovakia	44.2	22.0	25.9	22.2	6.3	6.3	27.1	27.2
DDR MONICA	38.2	17.5	31.9	32.5	N/A	N/A	26.3	25.8
Fruili	34.9	26.4	30.8	24.6	N/A	N/A	26.3	25.6
Ghent	42.7	25.0	7.6	4.5	6.1	5.9	26.1	25.2
Glasgow	52.4	50.2	27.5	21.5	6.2	6.4	25.4	25.5
Glostrup	44.6	43.7	11.3	6.6	6.2	6.1	25.4	23.5
Goteborg	32.3	34.5	N/A	N/A	6.1	6.0	25.0	23.6
Halle County	38.0	13.9	30.3	29.5	N/A	N/A	26.7	26.2
Haute-Garonne	36.5	17.4	21.9	13.0	5.9	5.7	25.5	23.6
Iceland	26.3	39.8	N/A	N/A	6.1	6.2	25.4	24.2
Karl-Marx-Stadt County	36.8	14.5	38.9	27.6	N/A	N/A	26.3	24.9
Kaunas	38.1	3.8	26.2	23.4	5.9	6.0	27.5	29.3
Kuopio Province	33.0	9.6	42.4	31.1	6.2	6.2	26.4	25.9
Luxembourg Province	42.6	17.8	10.3	11.3	6.4	6.3	25.6	25.1
Malta	48.8	10.2	29.1	29.3	N/A	N/A	27.1	28.6
Moscow (control)	48.3	12.2	34.4	31.5	N/A	N/A	25.6	27.8

Moscow (intervention)	46.2	8.7	24.9	21.5	N/A	N/A	25.7	28.0
Newcastle	32.9	23.3	17.8	13.4	5.7	5.6	26.0	24.5
North Karelia	29.4	8.2	34.8	29.7	6.3	6.2	26.7	26.2
Northern Sweden	23.7	26.5	15.2	12.7	N/A	N/A	25.6	24.7
Novi Sad	48.9	27.8	16.9	17.4	N/A	N/A	26.7	27.4
Novosibirsk (control)	58.8	3.4	27.5	26.8	N/A	N/A	25.7	28.9
Novosibirsk (intervention)	53.4	2.7	33.7	34.5	N/A	N/A	25.9	24.7
Pecs	48.5	24.3	N/A	N/A	N/A	N/A	26.1	26.4
Perth	32.8	21.9	19.9	11.5	5.8	5.7	25.5	23.8
Rhien-Necker Region	31.0	21.4	12.7	9.1	5.7	5.7	26.2	24.3
Stanford	40.0	36.8	15.8	8.6	5.3	5.2	25.6	23.5
Tarnobrzeg Voivodship	57.9	11.1	23.2	26.7	5.3	5.4	25.2	27.3
Ticino	38.2	24.1	15.3	11.6	5.5	5.2	26.8	24.2
Turku/Loimaa	30.2	17.5	31.3	19.4	6.1	6.0	26.5	25.2
Vaud/Fribourg	32.2	20.6	13.7	9.2	6.3	6.0	25.9	24.0
Warsaw	58.5	33.7	35.7	27.7	5.5	5.5	26.4	26.8

*Hypertension Defined as systolic blood pressure ≥140 mmHg or diastolic blood pressure ≥90 mmHg
†Not available.
Source: Adapted from the WHO MONICA Project.[3]

TABLE 2–8 Estimated Prevalence of Overweight, Obesity, and Hypercholesterolemia by Race/Ethnicity and Hypertension (Systolic > 140 mmHg or Diastolic >90 mmHg) by Race/Ethnicity and Gender, NHANES II and NHANES III*

	Men			Women		
Group	NHANES II (1976–80)	NHANES III (1988–94)	% Change	NHANES II (1976–80)	NHANES III (1988–94)	% Change
Non-Hispanic whites						
Overweight	51.5	59.6	15.7	37.4	45.5	21.7
Obesity	12.0	20.0	66.6	14.8	22.4	51.4
High cholesterol	24.7	17.3	−30.0	28.3	20.2	−28.7
Hypertension	43.9	24.4	−44.5	32.1	19.3	−39.9
Non-Hispanic blacks						
Overweight	48.9	57.5	17.6	60.2	66.5	10.5
Obesity	15.0	21.3	42.0	30.0	37.4	24.7
High cholesterol	24.0	15.7	−34.6	24.9	19.8	−20.5
Hypertension	48.7	35.0	−28.2	47.6	34.2	−28.2
Mexican-American						
Overweight	59.7	67.1	12.4	60.1	67.6	12.5
Obesity	15.4	23.1	50.0	25.4	34.2	34.6
High cholesterol	18.8	17.8	−5.4	20.0	17.5	−12.5
Hypertension	25.0	25.2	0.8	21.8	22.0	0.9
All racial and ethnic groups						
Overweight	51.4	59.3	15.4	40.8	49.6	21.6
Obesity	12.3	19.9	61.8	16.5	24.9	50.9
High cholesterol	24.6	17.5	−28.9	27.6	20.0	−27.6
Hypertension	44.0	25.3	−42.5	34.0	20.8	−38.9

*The following definitions were used: overweight (BMI ≥25 kg/m2); obesity (BMI >30 kg/m2); hypercholesterolemia (≥6.2 mmol/L); hypertension (SBP ≥140 or DBP ≥90 mmHg)

Source: Adapted from: Flegal et al.[14]

ranges from 22 percent in Oklahoma to 34.3 percent in Illinois (Table 2–9).[6]

Cigarette Smoking

Tobacco use has been linked to CVD mortality and subclinical CVD. Data from WHO MONICA populations indicate very high rates of cigarette smoking across the world[11] (Table 2–7). Population percentages of regular smokers (those reporting smoking cigarettes every day) for men aged 35 to 64 ranged from 23.7 percent in Northern Sweden to 58.8 percent in Novosibirsk, Russia, while the percentages in women ranged from 2.7 percent in Novosibirsk, Russia, to 50.2 percent in Glasgow, United Kingdom. Eight sites reported that over half their male population were regular cigarette smokers (Charleroi, Belgium; Budapest,

Hungary; Glasgow, United Kingdom; Novosibirsk, Russia (intervention); Tarnobrzeg Voivodship, Poland; Beijing, China; Warsaw, Poland; Novosibirsk, Russia). An additional 20 to 35 percent of the population in most of these sites were identified as ex-smokers.

International data on secular trends in smoking prevalence indicate declines in most populations. From 16 WHO MONICA sites, annual reductions in smoking prevalence from 1982 to 1985 to 1987 to 1990 of 0.02 to 1.92 percent were observed in 14 communities, while increases of 0.44 and 0.67 percent were observed in two communities. Not surprisingly, these were the only two communities that also observed increases in annual coronary disease death rates during this time period.[12]

In the United States, approximately 25 percent of adults (or 50 million persons) were considered

TABLE 2–9 State-specific Prevalence of Risk Factors for Cardiovascular Disease (High Blood Pressure, Overweight, High Cholesterol, Cigarette Smoking, Physical Inactivity among Adults), 1996–1997

State	High Blood Pressure*	Overweight**	High Cholesterol***	Cigarette Smoking#	Physical Inactivity##
Alabama	28.9	32.7	28.8	24.7	32.4
Alaska	22.6	34.1	25.5	26.5	25.4
Arizona	16.3	25.4	31.9	21.1	33.3
Arkansas	26.3	32.1	30.1	28.4	37.4
California	21.3	29.1	30.4	18.4	23.6
Colorado	20.4	25.1	27.9	22.6	20.2
Connecticut	20.6	29.1	24.3	21.6	25.6
Delaware	25.5	32.5	28.9	26.6	36.1
Florida	26.1	30.4	31.9	23.6	27.1
Georgia	21.4	30.8	24.1	22.4	51.4
Hawaii	24.0	26.6	31.5	18.7	21.0
Idaho	24.1	29.6	29.8	19.9	20.5
Illinois	24.3	32.0	34.3	23.2	24.9
Indiana	25.2	34.6	29.0	26.4	31.0
Iowa	23.4	33.3	28.1	23.1	26.9
Kansas	20.9	31.5	28.1	22.6	36.4
Kentucky	27.1	35.6	30.1	30.7	45.6
Louisiana	25.1	33.5	26.6	24.5	34.9
Maine	22.8	30.2	32.2	22.7	34.0
Maryland	23.8	31.2	28.6	20.4	33.8
Massachusetts	19.8	25.5	25.0	20.5	23.0
Michigan	23.3	34.9	31.2	26.0	23.3
Minnesota	21.2	29.7	31.2	21.9	23.6
Mississippi	34.4	35.1	28.8	23.1	39.5
Missouri	27.3	31.6	30.5	28.6	30.2
Montana	22.9	27.9	31.0	20.5	21.2
Nebraska	22.4	31.1	30.0	22.1	22.9
Nevada	24.1	26.2	29.6	28.0	22.7
New Hampshire	22.6	27.5	30.9	24.7	25.5
New Jersey	23.6	28.2	27.9	21.4	26.3
New Mexico	21.3	29.8	28.0	22.1	27.7
New York	22.7	28.4	28.0	23.1	30.4
North Carolina	23.3	32.4	26.5	25.9	40.7
North Dakota	25.5	32.9	29.8	22.3	33.9
Ohio	22.0	32.6	27.7	25.1	42.6
Oklahoma	21.7	28.4	22.0	24.6	38.2
Oregon	22.8	32.4	32.0	20.7	19.6
Pennsylvania	21.7	32.2	25.9	24.2	26.3
Rhode Island	22.5	28.1	28.1	24.3	26.7
South Carolina	26.9	31.8	24.5	23.4	29.7
South Dakota	20.6	31.1	25.7	24.3	34.8
Tennessee	27.8	31.6	29.5	26.9	40.8
Texas	23.1	32.8	28.7	22.6	27.9
Utah	22.5	27.0	26.4	13.8	17.1
Vermont	20.9	29.9	25.9	23.3	21.4
Virginia	24.5	30.0	29.5	24.4	29.2
Washington	23.2	29.1	25.6	23.8	19.1
West Virginia	28.3	36.3	32.2	27.4	42.7
Wisconsin	23.1	32.8	26.9	23.2	22.1
Wyoming	22.1	27.9	29.9	24.0	20.4

*Ever told blood pressure is high by a health professional
**Overweight defined as body mass index GE 27.8 for men and 27.3 for women
***Ever told cholesterol is high by a health professional
#Current smokers
##No reported leisure-time physical activity during previous month

Source: 1997 Behavioral Risk Factor Surveillance System (1996 for Physical Inactivity), Centers for Disease Control and Prevention

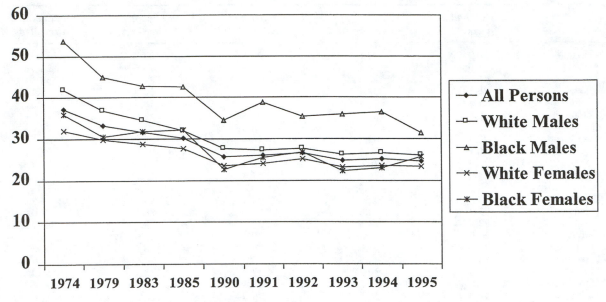

FIGURE 2–6 Age-adjusted prevalence of current cigarette smoking among adults age 25 years and older, by race and sex, 1974 to 1995. (Adapted from National Center for Health Statistics.[5])

current smokers.[2] Cigarette use is more common among persons of lower socioeconomic status across all racial/ethnic groups for men and women. Overall, cigarette smoking is higher among men (26.4 percent) than women (23 percent). In comparing smoking rates among four racial/ethnicity/gender groups, African-American men have the highest prevalence of current smoking (31.4 percent), followed by white men (26.0 percent). Between states, there is roughly a twofold variation in adult smoking prevalence, ranging from 30.7 percent in Kentucky to 13.8 percent in Utah. California, having an active smoking prevention program funded by tobacco tax monies, reports a smoking prevalence of 18.4 percent[6] (Table 2–9), and a noteworthy 26 percent decline (from 26 to 19.2 percent, $p < .001$) between 1984 and 1996.[13]

Cigarette smoking has been declining over the last three decades. According to data from the National Health Interview Survey (Fig. 2–6),[5] in 1974 the prevalence of current cigarette smoking among adults ≥25 years of age was 37.1 percent, a rate that is 50 percent higher than the 1995 estimate of 24.6 percent. Declines were greatest among black males;

53.8 percent of adult black men smoked in 1974 as compared with 31.4 percent in 1995, a decrease of approximately 41 percent.

Obesity

Obesity is a well-established risk factor for CVD and contributes to an increased prevalence of other CVD risk factors, such as hypertension, hypercholesterolemia, and diabetes mellitus. Table 2–7 presents age-standardized median body mass index (BMI) values for men and women across 44 WHO MONICA communities. Median BMI for men and women ranged from a low of 23.4 and 23.9 for men and women, respectively, in Beijing, China, to a high of 27.5 and 29.3 for men and women, respectively, in Kaunus, Lithuania.[11]

In the United States, approximately 66 million adults are overweight. Obesity is more common among persons of lower socioeconomic status and among some ethnic minority groups. According to data from the National Health and Nutrition Examination Survey (NHANES) III, prevalence of overweight, defined as BMI ≥ 25.0, varied across race/gender groups from 45.5 percent (white women) to 67.6 percent (Mexican-American women).[2] The prevalence of obesity, defined as BMI ≥ 30.0, ranged from 20 percent for non-Hispanic white men to 37.4 percent for African-American women. Between states, the prevalence of overweight, defined by a BMI of ≥ 27.8 kg/m^2 for men and ≥ 27.3 kg/m^2 for women, ranged from a high of 36.3 in West Virginia to 25.1 in Colorado. Similarly, there are great variations in the prevalence of no leisure-time physical activity (during the past month), ranging from 51.4 percent in Georgia to 17.1 percent in Utah (Table 2–9).[6]

These data also show that the prevalence of overweight and obesity is increasing. Flegal and colleagues[14] observed an increase in the prevalence of overweight from 46.0 to 54.4 percent (an 18 percent increase) from NHANES II (1976 to 1980) to NHANES III (1988 to 1994), while the prevalence of obesity increased from 14.5 to 22.5 percent (an increase of 55 percent) during the same time period. The greatest increase in overweight was observed for white women (22 percent increase), while the greatest increase in obesity was observed for white men (66 percent increase) (Table 2–8). Among California adults in 1996, more than one in four (26.7 percent) were considered overweight (defined as a BMI of 27.8 kg/m^2 or greater for men and 27.3 kg/m^2 or greater for women), a 50 percent increase since 1984 ($p < .0001$).[13]

Medical Care Trends

Substantial changes have occurred over the 1980s and 1990s in the medical care of CVD. Changes have occurred both in risk-factor reduction in high-risk groups and also in the treatment administered during and following acute CVD events. Over the past few decades, there have been dramatic improvements in awareness, treatment, and control of hypertension and elevated serum cholesterol levels in the United States; these have been linked to changes in medical evaluation and treatment. Increased use of pharmacologic as well as nonpharmacologic modalities to reduce risk factors for CVD

have been postulated to contribute to up to 50 percent of the observed decline in CHD mortality, while changes in medical care have been suggested to contribute the remaining 50 percent of the decline. There remains, however, room for significant improvement regarding the identification, management, and control of those with elevated cholesterol levels,[15,16] and hypertension,[17] as well as other risk factors.

Substantial changes have occurred in the treatment of cardiovascular disease. Figure 2–7 documents trends in cardiovascular operations and procedures in the United States from 1979–1995.[2] Specifically, the number of cardiac catheterizations has increased from approximately 300,000 per year in 1979 to more than 1.1 million in 1995. Likewise, similar increases in the number of coronary artery bypass graft procedures, number of percutaneous transluminal coronary angioplasty procedures, number of pacemaker implantations, and number of carotid endarterectomies have occurred. An important factor contributing to reductions in CVD burden in the United States is intervention targeted toward the high-risk subgroups that bear a disproportionate burden of the CVD morbidity/mortality.[2] Thus, the adoption of primary and secondary prevention strategies by the medical care system in the United States and other developed countries has contributed to the recent decline in CVD mortality rates.

Migrant Studies

As shown above, substantial differences in the CVD burden exist between different countries. These differences may be attributable to many factors, including country/regional differences in genotypes, gene-environment interactions, differences in health behaviors, and also differences in the awareness, diagnosis, and treatment of CVD risk factors and disease. Studies of individuals who migrate from areas of low CVD prevalence to areas of higher CVD prevalence provide valuable corroborating evidence to the observed ecological comparisons of countries.

Figure 2–8 shows mean cholesterol levels and corresponding CHD incidence rates among participants

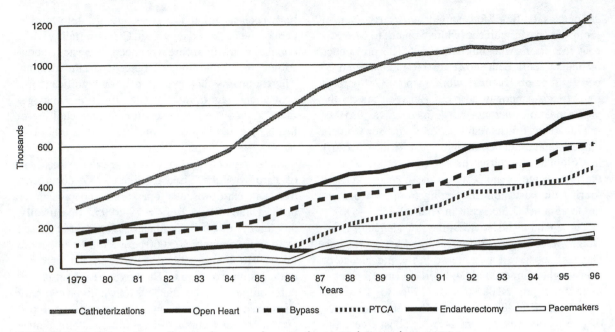

FIGURE 2–7 Trends in cardiovascular procedures in the United States from 1979 to 1995. (From American Heart Association,[2] with permission.)

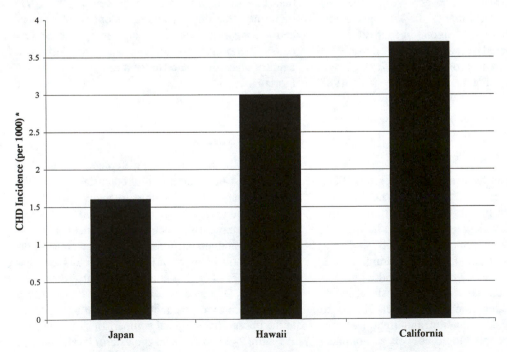

FIGURE 2–8 CHD Incidence in middle-aged Japanese men residing in Japan, Hawaii, and California. (Adapted from Robertson et al.[18])

in the Ni-Hon-San Study contrasting Japanese who remain in Japan with those who migrated to Hawaii and with those who migrated to the San Francisco Bay area. These data show that risk factor behaviors of the migrants become more similar to those observed in their newly adopted country.[18] Likewise, CVD morbidity and mortality in migrants to the U.S. mainland were observed to approach levels observed in U.S. Caucasian populations rather than remaining at the lower rates observed in individuals remaining in Japan (Figure 2–8). This information suggests that environmental factors likely play a key role in mediating some of the large differences observed between countries. It is unlikely that individuals genetically predisposed toward a more abnormal CVD risk profile and higher rates of CVD morbidity and mortality are more likely to migrate. Therefore, the adoption of new health behaviors by migrants likely mediates the majority of the increase in CVD burden. This is extremely important in the context of international CVD prevention. It suggests that increasing rates of CVD that are either currently occurring or projected to occur in countries with previously low rates of CVD are likely mediated to a great extent by the adoption of a more westernized lifestyle.

Changes in Age-Adjustment Standards

Age is one of the strongest predictors of increased prevalence of CVD risk factors, morbidity, and mortality. Therefore, age is an important confounder to consider when making comparisons across geographic-, gender-, and ethnic-specific groups. For the purpose of clarity, age-adjusted rates are used to potentially remove the effect of age differences between groups. The standard population used for age adjustment has varied between countries, continents, and study groups. For nearly 60 years, the official U.S. mortality statistics have used the 1940 U.S. population as their age-adjustment standard. In fact, many of the data cited in this chapter use this standard. However, since the demographics of the United States have changed markedly from 1940 through the late 1990s, using the 1940 population (with proportionally fewer older adults) results in age-adjusted rates

that are substantially lower than the actual disease rates for the major chronic diseases (CVD, cancer, etc.). All future versions of the U.S. mortality statistics will utilize the projected 2000 U.S. population as the standard population. As a consequence of using this population standard, the age-adjusted rates of heart disease will increase dramatically and will more closely approximate the current overall rates of CVD. As is shown in Fig. 2–9, the age-adjusted mortality rates for heart disease and cancer are nearly twofold higher when the 2000 U.S. population is used as the standard as compared with the 1940 U.S. population standard. It should be noted that the CVD time trends are affected very little by this change. A more detailed description of the statistical methodology incorporating this new population standard has been recently published.[19]

Future Trends in Cardiovascular Disease

Using currently observed trends in cardiovascular disease as a predictor of subsequent trends is a challenging task. There are, however, a number of key points that can be elucidated with some confidence. These include the following: (1) a continued unacceptably high burden of CVD is observed in developed countries, (2) a rapidly increasing CVD burden is occurring in emerging economies, and (3) the large number of known modifiable risk factors are identifiable and treatment is known to decrease CVD. Projections done by Murray and Lopez state that CVD will be the leading cause of death in both developed and developing regions of the world by the year 2020.[20] These projections are shown in Fig. 2–10, which contrasts the leading causes of death in developed and developing countries projected for 2020. In developed countries, ischemic heart disease and cerebrovascular disease are projected to account for nearly 37 percent of all-cause mortality, while in developing countries they are projected to account for only 25 percent of all-cause mortality. Importantly, both the endemically high rates of CVD in developed countries and the rapidly increasing rates of CVD in developing countries are linked to population levels of CVD risk factors. The remarkable declines

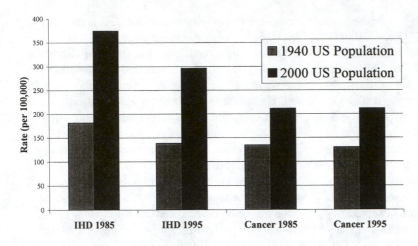

FIGURE 2–9 Age-adjusted heart disease and cancer mortality trends using 1940 and 2000 U.S. age distributions as population standard. (Adapted from Sorlie et al.,[19] with permission.)

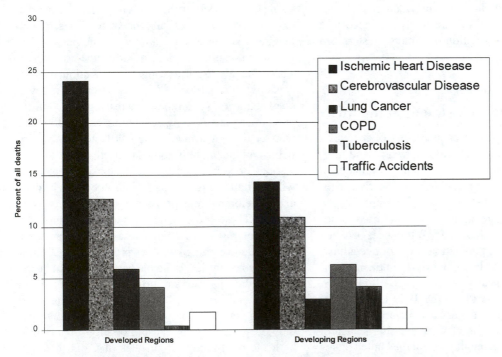

FIGURE 2–10 Projected leading causes of death in 2020 by region of the world. (From Murray and Lopez,[20] with permission.)

in cardiovascular mortality observed in Western countries over the last three decades are attributable in large measure to successful primary and secondary prevention of CVD disease. Despite these dramatic improvements in developed countries, substantial opportunities remain to further reduce CVD burden. For example, cigarette smoking continues to be a habit of more than 20 to 40 percent of adults in many of these countries. Further opportunities remain for identification and treatment of elevated blood pressure, dyslipidemia, and obesity. Although prognosis following myocardial infarction and stroke has shown dramatic improvements, further advances in the early detection and early treatment of these conditions would certainly be of great benefit. Therefore, while huge improvements in reducing CVD have been observed in developed countries, unacceptably large subgroups of the population remain at high risk for CVD events.

Conversely, in developing countries, less emphasis has been placed on chronic disease prevention due to economic pressures and the historically lower rates of CVD burden in these societies. Unless we are able to learn from the unfortunate lessons associated with the epidemic of CVD in developed countries, the developing countries will likely repeat the history of increasing CVD burden that was seen in the developed countries during much of the twentith century. As we have shown, many of these developing countries currently have high rates of cigarette smoking, increasing rates of obesity, and increasing rates of CVD risk factors. Ironically it is the ongoing adoption of Western lifestyles that puts individuals in the developing world at risk for chronic diseases. Active efforts are required even to maintain current levels of physical activity and healthy components of traditional diets in these countries. In addition, the development of effective prevention strategies for CVD, such as risk-factor screening/treatment and appropriate medical intervention for acute events, is necessary to reverse the current trend toward increasing burden from CVD.

Important steps should be taken to reduce the future burden of CVD in both developing and developed countries. In Western developed countries, specific steps should be taken to deal with the existing high burden of CVD. Primary prevention should be emphasized, including increased physical activity, the promotion of a heart-healthy diet, and a decreased prevalence of obesity. Interventions that focus on reducing the prevalence of traditional risk factors should continue to be emphasized as an important part of primary and secondary prevention efforts. Specific efforts will include the identification and treatment of hypertension, the identification and treatment of dislipidemia, and enhanced efforts to prevent smoking initiation and to encourage smoking cessation. Given the large number of high-risk individuals with existing cardiovascular disease in developed countries, secondary prevention efforts will be an important strategy to reduce subsequent CVD morbidity and mortality in high-risk individuals.

Although strategies for CVD interventions in developing countries are similar, they should be tailored to the specific needs of these emerging economies. In many of these settings, the current burden of CVD is relatively low, with the potential for a substantially higher future burden. In these countries, primary prevention of CVD will be a key part of these efforts. It is of paramount importance to encourage the maintenance of existing heart-healthy habits such as physical activity, a traditional (and healthier) diet, and the maintenance of low rates of obesity. A secondary strategy should be the identification and treatment of traditional risk factors. One very important risk factor in developing countries is a cigarette smoking rate that is often higher than in developed countries. Given the lower prevalence of CVD in these countries, secondary prevention efforts in these emerging countries are often less than in developed countries. However secondary prevention programs need to be initiated. Hopefully, the emerging economies will learn from the mistakes of developed countries and hence the epidemic of cardiovascular disease will be avoided.

Summary

Despite the fact that most countries have observed reductions in the prevalence of CVD risk factors in recent years, there remains tremendous international variation in the prevalence of major cardiovascular risk factors. The exception to the pattern of an improving CVD risk profile is the increasing rates of obesity, particularly in the United States. The overall reductions in CVD risk factors may explain in part the concordant reductions in CVD mortality and morbidity in the United States and in other developed countries.

This chapter has focused on describing recent trends in CVD in the United States and in other countries. Substantial heterogeneity exists in CVD mortality between countries. Encouraging improvements have been observed over the last few decades in some of the countries with the highest rates of CVD mortality, while less encouraging developments have occurred in regions of the world with lower rates of CVD, such as eastern Europe. In addition, projections suggest that developing countries in South Asia and in the Pacific Rim will have a rapidly increasing burden of CVD in the future. As would be expected, international trends in CVD morbidity and mortality are highly correlated with the presence or absence of health-promoting behaviors and traditional CVD risk factors.

Substantial opportunities exist to further reduce CVD burden in developed countries and to prevent further increases in CVD in developing countries. Subsequent chapters in this book focus on effective strategies for CVD prevention both in clinical and community settings. While implementation of these prevention and treatment strategies requires substantial allocation of human and monetary resources, the potential payoffs in reduction of death and disability make this effort essential.

References

1. The WHO MONICA Project: A worldwide monitoring system for cardiovascular disease. *World Health Stat Ann* 1989; 27:149.
2. American Heart Association: *Heart and Stroke Facts, 1998*. Dallas, AHA, 1998.
3. The WHO MONICA Project: Ecological analysis of the association between mortality and major risk factors of cardiovascular disease. *Int J Epidemiol* 1994; 23:505–516.
4. The WHO MONICA Project: Myocardial infarction and coronary deaths in the World Health Organization MONICA Project. *Circulation* 1994; 90:583–612.
5. National Center for Health Statistics: *Health, United States, 1998, with Socioeconomic Status and Health Chartbook*. Hyattsville, MD, NCHS, 1998.
6. Centers for Disease Control and Prevention: *Behavioral Risk Factor Surveillance System, National Summary Report, 1996 and 1997*. Atlanta, U.S. Department of Health and Human Services, Centers for Disease Control and Prevention, 1998.
7. National Heart, Lung, and Blood Institute: *Morbidity and Mortality: 1996 Chartbook on Cardiovascular, Lung, and Blood Diseases*. Bethesda, MD, National Institutes of Health, 1996.
8. The WHO MONICA Project: Stroke trends in the WHO MONICA Project. *Stroke* 1997; 28:500–506.
9. Kesteloot H, Joossens JV: Worldwide mortality changes from all causes and from cardiovascular diseases between 1968 and 1988. *Acta Cardiol* 1993; 48:421–439.
10. Rosamond WD, Chambless LE, Folsom AR, et al: Trends in the incidence of myocardial infarction and in mortality due to coronary heart disease, 1987 to 1994. *N Engl J Med* 1998; 339:861–867.
11. The WHO MONICA Project: Risk factors. *Int J Epidemiol* 1989; 18:S46–S55.
12. Dobson A, Filipiak B, Kuulasmaa K, et al: Relations of changes in coronary disease rates and changes in risk factor levels: methodological issues and a practical example. *Am J Epidemiol* 1996; 143:1025–1034.
13. Gazzaniga JM, Kao C, Cowling DW, et al: *Cardiovascular Disease Risk Factors Among California Adults, 1984–1996*. Sacramento, CA, CORE Program, University of California San Francisco and California Department of Health Services, 1988.
14. Flegal KM, Carroll MD, Kuczmarski RJ, Johnson CL: Overweight and obesity in the United States: prevalence and trends, 1960–94. *Int J Obesity* 1998; 22:39–47.
15. Stafford RS, Blumenthal D, Pasternak RC. Variations in cholesterol management practices by U.S physicians. *J Am Coll Cardiol* 1997; 29:139–146.
16. Danias PG, O'Mahony S, Radford M, et al: Serum cholesterol levels and underevaluated and undertreated. *Am J Cardiol* 1998; 81:1353–1355.
17. Joint National Committee on Prevention Detection Evaluation and Treatment of High Blood Pressure: The sixth report of the Joint National Committee on Prevention, Detection, Evaluation, and Treatment of High Blood Pressure. *Arch Intern Med* 1997; 157:2413–2446.
18. Robertson TL, Kato H, Rhoads GG, et al: Epidemiologic studies of coronary heart disease and stroke in Japanese men living in Japan, Hawaii and California. *Am J Cardiol* 1977; 39:239–243.
19. Sorlie PD, Thom T, Manolio T, et al: Age-adjusted mortality rates: consequences of the year 2000 standard. *Ann Epidemiol* 1999; 9:93–100.
20. Murray JL, Lopez AD: *The Global Burden of Disease: A Comprehensive Assessment of Global Mortality and Disability from Diseases, Injuries, and Risk Factors in 1990 and Projected to 2020*. Geneva, Switzerland, World Health Organization, 1996.

Part **II**

Screening for Cardiovascular Risk and Subclinical Disease

CHAPTER 3

Exercise Testing, Ankle-Brachial Index, and Coronary Calcium Screening

Terence M. Doherty
Robert C. Detrano
Michael H. Criqui
Nathan D. Wong

Every year in the United States alone, approximately 2 million people are hospitalized for coronary heart disease (CHD) and another one-half million die of this disease.[1] Historically, the medical community has tended to focus its efforts on treating patients after CHD has been established, but data from large multinational studies indicate that as many as 30 to 40 percent of all individuals who present with an acute coronary syndrome have had no prior warning symptoms to suggest the presence of the underlying disease.[2] Pathologic studies have demonstrated that coronary atherosclerosis is a ubiquitous condition among adult residents of industrialized nations,[3–5] but epidemiologic data indicate that most of those afflicted will never suffer a serious coronary event.[6,7] Before preventive measures can be useful, it is necessary to identify those at greatest risk for cardiovascular events, both through office- and clinic-based risk assessment.

Information from the medical history, physical examination, and routine laboratory tests[8] can be helpful in initial risk stratification.[9] Further screening tests for subclinical disease in asymptomatic persons will detect not only the presence of coronary atherosclerosis but also can distinguish those who are destined to suffer a catastrophic coronary event from those who will not. Also, in screening higher-risk patients for atherosclerotic cardiovascular disease (CVD), an often overlooked area is screening for pe-

ripheral arterial disease (PAD). In this chapter, we review the roles of exercise testing, radiographic coronary calcium screening, and screening for PAD in identifying those at increased CVD risk.

Considerations in the Implementation of a Screening Test

A screening test must provide maximal information at minimal cost and risk; if it entails significant risk or is inconvenient, it is probably not worth pursuing. Societal and cost issues aside, a proposed screening test must certainly yield a high level of case detection and a minimum of false positives. Furthermore, there must be effective treatment available for positive cases; without treatment, screening becomes a pointless pursuit and a waste of time and resources. Finally, there are definite and important issues to consider related to the risks of screening versus the likely benefits, and an implicit price attendant to proliferation of a screening test before scientific evidence demonstrates a clear benefit to its use;[10] experience with screening for breast cancer with mammography over the past quarter century[11,12] provides an instructive example. In this instance, commercially motivated recommendations not based on scientific evidence were later revised when mounting scientific data demonstrated not only a lack of benefit but potential harm from recommending annual screening in younger women.

Clearly, a proposed screening test to identify persons at risk of suffering a devastating coronary event must have a compelling body of scientific evidence demonstrating its effectiveness, safety, precision, and benefit in those same individuals in whom its use is proposed before that test is placed into widespread clinical use. Before any risk-assessment tool can be widely implemented, (1) all or most widely accepted measures of risk must be incorporated, (2) its usefulness must be validated in clinical practice, and (3) methods to facilitate incorporation of risk assessment into the busy clinician's practice must be developed.[9]

Exercise Testing as a Screening Tool

Physiologic Rationale for Exercise Testing

Exercise testing attempts to identify patients with coronary atherosclerosis of sufficient obstructive severity to cause, upon exercise, an inability of coronary flow to meet the metabolic demands of the myocardium. The resultant metabolic state of the myocardium—myocardial ischemia—can then be identified by characteristic electrocardiographic (ECG) changes. Since the metabolic requirements of the myocardium can be significantly increased with exercise, coronary obstructions that may cause no ischemia at all at rest may cause severe ischemia with vigorous exercise and the corresponding increased workload demands placed upon the heart.

Variable Ability of a Coronary Obstruction to Cause Ischemia

Lesions with less than 50 percent of their lumens obstructed by atherosclerotic plaque have been considered not severe enough to cause ischemia, even with exercise; however, recent work using positron emission tomography has shown that ischemia can sometimes occur with less severe lesions.[13] On the other hand, lesions with greater than 50 percent obstruction to coronary flow may not produce ischemia for a variety of reasons. Myocardial ischemia develops

when myocardial oxygen demand outstrips the supply of oxygen to the myocardium. Oxygen supply is determined not only by the extent of luminal compromise but also by the oxygen-carrying capacity of the blood and the presence or absence of collateral vessels. Thus, the severity of coronary luminal compromise is only one factor that affects the myocardial supply-demand balance.

Accuracy of Exercise Testing in the Diagnosis of Obstructive Coronary Artery Disease

The "accuracy" of the exercise ECG can be loosely defined as its ability to discriminate between those individuals with a flow-limiting coronary stenosis and those without such stenosis. Wide variation in sensitivity, specificity, and positive and negative predictive values has been reported for exercise ECG testing.[14–17] If too narrow a spectrum of diseased and nondiseased patients is included in a study (problem of spectrum) or if the interpretation of the test and the establishment of the true diagnosis are not independent processes (problem of bias), the test accuracy may be questioned. Additionally, technical factors—such as the type of exercise protocol, the definition of a positive test, and the definition of angiographic disease—can also contribute to variability in reported sensitivities and specificities.[15,18]

Benefit of Identifying High-Risk Asymptomatic Persons

A critical question facing any proposed screening test is: If higher-risk subjects can be identified, will that result in diminished coronary morbidity and mortality? The answer may not be self-evident. The Multiple Risk Factor Intervention Trial (MRFIT) randomized a large group of asymptomatic men with multiple cardiac risk factors to a "usual care" or a "special intervention" group.[19] The special intervention group received counseling on smoking cessation, dietary practices to lower blood cholesterol level, and stepped-care drug treatment for hypertension. There was a trend toward reduction in overall coronary heart disease mortality in the special inter-

TABLE 3–1   Survival at 4 Years According to Duke Treadmill Score

Treadmill Score	Low Risk, More than +5	Intermediate Risk, −10 to +4	High Risk, Below −10
Inpatients	98%	92%	71%
Outpatients	99%	95%	79%

Source: From Califf et al.,[8] with permission.

vention group, but this did not reach statistical significance. However, when a subanalysis of the subjects with positive exercise tests was performed, special intervention dramatically reduced events. Therefore, those identified through exercise testing as being at higher risk for cardiac events substantially benefited from risk-factor modification.

A standard treadmill test can be routinely performed in patients who are not taking digoxin or other drugs that can affect evaluation of the results, who are able to exercise, and who have a normal ECG at rest. The response to exercise can permit an assessment of the severity of underlying coronary artery disease. Investigators from Duke University have developed a treadmill score that can be calculated by the following formula and is associated with 4-year survival, as shown in Table 3–1:[20]

Treadmill score = duration of exercise (min) − [maximal ST-segment deviation (mm) during or after exercise × 5] − (treadmill angina index × 4)

where the angina index is as follows: no angina during exercise = 0, nonlimiting angina = 1, exercise-limiting angina = 2.

The risk of exercise testing is primarily determined by the clinical characteristics of the patient. However, exercise testing is, in general, quite safe, with a mortality in a nonselected population of less than 0.01 percent (1 in 10,000) and a morbidity of less than 0.05 percent (5 in 10,000).[21] Typical complications associated with exercise testing appear in Table 3–2 and contraindications to testing in Table 3–3.

Criteria for ST-Segment Abnormality

Many investigators define a positive test by the presence of 1 mm or more of horizontal or downsloping ST-segment depression measured 80 ms after the J point. The Lipid Research Clinics (LRC) and MRFIT studies both used the ST integral as a marker for ischemia.[22,23] An ST-segment depression integral of 16 mV-s or more during peak exercise with a

TABLE 3–2   Complications Resulting from Exercise Tests

Cardiac Complications

Frequent ectopic beats
- Supraventricular
- Ventricular

Bradyarrythmias
- Sinus bradycardia
- Atrioventricular junctional bradycardia
- Ventricular ectopic rhythm

Atrioventricular block

Asystole

Tachyarrhythmias
- Supraventricular tachycardia
- Atrial fibrillation
- Ventricular tachycardia

Sudden death (ventricular tachycardia/fibrillation)

Myocardial infarction

Congestive heart failure

Hypotension and shock

Noncardiac and Miscellaneous Complications

Musculoskeletal trauma

Severe fatigue

Dizziness

Fainting

General malaise

Body aches

Delayed ill feelings

Fatigue, sometimes persisting for days

TABLE 3–3 **Contraindications to Exercise Testing**

Unstable angina with recent resting chest pain

Uncompensated congestive heart failure

Acute myocarditis or pericarditis

Critical aortic stenosis

Severe hypertrophic obstructive cardiomyopathy

Uncontrolled hypertension

Untreated life-threatening cardiac arrhythmias

Advanced atrioventricular block

Acute systemic illness

Inability to exercise*

*Due to orthopedic problem, claudication, lung disease, marked obesity, neurologic impairment, etc.

resting value of less than 6 mV-s was considered a positive response. Note that this endpoint is independent of the ST-segment slope. In the LRC study, a test was considered positive if ST depression or elevation of greater than 1 mm was determined visually or a computer-determined ST integral fell or rose by at least 10 mV-s from its resting value.[23]

Heart Rate Adjustment

Risk stratification in the Framingham Offspring Study failed to demonstrate the prognostic significance of ST depression alone in predicting coronary events.[24] When the degree of ST depression was adjusted for heart rate recovery, the subjects could be separated into low-, intermediate-, and high-risk groups. Heart rate adjustment has also been extensively studied in symptomatic patients undergoing exercise testing and has been validated by some authors[25-28] but not by others.[29,30]

"Hard" versus "Soft" Events

One problem in interpreting studies investigating the prognostic significance of exercise testing involves the definition of a cardiac event. Studies often define a cardiac event as angina, myocardial infarction, or sudden cardiac death. Some studies may also use the performance of revascularization procedures

(coronary bypass or angioplasty) as an endpoint. "Hard" events are typically considered to be myocardial infarction and CHD death, whereas angina and the performance of revascularization are usually considered "soft" endpoints.

One advantage of including angina and revascularizations as endpoints is that many more "events" may be anticipated, thus decreasing the sample size, the follow-up period, or both required to achieve sufficient power to obtain significant results. Clearly, however, the impact of angina is not equivalent to that of infarction or sudden death. Exercise testing would be of greater value if it could predict myocardial infarction and sudden coronary death in addition to angina. Furthermore, angina reported by study participants could be affected by recall bias; patients who are told that their exercise test is positive may be more likely to report angina on follow-up questioning. The intensity of utilization of exercise testing itself can lead to increased "downstream" cardiac procedures; the impact of this additional testing on the occurrence of subsequent cardiac events is unclear.[31]

An additional problem with using angina as an endpoint in prognostic studies is that chest pain resulting from noncardiac causes may be reported and analyzed as angina pectoris. In the case of revascularizations, a positive test result may influence the subsequent treatment of a patient ("posttest" referral bias) so as to make it more likely that the patient undergoes subsequent revascularization. Studies utilizing angina or revascularization as endpoints are subject to these potential sources of bias, whereas studies utilizing hard endpoints, which are certainly much less equivocal, are less likely to be unduly affected by these sources of bias.

Independent Prognostic Information Provided by Exercise Testing

One of the earliest and largest studies to address the prognostic significance of a positive exercise test was the Seattle Heart Watch.[32] Of the 2365 subjects who underwent symptom-limited exercise ECG testing, 47 sustained subsequent cardiac events (sudden cardiac death, myocardial infarction, or angina). The presence of any conventional risk factors and any two positive exercise test parameters (chest pain, exercise duration less than 6 min, failure to achieve greater than 90 percent age-predicted heart rate, or ST depression of a horizontal or downsloping nature and persisting for 1 min or more into recovery) was associated with a relative risk of 2.9 for a major cardiac event. Ischemic ST-segment depression alone carried a 3.4-fold higher risk for an event. In those individuals with no conventional risk factors, however, exercise testing was of no predictive value;

however, there were only three cardiac events in this subgroup.[22] Similar results have been reported by many other investigators, and the relative risk for a coronary event associated with a positive exercise ECG result alone has been reported to vary from 1.2 (not significant) to 14.[22-24,33-52] Table 3–4 summarizes major studies that have reported on the prognostic significance of an abnormal exercise test in asymptomatic subjects.

Exercise testing also provides prognostic data that are independent of other information, such as car-

TABLE 3–4   Prognostic Significance of an Abnormal Exercise Test in Asymptomatic Subjects

Reference	Women Included?	n	Follow-up (Years)	Cardiac Events[a] per 1000 Patient-Years	Multivariate Adjustment?	Relative Risk
Froelicher, 1974[49]	No	1,390	6.3	5.2	No	14.3
Bruce, 1980[32]	No	2,365	5.6	3.5	No	3.4[b]; 29[c]
Cumming, 1975[48]	No	510	3	17	No	10.3
McHenry, 1984[45]	No	916	12.7	5.6	No	4.9
Bruce, 1983[58]	Yes	4,158	6.1	8	No	1.3 to 6.7[d]
Giagnoni, 1983[53]	Yes	510	6	n/a	Yes	5.6
Allen, 1980[50]	Yes	1,077	5	10.8	Yes	1.9 to 14.7[e]
Gordon, 1986[23]	No	3,260	8.4	2.1	Yes	5.0
Rautaharju, 1986[22]	No	6,438	7	2.5	Yes	3.8[f]
				16.9		1.6[g]
				4.7		1.2[h]
Flegg, 1990[59]	Yes	407	4.6	21	Yes	1.4 to 6.7[i]
Okin, 1991[24]	Yes	3,168	4.3	4.7	Yes	1.2 to 3.6[j]
Total		24,199	69			Range: 1.2 to 29 Unweighted average: 5

[a]Cardiac events consisted of angina pectoris, myocardial infarction, or sudden cardiac death.

[b]For ST-segment depression alone.

[c]For two exercise criteria.

[d]Exercise duration: 6.7 in men, 3.6 in women; chest pain: 3.5 in men, 3.3 in women; maximum heart rate: 2.4 in men, 1.8 in women; rate-pressure product: 2.4 in men, 1.3 in women; ST-segment depression: 2.6 in men, 6.7 in women.

[e]ST-segment depression: 2.4 in men, 1.9 in women; R-wave response: 2.7 in men, 1.9 in women; exercise duration: 5.6 in men, 14.7 in women.

[f]For coronary heart disease death.

[g]For angina pectoris.

[h]For myocardial infarction.

[i]Two positive criteria (ST depression and segmental thallium defect): 3.6; ST depression alone: 2.4; segmental thallium defect alone: 1.4.

[j]For ST-segment depression: 1.2; for ST-segment heart rate: 2.2; for recovery loop: 2.1; for combined criteria: 3.6.

diac risk factors. Several large studies support the prognostic significance of a positive exercise ECG for predicting hard endpoints.[22–24,53] Giagnoni and colleagues showed that among 135 subjects with positive exercise tests (matched for work community, age, sex, and coronary risk-factor index against 379 controls with normal exercise tests), the relative risk for a cardiac event (sudden cardiac death, myocardial infarction, or angina) was 5.5 in those individuals with a positive exercise test result.[53] Other investigators, using multivariate adjustment, have demonstrated similar results. Multivariate adjustment was performed in both the LRC and MRFIT studies.[22,23] For the endpoint of 1 mm of ST-segment depression and using an exercise protocol to achieve 90 percent of maximum predicted heart rate, Gordon and colleagues reported a relative risk for coronary death of 4.6 in the LRC cohort.[23] Similarly, utilizing an ST-segment integral of 16 mV-s as an endpoint, Rautaharju and colleagues reported a relative risk for CHD death of 3.8 in the MRFIT study.[22] McHenry and colleagues, however, using a maximal protocol and 1-mm horizontal or downsloping ST-segment depression as an endpoint, showed an increased relative risk (4.9) only for angina.[45] Epstein and colleagues attributed this result to the "protective effect" of ischemia: patients with flow-limiting lesions developed protective collaterals, diminishing the probability of myocardial infarction or sudden cardiac death even if the vessel eventually becomes totally occluded.[54]

These results indicate that exercise testing can predict hard coronary events and may therefore be of prognostic value, but this may only be true for some patient subgroups. In a study of low-risk asymptomatic or mildly symptomatic patients with exercise testing followed clinically for over 4 years, noninvasive measures of ischemia were of no prognostic significance.[55]

In post–myocardial infarction patients, two meta-analyses (comprising 52 studies and 20,944 patients over a 22-year period) suggest that exercise testing can be of some prognostic value.[56,57] Froelicher and coworkers found that only an abnormal systolic blood pressure response and poor exercise capacity were of some prognostic value.[56] Also, submaximal

or predischarge testing had greater predictive power than did postdischarge or maximal testing. Furthermore, exercise-induced ST-segment depression was predictive of increased risk only in patients with inferior-posterior infarctions.[56] However, Shaw and colleagues found that the positive predictive value of predischarge exercise testing is low (most noninvasive risk markers were < 0.10 for cardiac death and < 0.20 for death or reinfarction) and that ST-segment depression and angina identified morbid and fatal outcomes poorly.[57] Indicators of left ventricular dysfunction, such as exercise duration and blunted systolic blood pressure response, appeared to be better predictors of morbidity and mortality than indicators of myocardial ischemia.[57]

Exercise Duration

The duration of exercise has been found to have important prognostic significance. For example, Bruce et al. found that an exercise duration of less than 6 min using the Bruce protocol was associated with an unadjusted relative risk for a cardiac event of 6.7 in men and 3.6 in women.[58] Allen and colleagues reported a relative risk for a cardiac event of 5.6 for an exercise duration of less than 5 min on a maximal Ellestad protocol.[50] Female patients who could not complete at least 3 min on this protocol had a 14.7-fold higher risk than those who could. Since neither of these studies adjusted for confounding variables, it is not clear if this finding is independent of patient age. However, Fleg et al. did perform multivariate adjustment and also reported exercise duration to be significantly associated with coronary events.[59]

Conversion to a Positive Test

Although it has been hypothesized that individuals who have a negative exercise test but subsequently convert to a positive test would be at increased risk of a cardiac event by comparison with those whose initial test is positive, this does not appear to be the case. In a study involving serial maximal stress tests in asymptomatic male employees of the Indiana State Police Department[45] followed for 12.7 years, the 5.1

percent of the subjects who demonstrated conversion to an abnormal test from an initially normal test had a similar prognosis as those with initially positive tests. Also, in a study of serial exercise tests in healthy men and women participating in the Baltimore Longitudinal Study of Aging,[60] the incidence of events was nearly identical between those who were initially positive and those who converted.

The High-Risk Patient

The absolute risk of a cardiac event is a function of both conventional risk factors and the results of an exercise ECG: patients at highest risk for events have several conventional risk factors in addition to abnormal exercise tests. Exercise ECG abnormalities alone, in the absence of conventional risk factors, seem to have little predictive value. Bruce and colleagues[32] identified a very high risk subset on the basis of the presence of conventional risk factors and two or more exercise ECG abnormalities and found that in patients with at least one conventional risk factor, the presence of two or more exercise endpoints imparted a significantly higher risk for coronary events as compared with patients without risk factors. Others show, however, that regardless of risk factors, a "strongly positive" exercise test (2 mm or more ST depression, or onset in the first 6 min of the modified Bruce protocol) has additional prognostic value.[22]

Prognostic Value of Exercise Testing in Women

The accuracy of exercise testing in women is controversial. Some investigators have reported lower specificity for an exercise ECG in women as opposed to men,[61] but others have found no difference.[33,62] A recent meta-analysis encompassing 19 studies comprising 3872 female subjects found that the exercise ECG is less accurate in women than in men.[63] Estrogen replacement therapy or estrogen itself could possibly play a role in the development of false-positive responses,[64] since it has been shown to have vasoconstrictive properties[65] and could, therefore, alter the supply-demand balance and so influence the results of an exercise test. However, a causal role for estrogen in false-positive exercise ECG results has not been clearly established.

Although the majority of studies on prognosis in asymptomatic subjects have involved male subjects only, the limited data available do support the prognostic value of exercise ECG testing in women. The Seattle Heart Watch[56] followed 547 women and 3611 men for 10 years who had undergone symptom-limited exercise testing. The prognostic significance of 1 mm of ST depression was higher in women than in men (relative risks: 2.6 for men, 6.7 for women).[58] However, these results were not subjected to multivariate adjustment. Since women tended to be older (30 percent of women but only 15 percent of men were over 55 years of age), adjustment for age would likely lead to a reduction in the prognostic significance of the exercise ECG results in women as opposed to men. Several other studies involving asymptomatic subjects included women,[24,50,52,59] but, unfortunately, gender-specific analyses and comparisons were not performed. A recent population-based study of 1452 men and 741 women in Olmsted County, Minnesota, did include both multivariate analysis and gender comparisons.[33] Most patients (64 percent of men and 63 percent of women) were either asymptomatic or had atypical chest pain. These investigators found no gender difference in the association of positive exercise test results (exercise-induced angina, ECG changes, and achieved workload) with subsequent cardiac events. After adjustment with multivariate analysis, independent predictors of a cardiac event in both sexes included age, diminished workload capacity, and number or risk factors.[33]

Additional Uses of the Exercise Test as a Screening Tool

Besides being useful in the prognostic evaluation of both symptomatic patients with CHD and asymptomatic subjects with no history of CHD, exercise testing has been utilized in fitness assessment and in the evaluation of individuals employed in high-risk professions. The exercise test can be used not only to evaluate the safety of participating in an exercise program but also to help formulate an exercise prescription.[66] Certain high-risk individuals may be best evaluated in this controlled environment. In addition, for athletes in training, serial exercise testing can provide feedback on improvements in cardiovascular fitness that may influence athletic performance. This can be an effective means of providing incentive and motivation to such individuals,[67] since aerobic exercise training can increase maximal oxygen uptake by approximately 25 percent.[68]

Routine exercise testing of persons engaged in certain high-risk professions (airline pilots, bus drivers, firefighters, and police officers) is frequently performed; however, the American College of Cardiology/American Heart Association (ACC/AHA) Task Force indicates that there are insufficient data at present to justify this approach.[69,70] In some cases, such evaluations are performed for statutory reasons, and the reasoning is that public safety could be jeopardized if individuals in these professions were to sustain a sudden cardiac event while working. The U.S. Air Force screens all air crew members over 35 years of age with a resting ECG. Subjects with "potential coronary artery disease" are referred for symptom-limited treadmill testing. Ninety-five percent of these individuals, in one report, were asymptomatic;[71] nevertheless, cardiac catheterization is mandatory if the exercise test is positive and the individual wishes to continue flying.

Adjunctive Imaging Modalities to Exercise Testing

Many techniques have been utilized to attempt to improve the diagnostic and prognostic accuracy of the exercise test. These include echocardiographic monitoring during exercise, radionuclide testing (including gated blood pool imaging and myocardial perfusion imaging), and various pharmacologic adjuncts (in combination with one or more of the above modalities). Studies of pharmacologic stress echocardiography have shown that this technique is potentially valuable for enhancing risk stratification in women, showing ischemia to be a strong predictor of hard cardiac events, providing incremental value over that provided by clinical variables,[72] being

highly sensitive for detection of CHD,[73,74] and being effective for stratifying those with either a normal or abnormal treadmill stress test.[73] Exercise thallium tomography also appears to provide further value over that of treadmill exercise testing and clinical variables for the prediction of hard coronary events in both high-risk asymptomatic individuals[75] and those with known or suspected CHD.[76] From a practical standpoint, however, a screening test must be inexpensive before widespread implementation may be considered. The cost of these modalities varies from about twice to five times that of the standard exercise test.[77] This expense precludes serious consideration of their utilization as screening tests for coronary heart disease and they are therefore not within the scope of this chapter.

Radiographic Assessment of Coronary Artery Calcium

Exercise testing examines physiologic parameters related to blood-flow limitation. In contrast, radiographic scanning techniques that detect calcium deposits in the coronary arteries—cardiac fluoroscopy, electron beam computed tomography (EBCT), and helical computed tomography (HCT)—instead provide anatomic information. Thus, exercise testing and radiographic calcium scanning provide entirely different information, yet each may have prognostic value. In recent years, EBCT in particular has attracted much attention, primarily a result of the hope that detection of calcium deposits will make it possible to assess the risk of a future coronary event and do so with an accuracy superior to that of exercise testing or evaluation of coronary risk factors. This is based on the premise of a relationship between calcific deposits in atherosclerotic plaque and the natural history of atherosclerotic disease.

Coronary Calcium, Risk Factors, and Atherosclerosis

The presence of calcium in the coronary arteries appears invariably to indicate the presence of atherosclerotic plaque; however, atherosclerotic lesions do

TABLE 3–5 Mean (±SD), Total Calcium Score, and Prevalence of Detectable Calcium (Score > 0) in All Arteries of Patients with No Symptoms, by Age Group

Age (years)	Males			Females		
	Mean ± SD	>0	(n)	Mean ± SD	>0	(n)
<40	23.7 ± 86.4	15%	(75)	1.6 ± 4.1	30%	(10)
40–49	34.9 ± 94.8	45%	(240)	7.6 ± 21.2	30%	(50)
50–59	115.7 ± 274.7	67%	(212)	36.5 ± 119.4	27%	(63)
60–69	291.9 ± 504.3	83%	(120)	69.5 ± 130.3	71%	(51)
≥70	928.4 ± 1036.1	93%	(28)	137.3 ± 259.6	75%	(16)
Comparison across age groups:	$p < .0001$	$p < .001$	$p < .0001$	$p < .001$		

Source: Adapted from Wong et al.,[83] with permission.

not always contain calcium.[78–82] Calcium deposition may begin quite early in life, in some cases as early as the second decade, and may occur in lesions that are not advanced.[3,4,78–80] The association of increasing calcium deposition with increasing age and also with the presence and severity of coronary risk factors—including hypercholesterolemia, hypertension, and diabetes—has been documented by several investigators.[83–89]

Wong et al.[83] have shown, in a report of 800 high-risk asymptomatic individuals who underwent coronary artery screening by EBCT, that the prevalence of coronary calcium increased by age group from 15 percent in men under age 40 years to 93 percent in those aged 70 years and older ($p < .001$) and from 30 percent in women under age 40 to 75 percent in those aged 70 years or older ($p < .001$) (Table 3–5). Further, calcium prevalence is shown to increase with the number of risk factors (Table 3–6), and—from multiple logistic regression analysis—the likelihood of coronary calcium is associated with increasing age, male gender, hypertension, diabetes, hypercholesterolemia, and obesity (Table 3–7).

Potentially attractive is the ability to detect coronary artery calcification noninvasively so as to motivate healthful lifestyle changes before the onset of clinical events. In one study, patients demonstrating coronary calcium on an initial scan, versus those

TABLE 3–6 Mean (±SD) Total Calcium Score and Prevalence of Detectable Calcium (Score > 0) in All Arteries of Patients with No Symptoms by Number of Risk Factors

Number of Risk Factors*	Males			Females		
	Mean ± SD	>0	(n)	Mean ± SD	>0	(n)
0	79.1 ± 299.9	40%	(119)	35.3 ± 174.4	29%	(35)
1	158.2 ± 441.5	56%	(246)	24.9 ± 32.3	39%	(66)
2	128.0 ± 313.4	62%	(188)	33.3 ± 77.9	46%	(54)
3 or more	220.4 ± 494.0	74%	(86)	122.0 ± 320.1	64%	(28)
Comparison across number of risk factors:	$p < .0001$		$p < .001$	$p = .02$		$p = .03$

*Reported history of high blood pressure, high blood cholesterol, diabetes, smoking, and family history of premature myocardial infarction.

Source: Adapted from Wong et al.,[83] with permission.

TABLE 3–7 Indicators of Coronary Artery Calcium: Multiple Logistic Regression Analyses ($n = 800$)

Risk Factor	Coefficient	Risk Ratio	95% Confidence Interval
Intercept	−5.50		
Age (per 10 years)	1.04	2.82†	(2.33–3.43)
Female gender	−1.07	0.34†	(0.23–0.50)
Hypertension (yes vs. no)	0.42	1.53*	(1.03–2.25)
Diabetes (yes vs. no)	0.84	2.32*	(1.06–5.08)
Hypercholesterolemia (yes vs. no)	0.49	1.63†	(1.18–2.24)
Obesity (yes vs. no)	0.80	2.22†	(1.47–3.34)

*$p < .05$.
†$p < .01$.
Source: Adapted from Wong et al.,[83] with permission.

without calcium, were reported to be significantly more likely to begin new aspirin use, cholesterol-lowering medication, dietary fat reduction, and other risk-reducing therapies.[90]

Several investigators have proposed that serial EBCT calcium scanning may be useful to track the progression or regression of coronary atherosclerosis over time as well as the effects of medical treatment.[91,92] A recently published observational study showed that patients on cholesterol-lowering therapy demonstrated reduced progression of coronary calcium on serial radiographic evaluation with EBCT.[91]

However, before assessment of changes in plaque burden in individual patients may be seriously considered, it must first be demonstrated that the measurement technique is sufficiently reproducible that changes in measured calcium quantity may justify the conclusion that a change has, in fact, taken place. Interobserver and intraobserver reliability of EBCT scanning is within acceptable limits, but this merely indicates that two observers will give similar interpretations of scan data and that an individual observer will interpret the same scan similarly on separate occasions. However, the retest reproducibility (that is, the extent to which two scans of the same patient taken sequentially agree with one another) of EBCT scanning has been shown to be less than acceptable for purposes of clinical evaluation of disease progression in an individual patient[80] (Table

3–8). Although specialized scanning protocols[93] and image processing techniques[94] have been shown to improve reproducibility, these improvements have not been uniformly adopted by those performing EBCT scanning clinically. Furthermore, although changes in calcium quantity over time have been

TABLE 3–8 Retest Reliability of Electron Beam Computed Tomography Calcium Scanning

Author	Reference	Year	n	Variability[a]
Kajinami et al.	171	1993	25	34%
Bielak et al.[b]	110	1994	177	51%
Shields et al.[c]	172	1995	50	38%
Devries et al.	111	1995	42	49%
Wang et al.[d]	93	1996	72	29%
Wang et al.[e]	93	1996	77	14%
Callister et al.[f]	94	1998	52	35%
Callister et al.[g]	94	1998	52	22%

[a]Calculated as [(difference of two scans)/mean] × 100.
[b]Variability derived from Figure 3-4 of this report.
[c]Variability was calculated as the standard error of the estimate divided by the mean calcium score.
[d]3-mm slice thickness protocol.
[e]6-mm slice thickness protocol.
[f]Calcium score.
[g]Calcium volume score.

demonstrated in relatively large groups,[91] it is not known how these changes may be related to increases or decreases in the amount of plaque. Also, it is not known how changes in calcium quantity may alter risk of a coronary heart disease event. It is possible that risk-factor modification (particularly pharmacologic therapy), which may alter the stability of coronary plaque, may not be reflected by either the amount of plaque or the amount of calcium, or that the relationship between calcium quantity and plaque burden may vary with risk-factor modification and pharmacologic therapy.[78]

Coronary artery calcium deposits occur in the arterial intima and are an integral component of the lesion. This is not necessarily the case in peripheral and visceral arteries, which may exhibit calcium deposition in the media (Mönckeberg's calcinosis), and where calcium may be seen in areas with no atherosclerotic disease whatsoever.[95,96] Until recently, coronary calcium deposits were thought to be the result of a passive precipitation of hydroxyapatite mineral salts, but more current studies suggest instead that the process leading to calcium deposition is a complex, active, regulated process sharing many similarities to bone formation.[78,79,97,98]

The relationship of calcium to atherosclerosis has been extensively studied, with studies consistently showing coronary calcium to be a marker for atherosclerotic disease. Mautner et al. examined 4298 coronary artery segments from 50 hearts, and found a relationship between the amount of calcium deposition and the percent stenosis at that site, although that relationship was highly variable.[99] Rumberger et al. performed postmortem analysis of 13 hearts (522 separate sections from a total of 39 coronary arteries), and compared histopathologic findings (plaque area and percent lumen stenosis) with "calcium burden" assessed by EBCT for each section as well as for each artery and each of the 13 hearts.[100–102] Moderate correlations were found when the "calcium burden" was compared with the plaque volume ($r = .57$, $.69$, and $.76$ for the right, left circumflex, and left anterior descending coronary arteries, respectively).[100] Reanalysis of these data revealed that transformed and summed plaque areas and calcium areas were highly correlated

when an individual artery ($r = .90$) or an individual heart ($r = .93$) was assessed.[101] Only one study has directly compared the histopathologic quantity of atherosclerosis with the histopathologic quantity of calcium in the coronary arteries.[103] These investigators found a moderate correlation between the histopathologic amounts of atherosclerosis and calcium ($r = .52$), but there was very wide variability in the quantities of calcium associated with a particular amount of plaque.

Clinical and angiographic studies have produced similar results, consistently showing that patients with a history of coronary artery disease (CAD) have greater amounts of coronary calcium than did patients of comparable age without a history of CAD.[104–109] Rumberger and coworkers found that the magnitude of an individual's calcium score could be used in predicting associated stenosis within the epicardial coronary system.[106] Multiple studies have found that the absence of calcium indicated a low likelihood for the presence of significant luminal obstruction.[107–112] A common finding, however, was that the absence of coronary calcium did not always indicate the absence of disease, and that for a specific stenosis there was a variable amount of associated calcium. Table 3–9 summarizes conclusions that can be drawn based on a negative EBCT coronary calcium study (when no calcium is detected) and Table 3–10 provides guidelines for the interpretation

TABLE 3–9 Absence of Detectable Coronary Artery Calcification Using Electron Beam Computed Tomography (Negative Test)

Does not rule out the presence of atherosclerotic plaque, including unstable plaque or the possibility of a cardiovascular event

Highly unlikely in the presence of significant luminal obstructive disease

Observation made in the majority of patients who have had both angiographically normal coronary arteries and EBCT scanning

May be consistent with a low risk of a cardiovascular event in the next 5 years

Source: Modified from Wexler et al.,[80] with permission.

TABLE 3–10 Presence of Detectable Coronary Artery Calcification Using Electron Beam Computed Tomography (Positive Test)

Confirms the presence of coronary atherosclerotic plaque.

The greater the amount of calcification (i.e., calcium area, score, or volume), the greater the likelihood of obstructive disease, but there is no one-to-one relation, and findings may not be site-specific.

Total amount of calcification correlates best with total amount of atherosclerotic plaque, although the true "plaque burden" is underestimated.

A high calcium score may be more likely to demonstrate progression or be associated with a cardiovascular event or procedure over the next 5 years than a low or negative calcium score.

Source: Modified from Wexler et al.,[80] with permission.

of a positive scan (some calcium detected in at least one vessel).[80]

Diagnostic versus Prognostic Value of Calcium Detection

It is now undisputed that coronary events such as myocardial infarction, unstable angina, and sudden cardiac death are often precipitated by rupture or fissuring of an atherosclerotic plaque[113–116] and that the likelihood of a given plaque to rupture is unrelated to the quantity of atherosclerosis or the angiographic severity of obstruction.[117–121] The ability of calcium assessment to predict subsequent coronary events is dependent in large part on the relationship between the amount of calcium in a lesion and the likelihood of that plaque to fissure or rupture, causing coronary thrombosis and a resultant clinical event. At present, it is not known if calcium in a lesion tends to increase or decrease the probability of that lesion to rupture. There is some clinical and biomechanical evidence that calcium may, in fact, act to strengthen atherosclerotic plaques, rendering them less likely to fissure or rupture.[78,79] Nevertheless, radiographic studies reviewed below indicate a moderate relationship between the amount of coronary calcium and the probability of a subsequent coronary event. The explanation for this discrepancy has not been determined. It has been suggested that these paradoxical results may be secondary to the association of calcium quantity with the extent of coronary atherosclerosis and, more specifically, with the presence of unstable lipid-filled lesions somewhere in the coronary vasculature.[78,122]

Techniques for the Radiographic Assessment of Coronary Calcium

There are three major modalities of radiographic calcium detection: fluoroscopic imaging, EBCT (Figs. 3–1 to 3–3), and HCT. There are, in turn, two fluoroscopic methods that have been studied: cinefluoroscopy and digital subtraction cinefluoroscopy. Digital subtraction cinefluoroscopy possesses two advantages over standard cinefluoroscopy: first, stationary densities in the lungs and noncardiac thoracic soft tissues, including calcium deposits, are eliminated;[123,124] second, digital subtraction offers enhanced detection of objects with high spatial frequencies, which small calcium deposits exhibit.[125] There is a strong correlation between the calcium quantity detected by digital subtraction cinefluoroscopy and the measured calcium mass in excised coronary arteries,[126] and interobserver reproducibility is good.[127]

Additional—and not trivial—advantages of fluoroscopic techniques as well as HCT include their ready availability at virtually every major medical facility, the multiple uses of fluoroscopic equipment for purposes other than cardiac scanning, and their much lower cost in comparison to EBCT scanners. The advantages of EBCT, on the other hand, include superior resolution and sensitivity with respect to calcium detection. However, sensitivity is achieved partly at the expense of specificity, which is inferior to that of fluoroscopic techniques. In addition, EBCT possesses the ability to quantify coronary calcium, whereas fluoroscopic techniques provide only a semiquantitative estimate of the amount of coronary calcium. Although interobserver and intraobserver reliabilities are excellent, the retest reproducibility of an EBCT calcium scan is limited (Table 3–8), probably in large part owing to minute intrathoracic cardiac motion between the acquisition of successive tomographic scan slices.[93]

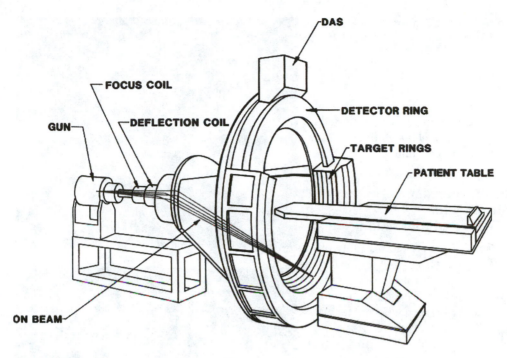

FIGURE 3–1 Schematic diagram of coronary calcium scanning performed by electron beam computed tomography (EBCT) scanner.

Total evaluation of coronary calcium content using EBCT or HCT can be performed in 10 to 15 min with only about 30 s of actual scanning time. EBCT and HCT are noninvasive, painless techniques that expose patients to minimal amounts of radiation,[112,128] can be performed in virtually any subject, and require no preparation or discontinuation of medications. As noted above, EBCT and HCT demonstrate a sensitivity with respect to calcium detection that is superior to that of fluoroscopic techniques, but with lower specificity. In addition, sites of calcium deposits identified by EBCT, and probably also with HCT, do not necessarily correspond with sites of angiographic stenosis.[129]

Prognostic Value of Fluoroscopic Techniques to Detect Coronary Calcium

Several investigators have examined the utility of fluoroscopic techniques to provide useful prognostic in-

formation. In a study of 800 symptomatic patients, Margolis and colleagues found that those with coronary calcium by cardiac fluoroscopy had a 5-year survival rate of only 58 percent, compared with 87 percent for those without detectable calcium.[130] On the other hand, Hudson and Walker assessed coronary calcium in 440 asymptomatic subjects, of whom 78 exhibited coronary artery calcium.[131] These investigators found no difference in 5-year survival between those with calcium and those without. These discrepant findings could indicate that symptomatic versus asymptomatic status might affect the usefulness of calcium in predicting future coronary events, but the small sample size in the study of asymptomatic subjects renders such a conclusion hazardous. Using digital subtraction cinefluoroscopy in 1461 asymptomatic subjects with coronary risk factors, Detrano and coworkers were able to show that individuals with coronary calcium had a 2.7 times greater risk of suffering a coronary event than

FIGURE 3–2 Examples of EBCT coronary calcium scans demonstrating (A) no coronary calcium, (B) minimal coronary calcium, and (C) moderate coronary calcium.

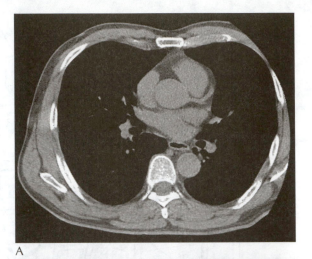

A

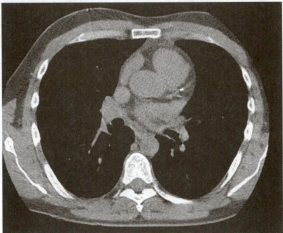

B

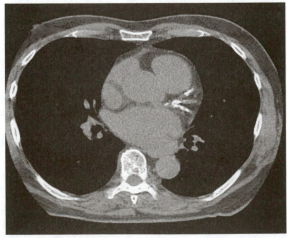

C

that of subjects with no calcium in analyses adjusted for major coronary risk factors, although five events did occur in persons with no calcium.[132,133]

Prognostic Value of Detection of Coronary Calcium with Electron Beam Computed Tomography

Two studies have examined the prognostic utility of EBCT in symptomatic subjects.[134,135] In the first, a multicenter angiographic study involving 422 symptomatic patients who underwent both EBCT and coronary angiography and were then followed for up to 45 months, a significantly higher event-free survival was observed in patients with initial EBCT calcium scores below 100.[134] Events (cardiac death or hospital admission for chest pain or suspected myocardial infarction) were more likely in those patients with the highest coronary calcium scores, and the calcium score, but not the number of angiographically diseased vessels, predicted cardiac events. In the second study, 91 patients who had received heart transplants underwent EBCT calcium scanning, coronary angiography, exercise testing, and exercise radionuclide ventriculography approximately $4\frac{1}{2}$ years after their transplantation.[135] These patients were then followed clinically for an additional 2 years. Those patients with no detectable calcium were significantly less likely to suffer an event during the follow-up period than those who had some calcium by EBCT ($p = .01$).

Published data on the ability of EBCT to predict events in asymptomatic individuals are limited, and show varied results.[136,137] Arad and coworkers[136] performed EBCT scans on 1173 self-referred subjects who were asymptomatic at the time of enrollment. These subjects were followed for an average of 19 months, and the occurrence of cardiac events was noted. Cardiac events included 17 revascularizations, 7 myocardial infarctions, and 1 cardiac

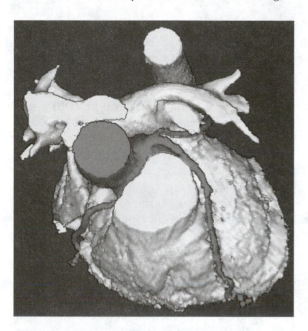

FIGURE 3–3 Example of three-dimensional volume reconstruction of coronary arteries by EBCT angiography demonstrating significant coronary calcium.

death. These investigators found that those individuals who suffered events had significantly higher coronary calcium scores by EBCT than those who remained event-free during the follow-up period. The positive predictive value of EBCT was poor (6 to 14 percent), but the negative predictive value was excellent (>99 percent). For a threshold calcium score of 100, sensitivity was 89 percent, but specificity was only 77 percent. Increasing this threshold calcium score to 680 resulted in an improvement in specificity (to 95 percent), but sensitivity declined to only 50 percent. All events were combined in the analysis, so the value of EBCT in predicting infarctions or cardiac death separately could not be determined.

Secci and colleagues assessed coronary calcium with EBCT in 326 asymptomatic subjects with coronary risk factors and followed these subjects for 2 years prior to EBCT and for an average of 32 months after calcium scanning, during which a total of 41 events occurred.[137] Events were three times more frequent in subjects with EBCT calcium scores

above the median, but there was no significant relationship between calcium score and hard coronary events (infarction or cardiac death), and only ECG evidence of left ventricular hypertrophy predicted events during the follow-up period. Coronary calcium score did, however, predict revascularizations.[137] Analysis of data obtained from a larger cohort ($n = 1196$) involving a longer follow-up period (average of 41 months) by these investigators has recently been reported.[138,139] These results, involving a larger number of cardiac events (17 cardiac deaths and 34 infarctions), showed a 2.2-fold greater incidence of myocardial infarction ($p < .01$) and the combined endpoint of myocardial infarction or coronary death ($p < .01$) among those above versus below the median of coronary calcium quantity. However, comparison of Receiver Operating Characteristic (ROC) curve areas indicated that combining EBCT calcium scores with risk-factor data provided no significant prognostic advantage over either risk-factor assessment alone or calcium score alone.[138] Moreover, 17 percent of infarctions and coronary deaths occurred in those with little or no coronary calcium (first tertile, or scores of 3 or less), and another 35 percent of events occurred in those with relatively mild coronary calcium (second tertile, or scores of 4 to 151).[138,139] In addition, a recent prospective fluoroscopic investigation also indicates that African Americans have a lower prevalence of coronary calcium than similar white subjects, yet they suffer more coronary heart events on follow-up,[140] raising the possibility that EBCT calcium scanning may predict coronary event risk differently in some ethnic groups. These results suggest that more investigation is needed before conclusions can be drawn and recommendations made regarding the utility of EBCT coronary calcium screening in selected high-risk or general populations.[80, 141]

Screening for Peripheral Artery Disease in Cardiovascular Risk Assessment

In screening higher-risk patients for atherosclerotic cardiovascular disease (CVD), an often overlooked area is screening for peripheral arterial disease (PAD). Historically as well as currently, the "gold standard" for PAD diagnosis is arteriography. However, this procedure would be inappropriate not only for asymptomatic persons but for symptomatic persons as well unless an interventional procedure were contemplated. Current technology allows rather sophisticated noninvasive assessment of PAD in symptomatic as well as asymptomatic persons. Major categories of evaluation, in descending order of ease and simplicity of assessment, are (1) segmental (e.g., ankle-brachial) blood pressure ratios, (2) flow velocity by Doppler ultrasound, (3) Doppler waveform analysis, and (4) duplex imaging and flow velocity evaluation. For office assessment of CVD risk in persons without leg symptomatology, the last three methods are probably not currently cost-effective, since each requires fairly sophisticated equipment and technical skill. Conversely, segmental blood pressure ratios are conceptually and operationally relatively straightforward, especially for measurement of the ratio of ankle systolic blood pressure (SBP) to SBP in the arm, or the ankle-brachial index (ABI). In terms of sensitivity, specificity, and positive and negative predictive value for significant PAD determined angiographically, the ABI gives most of the information that would be obtained by, in addition, measuring segment-to-arm SBP ratios at the upper thigh, above the knee, and below the knee.[142] However, measurement of the ratio of SBP at the toe to the arm, or the toe-brachial index (TBI), does provide incremental information and is discussed below. Procedures for measuring ABI and TBI appear in Table 3–11.

Relation of Ankle-Brachial and Toe-Brachial Indexes to Cardiovascular Risk

The ABI has been employed in clinical practice for over a half-century.[143] It is fairly simple to measure (Table 3–11) and shows good reproducibility, with the 95 percent confidence interval variability of a single measurement being about ± 16 percent.[144,145] The normalized reproducibility of the ABI is actually considerably better than that of many standard clinical, hematologic, and biochemical measurements, such as heart rate, white blood cell count, and blood urea nitrogen.[146] The ABI correlates highly with angiographically determined PAD.[147] Extensive data document the association of the ABI with traditional CVD risk factors, such as cigarette smoking, SBP and diastolic blood pressure (DBP), and dyslipidemia, particularly low high-density-lipoprotein (HDL) cholesterol and high triglycerides.[148–151] Other studies have shown ABI correlations with lipoprotein(a),[152,153] homocysteine,[154] and fibrinogen and blood viscosity.[155]

Cross-sectionally, PAD shows considerable overlap with CHD and cerebrovascular disease.[156] In the lower extremities, it has been shown that PAD, diagnosed by both segmental blood pressure and flow velocities, increased the risk of total mortality threefold and the risk of CVD mortality sixfold in both men and women.[157] Again, nearly all the segmental blood pressure information for prognosis was carried in the ABI alone.[142] In addition, CVD morbidity was also sharply increased in subjects with PAD.[158] Several other investigators have reported similar results for morbidity and mortality.[159,160] Also demonstrated is a clear dose-response relationship between the severity of PAD and CVD mortality,[157] with other severe cases being more likely to be symptomatic. Nonetheless, only one in five cases of PAD had any symptoms of claudication,[161] and even among completely asymptomatic PAD patients (i.e., true subclinical PAD), the relative risk (RR) for CVD mortality was fivefold and highly statistically significant. This study also showed the striking independence of PAD as a predictor of CVD mortality. Relative risks were little changed after exclusion of subjects with clinical CVD at baseline as well as after adjustment for CVD risk factors. An indication of the clinical importance of these findings was the use of these and related data to revise the National Cholesterol Education Program Adult Treatment Guidelines to treat patients with PAD, even if asymptomatic, as secondary prevention.[162]

Two other follow-up studies using the ABI alone to diagnose PAD have reported quite similar results.[163,164] In both these studies, the ABI predicted CVD mortality independent of both CVD diagnosed at baseline and CVD risk factors, and in a graded

TABLE 3–11   Measurement of Ankle-Brachial Index (ABI) and Toe-Brachial Index (TBI)

Measurement of ABI:

1. Patients should be studied in the supine position at rest.

2. When the ABI is measured alone, an appropriate-sized blood pressure cuff is used in the arm and a 12-cm cuff is nearly always the correct size at the ankle, although a few patients may have very large ankle circumferences and require larger ankle cuffs.

3. Six SBPs are recorded; the left arm, the right arm, two right ankle pressures, and two left ankle pressures. Each is recorded using a hand-held Doppler over the brachial artery at the antecubital fossa in the arm and over the posterior tibial artery at the ankle. If the posterior tibial pulse cannot be located, the dorsalis pedis is employed. If neither pulse can be located with the Doppler, the patient can be considered to have peripheral arterial disease (PAD).

4. The arm systolic blood pressure (SBP) is the average of the left and right arm SBPs unless the arms differ by >10 mmHg, in which case the higher arm pressure is used because of the possibility of stenosis in the arm with the lower pressure.

5. The right ankle SBP is the average of the two right ankle SBPs, and the left ankle SBP, similarly, is the average of the two left ankle SBPs.

6. Two pressures are averaged for both the numerator and denominator of each ABI to reduce the inherent moment-to-moment variability of SBP.

7. The most commonly used cutpoint defining an abnormal ABI is < 0.90, although cutpoints from 0.95 to 0.80 have been employed in various studies.

Measurement of ABI and TBI:

The same general principles outlined above apply when the ABI and TBI are measured together, but the procedure and equipment differ. Since the TBI can be influenced by cold, the feet should be covered with a blanket prior to evaluation and minimum room temperature should be 25°C.

1. Measurement of the TBI requires toe cuffs and a photoplethysmographic (PPG) sensor at the hands and toes.

2. Using PPGs on the middle finger of each hand (to assess brachial SBP) and on each great toe (to assess both ankle and toe SBP) and with cuffs on both arms, both ankles, and both toes, one can rapidly assess all six SBPs. This method is exactly comparable to using a Doppler for the ABI, but it is simpler and allows simultaneous measurement of the TBI.

3. Toe cuffs (2.5-cm) are employed and the PPGs are applied to both middle fingers and the plantar aspect of the great toes.

4. Tests can be readily done with an integrated system containing all equipment necessary for determination of the ABI and TBI. This equipment includes cuffs, PPGs, and a recorder.

5. Because transient vasomotor changes in small vessels can change the TBI, the cutpoint for abnormality is lower; it is normally defined as < 0.70.

dose-response fashion. Another study restricted to 422 patients with abnormal ABIs showed a strong ABI dose-response gradient for mortality,[165] and similarly a study of over 2000 PAD patients showed low ABI to independently predict all CVD events and total mortality.[166] Although ABI abnormalities increase sharply with age, even in adults aged 40 to 59, the ABI is abnormal in 2 to 3 percent of persons,[151,167] which highlights its potential importance in screening higher-risk middle-aged and older persons.

In summary, the ABI is noninvasive, simple to measure, highly reproducible, shows a strong correlation with angiographically determined PAD, and is strongly predictive of CVD events in middle-aged and older persons, suggesting its utility as a screening test in these age groups.

The TBI can be determined efficiently at the same time as the ABI; the procedures are presented in Table 3–11. The TBI may assess both structural and vasoactive components of small-vessel subclinical

CVD. After 10 years of follow-up of 565 subjects aged 38 to 82 years at baseline in our population study, subjects with isolated small-vessel disease, as manifest by TBI < 0.7 and/or prolonged pulse reappearance times but normal ABIs, had significantly elevated risks of death from CHD (RR = 2.6, 95 percent CI = 1.1 to 6.4), CVD (RR = 2.5, 95 percent CI = 1.2 to 5.1), and a nonsignificant increase in total mortality (RR = 1.2, 95 percent CI = 0.7 to 2.1)[148] (Table 3–12). Interestingly, the RRs were approximately half the magnitude for those with low ABIs in the same cohort. All of these RRs were adjusted for the potential confounding effects of CVD risk factors.

Why does the TBI predict mortality even when the ABI is normal? As is well known in vascular laboratories, some patients, particularly diabetics, may have falsely normal (false negative) ABIs due to rigid, calcified vessels; in these cases, the TBI will demonstrate the true reduced pressure.[168] However, only a small portion of low TBIs fit into this category. In a recent natural history study of vascular laboratory patients, change in limb classification was examined over an average of 5 years of follow-up.[169] In limbs with a normal ABI (>0.9) and a low TBI (< 0.7) at baseline, 33.1 percent progressed to an abnormal ABI, 28.2 percent were stable, and 38.7 percent showed a normal TBI and ABI at follow-up.

Thus some isolated low-TBI limbs have early large-vessel PAD, while some such limbs appear to reflect temporary vasomotor changes.

In summary, the TBI (1) independently predicts CVD mortality, (2) may reflect both structural and dynamic changes of subclinical PAD, and (3) may detect subclinical PAD in diabetics or other patients with false-negative ABIs.

Summary

Coronary atherosclerosis is the predominant cause of morbidity and mortality in the United States as well as most other industrialized nations. Appropriate treatment and minimization of the devastating consequences of coronary atherosclerosis depends in large measure on our ability to reliably distinguish those individuals who will suffer an event from those who will not. This task is made all the more difficult because coronary atherosclerosis is a ubiquitous condition among adults, yet many of those afflicted will not suffer its consequences and therefore require neither identification nor intervention. On the other hand, coronary atherosclerosis is a dynamic process, and the onset of a coronary event is frequently unheralded, sudden, and lethal. Furthermore, many events are caused by plaques of minimal or moderate severity, and patients with such lesions may have normal or near-normal angiograms and exercise tests.

Nevertheless, a large body of evidence has now established that exercise testing can be of prognostic value in some groups of patients with known coronary artery disease. In asymptomatic subjects, exercise testing is of limited prognostic value with the exception of those individuals with multiple coronary risk factors and a few special situations, such as those starting exercise programs and individuals employed in high-risk professions. The ACC/AHA Task Force Guidelines indicate that exercise testing is not useful in screening asymptomatic populations and may even be harmful.

While the basis of exercise testing or blood pressure–based assessment of peripheral artery disease is fundamentally physiologic, the basis of radio-

TABLE 3–12 Relative Risks* (and 95% Confidence Intervals) of Large-Vessel Peripheral Arterial Disease (LV-PAD) and Isolated Small-Vessel Disease (ISV-PAD) for Coronary, Stroke, All-Cardiovascular, and All-Cause Mortality: 10-Year Follow-up

Mortality	LV-PAD ($n = 67$)	ISV-PAD ($n = 90$)
Coronary	5.8 (2.5–13.0)	2.6 (1.1–6.4)
Stroke	1.0 (0.1–11.0)	2.3 (0.4–14.0)
All cardiovascular	5.1 (2.7–9.9)	2.5 (1.2–5.1)
All cause	3.0 (1.8–4.8)	1.2 (0.7–2.1)

*Compared with subjects free of peripheral arterial disease ($n = 408$). Adjusted for age, sex, blood pressure, pack-years of cigarettes, HDL cholesterol, LDL cholesterol, log triglyceride, fasting plasma glucose, and body mass index.
Source: Adapted from Criqui et al.,[149] with permission.

graphic techniques such as cardiac fluoroscopy or EBCT is instead anatomic. EBCT appears to be capable of diagnosing coronary atherosclerosis, but data are limited regarding the relationship between quantity of coronary calcium and event likelihood. The diagnostic and prognostic value of EBCT calcium scanning is controversial. The lack of uniform, consensus-based guidelines limits its role in clinical evaluation or risk stratification of the patient with either known, suspected, or unsuspected coronary atherosclerosis. Well-designed clinical studies, such as the ongoing National Institutes of Health-sponsored Multiethnic Study of Atherosclerosis (MESA[170]), will further define the role of EBCT and other screening modalities in cardiovascular risk assessment.[171,172]

References

1. American Heart Association: *1999 Heart and Stroke Statistical Update.* Dallas, American Heart Association, 1999.

2. WHO-MONICA Project: Myocardial infarction and coronary deaths in the World Health Organization Monica Project: registration procedures, event rates, and case-fatality rates in 38 populations from 21 countries in 4 continents. *Circulation* 1994; 90:583–612.

3. Stary HC: The sequence of cell and matrix changes in atherosclerotic lesions of coronary arteries in the first forty years of life. *Eur Heart J* 1990;11(suppl E):3–19.

4. Stary HC: Evolution and progression of atherosclerotic lesions in coronary arteries of children and young adults. *Arteriosclerosis* 1989; 9(suppl I):19–32.

5. Strong JP: Coronary atherosclerosis in soldiers: a clue to the natural history of atherosclerosis in the young. *JAMA* 1986; 256:2863–2866.

6. Lloyd-Jones DM, Larson MG, Beiser A, Levy D: Lifetime risk of developing coronary heart disease. *Lancet* 1999; 353:89–92.

7. United States National Heart, Lung and Blood Institute: Kannel W, Wolf P, Garrison R (eds): *Framingham Study: An Epidemiological Investigation of Cardiovascular Disease.* Publication Number 87–2284. Bethesda, MD, U.S. Department of Health, 1986.

8. Califf RM, Armstrong PW, Carver JR, et al: Task Force 5: stratification of patients into high, medium, and low risk subgroups for purposes of risk factor management. *J Am Coll Cardiol* 1996; 27:1007–1019.

9. Greenland P, Grundy S, Pasternak RC, Lenfant C: Problems on the pathway from risk assessment to risk reduction. *Circulation* 1998; 97:1761–1762.

10. Taylor AJ, O'Malley PG: Self-referral of patients for electron-beam computed tomography to screen for coronary artery disease. *N Engl J Med* 1998; 339:2018–2020.

11. Kerlikowske K, Grady D, Rubin SM, et al: Efficacy of screening mammography: a meta-analysis. *JAMA* 1995; 273:149–154.

12. Eddy DM: Breast cancer screening in women younger than 50 years of age: what's next? *Ann Intern Med* 1997; 127:1035–1036.

13. Uren NG, Melin JA, DeBruyne B, et al: Relation between myocardial blood flow and the severity of coronary artery stenosis. *N Engl J Med* 1994; 330:1782–1788.

14. Detrano R, Lyons KP, Marcondes G et al: Methodologic problems in exercise testing research: are we solving them? *Arch Intern Med* 1988; 148:1289–1295.

15. Philbrick JT, Horwitz RI, Feinstein AR: Methodologic problems of exercise testing for coronary artery disease: groups, analysis, and bias. *Am J Cardiol* 1980; 46:807–812.

16. Detrano R, Gianrossi R, Mulvihill D, et al: Exercise-induced ST segment depression in the diagnosis of multivessel coronary disease: a meta analysis. *J Am Coll Cardiol* 1989; 14:1501–1515 .

17. Ransohoff DF, Feinstein AR: Problems of spectrum and bias in evaluating the efficacy of diagnostic tests. *N Engl J Med* 1978; 299:926–929.

18. Detrano R, Janosi A, Lyons K, et al: Factors affecting sensitivity and specificity of a diagnostic test: the exercise thallium scintigram. *Am J Med* 1988; 84:699–710.

19. Risk Factor Intervention Trial Research Group: Exercise electrocardiogram and coronary heart disease mortality in the Multiple Risk Factor Intervention Trial. *Am J Cardiol* 1985; 55:16–24.

20. Mark DB, Hlatky MA, Harrell FE Jr, et al: Exercise treadmill score for predicting prognosis in coronary artery disease. *Ann Intern Med* 1987; 106:793–800.

21. Stuart RJ, Ellestad MH: National survey of exercise stress testing facilities. *Chest* 1980; 77:94–97.

22. Rautaharju PM, Prineas RJ, Eifler WJ, et al: Prognostic value of exercise electrocardiogram in men at high risk of future coronary heart disease: Multiple Risk Factor Intervention Trial experience. *J Am Coll Cardiol* 1986; 8:1–10.

23. Gordon DJ, Ekelund LG, Karon JM, et al: Predictive value of the exercise tolerance test for mortality in North American men: the Lipid Research Clinics mortality follow-up study. *Circulation* 1986; 74:252–261.

24. Okin PM, Anderson KM, Levy D, et al: Heart rate adjustment of exercise-induced ST segment depression: improved risk stratification in the Framingham Offspring Study. *Circulation* 1991; 83:866–868.

25. Simoons ML: Optimal measurements for detection of coronary artery disease by exercise ECG. *Comput Biomed Res* 1977; 10:483–484.

26. Klingfield P, Ameisen O, Okin PM: Heart rate adjustment of ST segment depression for improved detection of coronary artery disease. *Circulation* 1989; 79:245–255.

27. Haraphongse M, Kappagoda T, Tymchak, et al: The value of sum of ST segment depression in 12 lead electrocardiogram in relation to change in heart rate during exercise to predict the extent of coronary artery disease. *Cardiovasc Med* 1986; 2:64–67.

28. Deckers JW, Rensing BJ, Tijssen JGP, et al: A comparison of methods of analyzing exercise tests for diagnosis of coronary artery disease. *Br Heart J* 1989; 62:438–444.

29. Lachterman B, Lehmann KG, Detrano R, et al: Comparison of ST segment/heart rate index to standard ST criteria for analysis of exercise electrocardiogram. *Circulation* 1990; 82:44–50.

30. Thwaites BC, Quyyumi AA, Raphael MJ, et al: Comparison of the ST/heart rate slope with the modified Bruce exercise test in the detection of coronary artery disease. *Am J Cardiol* 1986;57:554–556.

31. Wennberg DE, Kellett MA, Dickens JD Jr, et al: The association between local diagnostic testing intensity and invasive cardiac procedures. *JAMA* 1996; 275:1161–1164.

32. Bruce RA, DeRouen TA, Hossack KF: Value of maximal exercise tests in risk assessment of primary coronary heart disease events in healthy men: five years experience of the Seattle Heart Watch Study. *Am J Cardiol* 1980; 46:371–378.

33. Roger VL, Jacobsen SJ, Pellikka PA, et al: Prognostic value of treadmill exercise testing. A population-based study in Olmsted County, Minnesota. *Circulation* 1998; 98:2836–2841.

34. Dubach P, Froelicher VF, Klein J, et al: Exercise-induced hypotension in a male population: criteria, causes, and prognosis. *Circulation* 1988; 78:1380–1387.

35. Degenais GR, Rouleau JR, Hochart P, et al: Survival with painless strongly positive exercise electrocardiogram. *Am J Cardiol* 1988; 62:892–895.

36. Klein J, Froelicher VF, Detrano R, et al: Does the rest electrocadiogram after myocardial infarction determine the predictive value of exercise-induced ST depression? A 2 year follow-up study in a veteran population. *J Am Coll Cardiol* 1989; 14:305–311.

37. Krone RJ, Dwyer EM Jr, Greenberg H, et al: Risk stratification in patients with first non-Q wave infarction: limited value of the early low level exercise test after uncomplicated infarcts. The Multicenter Post-Infarction Research Group. *J Am Coll Cardiol* 1989; 14:31–37; discussion, 38–39.

38. Mark DB, Hlatky MA, Harrell FE Jr, et al: Exercise treadmill score for predicting prognosis in coronary artery disease. *Ann Intern Med* 1987; 106:793–800.

39. Brunelli C, Cristofani R, L'Abbate A: Long-term survival in medically treated patients with ischaemic heart disease and prognostic importance of clinical and electrocardiographic data (the Italian CNR Multicentre Prospective Study ODI). *Eur Heart J* 1989; 10:292–303.

40. Weiner DA, Ryan TJ, McCabe CH, et al: Prognostic importance of a clinical profile and exercise test in medically treated patients with coronary artery disease. *J Am Coll Cardiol* 1984; 3:772–779.

41. Gohlke H, Samek L, Betz P, Roskamm H. Exercise testing provides additional prognostic information in angiographically defined subgroups of patients with coronary artery disease. *Circulation* 1983; 68:979–985.

42. Peduzzi P, Hultgren H, Thomsen J, Angell W. Veterans Administration Cooperative Study of medical versus surgical treatment for stable angina—Progress report. Section 8. Prognostic value of baseline exercise tests. *Prog Cardiovasc Dis* 1986; 28:285–292.

43. Hammermeister KE, DeRouen TA, Dodge HT: Variables predictive of survival in patients with coronary disease: selected by univariate and multivariate analyses from the clinical, electrocardiographic, exercise, arteriographic, and quantitative evaluations. *Circulation* 1979; 59:421–430.

44. MacIntyre NR, Kunkler JR, Mitchell RE, et al: Eight-year follow-up exercise electrocardiograms in healthy, middle-aged aviators. *Aviat Space Environ Med* 1981; 52:256–259.

45. McHenry PL, O'Donnell J, Morris SN, Jordan JJ: The abnormal exercise electrocardiogram in apparently healthy men: a predictor of angina pectoris as an initial coronary event during long-term follow-up. *Circulation* 1984; 70:547–551.

46. Bruce RA, Fisher LD, Hossack KF: Validation of exercise-enhanced risk assessment of coronary heart disease events: longitudinal changes in incidence in Seattle community practice. *J Am Coll Cardiol* 1985; 5:875–881.

47. Aronow WS, Cassidy J: Five year follow-up of double Master's test, maximal treadmill stress test, and resting and postexercise apexcardiogram in asymptomatic persons. *Circulation* 1975; 52:616–618.

48. Cumming GR, Samm J, Borysyk L, Kich L: Electrocardiographic changes during exercise in asymptomatic men: 3-year follow-up. *Can Med Assoc J* 1975; 112:578–581.

49. Froelicher VF Jr, Thomas MM, Pillow C, Lancaster MC: An epidemiological study of asymptomatic men screened with exercise testing for latent coronary heart disease. *Am J Cardiol* 1974; 34:770–776.

50. Allen WH, Aronow WS, Goodman P, Stinson P: Five-year follow-up of maximal treadmill stress test in asymptomatic men and women. *Circulation* 1980; 65:522–527.

51. Manca C, Dei Cas L, Albertini D, et al: Different prognostic value of exercise electrocardiogram in men and women. *Cardiology* 1978; 63:312–319.

52. Bruce RA, McDonough JR: Stress testing in screening for cardiovascular disease. *Bull NY Acad Med* 1969; 45:1288–1305.

53. Giagnoni E, Secchi MB, Wu SC, et al: Prognostic value of exercise testing in asymptomatic normotensive subjects: a prospective matched study. *N Engl J Med* 1983; 309:1085–1089.

54. Epstein SE, Quyyumi AA, Bonow RO: Sudden cardiac death without warning: possible mechanisms and implications for screening asymptomatic populations. *N Engl J Med* 1989; 321:320–324.

55. Mulcahy D, Husain S, Zalos G, et al: Ischemia during ambulatory monitoring as a prognostic indicator in patients with stable coronary artery disease. *JAMA* 1997; 277:318–324.

56. Froelicher VF, Perdue S, Pewen W, Risch M: Application of meta-analysis using an electronic spread sheet for exercise testing in patients after myocardial infarction. *Am J Med* 1987; 83:1045–1054.

57. Shaw LJ, Peterson ED, Kesler K et al: A meta-analysis of predischarge risk stratification after acute myocardial infarction with stress electrocardiographic, myocardial perfusion, and ventricular function imaging. *Am J Cardiol* 1996; 78:1327–1337.

58. Bruce RA, Hossack KF, DeRouen TA, et al: Enhanced risk assessment for primary coronary heart disease events by maximal exercise testing: 10 years' experience of the Seattle Heart Watch. *J Am Coll Cardiol* 1983; 2:565–573.

59. Flegg JL, Gertenblith G, Zonderman AB, et al: Prevalence and prognostic significance of exercise-induced myocardial ischemia detected by thallium scintigraphy and electrocardiography in asymptomatic volunteers. *Circulation* 1990; 81:428–443.

60. Josephson RA, Shefrin E, Flegg JL: Is conversion from negative to positive exercise ECG a specific marker for future coronary events in asymptomatic subjects? (abstr). *Circulation* 1988; 78(suppl 2):246.

61. Fletcher GF, Froehlicher VF, Hartley LH, et al: Exercise standards: a statement for health professionals from the American Heart Association. *Circulation* 1990; 82:2286–2322.

62. Tavel MB: Specificity of electrocardiogram stress test in women versus men. *Am J Cardiol* 1992;70:545–547.

63. Kwok Y, Kim C, Grady D, et al: Meta-analysis of exercise testing to detect coronary artery disease in women. *Am J Cardiol* 1999; 83:660–666.

64. Morise AP, Dalal JN, Devaul RD: Frequency of oral estrogen replacement therapy in women with normal and abnormal exercise electrocardiograms and normal coronary arteries by angiogram. *Am J Cardiol* 1993; 72:1197–1199.

65. Colucci WS, Gimbrone MA, McLaughlin MK, et al: Increased vascular catecholamine sensitivity and alpha-adrenergic affinity in female and estrogen-treated male rats. *Circ Res* 1982; 50:805–811.

66. Detrano R, Froelicher VF: Exercise testing: uses and limitations considering recent studies. *Prog Cardiovasc Dis* 1988; 31:173–204.

67. Patterson J, Naughton J, Pietra R: Treadmill exercise in the assessment of the functional capacity of patients with cardiac disease. *Am J Cardiol* 1972; 30:757.

68. Astrand PO, Rodahl K: *Textbook of Work Physiology: Physiological Bases of Exercise.* New York, McGraw-Hill, 1977.

69. ACC/AHA Task Force: Guidelines for exercise testing. A report of the American College of Cardiology/American Heart Association Task Force on Assessment of Cardiovascular Procedures (Subcommittee on Extensive Testing). *J Am Coll Cardiol* 1986; 8:725–738.

70. Gibbons RJ, Balady GJ, Beasley JW, et al: ACC/AHA guidelines for exercise testing: a report of the American College of Cardiology/American Heart Association Task Force on Practice Guidelines (Committee on Exercise Testing). *J Am Coll Cardiol* 1997; 30:260–315.

71. Loecker TH, Schwartz RS, Cotta CW, et al: Fluoroscopic coronary artery calcification and associated coronary disease in asymptomatic young men. *J Am Coll Cardiol* 1992; 19:1167–1172.

72. Cortigiani L, Dodi C, Paolini EA, et al: Prognostic value of pharmacological stress echocardiography in women with chest pain and unknown coronary artery disease. *J Am Coll Cardiol* 1998; 32:1975–1981.

73. Ho YL, Wu CC, Huang LJ, et al: Assessment of coronary artery disease in women by dobutamine stress echocardiography: comparison with stress thallium-201 single-photon emission computed tomography and exercise electrocardiography. *Am Heart J* 1998; 135:655–662.

74. Dionisopoulos PN, Collins JD, Smart SC, et al: The value of dobutamine stress echocardiography for the detection of coronary artery disease in women. *J Am Soc Echocardiogr* 1997; 10:811–817.

75. Blumenthal RS, Becker DM, Moy TF, et al: Exercise thallium tomography predicts future clinically manifested coronary heart disease in a high-risk asymptomatic population. *Circulation* 1996; 93:915–923.

76. Marie PY, Danchin N, Durand JF, et al: Long-term prediction of major ischemic events by exercise thallium-201 single-photon emission computed tomography. Incremental prognostic value compared with clinical, exercise testing, catheterization and radionuclide angiographic data. *J Am Coll Cardiol* 1995; 26:879–886.

77. Fletcher GF, Schlant RC: The exercise test. In: Alexander RW, Schlant RC, Fuster V, et al (eds): *Hurst's The Heart,* 9th ed. New York, McGraw-Hill, 1998; 535.

78. Doherty TM, Detrano RC, Mautner SL, et al: Atherosclerotic coronary calcification: the good, the bad, and the uncertain. *Am Heart J* 1999;137:806–814.

79. Doherty TM, Detrano RC: Coronary arterial calcification as an active process: a new perspective on an old idea. *Calcif Tissue Int* 1994; 54:224–230.

80. Wexler L, Brundage B, Crouse J, et al: Coronary artery calcification: pathophysiology, epidemiology, imaging methods and clinical implications. A statement for health

professionals from the American Heart Association. *Circulation* 1996; 94:1175–1192.

81. Blankenhorn DH: Coronary arterial calcification: a review. *Am J Med Sci* 1961; 42:1–49.

82. Blankenhorn DH, Stern D: Calcification of the coronary arteries. *Am J Roentgenol* 1959; 81:772–777.

83. Wong ND, Kouwabunpat D, Vo AN, et al: Coronary calcium and atherosclerosis by ultrafast computed tomography in asymptomatic men and women: relation to age and risk factors. *Am Heart J* 1994; 127:422–430.

84. Kennedy J, Shavelle R, Wang S, et al: Coronary calcium and standard risk factors in symptomatic patients referred for coronary angiography. *Am Heart J* 1998; 135:696–702.

85. Maher JE, Raz JA, Bielak LF, Sheedy PF II, et al: Potential of quantity of coronary artery calcification to identify new risk factors for asymptomatic atherosclerosis. *Am J Epidemiol* 1996; 144:943–953.

86. Levenson J, Giral P, Megnien JL, et al: Fibrinogen and its relation to subclinical extracoronary and coronary atherosclerosis in hypercholesterolemic men. *Arterioscler Thromb Vasc Biol* 1997; 17:45–50.

87. Mahoney LT, Burns TL, Stanford W et al: Coronary risk factors measured in childhood and young adult life are associated with coronary artery calcification in young adults: the Muscatine Study. *J Am Coll Cardiol* 1996; 27:277–284.

88. Hoeg JM, Feuerstein IM, Tucker EE: Detection and quantitation of calcific atherosclerosis by ultrafast computed tomography in children and young adults with homozygous familial hypercholesterolemia. *Arterioscler Thromb* 1994; 14:1066–1074.

89. Janowitz WR, Agatston AS, Kaplan G, Viamonte M Jr: Differences in prevalence and extent of coronary artery calcium detected by ultrafast computed tomography in asymptomatic men and women. *Am J Cardiol* 1993; 72:247–254.

90. Wong ND, Detrano RC, Diamond G, et al: Does coronary artery screening by electron beam computed tomography motivate potentially beneficial lifestyle behaviors? *Am J Cardiol* 1996; 78:1220–1223.

91. Callister TQ, Raggi P, Cooil B, et al: Effect of HMG-CoA reductase inhibitors on coronary artery disease as assessed by electron-beam computed tomography. *N Engl J Med* 1998; 339:1972–1978.

92. Wong ND, Teng W, Abrahamson D, et al: Noninvasive tracking of coronary atherosclerosis by electron beam computed tomography: rationale and design of the felodipine atherosclerosis prevention study (FAPS). *Am J Cardiol* 1995; 76:1239–1242.

93. Wang S, Detrano RC, Secci A, et al: Detection of coronary calcification with electron-beam computed tomography: evaluation of interexamination reproducibility and comparison of three image-acquisition protocols. *Am Heart J* 1996; 132:550–558.

94. Callister TQ, Cooil B, Raya SP, et al: Coronary artery disease: improved reproducibility of calcium scoring with an electron-beam CT volumetric method. *Radiology* 1998; 208:807–814.

95. Lachman AS, Spray TL, Kerwin DM, et al: Medial calcinosis of Mönckeberg: a review of the problem and a description of a patient with involvement of peripheral, visceral and coronary arteries. *Am J Pathol* 1966; 49:739–771.

96. Roberts WC, Waller BF: Effect of chronic hypercalcemia on the heart: an analysis of 18 necropsy patients. *Am J Med* 1981; 71:371–384.

97. Böstrom K, Watson KE, Stanford WP, Demer LL: Atherosclerotic calcification: relation to developmental osteogenesis. *Am J Cardiol* 1995; 75:88B–91B.

98. Demer LL, Watson KE, Bostrom K: Mechanism of calcification in atherosclerosis. *Trends Cardiovasc Med* 1994; 4:45–49.

99. Mautner GC, Mautner SL, Froehlich J, et al: Coronary artery calcification: assessment with electron beam CT and histomorphometric correlation. *Radiology* 1994; 192:619–623.

100. Simons DB, Schwartz RS, Edwards WD et al: Noninvasive definition of anatomic coronary artery disease by ultrafast computed tomographic scanning: a quantitative pathologic comparison study. *J Am Coll Cardiol* 1992; 20:1118–1126.

101. Rumberger JA, Simons DB, Fitzpatrick LA, et al: Coronary artery calcium areas by electron beam computed tomography and coronary atherosclerotic plaque area: a histopathologic correlative study. *Circulation* 1995; 92:2157–2162.

102. Rumberger JA, Schwartz RS, Simons B, et al: Relation of coronary calcium determined by electron beam computed tomography and lumen narrowing determined by autopsy. *Am J Cardiol* 1994; 74:1169–1173.

103. Sangiorgi G, Rumberger JA, Severson A, et al: Arterial calcification and not lumen stenosis is highly correlated with atherosclerotic plaque burden in humans: a histologic study of 723 coronary artery segments using nondecalcifying methodology. *J Am Coll Cardiol* 1998; 31:126–133.

104. Agatston AS, Janowitz WH: Coronary calcification: detection by ultrafast computed tomography. In: Stanford W, Rumberger JA (eds), *Ultrafast Computed Tomography in Cardiac Imaging: Principles and Practice.* Mt. Kisco, NY, Futura, 1992:77–95.

105. Wong ND, Vo A, Abrahamson D, et al: Detection of coronary artery calcium by ultrafast computed tomography and its relation to clinical evidence of coronary artery disease. *Am J Cardiol* 1994; 73:223–227.

106. Rumberger JA, Sheedy PF, Breen JF, et al: Electron beam computed tomography and coronary artery disease: scanning for coronary artery calcification. *Mayo Clin Proc* 1996; 71:369–377.

107. Mautner SL, Mautner GC, Froehlich J, et al: Coronary

artery disease: prediction with in vitro electron beam CT. *Radiology* 1994; 192:625–630.

108. Budoff MJ, Georgiou D, Brody A, et al: Ultrafast computed tomography as a diagnostic modality in the detection of coronary artery disease: a multicenter study. *Circulation* 1996; 93:898–904.

109. Fallavollita JA, Brody AS, Bunnell IL, et al: Fast computed tomography detection of coronary calcification in the diagnosis of coronary artery disease: comparison with angiography in patients <50 years old. *Circulation* 1994; 89:285–290.

110. Bielak LF, Kaufmann RB, Moll PP, et al: Small lesions in the heart identified at electron beam CT: calcification or noise? *Radiology* 1994; 192:631–636.

111. Devries S, Wolfkiel C, Fusman B, et al: Influence of age and gender on the presence of coronary calcium detected by ultrafast computed tomography. *J Am Coll Cardiol* 1995; 25:76–82.

112. Rumberger JA, Sheedy PF II, Breen JF, et al: Coronary calcium, as determined by electron beam computed tomography, and coronary disease on arteriogram: effect of patient's sex on diagnosis. *Circulation* 1995; 91:1363–1367.

113. Shah PK: New insights into the pathogenesis and prevention of acute coronary syndromes. *Am J Cardiol.* 1997; 79(12B):17–23.

114. Davies M: Stability and instability: the two faces of coronary atherosclerosis. The Paul Dudley White Lecture, 1995. *Circulation* 1996; 94:2013–2020.

115. Falk E, Shah P, Fuster V: Coronary plaque disruption. *Circulation* 1995; 92:657–671.

116. Libby P: Molecular bases of the acute coronary syndromes. *Circulation* 1995; 91:2844–2850.

117. Tousoulis D, Davies G, Crake T, et al: Angiographic characteristics of infarct-related and non-infarct-related stenoses in patients in whom stable angina progressed to acute myocardial infarction. *Am Heart J* 1998; 136:382–388.

118. Ambrose JA, Fuster V: Can we predict future acute coronary events in patients with coronary artery disease? *JAMA* 1997; 277:343–344.

119. Ambrose JA, Fuster V: The risk of coronary occlusion is not proportional to the prior severity of coronary stenoses. *Heart* 1998; 79:3–4.

120. Little WC, Applegate RJ: Coronary angiography before myocardial infarction: can the culprit site be prospectively recognized? *Am Heart J* 1998; 136:368–370.

121. Topol EJ, Nissen SE: Our preoccupation with coronary luminology: the dissociation between clinical and angiographic findings in ischemic heart disease. *Circulation* 1995; 92:2333–2342.

122. Doherty TM, Detrano RC: Coronary artery calcification (letter). *Radiology* 1995; 195:576–577.

123. Detrano R, Markovic D, Simpfendorfer C, Salcedo E: Digital subtraction fluoroscopy: a new method of detecting coronary calcification with improved sensitivity for the prediction of coronary disease. *Circulation* 1985; 71:725–732.

124. Mistretta CA, Crummy AB: Basic concepts of digital angiography. *Prog Cardiovasc Dis* 1986; 28:245–255.

125. Sprawls P: Digital blurred-mask subtraction enhancement of radiologic images. *Digital Radiogr* 1981; 314:102–109.

126. Molloi S, Detrano R, Ersahin A, et al: Quantification of coronary arterial calcium by dual energy digital subtraction fluoroscopy. *Med Phys* 1991; 18:295–298.

127. Tang W, Young E, Detrano R, et al: Reproducibility of digital subtraction fluoroscopic readings for coronary artery calcification. *Invest Radiol* 1994; 29:147–149.

128. Stanford W, Thompson BH, Weiss RM: Coronary artery calcification: clinical significance and current methods of detection. *AJR* 1993; 161:1139–1146.

129. Borman JL, Stanford W, Stengerg RG, et al: Ultrafast tomographic detection of coronary artery calcification as an indicator of stenosis. *Am J Card Imaging* 1992; 6:191–196.

130. Margolis JR, Chen JT, Kong Y, et al: The diagnostic and prognostic significance of coronary artery calcification: a report of 800 cases. *Radiology* 1980; 137:609–616.

131. Hudson NM, Walker JK: The prognostic significance of coronary artery calcification seen on fluoroscopy. *Clin Radiol* 1976; 27:545–547.

132. Detrano RC, Wong ND, Tang W, et al: Prognostic significance of cardiac cinefluoroscopy for coronary calcific deposits in asymptomatic high risk subjects. *J Am Coll Cardiol* 1994; 24:354–358.

133. Detrano RC, Wong ND, Doherty TM, Shavelle R: Prognostic significance of coronary calcific deposits in asymptomatic high-risk subjects. *Am J Med* 1997; 102:344–349.

134. Detrano R, Hsiai T, Wang S, et al:Prognostic value of calcification and angiographic stenoses in patients undergoing coronary angiography: a multicenter study. *J Am Coll Cardiol* 1996; 27:285–290.

135. Lazem F, Barbir M, Banner N, et al: Coronary calcification detected by ultrafast computed tomography is a predictor of cardiac events in heart transplant recipients. *Transplant Proc* 1997; 29:572–575.

136. Arad Y, Spadaro LA, Goodman K, et al: Predictive value of electron beam computed tomography of the coronary arteries: 19-month follow-up of 1173 asymptomatic subjects. *Circulation* 1996; 93:1951–1953.

137. Secci A, Wong N, Tang W, et al: Electron beam computed tomographic (EBCT) coronary calcium as a predictor of coronary endpoints: comparison of two protocols. *Circulation* 1997; 96:1123–1129.

138. Detrano RC, Wong ND, Doherty TM, et al: Coronary calcium does not accurately predict near-term coronary events in high risk adults. *Circulation* 1999; 99:2633–2638.

139. Doherty TM, Wong ND, Shavelle RM, et al: Coronary

heart disease deaths and infarctions in people with little or no coronary calcium. *Lancet* 1999; 353:41–42.

140. Doherty TM, Tang W, Detrano RC: Racial differences in the significance of coronary calcium in asymptomatic black and white subjects with coronary risk factors. *J Am Coll Cardiol* 1999. In press.

141. Wong ND, Detrano RC, Abrahamson D, et al: Coronary artery screening by electron beam computed tomography: facts, controversy, and future. *Circulation* 1995; 92:632–636.

142. Feigelson HS, Criqui MH, Fronek A, et al: Screening for peripheral arterial disease: the sensitivity, specificity, and predictive value of non-invasive tests in a defined population. *Am J Epidemiol* 1994; 140:526–534.

143. Winsor T: Influence of arterial disease on the systolic blood pressure gradients of the extremity. *Am J Med Sci* 1950; 220:117–126.

144. Osmundson PJ, O'Fallon WM, Clements IP, et al: Reproducibility of noninvasive tests of peripheral occlusive arterial disease. *J Vasc Surg* 1985; 2:678–683.

145. Fowkes FGR, Housley E, Macintyre CCA, et al: Variability of ankle and brachial systolic pressures in the measurement of atherosclerotic peripheral arterial disease. *J Epidemiol Commun Health* 1988; 42:128–133.

146. Johnston KW, Hosang MY, Andrews DF: Reproducibility of noninvasive vascular laboratory measurements of the peripheral circulation. *J Vasc Surg* 1987; 6:147–151.

147. Kiekara O, Riekkinen H, Soimakallio S, Lansimies E: Correlation of angiographically determined reduction of vascular lumen with lower-limb systolic pressures. *Acta Chir Scand* 1985; 151:437–440.

148. Criqui MH, Browner D, Fronek A, et al: Peripheral arterial disease in large vessels is epidemiologically distinct from small vessel disease: an analysis of risk factors. *Am J Epidemiol* 1989; 129:1110–1119.

149. Criqui MH, Langer RD, Fronek A, et al: Large vessel and isolated small vessel disease. In: FGR Fowkes (ed), *Epidemiology of Peripheral Vascular Disease.* London, Springer-Verlag, 1991.

150. Fowkes FGR, Housley E, Riermersma RA, et al: Smoking, lipids, glucose intolerance, and blood pressure as risk factors for peripheral atherosclerosis compared with ischemic heart disease in the Edinburgh Artery Study. *Am J Epidemiol* 1992; 135:331–340.

151. Hiatt WR, Hoag S, Hamman RF: Effect of diagnostic criteria on the prevalence of peripheral arterial disease. *Circulation* 1995; 91:1472–1479.

152. Tyrrell J, Cooke T, Reilly M, et al: Lipoprotein [Lp(a)] and peripheral vascular disease. *J Intern Med* 1992; 232:349–352.

153. Valentine RJ, Grayburn PA, Vega Gl, Grundy SM: Lp(a) lipoprotein is an independent, discriminating risk factor for premature peripheral atherosclerosis among white men. *Arch Intern Med* 1994; 154:801–806.

154. Malinow MR, Kang SS, Taylor LM, et al: Prevalence of hyperhomocyst(e)inemia in patients with peripheral arterial occlusive disease. *Circulation* 1989; 79:1180–1188.

155. Lowe DGO, Fowkes FGR, Dawes J, et al: Blood viscosity, fibrinogen, and activation of coagulation and leukocytes in peripheral arterial disease and the normal population in the Edinburgh Artery Study. *Circulation* 1993; 87:1915–1920.

156. Criqui MH, Denenberg JO, Langer RD, et al: The epidemiology of peripheral arterial disease: importance of identifying the population at risk. *Vasc Med* 1997; 2:221–226.

157. Criqui MH, Langer RD, Fronek A, et al: Mortality over a period of 10 years in patients with peripheral arterial disease. *N Engl J Med* 1992; 326:381–386.

158. Criqui MH, Langer RD, Fronek A, Feigelson HS: Coronary disease and stroke in patients with large vessel peripheral arterial disease. *Drugs* 1991; 42(suppl 5):16–21.

159. Ogren M, Hedblad B, Jungquist G, et al: Low ankle-brachial pressure index in 68-year-old men: prevalence, risk factors and prognosis. *Eur J Vasc Surg* 1993; 7:500–556.

160. Newman AB, Sutton-Tyrrell K, Vogt MT, Kuller LH: Morbidity and mortality in hypertensive adults with a low ankle/arm blood pressure index. *JAMA* 1993; 270:487–498.

161. Criqui MH, Fronek A, Klauber MR, et al: The sensitivity, specificity, and predictive value of traditional clinical evaluation of peripheral arterial disease: results from non-invasive testing in a defined population. *Circulation* 1985; 71:516–521.

162. Expert Panel on Detection, Evaluation and Treatment of High Blood Cholesterol in Adults: Summary of the Second Report of the National Cholesterol Education Program (NCEP) Expert Panel on Detection, Evaluation and Treatment of High Blood Cholesterol in Adults (Adult Treatment Panel II). *JAMA* 1993; 269:3015–3023.

163. McKenna M, Wolfson S, Kuller L: The ratio of ankle and arm arterial pressure as an independent predictor of mortality. *Atherosclerosis* 1991; 87:119–128.

164. Vogt MT, Cauley JA, Newman AB, et al: Decreased ankle/arm blood pressure index and mortality in elderly women. *JAMA* 1993; 270:465–469.

165. McDermott MM, Feinglass J, Slavensky R, Pearce WH: The ankle-brachial index as a predictor of survival in patients with peripheral vascular disease. *J Gen Intern Med* 1994; 9:445–449.

166. Violi F, Criqui M, Longoni A, Castiglioni C: Relation between risk factors and cardiovascular complications in patients with peripheral vascular disease: Results from the ADEP study. *Atherosclerosis* 1996; 120:25–35.

167. Criqui MH, Fronek A, Barrett-Connor E, et al: The prevalence of peripheral arterial disease in a defined population. *Circulation* 1985; 71:510–515.

168. Fronek A: Arterial system (evaluation of the lower and

upper extremities). In: *Noninvasive Diagnostics in Vascular Diseases.* New York, McGraw Hill, 1989:88–120.

169. Bird CE, Criqui MH, Fronek A, et al: Qualitative and quantitative progression of peripheral arterial disease by non-invasive testing. *Vasc Med.* In press.

170. National Heart, Lung, and Blood Institute, National Institutes of Health: NHLBI-HC-98-XX. *Subclinical Cardiovascular Disease Study.* Request for Proposals. 1998.

171. Kajinami K, Seki H, Takekoshi N, Mabuchi H: Quantification of coronary artery calcification using ultrafast computed tomography: reproducibility of measurements. *Coron Artery Dis* 1993; 4:1103–1108.

172. Shields JP, Mielke CH Jr, Rockwood TH, et al: Reliability of electron beam computed tomography to detect coronary artery calcification. *Am J Card Imaging* 1995; 9:62–66.

CHAPTER 4

Ultrasound, Magnetic Resonance Imaging, and Positron Emission Tomography

Julius M. Gardin
Nathan D. Wong

Although traditional methods of cardiac risk assessment from the physical examination, laboratory tests, and treadmill exercise testing are often clinically utilized in cardiovascular disease (CVD) risk-stratification,[1] evaluation of subclinical disease is often not taken into account. Persons with subclinical disease, regardless of whether other risk factors are present, are at a greater risk of future cardiovascular events than are those without subclinical disease.[2] The roles of exercise testing, radiographic coronary artery calcium assessment, and ankle-brachial blood pressure in cardiovascular risk assessment have been reviewed in Chap. 3.

High-resolution Doppler ultrasound of the carotid arteries and of the heart (echocardiography)[3–5] has been utilized for more than a decade in population-based epidemiologic follow-up studies and even longer clinically in cardiovascular risk assessment. More recently, brachial artery reactivity, as measured by ultrasound, has been shown to be highly correlated with traditional risk factors,[6,7] and there is also increasing interest in magnetic resonance imaging (MRI)[8] and positron emission tomography (PET) for evaluating coronary atherosclerosis.[9] This chapter reviews the evidence supporting measures derived from these modalities and their relation to cardiovascular risk as well as the appropriateness of their use at present for evaluation of subclinical disease.

Carotid B-Mode Ultrasonography

Multiple studies, including observational studies and clinical trials involving antiatherosclerotic agents, have helped to establish high-resolution B-mode ultrasound imaging as a valid and reliable technique for measuring baseline carotid wall thickness and changes in thickness.[10] Carotid artery intima–media thickness (IMT) and changes in thicknesses can be measured cost-effectively and conveniently in large numbers of persons (Fig. 4–1). Carotid wall thickness has been measured in large population-based epidemiologic studies over the past decade, providing significant insight into its role in cardiovascular risk assessment and as a measure of subclinical atherosclerotic disease.

Relation to Cardiovascular Risk Factors and Events

Over recent years, several studies have documented a relation of carotid atherosclerosis to the risk of coronary heart disease (CHD) events. A limited 1-year follow-up of 1257 middle-aged Finnish men showed an association between common carotid artery IMT and cardiac events.[11] More recently, a nested case-control study within the Rotterdam Elderly Study showed an association between common carotid artery IMT and the risk of myocardial infarction (MI) and stroke.[12]

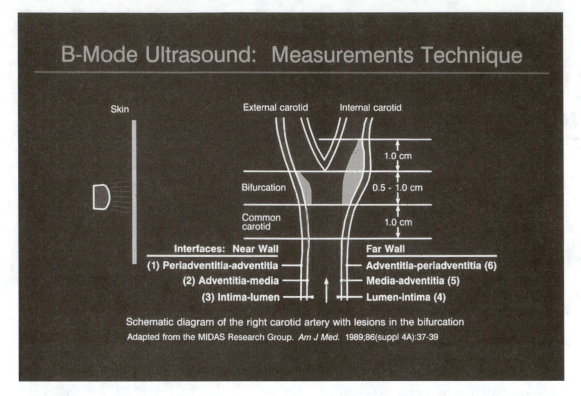

FIGURE 4–1 Schematic diagram of high resolution B-mode ultrasound showing measures of maximal intima-media thicknesses of the common carotid and internal carotid artery in the near and far walls.

Among nearly 13,000 men and women aged 45 to 64 at baseline participating in the Atherosclerosis Risk in Communities (ARIC) study, carotid IMT, consisting of the mean of B-mode ultrasound measurements at six sites in the carotid arteries, predicted CHD over years. For a mean IMT of 1 mm or greater compared to less than 1 mm, the relative risk (RR) for incident CHD was greater in women (RR = 5.07, 95 percent confidence interval (CI) = 3.08 to 8.36) than in men (RR = 1.85, 95 percent CI = 1.28 to 2.69).[13] A closer association in this study of low-density-lipoprotein cholesterol (LDL-C), compared to other lipid fractions, with carotid wall thickening suggested a particularly important role of LDL-C in earlier stages of atherosclerosis, while additional evidence suggests that other lipids may be more important in later stages.[14]

More recently, carotid B-mode ultrasonography was used in the multicenter, population-based Cardiovascular Health Study (CHS) to obtain a longitudinal image of the common carotid artery and three longitudinal images of the internal carotid artery. Readers at a central reading laboratory who were blinded to all clinical information performed all measurements obtained on over 5000 men and women aged 65 years and older who had been recruited at four field centers. The maximal rather than the mean IMT thickness was used as the key variable, based on comparisons of the strength of the relation of various thickness and diameter measurements with CHD risk factors. This IMT parameter was defined as the mean of the maximal IMT of the near and far wall, with measures obtained from both the left and right sides. The multiple measures of

IMT were summarized into two variables—one for the common carotid artery and another for the internal carotid artery.[15]

In elderly CHS participants who had no history of CVD, there was a closer association of internal carotid artery IMT—as opposed to common carotid artery IMT—and a history of CHD.[5] Moreover, a combined index of the sum of internal carotid artery and common carotid artery IMTs was more closely related to cardiovascular risk factors than was either measurement alone.

A recent report from CHS incorporating 6.2 years of follow-up data in this cohort showed, after adjustment for major risk factors, increased carotid IMT to be significantly associated with risk for MI or stroke.[15] Unadjusted rates of combined MI or stroke were directly related to quintile of IMT for all three measures (maximal common carotid IMT, maximal internal carotid IMT, and combined maxi-

mal common and internal carotid artery IMT) (Fig. 4–2). Relative risks (and 95 percent CIs) for second through fifth quintiles, compared to the first quintile, were 1.54 (1.04 to 2.28), 1.84 (1.26 to 2.67), 2.01 (1.38 to 2.91), and 3.15 (2.19 to 4.52), respectively, adjusted for major risk factors. Longitudinal analysis for MI and stroke paralleled these results. Cumulative event-free rates for a combined endpoint of MI and stroke were substantially less with increasing quintile of combined standardized average values of the maximal common carotid and internal carotid artery IMT (Fig. 4–3).

Patients with CHD have been demonstrated to have a significantly higher prevalence of atherosclerotic plaques in the carotid, femoral, and thoracic aorta, with extracoronary plaque being a stronger predictor of CHD than conventional CHD risk factors.[16] One recent study showed each 0.1-mm increase in common carotid artery IMT to be

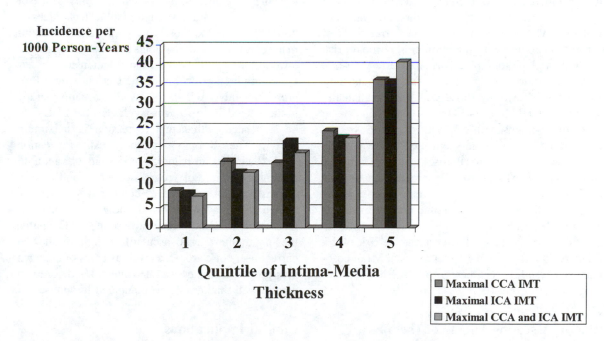

Incidence per 1000 Person-Years

Quintile of Intima-Media Thickness

■ Maximal CCA IMT
■ Maximal ICA IMT
■ Maximal CCA and ICA IMT

FIGURE 4–2 Unadjusted incidence of myocardial infarction or stroke according to quintile of carotid artery intima–media thicknesses (IMT). The rates were similar for quintiles of common carotid artery (CCA) IMT and internal carotid artery (ICA) IMT, but the gradient of increasing risk was slightly less pronounced than for the combined measure. The yearly incidence of the combined endpoint of myocardial infarction or stroke increased. (From O'Leary et al.,[15] with permission.)

FIGURE 4–3 Unadjusted cumulative event-free rates for the combined endpoint of myocardial infarction or stroke, according to quintile of combined IMT. The estimated cumulative rate of the combined endpoint for the fifth quintile of the combined measure was over 25 percent at 7 years, as compared with a cumulative rate of less than 5 percent for the first quintile. (From O'Leary et al.,[15] with permission.)

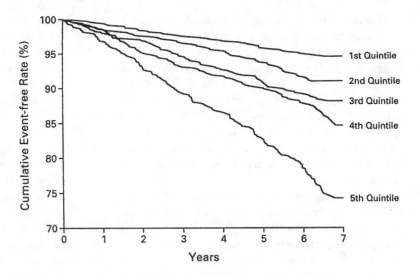

associated with a 1.91-fold (95 percent CI = 1.46 to 2.50) increased risk for positive exercise tests or CHD as defined by the electrocardiogram and medical history.[17] Although significant correlations of carotid thickening with the number of coronary risk factors[18] and angiographic coronary artery disease have been shown,[19,20] reported specificity and sensitivity for identifying those with angiographically significant CHD have not always been high.[20]

Among persons with a history of previous coronary artery bypass surgery enrolled in the Cholesterol-Lowering Atherosclerosis Study (CLAS), carotid artery IMT as well as progression in IMT predicted the risk of coronary events independently of that predicted by angiographic arterial measures and lipid levels. Each 0.03-mm increase per year in carotid arterial IMT conferred a relative risk of 2.2 (95 percent CI = 1.4 to 3.6) for nonfatal MI or coronary death and 3.1 (95 percent CI = 2.1 to 4.5) for any coronary event (both $p < .001$).[21]

Role in Assessing Effects of Therapy

There is great interest in examining whether use of certain preventive therapies may be related to altering the degree of progression of atherosclerosis, assessed using measures of subclinical disease, particularly in asymptomatic individuals free of CHD.

Practically, such a population can be studied only by utilizing a noninvasive assessment modality, as use of more invasive coronary angiographic techniques is normally limited to those with presumed or symptomatic coronary disease. Studies involving cholesterol-lowering therapy have been most demonstrative.[22,23] For example, the Asymptomatic Carotid Artery Progression Study (ACAPS) showed lovastatin therapy in those aged 40 to 79 years with elevated LDL-C to be associated with actual regression in maximum IMT.[22] The Kuopio Atherosclerosis Prevention Study[23] showed, in men 45 to 65 years of age, a 45 percent lower rate of progression of carotid atherosclerosis in those treated as compared to those not treated with pravastatin—with more pronounced effects the greater the degree of baseline IMT. Finally, the longitudinal Cardiovascular Health Study showed current users of estrogen as well as users of estrogen plus progestin to have smaller internal and common carotid wall thicknesses, as compared to nonusers.[24]

Clinical Implications

Although the degree of carotid atherosclerosis bears a relation to coronary atherosclerosis and the risk of CHD events and stroke, relative risks relating carotid atherosclerosis to coronary events are only modest, usually in the range of 1.5 to 3. With the advent of mobile "stroke" screening units, it should be realized that there are no established guidelines for routine screening of any population group involving carotid ultrasound, and some have questioned whether routine screening of the general population might cause more strokes (e.g., from unnecessary interventions) than it would prevent.[25,26] Although certain high-risk individuals with multiple risk factors or preexisting CHD may benefit from such assessment, which can be utilized in further risk stratification, a physician should determine the appropriate clinical indications before such testing is performed. The great advantages of carotid ultrasound imaging include its noninvasive nature and the relatively direct assessment it provides of parameters related to atherosclerosis; however, its principal limitation remains that measures of carotid wall thickness or progression may not directly relate to changes in coronary atherosclerotic burden.[27] Besides its established relation to clinical event risk, promising data[22,23] are emerging regarding its utility in tracking the effects of preventive therapies through serial measurements.

Brachial Artery Endothelial Reactivity

Background and Methodology

Endothelial dysfunction is an early physiologic event in atherogenesis.[28] In vitro studies have shown that endothelium is normal in the earliest stages of atherosclerosis, before plaques exist and before clinical detection of disease, and that endothelial injury predisposes to thrombosis, leukocyte adhesion, and proliferation of smooth muscle cells in the arterial wall.[29] An important functional consequence of endothelial dysfunction is the inability to release endothelium-derived relaxing factor (EDRF).[30] Coronary artery endothelial dysfunction has been demonstrated in vivo in response to various pharmacologic and physiologic stimuli—primarily in adults with symptoms of established coronary atherosclerosis.[31,32] These studies used invasive coronary angiography, which is not suitable for the investigation of either the early development of vascular damage in younger symptom-free subjects or for serial studies of progression or reversibility in these subjects.

A noninvasive method has been developed that uses high-resolution ultrasound to measure changes in brachial or superficial femoral artery diameter in response to increased flow or to sublingual nitroglycerin.[33] Increased flow can be induced as reactive hyperemia after 4 to 5 min of cuff occlusion of the brachial artery.[33] In arteries lined by healthy endothelium, increased flow causes dilatation of the vessel.[34-36] However, this vasodilatory mechanism fails to occur in the presence of endothelial dysfunction.[37] In contrast, the mechanism of action of nitroglycerin, which causes vasodilatation by direct action on the smooth muscle, is independent of the presence or the state of the endothelium.

Relation to Cardiovascular Risk Factors

Of interest, a number of risk factors for CHD have been shown to produce abnormalities in flow-mediated dilatation (FMD) of the brachial artery. For example, impaired FMD has been shown in insulin-dependent diabetes mellitus to be related to the duration of the disease and to LDL-C levels.[6] Brachial artery FMD was found to be significantly impaired in diabetic subjects [percent diameter change = 5.0 ± 3.7 percent (mean ± SD), compared to control subjects (9.3 ± 3.8 percent), $p < .001$]. Large-vessel atherosclerotic disease is the major cause of morbidity and mortality in diabetics.

FMD has also been shown to be significantly impaired in passive smokers (percent change = 3.0 ± 2.7 percent) and in active smokers (4.4 ± 3.1 percent) compared with control subjects (8.2 ± 3.1 percent, $p < .001$ compared with smoking groups). There was an inverse relation between the intensity of exposure to tobacco smoke and FMD ($r = -.67$, $p < .001$). These findings suggest that passive smoking is associated with dose-related impairment of endothelium-dependent dilatation in healthy young adults, suggesting early arterial damage. In 500 clinically well, nonhypertensive subjects, [252 men and 248 women, age (mean ± SD) 36 ± 15 years], multiple stepwise regression analysis revealed that reduced FMD of the brachial ($n = 454$) or superficial femoral ($n = 46$) artery was independently associated with cigarette smoking, older age, male gender, and larger vessel size ($p < .005$) but not with total cholesterol, blood pressure, or family history. A composite risk-factor score was independently related to FMD ($r = -.30$, $p < .0001$), suggesting risk-factor interaction. These findings suggest that loss of endothelium-dependent dilatation in the systemic arteries occurs in the preclinical phase of vascular disease and is associated with an interaction of traditional risk factors for atherosclerosis.[7]

In 238 subjects [103 men and 135 women, age (mean ± SD) 38 ± 17 years], reduced flow-mediated brachial arterial dilatation was related to older age ($r = ^-.34$, $p < .001$). In men, FMD was preserved in subjects 40 years of age or below but declined (at 0.21 percent per year) thereafter; in women, FMD was stable until the early fifties, after which it declined by 0.49 percent per year ($p = .002$, compared with men). These findings suggest that aging is associated with progressive endothelial dysfunction in normal humans, and this appears to occur earlier in men than in women. A steep decline in flow-mediated endothelial function in women commences at about the time of menopause, suggesting a protective effect of estrogens on the arterial wall.[38]

Clinical Relevance

Although the above data relating brachial FMD to cardiovascular risk factors are encouraging, further data, particularly relating FMD to cardiovascular endpoints in large populations, are needed before recommendations for routine assessment of selected populations can be made. This technique, however, represents a potentially important tool for the noninvasive assessment of subclinical CVD risk.

Echocardiography

Role of Echocardiography in Population-Based Studies

The role of cardiac ultrasound, in particular two-dimensionally (2D) guided M-mode echocardiography, in assessing subclinical disease risk has been a subject of several major population-based studies over the past two decades.[39–43] The Bogalusa[39] and Muscatine[40] studies in longitudinal cohorts of youth documented a relation of increased left ventricular mass measured by echocardiography to blood pressure. The Framingham Heart Study[41–43] was the first longitudinal study to extensively document the prognostic significance of echocardiographic measures, particularly left ventricular mass. The Coronary Artery Risk Development in Young Adults (CARDIA) study,[44] Cardiovascular Health Study (CHS),[4] and, most recently, the Strong Heart Study[45] involved multiple field centers performing echocardiography using a common protocol.

In CARDIA[44] and CHS,[4] baseline echocardiograms were recorded onto super-VHS tape using a standard protocol and equipment. Echocardiographic images were digitized and measures made at a centralized reading site using customized image-analysis software. Quality control measures included standardized training of echocardiography technicians and readers, periodic blind duplicate readings with reader review sessions, phantom studies, and quality-control audits.

Measures of interest in CHS and CARDIA involved those related to left ventricular anatomy and function. Specifically, 2D echocardiography was used to assess left ventricular global and regional systolic function. In addition, 2D-directed M-mode echocardiography was used to derive measures of left ventricular (LV) mass and its three component variables: ventricular septal thickness at end-diastole (VSTd), LV (internal) dimension at end-diastole (LVIDd), and LV posterior wall thickness at end-diastole (PWTd) (Fig. 4–4). Measurements in the CHS and CARDIA studies were performed according to conventions established by the American Society of Echocardiography (ASE),[46] with LV mass determined according to the formula described by Devereux et al.[47]: LV mass (in grams) = 0.80 × 1.04 [(VSTd + LVIDd + PWTd)^3 − (LVIDd)^3] + 0.6, where thickness and dimension measurements are expressed in centimeters. Key 2D directed M-mode echocardiographic measures performed as part of the CHS Echocardiography Reading Center protocol are shown in Table 4–1.[4]

Pulsed Doppler echocardiographic measurements of left ventricular diastolic function, including mitral

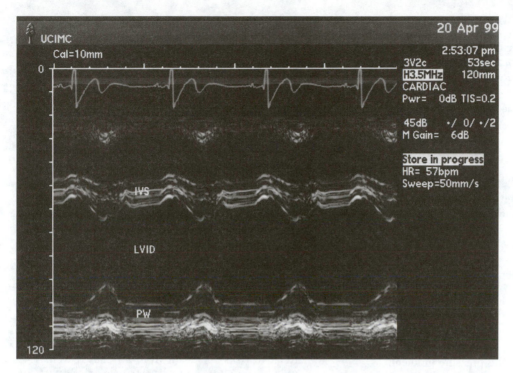

FIGURE 4–4 Two-dimensionally guided M-mode echocardiographic images demonstrating important components of the calculated left ventricular mass: left ventricular internal dimension at end-diastole (LVIDd), ventricular septal thickness at end-diastole (VSTd), and posterior wall thickness at end-diastole (PWTd). These measurements were all made at the onset of the QRS complex (*electrocardiogram at top*). Key: IVS = VSTd, LVID = LVIDd, PW = PWTd.

peak flow velocity in early and late diastole (PFVE and PFVA, respectively), as well as the PFVE/PFVA ratio, have also been described in various populations, including Framingham, CARDIA, and CHS. For example, Xie et al.[48] in the CARDIA study demonstrated that in Caucasian and African-American young adults, Doppler measures of LV diastolic filling were related to age, gender, body weight, blood pressure, heart rate, left ventricular systolic function, and lung function. Women tended to have significantly higher peak PFVE and PFVA than did men, independent of other variables. However, the PFVE/PFVA ratio did not differ between genders. In the Framingham Heart Study, Benjamin et al.[49] also found age to be a major determinant of Doppler left ventricular filling parameters.

Although data are not available to suggest that Doppler filling velocity patterns in healthy young adults can be used to predict subsequent CVD, there are data in patients who have had a previous MI or have dilated cardiomyopathies suggesting that mitral diastolic velocity parameters—e.g., early diastolic deceleration time—can be used to predict subsequent CVD events and prognosis.[50,51] Among the elderly subjects of the Cardiovascular Health Study, men with congestive heart failure (CHF) had the highest PFVE/PFVA ratio (1.19), while the subgroup with hypertension had the lowest ratio (0.89 and 0.87 in females and males, respectively). The authors concluded that the hypertensive subjects most likely exhibited an abnormal left ventricular relaxation pattern, whereas patients with CHF had a Doppler

TABLE 4–1 Two-Dimensionally-Directed M-mode Echocardiographic Measures Performed in the Cardiovascular Health Study

Left ventricular internal dimension in diastole (LVIDd)

Left ventricular internal dimension in systole (LVIDs)

Ventricular septal thickness in diastole (VSTd)

Ventricular septal thickness in systole (VSTs)

LV posterior wall thickness in diastole (LVPWTd)

LV posterior wall thickness in systole (LVPWTs)

Left atrial dimension (LA)

Aortic root dimension (Ao)

LV % fractional shortening (LVFS) (calculated)

LV end-systolic stress (LVESS) (calculated)

LV mass (grams) (calculated) = 0.80 {1.04[(VSTd + LVIDd +
   PWTd)^3 − (LVIDd)^3]} + 0.6

Relation of Left Ventricular Mass to Atherosclerosis and Risk Factors

Although increased LV mass may be a consequence of hypertensive heart disease, among other causes, and is not a direct measure of subclinical atherosclerosis, it does bear a relation to atherosclerosis and the risk of CVD events. In subjects primarily free of clinical coronary disease, measures of LV mass relate to common carotid artery diameter and IMT (r = .40 and .20, respectively, p < .01).[52]

Further, measurements of echocardiographic LV mass bear a strong relation to important risk factors for CHD. In the CHS cohort of elderly men and women, factors positively associated with LV mass included body weight, male gender, systolic blood pressure, present smoking, major and minor electrocardiographic abnormalities, and treatment for hypertension, whereas diastolic blood pressure, bioresistance (a measure of adiposity), and high-density-lipoprotein cholesterol (HDL-C) were inversely related to LV mass. Further, pulse pressure was positively related to LV mass.[53] In younger adults, LV mass has been shown to be independently associated with body mass index (or subscapular skinfold thickness) and systolic blood pressure.[44]

Echocardiographic Left Ventricular Mass and Prognosis

Increased LV mass, as well as LV hypertrophy as defined by echocardiography, has been shown to be associated with an increased incidence of subsequent CHD events and mortality. Findings from the Framingham Heart Study originally established the prognostic significance of increased LV mass.[41] In a 4-year follow-up study of 3220 subjects 40 years of age and older who were initially free of cardiovascular disease, a 50 g/m increment in LV mass divided by height, adjusted for other risk factors, was found to be associated with a relative risk of new CVD events of 1.49 (95 percent CI = 1.20 to 1.85) in men and 1.57 (95 percent CI = 1.20 to 2.04) in women. Relative risks for death from all causes were 1.49 (95 percent CI = 1.14 to 1.94) in men and 2.01 (95 percent CI = 1.44 to 2.81) in women.[41] Among the subgroup of elderly subjects aged 59 to 90 years, similar increases in risk for new coronary events were seen with increased LV mass.[42] Cutoff values of LV mass/height of 143 g/m for men and 102 g/m for women have been used to define LV hypertrophy by the Framingham Heart Study.[43]

Preliminary data from the Cardiovascular Health Study suggest that, among elderly subjects without prevalent CVD at baseline, the highest quartile of LV mass conferred a relative risk of 3.35—compared to the lowest quartile—for incident CHF. Furthermore, eccentric and concentric LV hypertrophy, respectively, defined using a ratio of 2 × (LV diastolic wall thickness) to internal dimension, conferred adjusted hazards ratios, compared to normal LV geometry, of 2.05 and 1.61 for incident CHD and 2.95 and 3.32 for incident CHF.[54]

In a 10-year follow-up study of 151 hypertensive patients who had repeat echocardiography, Muiesan et al.[55] reported that those without reduction in LV mass indexed for body surface area (g/m^2) were at a greater risk for nonfatal cardiovascular events than

pattern suggesting an increased early diastolic left atrial–left ventricular pressure gradient.[51]

those with regression of LV hypertropy (relative risk of 3.52 versus 1.38, $p < .0001$).

Other Echocardiographic Measures and Cardiovascular Risk

Other measures obtained from M-mode and 2D echocardiography, such as decreased LV ejection fraction (LVEF) and abnormal segmental wall motion, are also associated with a higher incidence of cardiovascular morbidity and mortality.[56,57] Various measures of LV diastolic dysfunction obtained from Doppler echocardiography—e.g., early diastolic deceleration time—may also relate to an increased risk of cardiovascular events.[50,51] Echocardiographic measures such as left atrial dimension and the presence of mitral annular calcification have been reported to be related to the risk of stroke.[58,59]

Only recently have population studies, including the Cardiovascular Health Study and CARDIA, begun to evaluate the distribution and risk-factor correlates of LV systolic and diastolic function measures.[60–62] In elderly participants of the CHS, decreased LV ejection fraction and LV segmental wall motion abnormalities were more prevalent in men than in women.[60] In CHS, an abnormal LVEF was one of several risk and subclinical disease factors found to be associated with an increased risk of mortality over 5 years.[61] Decreased LVEF has recently been associated with prevalent CHD in this cohort (RR = 1.9, 95 percent CI = 1.1 to 3.3).[62] However, approximately three-fourths of those with clinical CHF have systolic function that is intact, but mortality remains high, regardless of whether systolic function is impaired (RR = 6.3, 95 percent CI = 4.3 to 9.3) or intact (RR = 3.2, 95 percent CI = 2.5 to 4.2) in those with CHF as compared to those with intact LVEF and no CHF.[63]

Among young adults 23 to 35 years of age, male gender, history of hypertension, and current smoking were each independently associated with about a 1 percent lower LVEF.[64] The prognostic significance of lower levels of LVEF among young adults in CARDIA will not be known unless and until a sufficient number of CVD events have occurred.

Clinical Recommendations Regarding Echocardiography in Cardiovascular Risk Assessment

Although selected echocardiographic measures, such as increased LV mass or decreased LV ejection fraction, undoubtedly relate to an increased risk of CVD events, there are presently no guidelines for routine echocardiographic assessment in general population groups. Echocardiographic assessment is part of the standard evaluation of patients with known or suspected, cardiac disease, but high-risk asymptomatic patient groups do not routinely undergo such testing. Recently, however, some select patient groups, such as hypertensives, have been recommended as candidates for low-cost limited and focused (e.g., on the left ventricle and left atrium) echocardiographic screening.[65] Also, the issue has been raised whether individuals taking certain medications (such as weight-reducing drugs) should have echocardiograms to screen for possible subclinical heart valve disease, pulmonary hypertension, or other problems.[66,67]

Magnetic Resonance Imaging (MRI)

Promising data are emerging regarding the possible role of magnetic resonance imaging (MRI) in assessing atherosclerosis. Experimental studies in rabbit abdominal aortas show the ability of MRI to image the lumen and arterial wall with high resolution and to detect progression as measured by increased lesion mass, decreased arterial lumen or increased stenosis, or the development of intralesion abnormalities. Lesion characteristics such as a fibrous cap, necrotic core, and lesion fissures can also be identified by MRI.[68] More recent reports show a high degree of correspondence between MRI measurements of wall area versus histopathology.[69] MRI has been shown to characterize (as to presence of a lipid core, fibrous cap, calcium, thrombus, and intraplaque hemorrhage) atherosclerotic carotid arteries, and, more recently, thoracic aortic plaque morphology and composition.[70]

Technical advantages of MRI include its excellent spatial resolution, ability to differentiate infarcted from normal myocardial tissue, and the potential for three-dimensional (3D) imaging.[71] In addition, MRI does not require the use of ionizing radiation or injection of contrast material. A signal is generated from flowing blood to create tomographic images of the bloodstream in coronary arteries, images of which resemble conventional contrast-enhanced x-ray angiograms. More rapid pulse sequences, dedicated radiofrequency receiver coils, and cardiac and respiratory gating techniques serve to improve the quality of images obtained. These enhancements in image quality are essential, given the tortuosity, small diameter, and motion of the coronary arteries. Approaches such as repetitive breath-holding facilitate imaging of the coronary artery tree, including most of the proximal and middle portions of the arteries.

Relation to Established Measures of Atherosclerosis

The ability of MRI to quantitate flow in the coronary arteries noninvasively may permit assessment of the function and physiologic implications of significant stenoses.[72] Clinically, MRI can, through noninvasive magnetic resonance angiography (MRA), identify pathology in the left main, left anterior descending, circumflex, and right coronary arteries.[73] However, the sensitivity and specificity for detecting significant stenoses (50 percent or more of luminal diameter) vary substantially by artery, with reported values for sensitivity for the circumflex, left anterior descending, right, and left main coronary arteries of 0, 53, 71, and 100 percent, respectively. Specificities ranged from 73 percent for the left anterior descending to 96 percent for the circumflex.[74] Another study reported 3D MRI to be highly sensitive (83 percent) and specific (94 percent), with high positive and negative predictive values (87 and 93 percent, respectively) for detecting significant stenosis (50 percent or greater as measured by conventional contrast coronary angiography).[75] One comparative report, however, showed the sensitivity of MRA in correctly identifying coronary artery bypass graft patency to be substantially lower (67 percent) than that of electron-beam computed tomography (96 percent).[76] Protocols incorporating breath-holding and multiple slices may help to enhance the reproducibility of MRI.[77,78]

Clinical Considerations

The role of MRI in screening for coronary artery lesions is not yet established. Nonetheless, significant progress is being made in addressing important technical problems that need to be resolved before its role as a noninvasive screening tool can be established.[79] Among persons with ischemic heart disease, MRI, including MRA, is positioned to play an increasingly greater role in providing, from a single examination, multiple pieces of information necessary for CHD risk stratification.[80] Specifically, given the high resolution and noninvasive nature of MRI, there is the potential for serial studies of atherosclerosis and for further investigation of plaque formation, rupture, and stabilization.[81] Further studies are needed to evaluate whether the coronary atherosclerosis (and its progression) measured by MRI is associated with cardiac risk factors or prognosis. Moreover, the cost-effectiveness of MRI in screening selected risk groups and its value in cardiac risk stratification needs to be established before any recommendations can be made regarding the general clinical utility in cardiac risk assessment.

Positron Emission Tomography

One of the most accurate methods for identifying and noninvasively assessing the severity of coronary artery stenosis is positron emission tomography (PET).[9] Myocardial perfusion, metabolism, and cell membrane function can be evaluated. The technique assesses the severity and location of coronary artery disease using radionuclides such as nitrogen-13, ammonia, and rubidium-82. Fluorine-18 fluorodeoxyglucose can be used to identify impaired but viable myocardium.[82]

A large study involving 1460 patients undergoing coronary angiography and PET showed sensitivities and predictive accuracies of (1) 87 and 88 percent, respectively, for identifying angiographic stenoses exceeding 67 percent diameter, and (2) 92 and 91 percent, respectively, for identifying stenoses of greater than 90 percent diameter.[83] Coronary flow reserve (CFR), a measure of vascular integrity using PET, has been reported to be inversely related to total cholesterol (TC), LDL-C, and the ratio of TC to HDL-C, suggesting its utility in identifying possible alternations in vascular reactivity as a marker of subclinical atherosclerosis. This technique may help provide a basis for modification or elimination of risk factors, thereby potentially slowing, retarding, or even reversing the progression of coronary artery disease.[84]

One of the most important potential uses of PET lies in tracking the progression of atherosclerosis and the effects of medical therapy aimed to retard or reverse atherosclerosis. In a study of patients with CHD assigned to aggressive cholesterol-lowering therapy for 90 days, myocardial perfusion as measured by serial dipyridamole PET scanning improved while patients were on the lipid-lowering therapy but deteriorated after withdrawal from therapy.[85]

The prognostic implications of myocardial perfusion imaging using rubidium-82 PET have been evaluated. In one study of 685 patients, the presence and extent of perfusion defects determined by PET performed at rest before and during dipyridamole stress testing were independent predictors of cardiac death and total cardiac events.[86]

As is the case with other imaging modalities, the clinical utility of PET scanning will depend not only on the results of further investigation establishing its role in risk assessment and stratification but also on its cost-effectiveness, given more currently established, available, and lower-cost office-based measures.

Combined Measures for Subclinical Disease Assessment

Considering that atherosclerosis is systemic rather than limited to a single vascular bed, measurements made from several vascular beds combined with other markers of subclinical CVD may provide better prediction of CHD risk than do single measures. A combined subclinical disease index—consisting of measures of ankle-brachial blood pressure, carotid artery stenosis and wall thickness, electrocardiographic and echocardiographic abnormalities, and a positive response to the Rose Angina and Claudication Questionnaire—has been applied to the large elderly population–based Cardiovascular Health Study (CHS) to address this question[2] (Table 4–2). Independent of other coronary risk factors, the presence of subclinical disease was associated with an increased incidence, over a mean 2.4-year follow-up, of total CHD in both sexes, and of total mortality in

TABLE 4–2   Criteria for Clinical and Subclinical Disease in the Cardiovascular Health Study

Clinical Disease Criteria	Subclinical Disease Criteria
Atrial fibrillation or pacemaker	Ankle-arm index of 0.9 or less
History of intermittent claudication or peripheral vascular surgery	Internal or common carotid wall thickness >80th percentile
History of congestive heart failure	Carotid diameter stenosis >25%
History of stroke, transient ischemic attack, or carotid surgery	Major ECG abnormalities* or abnormal ejection fraction
History of CABG or PTCA	Abnormal wall motion on echocardiogram
History of angina or use of nitroglycerin	Positive Rose questionnaire for claudication or angina pectoris
History of myocardial infarction	

Key: CABG, coronary artery bypass graft; PTCA, percutaneous transluminal coronary angioplasty.

*According to the Minnesota Code, ventricular conduction defects (7-1, 7-2, 7-4), major Q/QS abnormalities (1-1, 1-2), left ventricular hypertrophy (high-amplitude R waves with major or minor ST-T abnormalities) (3-1, 3-3, and 4-1 to 4-3 or 5-1 to 5-3), and isolated major ST/T-wave abnormalities (4-1, 4-2, 5-1, 5-2).

Source: Adapted from Kuller et al.,[2] with permission.

men—but not with MI in either sex or with total mortality in women[2] (Table 4–3). More extensive follow-up data reported from CHS showed that among 20 characteristics significantly associated with 5-year mortality, several risk factors and measures of subclinical or clinical disease were included—specifically, high brachial (>169 mmHg) and low tibial (≤127 mmHg) systolic blood pressure, low forced vital capacity (≤206 mL), aortic stenosis (moderate or severe), abnormal left ventricular ejection fraction (by echocardiography), major electrocardiographic abnormality, and stenosis of the internal carotid artery (by ultrasound). Increased left ventricular mass by echocardiography, however, was not a significant predictor of mortality after these other factors were considered.[61]

These findings suggest that subclinical disease assessment utilizing a combined set of measures representing several vascular beds may provide improved risk prediction over and above standard CHD risk factors.[2] At least in older individuals—from whom these data were derived—assessment of subclinical disease may provide an approach for identifying high-risk individuals who may be candidates for more active intervention to prevent clinical disease. Measurements of subclinical disease from these tests can be done by trained technicians under the supervision of physicians. The costs of performing one or more of these tests in the office-based health care setting, which continue to decrease, will help determine the practical application of such tests in risk-stratification for the population as a whole. Further follow-up of the cohort in CHS and other studies incorporating subclinical disease assessment—such as the recently initiated National Institutes of Health–sponsored Multiethnic Study of Atherosclerosis (MESA)—should help determine the best combination of measures to efficiently identify those at highest risk of clinical disease outcomes.[87]

Conclusions

Over the past decade, evidence from large population-based studies has established the prognostic value for CVD of several noninvasive subclinical disease measures, including carotid artery IMT measured by ultrasound; echocardiographic LV mass and hypertrophy; and LV global systolic function (ejection fraction). Although these measures do show predictive value over and above standard risk-factor assessment, their utility in screening general or selected population groups has yet to be determined, and no consensus regarding such screening currently exists. Newer noninvasive measures of subclinical disease assessment—including brachial artery function, coronary artery evaluation involving magnetic resonance imaging and angiography, and positron emission tomography (PET)—are being developed. In certain circumstances, these techniques appear promising in their ability to detect significant clinical and subclinical disease.

TABLE 4–3   Multivariate Assessment of Group Differences in Incident Clinical Cardiovascular Diseases: Subclinical Disease Compared with No Subclinical Disease Group*

	Men and Women		*Men Only*		*Women Only*	
Incident Disease	**Or**	**95% CI**	**OR**	**95% CI**	**OR**	**95% CI**
Total CHD	1.99	1.33–3.00	1.84	1.09–3.09	2.41	1.26–4.62
Total MI	1.32	0.75–2.32	0.93	0.47–1.84	2.54	0.87–7.43
Total Mortality	1.82	1.08–3.08	2.52	1.18–5.37	1.21	0.57–2.57

Key: OR, odds ratio; CI, confidence interval; CHD, coronary heart disease; MI, myocardial infarction.

*Included in model: age, systolic blood pressure, LDL cholesterol level, HDL cholesterol level, triglyceride level, diabetes, hypertension, weight, and current smoking status.

Source: Adapted from Kuller et al.,[2] with permission.

The ability of these newer tests to predict prognosis in high-risk asymptomatic groups, however, has yet to be determined. More importantly, the utility of these newer tests in risk stratification in relation to other, more established measures of subclinical disease assessment is not yet defined. A major challenge will be to establish consensus on a limited set of indicators or measures of subclinical disease that are not only cost-effective and efficiently implementable in the office-based setting but also provide information over and above standard CHD risk-factor assessment.

References

1. Califf RM, Armstrong PW, Carver JR, et al: 27th Bethesda Conference: matching the intensity of risk factor management with the hazard for coronary disease events. Task Force 5. Stratification of patients into high, medium and low risk subgroups for purposes of risk factor management. *J Am Coll Cardiol* 1996; 27:1007–1019.

2. Kuller LH, Shemanski L, Psaty BM, et al: Subclinical disease as an independent risk factor for cardiovascular disease. *Circulation* 1995; 92:720–726.

3. Celermajer DS: Noninvasive detection of atherosclerosis (editorial). *N Engl J Med* 1998; 339:2014–2015.

4. Gardin JM, Wong ND, Bommer W, et al: Echocardiographic design of a multicenter investigation of free-living elderly subjects: the Cardiovascular Health Study. *J Am Soc Echocardiogr* 1992; 5:63–72.

5. O'Leary DH, Polak JF, Kronmal RA, et al: Thickening of the carotid wall: A marker of atherosclerosis in the elderly? Cardiovascular Health Study Collaborative Research Group. *Stroke* 1996; 27:224–231.

6. Clarkson P, Celermajer DS, Donald AE, et al: Impaired vascular reactivity in insulin-dependent diabetes mellitus is related to disease duration and low density lipoprotein cholesterol levels. *J Am Coll Cardiol* 1996; 28:573–579.

7. Celermajer DS, Sorensen KE, Bull C, et al: Endothelium-dependent dilatation in the systemic arteries of asymptomatic subjects relates to coronary risk factors and their interaction. *J Am Coll Cardiol* 1994; 24:1468–1474.

8. Pohost GM, Fuisz AR: From the microscope to the clinic: MR assessment of atherosclerotic plaque. *Circulation* 1998; 98:1477–1478.

9. Gould KL: Identifying and measuring severity of coronary artery stenosis: quantitative coronary arteriography and positron emission tomography. *Circulation* 1988; 78:237–245.

10. Mercuri M: Noninvasive imaging protocols to detect and monitor carotid atherosclerosis progression. *Am J Hypertens* 1994; 7(pt 2):23S–29S.

11. Salonen JT, Salonen R: Ultrasonographically assessed carotid morphology and the risk of coronary heart disease. *Arterioscler Thromb* 1991; 11:1245–1249.

12. Bots ML, Hoes AW, Koudstaal PJ, et al: Common carotid intima–media thickness and risk of stroke and myocardial infarction: the Rotterdam Study. *Circulation* 1997; 96:1432–1437.

13. Chambless LE, Heiss G, Folson AR, et al: Association of coronary heart disease incidence with carotid arterial wall thickness and major risk factors: the Atherosclerosis Risk in Communities (ARIC) Study, 1987–1993. *Am J Epidemiol* 1997; 146:483–494.

14. Sharrett AR, Patsch W, Sorlie PD, et al: Associations of lipoprotein cholesterols, apolipoproteins AI nd B, and triglycerides with carotid atherosclerosis and coronary heart disease. The Atherosclerosis Risk in Communities (ARIC) Study. *Atherioscler Thromb* 1994; 14:1098–1104.

15. O'Leary DH, Polak JF, Kronmal RA, et al for the Cardiovascular Health Study Collaborative Research Group: Carotid-artery intima and media thickness as a risk factor for myocardial infarction and stroke in older adults. Cardiovascular Health Study Collaborative Research Group. *N Engl J Med* 1999; 340:14–22.

16. Khoury Z, Schwartz R, Gottlieb S, et al: Relation of coronary artery disease to atherosclerotic disease in the aorta, carotid, and femoral arteries evaluated by ultrasound. *Am J Cardiol* 1997; 80:1429–1433.

17. Nagai Y, Metter J, Earley CJ, et al: Increased carotid artery intima–media thickness in asymptomatic older subjects with exercise-induced myocardial ischemia. *Circulation* 1998; 98:1504–1509.

18. Gnasso A, Irace C, Mattioli PL, Pujia A: Carotid intima–media thickness and coronary heart disease risk factors. *Atherosclerosis* 1996; 119:7–15.

19. Visona A, Pesavento R, Lusiani L, et al: Intima medical thickening of common carotid artery as indicator of coronary artery disease. *Angiology* 1996; 47:61–66.

20. Adams MR, Nakagomi A, Keech A, et al: Carotid intima–media thickness is only weakly correlated with the extent and severity of coronary artery disease. *Circulation* 1995; 92:2127–2134.

21. Hodis HN, Mack WJ, LaBree L, et al: The role of carotid arterial intima–media thickness in predicting clinical coronary events. *Ann Intern Med* 1998; 128:262–269.

22. Furberg CD, Adams HP, Applegate WB, et al: Effect of lovastatin on early carotid atherosclerosis and cardiovascular events. Asymptomatic Carotid Artery Progression Study (ACAPS) Research Group. *Circulation* 1994; 90:1679–1687.

23. Salonen R, Nyyssonen K, Porkkala E, et al: Kuopio Atherosclerosis Prevention Study (KAPS). A population-based primary prevention trial of the effect of LDL-lowering on atherosclerotic progression in carotid and femoral arteries. *Circulation* 1995; 92:1758–1764.

24. Jonas HA, Kronmal RA, Psaty BM, et al: Current estrogen-progestin and estrogen replacement therapy in elderly women: association with carotid atherosclerosis. CHS Collaborative Research Group: Cardiovascular Health Study. *Ann Epidemiol* 1996; 6:314–324.

25. Whitty CJ, Sudlow CL, Warlow CP: Investigating individual subjects and screening populations for asymptomatic carotid stenosis can be harmful. *J Neurol Neurosurg Psychiatry* 1998; 64:619–623.

26. Perry JR, Szalai JP, Norris JW: Consensus against both endarterectomy and routine screening for asymptomatic carotid artery stenosis. Canadian Stroke Consortium. *Arch Neurol* 1997; 54:25–28.

27. Wong ND, Gardin JM: Noninvasive assessment of and newer therapies for influencing atherosclerosis progression and regression. *Atheroscler ID Res* Alert 1997; 2:141–148.

28. Healy B: Endothelial cell dysfunction: An emerging endocrinopathy linked to coronary disease. *J Am Coll Cardiol* 1990; 16:357–358.

29. Ross R: The pathogenesis of atherosclerosis—an update. *N Engl J Med* 1986; 8:488–500.

30. Furchgott R, Zawadzki D: The obligatory role of endothelial cells in the relaxation of arterial of smooth muscle by acetycholine. *Nature* 1980; 288:373–376.

31. Ludmer PL, Selwyn AP, Shook TL, et al: Paradoxical vasoconstriction induced by acetylcholine in atherosclerotic coronary arteries. *N Engl J Med* 1986; 315:1046–1051.

32. Nabel EL, Selwyn AP, Ganz P: Large coronary arteries in humans are responsive to changing blood flow: an endothelium-dependent mechanism that fails in patients with atherosclerosis. *J Am Coll Cardiol* 1990; 16:349–356.

33. Celermajer DS, Sorensen KE, Gooch VM, et al: Noninvasive detection of endothelial dysfunction in children and adults at risk of atherosclerosis. *Lancet* 1992; 340:1111–1115.

34. Laurent S, Lacolley P, Brunel P, et al: Flow-dependent vasodilatation of brachial artery in essential hypertension. *Am J Physiol* 1990; 258:H1004–1011.

35. Rubanyi RM, Romero C, Vanhouette TM: Flow-induced release of endothelium-derived relaxing factor. *Am J Physiol* 1986; 250:1115–1119.

36. Pohl U, Holtz J, Busse R, Bassenge E: Crucial role of endothelium in the vasodilator response to increased flow in vivo. *Hypertension* 1986; 8:37–44.

37. Wendelhag I, Gustavsson T, Suurkula N, et al: Ultrasound measurement of wall thickness in the carotid artery; fundamental principles and description of computerised analysing system. *Clin Physiol* 1991; 11:565–577.

38. Celermajer DS, Sorensen KE, Spiegelhalter DJ, et al: Aging is associated with endothelial dysfunction in healthy men years before the age-related decline in women. *J Am Coll Cardiol* 1994; 24:471–476.

39. Burke GL, Arcilla RA, Culpepper WS, et al: Blood pressure and echocardiographic measures in children: the Bogalusa Heart Study. *Circulation* 1987; 75:106–114.

40. Mahoney LT, Schieken RM, Clarke WR, Lauer RM: Left ventricular mass and exercise responses predict future blood pressure: the Muscatine Study. *Hypertension* 1988; 12:206–213.

41. Levy D, Garrison RJ, Savage DD, et al: Prognostic implications of echocardiographically determined left ventricular mass in the Framingham Heart Study. *N Engl J Med* 1990; 322:1561–1566.

42. Levy D, Garrison RJ, Savage DD, et al: Left ventricular mass and incidence of coronary heart disease in an elderly cohort: the Framingham Heart Study. *Ann Intern Med* 1989; 110:101–107.

43. Levy D, Savage DD, Garrison RJ, et al: Echocardiographic criteria for left ventricular hypertrophy: the Framingham Heart Study. *Am J Cardiol* 1987; 59:956–960.

44. Gardin JM, Wagenknecht LE, Anton-Culver H, et al: Relationship of cardiovascular risk factors to echocardiographic left ventricular mass in healthy young black and white adult men and women: the CARDIA Study. *Circulation* 1995; 92:380–387.

45. Devereux RB, Roman MJ, de Simone G, et al: Relations of left ventricular mass to demographic and hemodynamic variables in American Indians: the Strong Heart Study. *Circulation* 1997; 96:1416–1423.

46. Sahn DJ, DeMaria A, Kisslo J, et al: The Committee on M-mode Standardization of the American Society of Echocardiography: Recommendations regarding quantitation in M-mode echocardiography: results of a survey of echocardiographic methods. *Circulation* 1978; 58:1072–1083.

47. Devereux RB, Alonso DR, Lutas EM, et al: Echocardiographic assessment of left ventricular hypertrophy: comparisons with necropsy findings. *Am J Cardiol* 1986; 57:450–458.

48. Xie X, Gidding SS, Gardin JM, et al: Left ventricular diastolic function in young adults: the Coronary Artery Risk Development in Young Adults Study. *J Am Soc Echocardiogr* 1995; 8:771–779.

49. Benjamin EJ, Levy D, Anderson KM, et al: Determinants of Doppler indices of left ventricular diastolic function in normal subjects: the Framingham Heart Study. *Am J Cardiol* 1992; 70:508–515.

50. Oh JK, Ding JB, Gersh BJ, et al: Restrictive left ventricular diastolic filling identifies patients with heart failure after acute myocardial infarction. *J Am Soc Echocardiogr* 1992; 5:497–503.

51. Ortiz J, Matsumoto AY, Ghefter CGM, et al: Prognosis in dilated myocardial disease: influence of diastolic dysfunction and anatomical changes. *Echocardiography* 1993; 10:247–253.

52. Kronmal RA, Smith VE, O'Leary DH, et al: Carotid artery measures are strongly associated with left ventricular mass in older adults (a report from the Cardiovascular Health Study). *Am J Cardiol* 1996; 77:628–633.

53. Gardin JM, Arnold A, Gottdiener JS, et al: Left ventricular mass in the elderly: the Cardiovascular Health Study. *Hypertension* 1997; 29:1095–1103.

54. Gardin JM, McClelland R, Kitzman D, et al: M-mode echocardiographic predictors of six-to-seven year incidence of coronary heart disease, stroke, congestive heart failure, and mortality of an elderly cohort: the Cardiovascular Health Study (abstr). *Circulation* 1999 (in press).

55. Muiesan ML, Salvetti M, Rizzoni D, et al: Persistence of left ventricular hypertrophy is a stronger indicator of cardiovascular events than baseline left ventricular mass or systolic performance: 10-years of follow-up. *J Hypertens* 1996; 14(suppl):S43–S49.

56. Taylor GJ, Humphries JO, Mellits ED, et al: Predictors of clinical course, coronary anatomy, and left ventricular function after recovery from acute myocardial infarction. *Circulation* 1980; 62:960–970.

57. Ong L, Green S, Reiser P, Morrison J: Early prediction of mortality in patients with acute myocardial infarction: a prospective study of clinical and radionuclide risk factors. *Am J Cardiol* 1986; 57:33–38.

58. Benjamin E, Levy D, Plehn J, et al: Left atrial size and the risk of stroke and death: the Framingham Heart Study. *Circulation* 1995; 92:835–841.

59. Aronow WS, Koenigsberg M, Kronzon I, Gutstein H: Association of mitral annular calcium with new thromboembolic stroke and cardiac events at 39-month follow-up in elderly patients. *Am J Cardiol* 1990; 65:1511–1512.

60. Gardin JM, Siscovick D, Anton-Culver H, et al: Sex, age, and disease affect echocardiographic left ventricular mass and systolic function in the free-living elderly. The Cardiovascular Health Study. *Circulation* 1995; 91:1739–1748.

61. Fried LP, Kronmal RA, Newman AB, et al: Risk factors for 5-year mortality in older adults: the Cardiovascular Health Study. *JAMA* 1998; 279:585–592.

62. Gottdiener JS, Arnold AM, Marshall RJ, et al: LV function and congestive heart failure in the elderly: relevance to therapeutic trials: the Cardiovascular Health Study (abstr). *Circulation* 1998; 98:I-718.

63. Marshall RJ, Gottdiener JS, Shemanski L, et al: Influence of LV function on mortality in elderly with congestive heart failure: the Cardiovascular Health Study (abstr). *Circulation* 1998; 98:I-205.

64. Wong ND, Gardin JM, Kurosaki T, et al: Echocardiographic left ventricular systolic function and volumes in young adults: distribution and factors influencing variability. *Am Heart J* 1995; 129:571–577.

65. Black HR, Weltin G, Jaffe CC: The limited echocardiogram: a modification of standard echocardiography for use in the routine evaluation of patients with systemic hypertension. *Am J Cardiol* 1991; 67:1027–1030.

66. Schreiner PJ, Lewis CE, Gardin JM, et al: Correlates of fen-phen use in young women: the CARDIA Study (abstr). *Circulation* 1998; 98:I-375.

67. Bonow RO, Carabello B, de Leon AC Jr, et al: ACC/AHA guidelines for the management of patients with valvular heart disease: a report of the American College of Cardiology/American Heart Association Task Force on Practice Guidelines (Committee on Management of Patients with Valvular Heart Disease). *J Am Coll Cardiol* 1998; 32:1486–1588.

68. Skiner MP, Yuan C, Mitsumori L, et al: Serial magnetic resonance imaging of experimental atherosclerosis detects lesion fine structure, progression, and complications in vivo. *Nature Med* 1995; 1:69–73.

69. Fayad ZA, Fallon JT, Shinnar M, et al: Noninvasive in vivo high-resolution magnetic resonance imaging of atherosclerotic lesions in genetically engineered mice. *Circulation* 1998; 98:1541–1547.

70. Fayad ZA, Nahar T, Badimon JJ, et al: In vivo MR characterization of plaques in the thoracic aorta (abstr). *Circulation* 1998; 98:I-515.

71. Van der Wall EE, Vliegan HW, de Roos A, Bruschke AV: Magnetic resonance imaging in coronary artery disease. *Circulation* 1995; 92:2723–2729.

72. van Rossum AC, Post JC, Visser CA: Coronary imaging using MRI. *Herz* 1996; 21:97–105.

73. McConnell MV, Ganz P, Selwyn AP, et al: Identification of anomalous coronary arteries and their anatomic course by magnetic resonance coronary angiography. *Circulation* 1995; 92:3158–3162.

74. Post JC, van Rossum AC, Hofman MB, et al: Clinical utility of two-dimensional magnetic resonance angiography in detecting coronary artery disease. *Eur Heart J* 1997; 18:426–433.

75. Muller MF, Fleisch M, Kroeker R, et al: Proximal coronary artery stenosis: three-dimensional MRI with fat saturation and navigator echo. *J Mag Reson Imaging* 1997; 7:644–651.

76. von Smekal A, Knez A, Seelow KC, et al: A comparison of ultrafast computed tomography, magnetic resonance angiography, and selected angiography for the detection of coronary bypass patency. *Bildgebenden Verfahren* 1997; 166:185–191.

77. Scheidegger MB, Muller R, Boesinger P: Magnetic resonance angiography: methods and its implications to the coronary arteries. *Tech Health Care* 1994; 2:255–265.

78. Pennell DJ, Keegan J, Firmin DN, et al: Magnetic resonance imaging of coronary arteries: technique and preliminary results. *Br Heart J* 1993; 70:315–326.

79. Duerinckx AJ: MRI of coronary arteries. *Int J Cardiac Imaging* 1997; 13:191–197.

80. Blackwell GG, Pohost GM: The evolving role of MRI in the assessment of coronary artery disease. *Am J Cardiol* 1995; 75:74D–78D.

81. Pohost GM, Fuisz AR: From the microscope to the clinic: MR assessment of atherosclerotic plaque (editorial). *Circulation* 1998; 98:1477–1478.

82. Bratton NG: Positron emission tomography in the diagnosis and management of coronary artery disease. *J Louisiana State Med Soc* 1995; 147:193–196.

83. Williams RB, Mullani NA, Jansen DE, Anderson BA: A retrospective study of the diagnostic accuracy of a community hospital–based PET center for the detection of coronary artery disease using rubidium-82. *J Nucl Med* 1994; 35:1586–1592.

84. Dayanikli F, Grambow D, Muzik O, et al: Early detection of abnormal coronary flow reserve in asymptomatic men at high risk for coronary artery disease using positron emission tomography. *Circulation* 1994; 90:808–817.

85. Gould KL, Martucci JP, Goldberg DI, et al: Short-term cholesterol lowering decreases size and severity of perfu-

sion abnormalities by positron emission tomography after dipyridamole in patients with coronary artery disease: a potential noninvasive marker of healing coronary endothelium. *Circulation* 1994; 89:1530–1538.

86. Marwick TH, Shan K, Patel S, et al: Incremental value of rubidium-82 positron emission tomography for prognostic assessment of known or suspected coronary artery disease. *Am J Cardiol* 1997; 80:865–870.

87. National Heart, Lung, and Blood Institute, National Institutes of Health: NHLBI-HC-98-XX. *Subclinical Cardiovascular Disease Study.* Request for Proposals, 1998.

Part III

Risk Factors: Evidence, Assessment, and Intervention

CHAPTER 5

Family History and Genetic Factors

Paul N. Hopkins
Steven C. Hunt
Lily L. Wu
Roger R. Williams

Cardiovascular disease (CVD) accounts for a large proportion of deaths each year in the United States and other Western nations. When heart attacks and strokes occur at a relatively early age, a large fraction can be attributed to inherited or familial predisposition. Knowledge of an individual's family history can help guide preventive efforts. Genetic contributions to risk factors for atherosclerosis continue to be reported at accelerating rates. We are currently witnessing a great increase in the understanding of how genetic factors promote or prevent atherosclerosis. This chapter reviews some of the major genetic disorders affecting cardiovascular risk and helps us consider how to apply the growing knowledge of genetics so we can start practicing now the preventive medicine of the future.

Approaches to Understanding Genetic Contributions to Premature Coronary Heart Disease

There are several fundamental approaches to studying familial or genetic contributions to premature coronary heart disease (CHD), including (1) family studies to establish and quantify aggregation of premature disease or a phenotype within families, (2) quantitative methods to study phenotype transmission in families (complex segregation analysis and path analysis), and (3) examination of specific genes and their effect on phenotype either through linkage analysis or in association studies. A general review of these approaches was recently published.[1] In this section we provide some specific examples of these approaches with important applications relevant to the screening and prevention of CHD.

Family Studies

Family studies fall into two general categories. The first examines the presence or absence of a disease in family members, such as in comparing family history of CHD in cases and controls. Recall bias appears to have only a small impact on estimates of risk from such studies.[2] These studies are critical to document the extent to which disease aggregates in high-risk families. Without such information, public health planning regarding the potential utility of family history collection, risk assessment, and directed intervention would be impossible. The second approach examines degree of family aggregation of a quantitative trait—for example by examining sibling or twin correlations of blood pressure and calculating heritability.

As an example, hospital charts of married men who had died by age 45 of CHD were examined. Surviving spouses or relatives were contacted and family history of CHD in the men's families was compared with either the spouses' families or the spouses of other family informants. There was an approximate threefold increase in risk for CHD (most striking for early disease, with relative risks up to

TABLE 5–1 Relative Risk for CHD by Family History in 15,200 Utah Families: Data for 94,292 Persons

CHD FHx Definition	Prevalence	Relative Risk at Ages		
		20–39	50–59	70+
1+ Affected	38%	2.9	1.3	1.3
1+ Age <55	13%	3.9	1.5	1.1
2+ Affected	8%	5.9	1.8	2.0
2+ Age <55	2%	12.7	2.9	0.7
FHx score >1.0	6%	6.9	2.0	3.0
FHx score >2.0	3%	9.1	2.5	4.2

Key: 1+, one or more relatives affected; 2+, two or more relatives affected.

fivefold).[3] In a 2.5-year prospective follow-up of 1196 men and women, there was a significant increase in risk for newly diagnosed CHD associated with a positive family history, independent of all measured risk factors.[4] At least 10 other investigators have reported an independent contribution to risk assessment of positive family history.[5–7] Perhaps most impressive was a 26-year follow-up of 21,004 Swedish twins. Among men, when a twin died of CHD before age 55, the relative risk was 8.1 for monozygous twins and 3.8 for dizygous twins. For women, relative risks of 15.0 and 2.6, respectively, were reported. The earlier the death of the first twin, the greater the relative risk to the remaining twin.[8]

To obtain a population perspective of the extent of CHD familial aggregation, risk to remaining siblings was studied as a function of CHD experience of older siblings in 15,200 Utah families (Table 5–1).[9] Up to 12-fold increases in risk were seen for surviving siblings when two or more siblings had already experienced early-onset of CHD. In the Family Heart Study, sponsored by the National Heart Lung and Blood Institute, participating centers in Minneapolis, Minnesota; Forsyth County, North Carolina; Framingham, Massachusetts; and Salt Lake City, Utah collected information on 122,155 families, providing a net experience of 16,602 early CHD cases and 54,182 cases of CHD at any age. Family history scores, the ratio of (observed-expected)/expected with a continuity correction were calculated for each family. The score is progressively more positive with increasing numbers of coronary cases in a family above the cumulative number expected based on the number of family members and their ages. As shown in Table 5–2, an impressive 35 percent of all early CHD aggregated in just 3.2 percent of families.

Heritability (h^2) is an estimate of the fraction of the variance of a quantitative trait in the population

TABLE 5–2 Aggregation of CHD in Families by Family History Score in the NHLBI Family Heart Study

Family History Score	Percent of Families	Percent of Early CHD	Percent of All CHD
≥0.5	14	72.1	48.4
≥1.0	3.2	34.7	17.6
≥2.0	1.0	16.8	6.3

explained by inheritance. An h^2 of 1.0 would mean all of the variance was explained by inherited factors. Estimates above 0.3 to 0.4 suggest strong heritability. Most estimates assume a polygenic inheritance (as is likely true with height and several other traits). In twin studies, the classic estimate of heritability is $2(r_m - r_d)$, where r_m is the correlation coefficient between monozygous twins (for example, the systolic blood pressure in twin 1 versus twin 2) and r_d is the correlation coefficient between dizygous twins. This estimate assumes that monozygous and dizygous twins share the environment to a similar degree. In actuality, studies have shown that a number of environmental factors are more similar for monozygous twins than for dizygous twins. Therefore, environment cannot be entirely extracted from genetic effects in these estimates. Nevertheless, a highly heritable trait is most likely strongly influenced by genes.

Heritability of a variety of traits related to CHD were estimated in Utah families using both pedigree and twin methods (Table 5–3).[10,11] In this table, c^2 is an estimate of the shared household effect or "cultural heritability" for the trait. As may be seen, approximately half the variance of blood pressure and lipids can be explained by inherited (primarily genetic) factors. Estimates of heritability from twin studies tend to be higher than those from pedigree studies. This suggests that risk factors aggregate in families because of genetic factors, suggesting the usefulness of a public health approach that focuses attention on high-risk families.

Complex Segregation Analysis

In complex segregation analysis, evidence is sought for the transmission of major gene traits in families using purely statistical inference. Finding bimodality can be a tipoff for a segregating major gene. For example, plasma low-density-lipoprotein (LDL) levels are distributed into two distinct modes in familial hypercholesterolemia, a dominantly transmitted trait. Complex segregation analysis can provide evidence for such a trait and test for the most likely type of transmission (dominant, recessive, polygenic, random, or not genetically transmitted).

In 98 extended Utah high-risk families examined for several traits potentially related to hypertension, a recessive gene explained 34 percent of the variance of sodium-lithium countertransport (SLC) (polygenic inheritance accounted for another 46 percent of the variance).[12] Follow-up of the 5 percent of the population inferred to have the recessive trait for high SLC revealed a fourfold increased risk for developing newly identified hypertension.[13] In these same families, a major gene with additive effects was inferred to explain 51 percent of the variance in urinary kallikrein activity, with polygenic effects explaining another 27 percent. High homozygotes excreted urinary kallikrein at levels 1 SD above the general population mean, while low homozygotes excreted urinary kallikrein 1 SD below the mean.[14] Offspring of hypertensive patients had lower kallikrein excretion as compared to offspring of normotensives. The 50 percent of the population who were inferred to be heterozygotes for this trait showed evidence for interaction with dietary potassium. Those with a high intake of potassium showed protective high levels of urinary kallikrein (similar to high homozygotes), while, conversely, those on low-potassium diets had low urinary kallikrein (similar to low homozygotes).[15] Other relevant findings

TABLE 5–3 Heritability (h^2) of Selected Traits in Twins and Pedigrees*

	h^2 Twins	h^2 Pedigrees	c^2 Pedigrees
Standing height	—	0.75	0.11
BMI	0.54	0.24	0.00
Scapular skinfold	—	0.32	0.03
Sitting systolic BP	0.42	0.17	0.07
Sitting diastolic BP	0.46	0.22	0.03
Total cholesterol	0.61	0.45	0.08
Triglycerides	0.81	0.37	0.06
HDL cholesterol	0.74	0.45	0.15

*Includes 146 male MZ twins, 162 male DZ twins, and 1102 adults in 67 Utah pedigrees.

Key: c^2, shared household effect or "cultural heritability" for the trait.

Sources: From Hunt et al.[10] and Williams et al.,[11] with permission.

from this population were evidence for recessive genes affecting fasting plasma insulin[16] and a fat pattern index.[17] For complex traits with multiple features, such as the multiple metabolic syndrome (see below), factor analysis may be applied to identify statistical groupings of various measurements into "factors," followed by complex segregation analysis to study transmission of these factors in pedigrees. In Utah pedigrees, evidence was found for major gene transmission of a multiple metabolic syndrome factor as well as other factors.[18]

Linkage Analysis and Genetic Association Studies

Linkage studies are primarily concerned with finding new gene loci associated with phenotypic traits. These studies take advantage of family structure to ask whether sequence variations in or near a gene locus are found in affected family members (as compared to unaffected family members) more frequently than expected by chance. In contrast, association studies simply divide a population by genotype and examine differences in phenotype without regard for family structure. Association studies probably should be considered primarily an approach to determine the phenotypic impact of known, functional gene variations at candidate gene loci. The distinction can be subtle. Of the two approaches, linkage studies generally provide more definitive evidence for a genotypic effect. Association studies run the risk that factors other than the gene locus are actually associated with phenotypic variation rather than the gene itself. Assume, for example, that ethnic origin was associated with differences in serum cholesterol (for example, because of different dietary habits). Also, assume that the ethnic groups had different prevalences of a particular polymorphism. If subjects from multiple ethnic origins were included in an association study, it may be impossible to determine whether an apparent difference in serum cholesterol by genotype was due to the gene or to differences in diet associated with ethnic group. An approach to compensate for this kind of population stratification using multiple markers at loci unrelated to the trait of interest has been proposed.[19]

Linkage for relatively rare traits with striking phenotypes is typically much easier to demonstrate than for common traits. For example, linkage to the LDL receptor is usually readily demonstrable in sufficiently large families manifesting heterozygous familial hypercholesterolemia (FH).[20] On the other hand, even when some FH patients are present, linkage to the LDL receptor in a large cross section of the general population is generally not possible. In this situation, heterogeneity greatly reduces the power to find linkage at any one locus. For blood pressure or hypertension, the problem may be even greater. Examples of key findings from linkage studies for hypertension are reviewed below.

As mentioned above, heterogeneity can greatly diminish the power of linkage studies. Four types of heterogeneity must be considered. *Clinical heterogeneity* exists when different clinical manifestations of the same disease can be identified (for example FH patients with and without tendon xanthoma, or different blood pressures in patients with glucocorticoid-remediable aldosteronism). *Genetic heterogeneity* refers to a disorder with apparently different transmission patterns (for example, type III hyperlipidemia has both recessive and dominant forms). *Locus heterogeneity* occurs when mutations at different loci lead to the same clinical phenotype. Long-QT syndrome displays this kind of heterogeneity,[21] as does hypertension. Allelic heterogeneity occurs when different mutations at the same locus can result in the same phenotype. As an example, over 600 mutations in the LDL receptor gene causing FH have been identified to date.

Although linkage studies tend to have limited power to find effects of rare genes on common traits, they may be very useful to rule out strong effects from a gene locus. For example, genetic variation of the amiloride-sensitive epithelial sodium channel, the gene that causes Liddle's syndrome (a rare form of severe, dominantly transmitted hypertension; see below), showed no linkage with essential hypertension.[22] Similarly, significant contributions to essential hypertension from other candidate gene loci have been effectively ruled out by linkage studies.[23-26] Linkage can also effectively rule out a genetic locus as the cause of a strong, dominantly transmitted phenotype. In one large Utah pedigree with a familial hypercholesterolemia phenotype, linkage to the LDL receptor and Apo-B loci was ruled out, proving the existence of another, as yet unidentified gene that can be responsible for severe, dominantly transmitted cholesterol elevations.[27] Similar results in several pedigrees were also published by a French group.[28]

Genetic Lipid Disorders

In the following discussion, important, recognized lipid disorders are briefly presented with an emphasis on how they have led to an increased understanding of lipoprotein metabolism and attendant cardiovascular risks. Understanding the underlying pathophysiology of a lipid disorder may lead to more appropriate intervention.

Disorders of Very Low Density Lipoprotein and Chylomicron Synthesis

Abetalipoproteinemia Absence of chylomicra, very low density lipoprotein (VLDL), and LDL has been termed *abetalipoproteinemia*. This is a rare recessive disorder. Obligate heterozygotes have entirely normal (not half normal) lipid levels. Affected homozygous patients are unable to secrete any Apo-B–containing lipoprotein. Total cholesterol levels in plasma are only 20 to 45 mg/dL, while triglyceride concentrations are even lower. Patients with this condition probably have a low risk for CHD. There is fat malabsorption, which can be severe, and fatty liver. Defective transport of fat-soluble vitamins (particularly vitamin E) can lead to pigmented retinopathy, hemolytic anemia, loss of deep tendon reflexes and proprioception; later, selective loss of large myelinated nerve fibers results in spinocerebellar degeneration, ataxia, and muscle dystrophy.[29]

Abetalipoproteinemia was relatively recently shown to be due to a deficiency of microsomal transfer protein (MTP), with resultant inability to transport triglycerides into Golgi apparatus and failure to produce Apo-B–containing particles.[30] MTP inhibitors offer enormous potential for lipid-lowering. Use of one of these agents in Watanabe heritable hyperlipidemic rabbits (with homozygous genetic de-

ficiency of the LDL receptor and severe hypercholesterolemia) resulted in normalization of lipid levels.[31] Given the severe consequences of abetalipoproteinemia, these agents will likely have a relatively narrow margin of safety.

Hypobetalipoproteinemia At least 35 defects in Apo-B gene structure, mostly truncations, have been found to result in diminished serum levels of Apo-B–containing lipoproteins due to reduced synthesis. However, these apparently do not account for the majority of families with very low LDL-cholesterol (LDL-C).[32] A range in plasma total cholesterol levels among heterozygotes has been reported (from 40 to 180 mg/dL), but on average, plasma LDL and VLDL lipid concentrations are 50 percent lower than in unaffected first-degree relatives. Generally, heterozygotes are asymptomatic. Rare, severely affected hypobetalipoproteinemia homozygotes, such as those with so-called normotriglyceridemic abetalipoproteinemia, can suffer from symptoms of vitamin E deficiency.[33] In one family, two compound heterozygotes (patients with both Apo–B alleles truncated but a different mutation on each allele) had total cholesterol levels of 39 and 50 mg/dL and Apo-B levels of 1 and 2 mg/dL, respectively. They were entirely asymptomatic. In other family members, either allele acting singly resulted in an approximately 50 percent reduction of LDL and VLDL lipids.[34] Patients with hypobetalipoproteinemia appear to be protected from premature CHD. Furthermore, the lack of adverse clinical effects for most patients with hypobetalipoproteinemia suggests that low LDL-C levels achievable with lipid-lowering agents such as statin drugs are unlikely to have significant adverse consequences.

Defects in Very Low Density Lipoprotein and Chylomicron Removal

Fasting plasma triglyceride levels above 2000 mg/dL define the chylomicronemia syndrome. However, chylomicra are usually present when fasting plasma triglycerides are above 800 mg/dL (9.0 mmol/L) and are almost always present when levels rise above 1200 mg/dL (13.5 mmol/L).[29] VLDL are usually markedly elevated when triglycerides are in this range (type V hyperlipidemia), but may rarely be normal (type I hyperlipidemia).

Acute pancreatitis is the major clinical concern when plasma triglycerides rise above about 1000 mg/dL and especially above 2000 mg/dL. Approximately 20 percent of cases of acute pancreatitis can be attributed to severe hypertriglyceridemia.[35] Eruptive xanthomas can occur when chylomicra or VLDL are engulfed by skin macrophages. A unique receptor on monocyte-macrophages was recently identified that recognizes a site on Apo-B common to both Apo-B–48 and Apo-B–100. Unmodified triglyceride-rich lipoproteins can be taken up rapidly and lead to foam cell formation.[36] This suggests the possibility of excess coronary risk if these particles are small enough to penetrate the arterial endothelial barrier. However, severe hypertriglyceridemia actually *protected* diabetic, cholesterol-fed rabbits from arterial atherosclerotic changes. Lipoproteins larger than large VLDL were shown to be incapable of penetrating the artery wall.[37] These findings may help explain why CHD risk appears to be low in severe hypertriglyceridemia (chylomicronemia), while pancreatitis risk is high.[38,39]

Causes of chylomicronemia are usually impossible to ascertain with certainty. Most cases are associated with acquired hypertriglyceridemia; a specific genetic cause, frequently apparent in families, can usually not be found.[35] A minority are due to reduced lipoprotein lipase (LPL) activity (15 to 17 percent), homozygous LPL deficiency, or Apo-CII deficiency (both very rare).[40] There is evidence for a substantial effect on plasma triglycerides from variation at the Apo-CIII gene locus.[41] Another study, however, failed to find linkage to any of these loci among several families with hypertriglyceridemia.[42] Apo-CIII inhibits removal of triglyceride-rich particles and relatively small increases can lead to hypertriglyceridemia.

Traditionally, only homozygous lipoprotein lipase (LPL) deficiency was clearly defined—a rare condition occurring in an estimated 1 in 10^6 persons. Studies in heterozygotes were hampered until relatively recently because marked overlap in lipoprotein lipase activity between normals and obligate heterozygotes prevented clear assignment of carrier status. Developments in molecular methods have overcome this obstacle. At least 38 functional mutations of the LPL gene have been described affecting the production of end-product, active site, conformation, and ability to self-dimerize.[43]

Heterozygous carriers of a LPL mutation from a large Utah pedigree have been characterized. The proband was homozygous for a mutation of Gly188 to Glu (the parents were unrelated). Unambiguous identification of carriers was achieved by allele-specific oligonucleotide hybridization (dot blots). Age was found to have a major impact on the phenotypic manifestations of the heterozygous state. Surprisingly, carriers under age 40 showed no statistically significant differences with noncarriers for any lipid. Those aged 40 and older, however, displayed higher triglycerides (mean $\pm$ SD in carriers of 441 $\pm$ 267 versus 195 $\pm$ 88 mg/dL in normals) but lower LDL-C and HDL cholesterol (HDL-C) levels.[44] Factors besides age associated with increased expression of the phenotype were increasing body mass index, higher insulin, higher blood pressure, and uric acid. When carriers were clearly marked, it became clear that persons with elevated LDL-C were generally not carriers. In fact, among carriers, there was a strong *inverse* relationship between plasma LDL-C and VLDL cholesterol (VLDL-C). This study suggests that many persons with moderately elevated triglycerides may be carriers for an LPL mutation.[44]

Given the lower HDL-C (together with high triglycerides in older family members) found among persons with heterozygous LPL deficiency, increased risk for associated premature CHD might be expected. Several studies have suggested increased risk.[45–48] However, there is inconsistency among the studies regarding the particular mutation associated with risk. The apparent association of hypertension with heterozygous LPL deficiency in the above pedigree led to further evaluation of this hypothesis. In a large U.S. population, linkage of hypertension to the LPL locus was essentially ruled out.[49]

Type III Hyperlipidemia or Familial Dysbetalipoproteinemia

Type III hyperlipidemia is characterized by the presence of significant concentrations of abnormal chylomicron and VLDL remnants, often called β-VLDL. Persons with type III hyperlipidemia have long been noted to be at severely increased risk for premature CHD.[50,51] The most objective estimates of the prevalence (0.4 percent in men, 0.2 percent in women) of type III hyperlipidemia come from the Lipid Research Clinics Prevalence Study.[52] Type III hyperlipidemia accounts for as much as 5 percent of early CHD (defined as a measured VLDL-C/total triglycerides $\geq$0.30).[53–55] An increased risk is also seen for persons with "possible" hyperlipidemia (measured VLDL-C/total triglycerides = 0.25 to 0.30). Together, these were found in at least 10 percent of early-onset familial CHD cases.[56]

Abnormal remnant accumulation is relatively difficult to quantify and various definitions for type III hyperlipidemia have been suggested. These abnormal lipoproteins were historically detected by the presence of a "broad β" band [continuous between the β (normally only LDL) and pre-β (VLDL) bands] on paper or gel electrophoresis of total plasma. A more accurate assessment of β-VLDL is obtained by combining gel electrophoresis and ultracentrifugation. The presence of a β band in the density above 1.006 (top) fraction of ultracentrifuged fasting plasma may be considered diagnostic for type III. A measured VLDL-C/plasma triglyceride ratio of 0.30 or higher is a highly specific (though not very sensitive) index for the presence of β-VLDL when plasma triglycerides are between 150 and 1000 mg/dL. A ratio of 0.25 to under 0.30 was considered "possible" type III hyperlipidemia.[50] Later investigators suggested that over 90 percent of patients with type III hyperlipidemia also have an Apo-E 2-2 genotype.[57] A quantitative estimate of β-VLDL can be derived from the composition of normal VLDL and reported composition of β-VLDL with estimated β-VLDL = [VLDL-C − 0.17 (total TG)]/0.521.[58] An estimated β-VLDL-C above 40 mg/dL is abnormal and highly suggestive of type III hyperlipidemia.[58] A newly developed immunoabsorption assay for remnant particles[59] supports the validity of this estimate.[56]

Clinical features of type III hyperlipidemia may include tuberous xanthomas (specific but insensitive), palmar striae (frequently present and specific),

and xanthelasma (nonspecific and insensitive). Cholesterol and triglycerides are elevated together (both usually above 300 mg/dL untreated). Remarkable reductions in serum lipids may be seen with treatment. Often, weight loss alone will result in 50 percent or greater reduction in both cholesterol and triglycerides. These patients are often responsive to niacin, fibrates, or (as second-line agents) statins.[60] Note that this disorder, in the absence of pathognomonic palmar striae or tuberous xanthomas, cannot be diagnosed with a simple lipid panel in which LDL-C and VLDL-C levels are calculated. A typical case of type III hyperlipidemia is presented in Table 5–4.

There are three common alleles for Apo-E, designated ϵ2, ϵ3, and ϵ4, with gene frequencies of approximately 10, 75, and 15 percent, respectively, in Caucasian populations. An allele from each parent is inherited in simple Mendelian fashion, resulting in six common genotypes. Compared with the Apo-E3 protein, Apo-E2 displays markedly lower binding to the LDL receptor while Apo-E4 shows slightly greater binding. The 1 percent of the population homozygous for ϵ2 (also designated Apo-E 2-2) have a greatly increased risk for displaying the type III phenotype. Nevertheless, only a fraction of these apparently ever develop overt or more severe type III hyperlipidemia. The basis for type III hyperlipidemia with the Apo-E 2-2 genotype (and in the less common dominant forms) is a marked deficiency in binding of the Apo-E apoprotein to the LDL receptor and to the remnant receptor (LRP). Actual expression of type III appears to depend on factors that may increase production or further impede removal of lipoproteins such as obesity, hypothyroidism, increasing age, estrogen deficiency, deficiency of LDL receptors as in FH, or genetically mediated excess VLDL synthesis as in familial combined hyperlipidemia.[60] A near universal expression of type III hyperlipidemia is seen among patients with FH and Apo-E 2-2. Approximately one-fourth of FH patients with even a single ϵ2 allele display lipids consistent with type III hyperlipidemia.[58,61] The severe atherogenicity of remnant particles collecting in type III appears to relate to their sheer excess and ability to promote foam cell formation without modification,[60,62] possibly

TABLE 5–4   A Case of Type III Hyperlipidemia

A 43-year-old male was first seen in our lipid clinic after his cardiologist noted abnormal lipids, with total cholesterol of 223 mg/dL, triglycerides of 333 mg/dL, HDL cholesterol of 32 mg/dL, and calculated LDL of 124 mg/dL. He was taking 20 mg of lovastatin twice daily at the time of the blood draw. He had experienced his first myocardial infarction at age 31, with recurrent infarcts at ages 38 and 40. After angiography disclosed diffuse coronary disease, he underwent coronary artery bypass grafting at age 40 but was being evaluated for worsening angina. A call to his primary care physician provided some important insights. The following information was obtained:

Age	Serum Total Cholesterol	Serum Triglycerides	Comments
31	215	328	Lipids at time of first MI
40	461	688	No treatment
40.5	377	395	Low-fat, low-cholesterol diet
41	371	503	Started lovastatin
41.5	306	410	On lovastatin 20 mg bid
42	256	418	On lovastatin 20 mg bid

HDL cholesterol levels were consistently between 30 and 39 mg/dL. The parallel and marked changes in total cholesterol and triglycerides suggested type III hyperlipidemia. After the initial consultation at our lipid clinic, the patient stopped (but then restarted) lovastatin and began a strict weight-loss diet. After a 13-lb weight loss and while taking lovastatin 20 mg/day, his lipids were analyzed with ultracentrifugation and his Apo-E phenotype was determined. Total cholesterol had fallen to 176 mg/dL, triglycerides were 209 mg/dL, HDL cholesterol was 35 mg/dL, measured LDL cholesterol was 45 mg/dL, and measured VLDL cholesterol was 93 mg/dL. Virtually 100% of this VLDL was estimated to be β-VLDL, a highly atherogenic lipoprotein characteristic of type III hyperlipidemia. He was found to have an Apo-E phenotype of 2-2, confirming the diagnosis of type III hyperlipidemia. Adding niacin to his regimen (increasing gradually to 1000 mg bid), resulted in a dramatic reduction in his lipids. Subsequent total cholesterol levels have remained under 144 mg/dL and triglycerides remained consistently below 120 mg/dL.

This is an example of typical type III hyperlipidemia. However, this patient never had xanthomas, and a diagnosis of type III hyperlipidemia would not have been possible at the time of initial consultation without making use of ultracentrifugation and Apo-E phenotyping. The historical lipids certainly pointed to the diagnosis, but many physicians do not take the time to obtain a complete record. Focusing only on calculated LDL cholesterol levels (which in this case were entirely misleading) had contributed to the inappropriate treatment (gemfibrozil or niacin would have been more appropriate as single initial agents). The marked reduction of lipids when niacin was added to the regimen is typical of type III hyperlipidemia.

mediated by way of a newly identified receptor found on macrophages that mediates uptake of triglyceride-rich lipoproteins.[36]

Hepatic Lipase Deficiency

Only three pedigrees with hepatic lipase deficiency have been described.[63-65] Some of the affected individuals had premature coronary disease. Serum lipids of affected individuals range from 260 to 1495 mg/dL for total cholesterol and 350 to 8200 mg/dL for triglycerides. Such individuals can respond to a strict metabolic diet restrictive in calories, saturated fat, and cholesterol. On electrophoresis, large amounts of β-VLDL were present in all cases, but the ratio of measured VLDL cholesterol/plasma triglycerides was normal. This surprising finding was

due to four- to eightfold elevations in the triglyceride content of HDL and LDL fractions. The major HDL subfraction present was HDL_2 with reduction in HDL_3, suggesting that hepatic lipase is required for recycling of HDL_2. The presence of β-VLDL and markedly reduced conversion of VLDL to LDL supports a role for hepatic lipase in remnant clearance.[66]

Familial Hypercholesterolemia

Familial hypercholesterolemia (FH) is one of the most common and best studied genetic diseases known, with one of the more than 600 LDL receptor mutations, affecting at least 1 heterozygote in 500 persons in most populations.[67,68] A representation of how the several mutations affect LDL receptor function is shown in Fig. 5–1. The dominant

FIGURE 5–1 Structure of the low-density-lipoprotein (LDL) receptor and consequences of defined mutations. Five functional classes of LDL-receptor mutations have been identified. Null alleles produce no protein product. Transport defective alleles (due mostly to abnormal protein folding) display impaired movement of protein product from endoplasmic reticulum to Golgi. Binding defective alleles bind reduced amounts of LDL (some bind normally to beta-very low density lipoprotein). Recycling deficient alleles do not release LDL normally in endosomes in the presence of acid pH. Internalization defective alleles do not group normally in clathrin-coated pits and do not internalize LDL. (Adapted from Hobbs et al.,[67] with permission.)

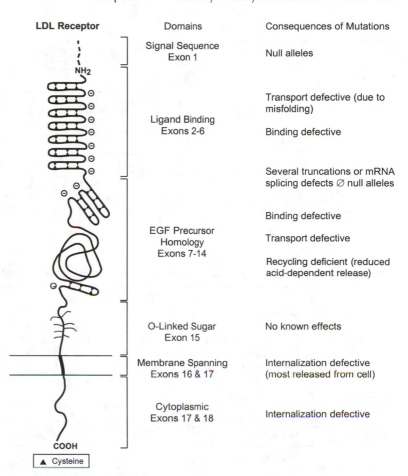

LDL Receptor	Domains	Consequences of Mutations
	Signal Sequence Exon 1	Null alleles
	Ligand Binding Exons 2-6	Transport defective (due to misfolding) Binding defective
	EGF Precursor Homology Exons 7-14	Several truncations or mRNA splicing defects ∅ null alleles Binding defective Transport defective Recycling deficient (reduced acid-dependent release)
	O-Linked Sugar Exon 15	No known effects
	Membrane Spanning Exons 16 & 17	Internalization defective (most released from cell)
	Cytoplasmic Exons 17 & 18	Internalization defective

▲ Cysteine

transmission and very early penetrance (essentially at birth) of severely elevated plasma LDL-C makes pedigree tracing relatively easy (see Fig. 5–2). Since about two-thirds of LDL is normally removed by way of the LDL receptor pathway and because LDL receptors affect the fraction of VLDL converted to LDL (and possibly net VLDL production), a 50 percent reduction in activity due to one nonfunctional allele results in an approximately twofold elevation of LDL-C. Thus, in untreated adults, total cholesterol is generally above 350 mg/dL (LDL-C above 260 mg/dL). With a diet very low in cholesterol and fat, serum total cholesterol may fall to as low as 250 mg/dL. However, for most patients, it remains above 300 mg/dL even with careful diet. In FH children there is less change in serum cholesterol with age, and it not unusual to find affected children (or infants) with total cholesterol levels above 300 mg/dL. Triglycerides are generally normal but may be elevated (as in those with E2-containing phenotypes, as noted above).

Tendinous xanthomata increase in prevalence with age [prevalence (percent) approximated by the age minus 10].[69] Presence of a tendinous xanthoma is, therefore, a very insensitive sign for a diagnosis of FH. Homozygotes are rare (1 in 10^6) and are affected much more severely with total cholesterol levels generally well over 600 mg/dL. A reasonably secure diagnosis of heterozygous FH can be made (without resorting to special testing such as fibroblast studies) if the criteria in Table 5–5 are met.[69]

FIGURE 5–2 Familial hypercholesterolemia pedigree.

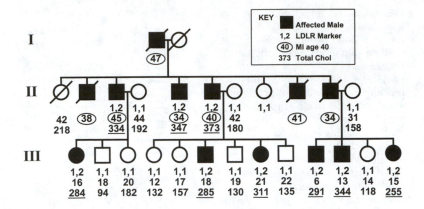

TABLE 5–5 Criteria for Diagnosis of Heterozygous Familial Hypercholesterolemia

Individual Criteria
1. Very high LDL-Cholesterol
Cut points for total cholesterol (LDL cholesterol in parenthesis) in mg/dL used in the U.S. MEDPED program for diagnosing FH. Patients with levels greater than or equal to cut points qualify. First-degree relatives are parents, offspring, brothers, and sisters. Second-degree relatives are aunts, uncles, grandparents, nieces, nephews, and half-siblings. Third-degree relatives are first cousins, siblings of grandparents, etc. LDL levels alone are given for the "100%" probability category.

| Age Group | Degree of Relatedness to Closest FH Relative | | | General Population | "100%" Probability |
	First	Second	Third		
<20	220 (155)	230 (165)	240 (170)	270 (200)	(240)
20–29	240 (170)	250 (180)	260 (185)	290 (220)	(260)
30–39	270 (190)	280 (200)	290 (210)	340 (240)	(280)
40+	290 (205)	300 (215)	310 (225)	360 (260)	(300)

2. No secondary cause (nephrosis, pregnancy, etc.)

Family Criteria:
3. Tendon xanthoma or youth meeting LDL criteria
4. Bimodal LDL cholesterol (usually a gap of 70–100 mg/dL)

Note: Because of higher a priori probability of having FH, relatives can be diagnosed with FH using lower LDL cholesterol criteria than persons evaluated as new index cases not known to be part of a family with FH.[4]

FH is a clinically important cause of very early CHD death and disability. The tenfold or higher relative risks for CHD that accompany FH are well documented[70,71] and constitute the major threat to survival in these patients. FH is an excellent model of clinical hypercholesterolemia because of its diversity of presentation, severity, and responsiveness to treatment, with regression of coronary atherosclerosis.[72,73] Indeed, clinical CHD may occur as early as the twenties in some nonsmoking FH heterozygotes or be delayed into the seventies in others with similar plasma total or LDL-C levels.[20] Some of the diversity is likely environmental, but in many cases it cannot be attributed to factors such as smoking, diet, or easily measured standard CHD risk factors. Significant correlation for age at coronary death between sibling pairs with FH from different families has been reported.[74] Less severe atherosclerosis was evident in FH homozygotes with LDL-receptor mutations having some residual activity, compared to those with no activity.[68]

Familial Defective Apo-B–100

Dominantly transmitted hypercholesterolemia (total cholesterol levels of approximately 300 mg/dL and normal triglycerides) with normal LDL-receptor activity in cultured fibroblasts led to the discovery of abnormal LDL Apo-B in affected family members that bound poorly to normal LDL receptors. Radioactively labeled LDL from carriers was cleared more slowly when given intravenously to normal volunteers. Normal LDL was cleared from carrier's plasma at a normal rate. Further investigation disclosed a substitution of Arg 3500 to Gln in Apo-B–100, which virtually abolished Apo-B–100 binding to the LDL receptor. The condition was named *familial defective Apo-B–100* (FDB).[75,76] At least two other mutations in Apo-B causing a similar syndrome have now been identified.[77] The defect in FDB, rather than affecting the LDL receptor binding site itself, involves malfunction of the tail the Apo-B protein that normally moves after VLDL lipolysis to reveal the LDL receptor binding site.[78,79] The frequency of FDB is about half that of FH. Compared to those with FH, FDB patients may be at lower risk for premature atherosclerotic disease even with similar LDL levels, possibly due to less remnant accumulation.[80] Within FDB families, carriers display lower average LDL-C than FH patients and a much wider range of LDL-C levels are expressed (from normal to severely elevated).[77]

Severe Low-HDL Syndromes

Several rare recessive, severe HDL-deficiency syndromes have been described.[81] These syndromes account for only a tiny proportion of the cases of low HDL-C associated with early-onset CAD. Surprisingly, some severe deficiencies of HDL are associated with premature coronary disease while others are not. It has been suggested that low HDL-C due to decreased production is associated with early CHD (especially if production of small HDL is impaired), while syndromes resulting in increased catabolism are not necessarily atherogenic.[82] Thus, Tangier disease and Apo-A–I Milano, associated with increased Apo-A–I removal but normal production, results in low or absent HDL-C yet little increased risk for CHD. In contrast, among families or cases with deficient A-I production (such as absent A-I/C-III), early CHD risk is high. Theoretically, if sufficient HDL is present to promote reverse cholesterol transport, then increased catabolism will not be atherogenic. In fact, increased catabolism may contribute to cholesterol transport by way of the prematurely removed HDL. The causal gene for Tangier disease, a defect in a transmembrane cholesterol transporter, has recently been identified (Brian Brewer, personal communications, June 1999).

Deficiency of Cholesterol Ester Transfer Protein

In animals, cholesterol found in nascent VLDL is primarily unesterified.[83] Cholesterol ester is transferred to VLDL from HDL by way of the cholesterol ester transfer protein (CETP) reaction. In kinetic studies in humans, up to 50 mg/kg per day is transferred from HDL to VLDL by this reaction,[84] similar to estimates for the total rate of esterification of free cholesterol by lecithin-cholesterol acyltransferase (LCAT).[85] Animals such as rats, which lack CETP, have high HDL-C and low LDL-C and are resistant to atherosclerosis. In contrast, rabbits with abundant CETP have much lower plasma HDL-C levels and are more susceptible to atherosclerosis. In humans, mutations of the CETP gene, particularly common in Japan, result in substantial elevations in HDL-C (164 mg/dL in homozygotes, 66 mg/dL in heterozygotes). LDL-C tended to be low, with relative increase in LDL triglyceride content.[86,87] Surprisingly, however, recent findings of higher CHD rates with

CETP deficiency in Japan raise the possibility that CETP deficiency interferes with reverse cholesterol transport despite the increased levels of HDL-C.[88]

Elevated Lipoprotein(a)

Lipoprotein(a) [Lp(a)] particles are formed by the covalent disulfide linkage of the glycoprotein apoprotein(a) to apoprotein B of LDL. Nearly all the population variance of plasma Lp(a) can be explained by genetic variability at the apoprotein(a) locus.[89] Renal disease can result in substantial elevations, while estrogen lowers Lp(a).[90,91] Plasma concentration of Lp(a) above 30 to 40 mg/dL (approximately the 90th percentile) have generally been associated with modestly increased risk for premature CHD (relative odds 2 to 4) in numerous retrospective case-control and angiographic studies among white subjects and in most prospective studies.[90,92,93] In contrast, the relative odds associated with high Lp(a) has been reported to be much higher in persons with familial hypercholesterolemia.[94,95] Yet, an elevated Lp(a) imparted little excess risk among participants of the Physicians Health Study, a group with relatively low serum cholesterol concentrations.[96] Furthermore, Maher et al.[97] found that in persons with a 10 percent or greater reduction in LDL-C during a vigorous lipid-lowering intervention, Lp(a) was not predictive of atherosclerosis progression or CHD events (only 9 percent incidence of new events in those with high Lp(a) and ≥10 percent LDL reduction), while in those with little change in LDL-C, Lp(a) remained a strong predictor of progression and events [with a 39 percent incidence in those with high Lp(a) and <10 percent LDL reduction].

These findings led to the hypothesis that Lp(a) is a risk factor primarily when serum cholesterol or LDL-C is elevated. Results from limited observational and intervention studies were consistent with this hypothesis when, in meta-analysis, relative odds reported in each study were plotted against average study LDL-C levels.[98] Nevertheless, few studies have examined this issue directly.[99–101] This interaction was recently confirmed in two large case-control studies.[92,93] In both studies, odds ratios associated with 90th percentile elevations in Lp(a) (approximately 40 mg/dL for the most commonly used assay) were associated with modest twofold increases in risk when considered in univariate analysis. However, in persons with total/HDL-C ratios above 5.8 (approximately equal to a total cholesterol of 200 mg/dL and an HDL-C of 35 mg/dL) risks for the same elevation in Lp(a) were elevated 10- to 35-fold compared to the group with more normal total and HDL-C and Lp(a). An interaction term was significant in both studies. The clinical implications of these findings may be important. Persons with total/HDL-C ratio above 5.8 (a modest elevation) may particularly benefit from measurement of Lp(a) and aggressive management of lipids if Lp(a) is elevated.

Common Familial Lipid Syndromes of Uncertain Etiology

The most common familial dyslipidemias, including polygenic hypercholesterolemia, familial combined hyperlipidemia (FCHL), familial hypertriglyceridemia, and most familial low HDL are poorly understood and probably represent heterogeneous entities due to the effects of multiple genes interacting with diverse environmental influences (Fig. 5–3). These syndromes are strongly associated with early familial CHD. Their frequency in cases of early familial CHD seems to be quite similar comparing data from Utah,[55,102] Boston,[103,104] and Seattle.[53,54,105] Frequencies of several familial syndromes and concordant risk factors (present in two or more siblings with early-onset CHD) were as follows: FH, 3 to 4 percent; type III hyperlipidemia, 0.5 to 3 percent (not reported in Boston); low HDL, 20 to 30 percent (not reported in Seattle); FCHL, 18 to 36 percent; familial hypertriglyceridemia, 18 to 20 percent; high Lp(a), 16 to 19 percent (not reported in Seattle); high homocyst(e)ine, 12 to 30 percent (not reported in Seattle); diabetes, 8 percent; hypertension, 24 percent (half of these had lipid abnormalities); and cigarette smoking, 37 percent. Few families had no known concordant risk factors. Classifications for FCHL varied by study, being based on 90th percentile elevations of plasma total or LDL-C and triglycerides and 10th percentile levels of HDL-C in

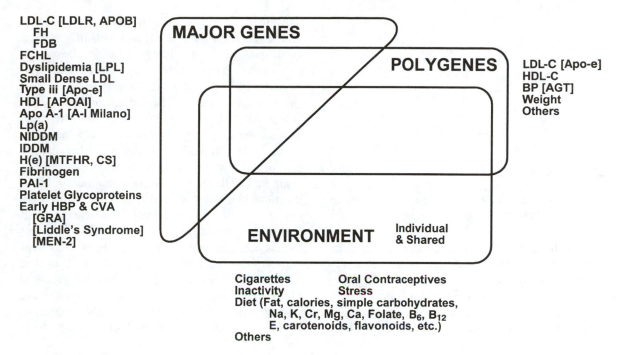

LDL-C [LDLR, APOB]
  FH
  FDB
FCHL
Dyslipidemia [LPL]
Small Dense LDL
Type iii [Apo-e]
HDL [APOAI]
Apo A-1 [A-I Milano]
Lp(a)
NIDDM
IDDM
H(e) [MTFHR, CS]
Fibrinogen
PAI-1
Platelet Glycoproteins
Early HBP & CVA
  [GRA]
  [Liddle's Syndrome]
  [MEN-2]

MAJOR GENES

POLYGENES

LDL-C [Apo-e]
HDL-C
BP [AGT]
Weight
Others

ENVIRONMENT Individual & Shared

Cigarettes   Oral Contraceptives
Inactivity   Stress
Diet (Fat, calories, simple carbohydrates,
    Na, K, Cr, Mg, Ca, Folate, B_6, B_{12}
    E, carotenoids, flavonoids, etc.)
Others

FIGURE 5–3   Overlapping domains represent combined (additive or multiplicative) effects of monogenic, polygenic, and environmental factors promoting atherosclerosis.

both the Boston and Utah studies. The Seattle study required combinations of 95th and 99th percentile elevations in its definitions of FH and FCHL.

Polygenic hypercholesterolemia   The most common cause of type IIa hyperlipidemia (elevation of LDL-C only) with serum total cholesterol between 240 and 350 mg/dL is probably polygenic predisposition, often aggravated by a poor diet, increased adiposity with age, and other poorly defined factors. Mechanisms for such elevations probably include both increased production and, to a lesser extent, decreased removal of LDL-C.[106–108] Heritability estimates for total cholesterol in Utah twins was 61 percent, while in family studies the estimate was 45 percent, with only 8 percent of the variance attributable to the effects of a common household (Table 5–3). Figure 5–4 depicts a sibship with polygenic hypercholesterolemia.

Genes contributing to polygenic hypercholesterolemia are largely unknown. A prototype, how-

ever, is Apo-E. About 7 to 14 percent of population variance has been attributed to the combined effects of Apo-E2, E3, and E4.[109,110] Persons with the Apo-E3-2 genotype have approximately 10 percent lower total and LDL-C compared with persons having the Apo-E3-3 genotype. The presence of an Apo-E4 allele raises total and LDL-C approximately 7 percent. Some have suggested that the lesser affinity of Apo-E2 for the LDL receptor results in reduced deposition of cholesterol ester–rich particles in the liver, with subsequently less downregulation of LDL receptors. The converse occurs with Apo-E4. Several investigators have reported increased risk of CHD associated with Apo-E4.[60]

Familial combined hyperlipidemia, hyperapobetalipoproteinemia, and the atherogenic lipoprotein phenotype   Familial combined hyperlipidemia (FCHL) is characterized by the presence of hypercholesterolemia (type IIa), hypertriglyceridemia (type IV), or both (type IIb), with two or more of

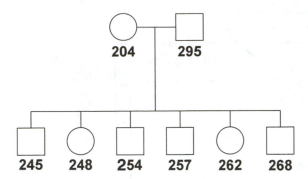

FIGURE 5–4 Sibship illustrating common polygenic hypercholesterolemia.

these patterns present among first-degree relatives. A recent review provides an excellent overview of FCHL and findings of genetic studies.[111] Typically the hyperlipidemia is in the 90th to 95th percentile range and thus is not nearly as striking as in familial hypercholesterolemia. Age dependency of expression is a prominent feature. Affected persons are generally not recognizable until the third decade, though in some families affected children can be identified by reference to age-specific percentiles.[112] Estimates of FCHL prevalence in the general population range from 0.5 to 2 percent or higher, depending on cut points used. When originally described, FCHL was thought to result from a single dominant allele. Subsequent segregation analyses have yielded conflicting results and the transmission of this trait remains unclear.[111]

Several investigators have reported increased VLDL Apo-B (and/or triglyceride) production as the underlying kinetic mechanism leading to multiple phenotypes in FCHL, based primarily on observations in unrelated individuals. While most investigators consider overproduction of Apo-B to be a sufficient explanation for FCHL, the only extensive family study to examine this issue provides a divergent view. More first-degree relatives of FCHL probands had decreased VLDL fractional catabolic rates rather than increased production.[113] More recently, a FCHL family with clearly impaired VLDL and LDL Apo-B catabolism as the major defect, further illustrating the heterogeneity of FCHL.[114]

Although increases in LDL cholesterol are expected in at least some family members in any given FCHL pedigree, some definitions of FCHL require only elevations of total cholesterol and triglycerides. Given such a definition, LPL or Apo-C–II deficiency could cause a FCHL pattern. Indeed, by investigating LPL activity and immunoreactive mass in the adipose tissue of relatives of LPL-deficient subjects, Babirak and coworkers suggested that the heterozygous state for LDL deficiency could account for FCHL observed in some families.[115] Modifications in the ability of LPL to promote direct removal of triglyceride-rich particles could theoretically lead to an FCHL pattern.[116,117] Nevertheless, linkage studies have not been consistent with an important role for LPL in FCHL.[111] In fact, no gene locus has yet been consistently linked to FCHL except possibly for two loci on chromosome 1 in Finnish FCHL families.[111] Locus heterogeneity may be contributing to conflicting results from linkage studies.

FCHL is also associated with small, dense LDL. Hyperapobetalipoproteinemia, defined as elevated LDL Apo-B with relatively normal LDL-C, is essentially the same entity.[118,119] A pattern of predominantly small, dense LDL [pattern B or atherogenic lipoprotein phenotype (ALP)] appears to be dominantly transmitted and has been linked to several loci including the LDL receptor, CETP, manganese superoxide dismutase, and the AI-CIII-AIV gene cluster.[111] Small, dense LDL has been reported as a risk factor for premature CHD by several investigators, usually with modest odds ratios of 2 to 3.[120–126] Some have found the associated risk independent of HDL-C and triglycerides;[122,125,126] others have not.[123,124] A plausible mechanism for accelerated atherosclerosis is the increased susceptibility to oxidation of small, dense LDL.[127] The expression of small, dense LDL is strongly dependent on plasma triglycerides; most persons will have pattern B when triglycerides are above 200 mg/dL (2.26 mmol/L). Although some support its clinical utility,[128] most lipid specialists consider determination of LDL particle size a research tool at the present time owing to technical difficulties or expense.

Familial dyslipidemic hypertension and the multiple metabolic syndrome In 1988, a syndrome descriptively named *familial dyslipidemic hypertension* (FDH) was described.[129] After screening the first 131 participants in a Utah study of familial hypertension selected *only* on the basis of early hypertension present in two or more siblings, a very high prevalence of lipid abnormalities (65 percent of individuals, concordant in 48 percent of sibships) was noted, with high triglycerides (30 percent) and low HDL-C (39 percent) being most common. High LDL-C (19 percent) was also more prevalent than the 10 percent expected for each abnormality. Further studies demonstrated a pattern of familial combined hyperlipidemia in approximately half those with FDH, while the other half had elevated triglycerides and/or low HDL-C, without elevated LDL-C. Both FDH groups had elevated fasting plasma insulin concentrations.[130] Follow-up in over 300 participants in this study confirmed and strengthened these initial findings and clearly placed FDH in the same realm as multiple metabolic syndrome or so-called insulin resistance syndrome.[131]

The combination of insulin resistance, hypertriglyceridemia, central obesity, and hypertension has been termed "the deadly quartet."[132] Very possibly, central or visceral obesity is the central causative feature of this syndrome rather than insulin resistance.[131,133] This model would be consistent with detailed genetic analysis of the multiple metabolic syndrome in a group of 289 Swedish twins.[134] In a study of twins by the National Heart, Lung, and Blood Institute, exaggerated risks of CHD were evident when hypertension and dyslipidemia were present jointly (Fig. 5–5). Furthermore, the combination of hypertension and dyslipidemia did appear to be genetically determined.[135] Approximately 12 percent of early familial CHD is associated with dyslipidemic hypertension.[136]

There are several practical implications from these observations. First, in persons with hypertension, lipid profiles including total cholesterol, triglycerides, and HDL-C should be obtained to assess risk more fully. Second, antihypertensive medications that do not adversely affect lipids should be utilized in persons with dyslipidemic hypertension. Finally, other family members of persons with dyslipidemic hypertension should be screened for both hypertension and dyslipidemia and treated accordingly.

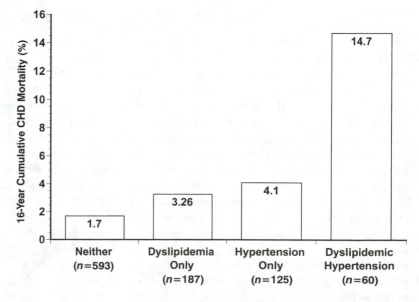

FIGURE 5–5 National Heart, Lung and Blood Institute Study of twins showing exaggerated risks of CHD when hypertension and dyslipidemia were present jointly. (Adapted from Selby et al.,[135] with permission.)

Nonlipid Genetic Disorders

Rare Monogenic Hypertension Syndromes

Two severe, dominant, but rare forms of hypertension—glucocorticoid-remediable hyperaldosteronism (GRA) and Liddle's syndrome—lead to early, severe hypertension and strokes. Although these are not important contributors to common or essential hypertension, new insights into these syndromes serve to illustrate potential mechanisms whereby less severe genetic variations could contribute to hypertension. In families affected by these disorders, informative diagnostic tests can now be performed and effective therapy prescribed that is tailored to the specific pathophysiology. In the future, a similar tailored approach may be available for essential hypertension.

GRA results from a dominant "gain of function" mutation on chromosome 8. The mutation induces high levels of abnormal adrenal steroids, 18-hydroxy cortisol, and 18-oxocortisol.[137] This unusual chimeric mutation derives from the combination of fragments of two genes, the aldosterone synthase gene and the steroid 11-beta-hydroxylase gene. The DNA sequences of these two genes are 95 percent identical, the genes have identical intron-exon boundaries, and the genes are located next to each other on chromosome 8. During recombination, unequal crossing over has occurred, producing a mutant gene having aldosterone synthase activity under the control of the steroid 11-beta-hydroxylase promoter. Lack of steroid 11-beta-hydroxylase activity impairs cortisol production, with subsequent elevation of adrenocorticotropic hormone (ACTH). The ACTH, acting on the chimeric gene, stimulates aldosterone synthesis, leading to hyperaldosteronism, excessive sodium resorption, and severe hypertension. Administration of exogenous glucocorticoids (like dexamethasone) can suppress aldosterone and abnormal steroid production and also normalize blood pressure. Persons with the gene for GRA may have early severe hypertension with death from cerebral hemorrhage by age 40. Because this is a dominantly transmitted trait, close relatives will have similar histories. GRA is also reported to fail to respond to ordinary antihypertensive medications, but can respond to prednisone (which will suppress hormone production), spironolactone (which will competitively inhibit the aldosterone receptor) or amiloride (which will inhibit distal renal epithelial sodium channel response to mineralocorticoid action).

Liddle's syndrome results from dominant mutations at a locus coding for the beta subunit of the epithelial sodium channel on chromosome 16p.[138] Mutations in other subunits resulting in a similar syndrome have also been described.[139] A genetically activated channel cannot be maintained in a properly closed state.[138] Low plasma renin activity and variable hypokalemia are seen in this syndrome as in GRA. However, Liddle's syndrome causes suppressed aldosterone secretion, in contrast to the hyperaldosteronism seen in GRA. Excessive reabsorption of sodium in exchange for potassium in the distal nephron probably accounts for the hypertension and hypokalemia. Both of these features of Liddle's syndrome are responsive to triamterene or amiloride, both of which specifically inhibit the epithelial sodium channel. Unlike GRA, this syndrome is not responsive to spironolactone, which inhibits the mineralocorticoid receptor. Kidney transplant also seems to eliminate the problem.

Common Essential Hypertension

Essential hypertension may be considered the result of interactions between genes and environment. The environmental effects are powerful and probably explain most or all of the substantial blood pressure differences between different populations. Genetic effects explain much of blood pressure distribution in populations with homogeneous nutrient intakes. One of the most powerful influences is body weight or obesity (itself largely genetically determined). Central or upper-body obesity is the major contributor in this relationship. An impressive 80 percent of all new-onset hypertension could be explained by subscapular skinfolds above the lowest quintile in the Framingham study.[140] Salt has a lesser but probably important effect.[141–145] Alcohol, physical activity, potassium intake (especially in fruits and vegetables), and possibly psychosocial stress are other potentially important environmental factors.[146,147] The mechanism of interaction probably involves how effectively the kidneys modulate changes in salt intake.[148] Indeed, the hypertension in virtually every genetically hypertensive animal model can be reversed by transplantation of the kidneys of a normotensive animal.[148]

The nature of the genetic contribution to blood pressure in humans was in dispute until relatively recently.[149] A key finding was that in human populations, even among first-degree relatives of hypertensive patients, blood pressure appears to be a unimodal trait.[149–152] This finding and studies in animals[153] argues for a polygenic or oligogenic model for blood pressure, wherein susceptibility imparted by any single genetic variation is modest and quantitative. Such gene variations would be expected to modulate response to environmental exposure and may only achieve significance through cumulative integration of lifetime experience. Although this scenario greatly complicates the task of the genetic epidemiologist, major studies are currently under way in several countries and are likely to produce a list of common genes contributing to hypertension.

The first gene to be linked to common, essential hypertension in a human population was the angiotensinogen gene (*AGT*) on chromosome 1. An association between the *AGT* 235T allele and hypertension was also demonstrated.[154] Most subsequent studies have confirmed the original association or linkage findings.[155–165] A recent meta-analysis of 12 studies reported a statistically highly significant 20 percent increase ($p < .0001$) in hypertension in persons with at least one *AGT* 235T allele and concluded that it would take an additional 38 studies with negative results to overturn this conclusion.[166] Nevertheless, some negative findings also continue to be reported.[167] Several studies suggest a significant effect of *AGT* genotype on plasma angiotensinogen levels.[154,168,169] Angiotensinogen levels have, in turn, been associated with blood pressure on the population level.[170] Increased angiotensinogen substrate might lead to excess angiotensin II production, especially at the tissue level. Consistent with this hypothesis, homozygous carriers of this *AGT* variant show blunting of renal response to infused an-

giotensin II (thought by some to be a sign of "salt-sensitive" hypertension).[171] The high-risk 235T allele is probably not, itself, causal, but is in complete association with a variant in the promoter region (at position −6), resulting in a modest but highly significant increase in function potentially leading to increased angiotensinogen production.[160]

The issue of salt sensitivity is controversial and complex. Nevertheless, if a gene test could be devised that allowed rational, focused intervention in those individuals who, because of genetic predisposition, would stand to benefit most from intervention, clinical implications would be enormous. Identifying such a susceptible subgroup could have a profound influence on patient compliance. Those having definite susceptibility would be much more motivated to reduce salt intake over the years necessary to have a substantial impact on the likelihood of hypertension and target organ damage. Initial studies suggest that *AGT* may be such a gene.

In the Trials of Hypertension Prevention (TOHP), 378 middle-aged adults with diastolic blood pressure between 83 and 89 mmHg were randomly assigned to sodium-reduced diets (average 25 percent reduction at 36 months) and were then compared to 384 similar participants assigned to "usual care."[172] New hypertension occurred in 34 percent of the sodium-reduction group compared to 39 percent of the usual care group ($p = .09$).[172] However, when these participants were subdivided according to their angiotensinogen genotype, those with the most "salt-sensitive" genotype (−6 AA) had the most hypertension in the usual-care group (45 percent) and the least hypertension in the sodium-reduction group (28 percent).[173] Increased salt sensitivity was also reported to be associated with a −6 A *AGT* allele in a Dutch salt intervention study among hypertensives.[174]

Another gene with accumulating evidence for an effect on blood pressure and salt sensitivity is alpha-adducin.[175] Variants in this gene, whose product is a cytoskeleton protein, may modify the activity of the sodium-potassium ATPase, affect renal salt resorption, and thereby influence blood pressure.[176,177] Several studies support an association or linkage in human populations.[175,177,178] Others fail to find an association with blood pressure or effects on salt metabolism.[179–182] It is possible that combinations of genes—including angiotensinogen, adducin, kallikrein, and others—would more accurately predict susceptible individuals.

Type 2 Diabetes

Diabetes is a major risk factor for CHD, resulting in three- to fivefold elevations in risk in numerous studies.[183] Both type 1 and type 2 diabetes are associated with increased risk, but the excess prevalence of lipid abnormalities and hypertension both accompanying and preceding type 2 diabetes may help explain the strong cardiovascular risk associated with this disorder.[184] The genetics of type 1 diabetes is much better understood, with genes now known to contribute 60 to 65 percent of the susceptibility to type 2 diabetes. Most cases involve a predisposition to autoimmune destruction of the pancreatic beta cells.[185] Type 1 diabetes is not discussed further here. A strong genetic component for type 2 diabetes has long been recognized. Concordance in monozygous twins ranges from 20 to 90 percent, compared with only about 9 percent in dizygous twins, consistent with very high heritability.[186] Like hypertension, type 2 diabetes is a complex quantitative disease with varying degrees of genetic and environmental contributions, depending on the patient or family.

Environmental effects are well illustrated by the Pima Indians. Pimas in Mexico living a traditional lifestyle in a remote mountainous area are lean [mean body-mass index (BMI), 24.9] and physically active; they have about the same prevalence of diabetes as the general U.S. population (about 6 percent).[187,188] In contrast, Pimas in southern Arizona are, on average, 26 kg heavier (mean BMI, 33.4) and have an exceedingly high frequency of diabetes, approximately 37 percent in women and 54 percent in men.[187] The interaction of weight and genetic predisposition is perhaps best illustrated in Fig. 5–6 by the strongly increasing gradient of risk associated with higher BMI among offspring of one and especially two diabetic parents. Higher BMI only modestly increased risk if family history of diabetes was negative.[189] This finding provides one of the most clinically useful messages for prevention of diabetes: if you have a family history of type 2 diabetes, get lean and stay lean.

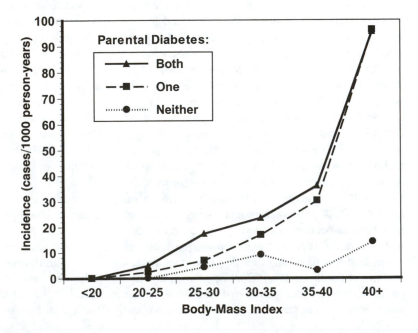

FIGURE 5–6 Interaction of weight and genetic predisposition to diabetes with incidence of diabetes, showing strongly increased gradient of risk associated with higher BMI among offspring of one, and especially two diabetic parents. (Adapted from Knowler et al.,[189] with permission.)

The emergence of diabetes among Pimas and several other populations after changing from a spartan traditional lifestyle to one in which food is more abundant has been attributed to a "thrifty genotype"; a gene or set of genes favoring efficient storage of body fat, thereby increasing survival in times of famine.[190] In times of relative abundance, however, the deposition of excess fat, particularly visceral fat, promotes insulin resistance.[131] Insulin resistance is probably the precursor of much, if not most diabetes,[191,192] leading to overt diabetes if superimposed on a primarily genetic failure of the beta cell to compensate adequately.[193,194] Not surprisingly, a few gene loci have been suggested to be involved with development of both diabetes and obesity, including the beta$_3$-adrenergic receptor,[195,196] the beta$_2$-adrenergic receptor,[197] glycogen synthase (also associated with hypertension, possibly aggravated by a high-fat diet),[198–200] the sulfanylurea receptor,[201] and a human uncoupling protein (UCP2).[202] Subsequent studies have not confirmed the association with UCP2.[203–206]

Interestingly, less than one-third of the tenfold variation seen in insulin sensitivity among young, healthy individuals can be explained by obesity and other known environmental factors.[207] Much of the remainder is likely to involve genetic variation. Several examples have begun to be identified, particularly involving the insulin signaling cascade, including mutations or variants of the insulin receptor substrate-1 (IRS-1), the p85 subunit of the phosphatidylinositol-3 (PI3)-kinase, and the regulatory subunit of glycogen-associated protein phosphate-1 (PP1G).[207] However, whether these are actually involved in the development of type 2 diabetes is questionable.[208] Several rare, severe, inherited forms of insulin resistance have been explained by mutations of the insulin receptor.[209,210] In one study three of 51 Japanese patients with ordinary type 2 diabetes had insulin receptor mutations that may have explained their disease.[211]

The genetic bases of other rare syndromes causing severe or early-onset type 2–like diabetes have been described. Examples include maturity-onset diabetes of the young (MODY), with MODY2 caused by defects in the glucokinase gene;[212,213] MODY1

caused by mutations hepatocyte nuclear factor 4α (HNF-4α); MODY3 caused by hepatocyte nuclear factor 1α (HDF-1α);[213] and maternally inherited diabetes and deafness (MIDD) caused by a mutation in the mitochondrial DNA.[214,215] No evidence of linkage to older-onset diabetes has been demonstrated for the glucokinase.[216] In fact, efforts to identify linkage or association with more than 250 candidate genes have largely been unsuccessful,[186,217–220] despite evidence for segregation of a major gene for type 2 diabetes in Pimas[221] and segregation of fasting insulin levels in Utah type 2 diabetes families.[16]

This relative lack of success may be due not only to incorrect candidates but also to the marked heterogeneity of type 2 diabetes. Although some of the problems of heterogeneity might theoretically be reduced by defining intermediate phenotypes, the cost and complexity involved in such phenotyping efforts (such as glucose-clamp studies) can be prohibitive. Another approach may be identification of new, novel candidate genes.[222] Others advocate genome-wide scans for type 2 diabetes susceptibility genes. One such scan in Mexican Americans found evidence for a major susceptibility locus on chromosome 2.[223] Another scan in Utah families failed to confirm the chromosome 2 site but did identify another possible site on chromosome 1q21–1q23.[224] A scan linked to prediabetic traits in Pima Indians (such as fasting plasma insulin, 2-h insulin after oral glucose challenge, and fasting glucose) revealed yet other possible loci.[225] The complexity of type 2 diabetes mellitus will continue to challenge geneticists. Nevertheless, this should not deter efforts directed at prevention through achieving and maintaining a lean body habitus through diet and exercise, particularly in persons with apparent familial predisposition.

Obesity

Obesity is a major determinant of hypertriglyceridemia, low HDL-C, small, dense LDL-C, hypertension, and diabetes. Coupled with genetic predisposition to these problems, excess body fat can have far more severe consequences for the individual than might be suggested by general population surveys. Such individuals will also benefit more by weight loss than the overweight individual without these risk factors. Although the incentive for achieving and maintaining optimal body weight for susceptible individuals is powerful, weight loss remains among the most difficult goals to attain, even for the highly motivated. Greater understanding of the powerful genetic determination of obesity and recognition of the limited long-term success of most interventional efforts should engender empathy for the overweight patient.

Obesity is a highly heritable trait.[226] In Utah twins, heritability was estimated to be 54 percent for BMI (Table 5–3). Others have reported similar heritability estimates. Interestingly, segregation analysis shows stronger major gene effects for younger persons, while multifactorial factors predominated in older individuals.[227] Perhaps this explains the extraordinarily high heritability of 80 percent for BMI in a large series of Finnish twins aged 16 to 17 years.[228] One of the most persuasive arguments for the strong heritability of body mass is the finding that the BMI of twins reared apart resembled that of their biological parents much more closely than that of their adoptive parents.[229] The biological reasons for this heritability are beyond the scope of this chapter, but of great interest is the finding of a wide range of weight gains between monozygous twin pairs fed excess calories, with a high correlation of weight gain within the twin pairs.[230]

Fat patterning is also highly heritable in humans.[17,231] Accumulation of visceral fat was one of the most heritable changes in body composition observed in studies of overfeeding among monozygous twins.[226,230] Evidence of a major recessive gene causing increased accumulation of truncal fat was recently presented.[232] Increased sharing of alleles on chromosome 1 was seen in sibling pairs with more similar BMI and waist/hip ratios in a recent preliminary study from Muscatine, Iowa.[233] Increased waist/hip ratios are also associated with a polymorphism of the angiotensinogen gene on chromosome 1 among Hutterites.[234] The authors suggested that another gene near the angiotensinogen locus on chromosome 1 may be related to control of abdominal obesity in humans. In the pig, a locus corresponding to chromosome 1 in humans has recently been described, which does control abdominal and back fatness.[235] The β_3-adrenergic receptor gene is an important candidate for central obesity and ensuing features of the multiple metabolic syndrome.[236]

Recently, a substantial research effort has been directed to finding causal genes for obesity. There is a small handful of patients (some two to three dozen in the cumulative world literature) with rare, severe obesity for which a specific gene mutation has been identified. These same gene loci, however, have generally not been found to be linked to common obesity.[237] For instance, these include just two patients with obesity due to leptin mutations. Because of the great complexity in metabolic pathways potentially leading to excess fat accumulation, genomewide scans have become the preferred approach among geneticists. Of particular note is the linkage to chromosome 20q13 found in a series of 92 nuclear families.[238] Others have found other candidate regions.[237,239–241] Most of these findings remain in the realm of gene finding. Indeed, very few candidate genes linked to obesity in one population have been confirmed to link in a separate population.[237] The incentive to find genes for obesity remains strong, with the hope of identifying metabolic pathways that could be amenable to pharmacologic treatment.

Hyperhomocysteinemia

Original observations of atherosclerotic changes in the arteries of young persons dying of severe recessive forms of homocystinuria can be attributed to McCully.[242] Subsequently, other investigations, including studies in Utah,[243,244] have found modest elevations in plasma homocysteine to be an important independent risk factor for premature CHD.[245] In the Utah series, 10 to 14 percent of early-onset, familial CAD could be attributed to elevated total homocysteine.[243] Modest doses of B vitamins, primarily folate, can significantly lower plasma homocysteine.[246]

Severe elevations of plasma homocysteine are associated with recessive defects in enzymes of homocysteine, folate, and vitamin B_{12} metabolism. Nevertheless, genetic contributions to more common hyperhomocysteinemia are poorly understood. A common mutation of the methylenetetrahydrofolate reductase gene is associated with greater sensitivity to low folate[247,248] but has generally not been found to be associated with premature CHD.[247,249–251] The cystathionine beta-synthase gene is another important candidate and has been related to moderately to severely elevated homocysteine in a number of studies.[252,253] It is currently unknown whether these loci sufficiently explain the excess familial aggregation of homocysteine, which is seen particularly in close relatives of patients with premature vascular disease.[254]

Applying Genetic Principles in a Clinical Setting

Practical Differences between Monogenic and Polygenic Factors

Genetic influences on phenotypes can be classified as monogenic or polygenic. Both types of phenotypic determinations can contribute to a person's susceptibility or resistance to atherosclerosis, as illustrated in Fig. 5–3. Polygenic traits (like the LDL-C in most of us) show a continuous blending effect. Offspring generally have a polygenically determined cholesterol level approximately halfway between the levels of the two parents when values are measured at about the same age for both generations. Classic polygenic traits lead to sibling similarity. If we find a patient with a polygenically high cholesterol level, all siblings will have a similarly elevated cholesterol level, as shown in Fig. 5–4. This finding leads to a practical application: when a patient meets the criteria for treatment of a polygenically elevated LDL cholesterol level (the most common cause), we should routinely arrange for siblings, who will generally also have elevated levels, to be tested in order to identify those who need treatment.[255] HDL cholesterol, blood pressure, and weight are examples of other common risk factors showing strong polygenic effects.

Monogenic traits such as heterozygous familial hypercholesterolemia (FH) have Mendelian inheritance (dominant for FH heterozygotes). If one parent carries a dominant gene, half of the offspring, on average, will receive the gene and half will not, causing *segregation* or *bimodal separation* of the offspring into two groups: those with twofold elevated LDL-C levels and those with normal LDL cholesterol levels. Monogenic separation is very evident in the two sibships shown in Fig. 5–7, from families with heterozygous FH. DNA markers for the LDL receptor locus on the short arm of chromosome 19 can be used to genetically diagnose the presence or absence of FH in these two sibships, as indicated. In the upper sibship of Fig. 5–7, siblings, sorted in order of increasing total cholesterol level, show an increase of almost 100 mg/dL (2.6 mmol/L) between the sibling with the highest normal reading and the sibling with the lowest reading and the FH gene. In the second FH sibship, shown at the bottom of Fig. 5–7, a similar large "gap" of 71 mg/dL or 1.8 mmol distinguishes FH gene carriers from noncarriers. Separation into distinct groups ("bimodality") is characteristic of a monogenic trait. These principles have been summarized into diagnostic criteria for FH in Table 5–4.[69,256]

Table 5–6 lists other monogenic risk factors for atherosclerosis, including familial defective apolipoprotein B (FDB), dominant and recessive variants of Apo-E causing type III hyperlipidemia, glucocorticoid remediable aldosteronism (GRA), Liddle's syndrome, and multiple endocrine neoplasia type II (MEN-II).[137,138,257]

Diabetes, familial combined hyperlipidemia (FCHL), and low HDL cholesterol are clinical atherogenic syndromes that exhibit some of the characteristics of major gene traits (bimodality and vertical transmission in multigenerational pedigrees). However, genetic studies of these traits suggest that they result from more than one gene and are sometimes referred to as *oligogenic traits* (i.e., traits involving a few genes).

A polygenic background influences phenotypic expression of a major gene. As illustrated in Fig. 5–7, polygenic influence has shifted the entire upper sibship toward higher background cholesterol and the entire lower sibship toward lower cholesterol without confounding the major gene effects between the non-FH and FH siblings. This interesting result illustrates how overlap can occur between the

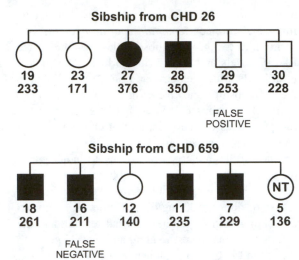

FIGURE 5–7 Two FH sibships demonstrate monogenic bimodality [from low-density-lipoprotein (LDL)-receptor defect] and polygenic effects, shifting the entire sibship toward higher cholesterol levels in the upper sibship and toward lower levels in the bottom sibship. Age and serum total cholesterol (mg/dL) are shown below each symbol. Shaded symbols represent DNA-diagnosed FH, while persons represented by clear symbols did not carry FH. NT indicates that no DNA testing was performed. In the sibship from CHD 659, the falsely negative sibling had total cholesterol levels much closer to the higher cholesterol mode in the sibship. The converse was true in the sibship from CHD 26. Interestingly, the false-positive case (non-FH carrier) from CHD 26 actually had higher serum cholesterol levels than the false-negative FH carrier from CHD 659.

cholesterol values of carriers and noncarriers in the general population. In these two sibships, carriers of the FH gene in the lower sibship have lower cholesterol levels than the noncarriers in the upper sibship.

Recognizing bimodality in sibships establishes a "cut point" between gene carriers and noncarriers in families with monogenic traits like FH. Applying this practical knowledge to the two sibships in Fig. 5–7 helps us to infer, correctly, that the 29-year-old male in the top sibship with a cholesterol of 253 does not carry the gene for FH, while the 16-year-old male in the bottom sibship with a cholesterol of 211 does carry the gene for FH.

Interaction between Genes and Environment

Environmental risk factors can have an exaggerated adverse effect in patients with genetic susceptibility,[3] as illustrated in Fig. 5–8. Among persons 30 to 49 years of age, cigarette smoking shows a multiplicative interaction with genetic predisposition, detected in this case by using family history of early CHD. A CHD relative risk of 4 for smokers with a strong positive family history (+FHx) compares to the usual relative risk of 2 for smokers with a negative family history (−FHx). (This difference in risk translates into a 10- to 14-year increase in life span for those who quit smoking and have genes like FH, compared to about 2 to 4 years of added longevity for those in the general population who quit.) A better understanding of the interactions between genes and the environment should lead to practical applications. In this case, vigorous smoking avoidance and smoking cessation projects should be especially beneficial when offered to genetically susceptible persons, such as those with familial lipid disorders or diabetes, because these people can benefit even more than the average person from risk reduction.

Some genetic factors may be hidden in many people unless they are also exposed to some necessary environmental factors. Homocysteine levels above 12 μmol/L seem to promote coronary atherosclerosis,[244] as illustrated in Fig. 5–9. The level of homocysteine can be affected by a common "heat-labile" mutation of the gene for methylene tetrahydrofolate reductase (MTHFR) as well as by dietary intake of a common vitamin, folic acid. Persons who were homozygous for the MTHFR heat-labile mutation *and* had low folic acid intake (as reflected in serum levels) had greatly elevated homocysteine levels.[258] The data in Fig. 5–10 suggest that neither low folate intake nor homozygous MTHFR mutation status alone would confer the strong risk of hyperhomocysteinemia and early CHD, but that *both* genetic and environmental ex-

TABLE 5–6 Treatable Dominant Cardiovascular Diseases

Genetic Trait	Description	Clinical Diagnosis	Genetic Diagnosis	Treatment or Prevention
Familial hypercholes-terolemia (FH)	High LDL cholesterol and very early heart attack deaths.	LDL cholesterol and xanthoma. Quite reliable.	LDL receptor gene tests (>400 causal mutations).	Drugs reduce cholesterol, and likely extend life 10–30 years.
Familial defective Apo-B (FDB)	High Apo-B and cholesterol with early heart attack deaths.	High cholesterol can mimic FH, but some levels are lower than FH.	Two specific causal mutations.	Same as for FH for those with very high cholesterol.
Dominant type III hyperlipidemia	Very high beta-VLDL cholesterol with early heart attack deaths.	High triglyceride and abnormal triglyceride/VLDL ratio.	Several specific causal mutations.	Specific medications can often normalize levels and prolong life.
Long-QT syndrome	High risk for sudden arrhythmic death in youth and young adults.	Long duration of QT interval on electro-cardiogram.	Linkage found and mutations being sought.	Medication can lower risk of sudden death and prolong life.
GRA hypertension	Severe high blood pressure and early stroke.	Abnormal steroid hormones. BP normal after dexamethasone.	Several specific causal mutations.	Suppress abnormal steroids with hormones like dexamethasone.
Liddle's syndrome	Severe high blood pressure and early stroke	Selective BP response to amiloride and triamterene	Causal mutations.	Amiloride or triamterene.
MEN II	Pheochromo-cytoma and other endocrine neoplasia.	MRI and CT scans for tumors.	Causal mutations.	Surgical removal of endocrine tumors.

Key: GRA, glucocorticoid remediable aldosteronism; MEN-II, multiple endocrine neoplasia II.

posures are required for an increased risk of CHD. Interestingly, most studies have failed to find an increased CHD risk associated with the MTHFR heat-labile mutation.[247,250,251,259]

Meaningful synergy has been suggested for selected environmental factors with other inherited atherogenic syndromes. Restricting saturated fat and cholesterol helps lower cholesterol for persons with FH. Weight loss, while potentially useful for the FH patient,[260] can be essential for patients with diabetes or hypertriglyceridemia who are overweight. Similarly, restricting simple carbohydrates may not be particularly helpful for FH patients but can substantially improve lipids in diabetics and persons with hypertriglyceridemia. Physical activity without weight reduction is relatively ineffective in altering lipids.[261] In fact, LDL-C is generally resistant to exercise, while increasing physical activity can help with weight reduction, lowering triglycerides, and raising HDL-C (among other benefits).[262–264] The angiotensinogen gene variant promoting hypertension identifies a subset in whom sodium restriction may be especially beneficial. A generous intake of B vitamins and folate seems

FIGURE 5–8 CHD incidence rates by family history and smoking status illustrates a multiplicative interaction, especially in the younger two age groups.

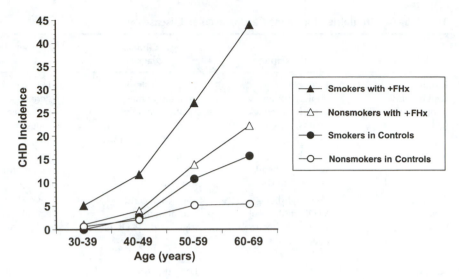

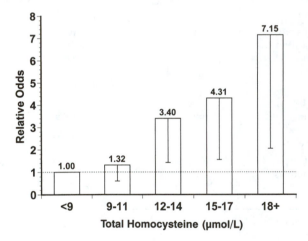

FIGURE 5–9 Relative odds of coronary disease according to plasma levels of homocysteine in 162 men and women with early coronary heart disease compared to 155 age- and sex-matched controls without coronary heart disease. Increased risk of CHD is prominent for persons with homocysteine levels above 13 μmol/L. (From Hasstedt et al.,[12] with permission.)

particularly important for persons carrying genes that promote hyperhomocysteinemia. Thus, a genetic diagnosis should lead to more effective risk reduction by identifying interventions that focus on specific environmental factors found to have a strong interaction with each person's particular genetic makeup.

Future Application of Genes for Sodium Sensitivity

Suppose you had a patient who has borderline diastolic blood pressure (83 to 89 mmHg) whom you were planning to ask to adhere to a reduced-sodium diet for the next several decades in order to help delay or even prevent hypertension. Would you like to be able to order tests to evaluate for the presence of the angiotensinogen gene and other genes, which together may define the degree of success your patient could hope to achieve with a reduced-sodium diet? Would your attitude toward prescribing a long-term low-sodium diet be different if you knew that the patient had multiple "sodium-sensitive" genotypes? What if the patient were found to have a sodium-resistant genotype? Researchers are currently trying to confirm the findings of the TOHP and Dutch mineral salt studies[173,174] and to extend findings on salt sensitivity associated with other genes in order to better predict individual responses to salt-lowering diets.

FIGURE 5–10   Plasma homocysteine levels [mean H(e) ± SEM)], according to presence (+) or absence (−) of the MTHFR mutation and folate intake levels. Levels associated with substantially increased risk for CHD (i.e., above 13 μmol/L) are limited to those with *both* homozygous MTHFR deficiency *and* low folate intake. (From Hunt et al.,[13] with permission.)

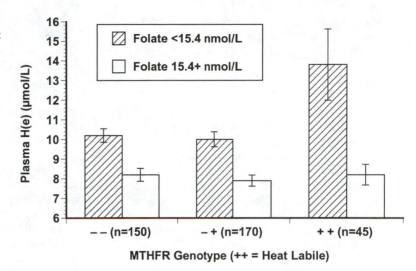

Genetic Effects beyond the Usual Effects of Environment

If we assume a "normal" cholesterol level to be about 200 mg/dL (5.2 mmol/L) and a maximum effect of a low-fat diet reducing cholesterol levels by about 20 to 30 percent,[265,266] then the maximum effect of a high-fat diet would elevate cholesterol about 20 to 30 percent, to about 240 to 260 mg/dL or about 6.0 to 6.5 mmol/L. Therefore, persons who have a cholesterol level above approximately 260 mg/dL (6.5 mmol/L) are likely to have dyslipidemia attributable, at least in part, to a genetic etiology. Whether their underlying genetic predisposition is monogenic or polygenic, they will likely have siblings who are in need of screening and treatment, suggesting that most patients with lipid levels high enough for drug treatment are also probands for family screening.

Obesity is another prominent factor in atherosclerosis. Although diet and exercise obviously play an important role, genes also play a strong role, especially for those who are extremely obese. Major research efforts are currently under way to map and understand genes for obesity. Future medications will likely include drugs to normalize weight for morbidly obese patients, just as potent statins now help patients with FH to normalize their cholesterol levels. These developments illustrate another practical benefit of applying genetics to disease prevention and control. The ongoing discovery of genes that promote disease is leading medical professionals to new and better diagnostic and therapeutic approaches.

Genetic Considerations in Case Studies

A lipid case history   Assume you are caring for a 45-year-old man with a fasting total cholesterol of 310 mg/dL, normal triglycerides (125 mg/dL), relatively low HDL-C (33 mg/dL), and high calculated LDL-C (252 mg/dL). He does not have any secondary causes such as hypothyroidism or nephrosis. His father and brother both had myocardial infarctions before age 55. The lipid levels in relatives are not known to the patient.

Questions regarding this lipid patient:

1. Is this patient's high LDL-C most likely due to genes, environment, or both?
2. What would be the differential diagnosis?
3. What would be required to determine the exact genetic diagnosis?
4. Will you likely prescribe medication for this patient's cholesterol regardless of the genetic causes?
5. If so, are there any important practical reasons for making the genetic diagnosis?

6. The patient's 43-year-old brother has similar lipid levels and asks you what he should do about diet and exercise. What do you tell him?

Answers:

1. The magnitude of this cholesterol elevation (55 percent above the median for the patient's age) strongly suggests an underlying genetic factor.

2. Heterozygous familial hypercholesterolemia (FH), familial combined hyperlipidemia (FCHL), and polygenic hypercholesterolemia (PH) are all possibilities. Probabilities that the true lipid syndrome was FH are high to moderate, moderate for PH, and low to moderate for FCHL. Individuals with PH and FH usually have normal triglycerides. Although 75 percent of affected persons in families with FCHL have high triglycerides, about 25 percent will have high LDL and normal triglycerides. LDL-C levels are not normally this high in families with FCHL.

3. First, examine the patient for tendon xanthomas, which would establish the diagnosis of FH. In the absence of tendon xanthomas, obtain lipid levels in siblings, children, aunts and uncles, and nieces and nephews to help distinguish the diagnosis. A "family lipid history" (Appendix 5–1) is a key tool for diagnosing familial lipid disorders as well as for finding affected relatives who need treatment. High triglyceride levels as well as high cholesterol levels in siblings support the diagnosis of FCHL. Bimodal, pure LDL-C elevations and very high LDL-C in children indicate FH. Both a blending effect that produces similar cholesterol elevations in siblings and an absence of severe pediatric hypercholesterolemia support PH.

4. An LDL-C level of 252 mg/dL is not likely to drop below 200 mg/dL, even with good compliance to a step 1 or 2 diet. A careful diet history may reveal that this patient had already implemented substantial changes and that prior LDL-C levels were considerably higher, making a diagnosis of FH much more likely and diminishing the chance that further dietary changes would substantially alter his lipids. This 45-year-old male with low HDL and a positive family history for CHD meets the guidelines of the National Cholesterol Educa-tion Panel for medication. The goal should be to reduce the LDL-C level to below 130 mg/dL. Drug therapy will be indicated regardless of whether the diagnosis is FH, PH, or FCHL.

5. Distinguishing between FH, PH, and FCHL can lead to different tailored approaches regarding relative screening, cardiology workup, exercise recommendations, and dietary prescription. (Perhaps only the choice of medication, often a potent statin, would be the same regardless of diagnosis.) If we extend cardiovascular disease prevention and control beyond isolated drug therapy to a more comprehensive approach, then the correct diagnosis does make a difference. An approach as follows could be recommended:

a. Screening of relatives based on genetic diagnosis. Screening lipids in relatives is necessary to help make the diagnosis. At the same time, it will identify other persons requiring treatment for FH, or PH, or FCHL. Extended relative screening is not recommended for PH but is recommended for FH and FCHL. If this patient has FH, *screening should extend to third-degree or more distant relatives and include children.* For PH, only siblings and adult children need screening. In some FCHL families, distant adult relatives may be found that need treatment, though lipid abnormalities tend not to be found in FCHL families as consistently as in FH families.

b. Cardiology workup tailored to a genetic diagnosis. Even in the absence of symptoms, some FH experts recommend a treadmill test or other noninvasive tests for CHD for FH men in their forties. Silent CHD is frequently found in FH patients.[267] Though few would recommend revascularization even with relatively advanced disease in the absence of symptoms (left main disease is rarely asymptomatic), results from such testing may be strongly motivating. It is important to remember that the very high cholesterol level in this 45-year-old FH patient has been present for over four decades, in contrast to men the same age with PH or FCHL, whose cholesterol levels may have been equally high for only one or two decades.

c. Exercise prescription tailored to a genetic diagnosis. Beginning a new jogging routine (or other moderate aerobic activity) without safety testing by a treadmill test could be dangerous for a middle-aged, sedentary man with FH. Perhaps in this case walking would be a more prudent form of exercise. Exercise may pose less risk and offers more benefit for men in their forties with FCHL than for those with FH. Therefore, jogging (or a similar activity) should be encouraged if this patient has FCHL and passes a treadmill electrocardiogram test. FCHL patients who do regular aerobic exercise will often see improvement in conditions such as hyperinsulinemia, obesity, high triglycerides, low HDL-C, and high blood pressure, though these benefits may be dependent on weight change.[261] Jogging is less dangerous and more beneficial for persons with PH than for those with FH. It may be less markedly beneficial for those with PH than for those with FCHL.

d. Genetically based dietary prescription. Dietary prescriptions can also be tailored to a specific genetic diagnosis. Patients with FCHL often need a diet like that prescribed for diabetics: low in calories, simple carbohydrates, and fat. For patients with polygenic hypercholesterolemia, a diet similar to the one for FH is appropriate (see Chap. 13).

6. The recommendation for an affected brother will be the same as for the patient and will depend on which genetic diagnosis is present in this family: FH, FCHL, or PH.

A hypertension case history Assume you are caring for a 40-year-old man with a resting blood pressure of 210/135 mmHg that has not responded to diuretics, beta blockers, angiotensin-converting enzyme (ACE) inhibitors, or calcium channel blockers. The patient has normal renal function and no evidence of renal artery stenosis. His older brother died of a stroke when he was 45 years of age. The patient's 16-year-old daughter has a blood pressure of 160/95 mmHg.

Practical questions regarding a severely hypertensive patient:

1. What possible genetic diagnoses should be considered?

2. What could be done to establish or rule out one of the dominant hypertension syndromes?

3. How could the screening of relatives help prevent early strokes? Which relatives should be screened?

4. How specifically should the medications be tailored to genetic diagnoses for these dominant hypertension syndromes?

Answers:

1. Glucocorticoid remediable aldosteronism (GRA) and Liddle's syndrome are both dominant hypertension syndromes that lead to early severe hypertension and stroke. Both are unresponsive to the ordinary antihypertensive medications listed above.

2. GRA often responds to a trial with spironolactone or dexamethasone, both of which address the two problems of abnormal steroids: hyperaldosteronism and severe hypertension. Severe hypertension with Liddle's syndrome responds to amiloride or triamterene. If there are clinical reasons to suspect a dominant hypertension syndrome, specific diagnoses may be made by testing blood and urine for the endocrine abnormalities described above. DNA testing can often identify a specific causal mutation for these disorders.

3. All first- and second-degree relatives should be screened for hypertension or diagnostic endocrine abnormalities. If specific mutations are known for a given family, other relatives can be sequentially screened and given a definitive result (gene present or absent) from a single blood sample. It is important to make the diagnosis and institute effective treatment as early as possible. If hypertension is undiagnosed and untreated for too long, it generates vessel and renal changes that cause irreversible hypertension, even with proper medication. Tracing families with GRA and Liddle's syndrome can save relatives from early strokes and premature death. All easily found relatives on the affected side of the family—including siblings, offspring, parents, aunts, and uncles—should be screened. If any affected second-degree relatives are found, their offspring should also be screened.

4. GRA and Liddle's syndrome are two excellent examples of clinical settings in which very

specific medications can be chosen to match a specific genetic mechanism. Steroids or spironolactone are specific for GRA. Triamterene, amiloride, or renal transplantation are specific treatments for Liddle's syndrome.

MEDPED: A Genetically Oriented Public Health Approach for High-Risk Pedigrees

Unfortunately, even well-understood and very treatable dominant disorders like FH are not diagnosed or treated in most gene carriers.[268] For relatively uncommon gene traits like FH, FDB, GRA, and Liddle's syndrome, more cases can be found efficiently by screening relatives of known probands and initiating treatment to normalize levels and prevent or delay early CHD or stroke.

MEDPED (Make Early Diagnoses to Prevent Early Deaths in medical pedigrees) is a nonprofit humanitarian project organized in 38 collaborating countries to collect all known index cases with FH or FDB. Investigators contact relatives for screening and treatment in both close and distant medical pedigrees. From one index case, 5 to 15 new FH cases can often be found among "close relatives" (siblings, parents, offspring, aunt, uncles, nieces, nephews, first cousins, and their offspring). In some families, hundreds of FH cases have been found by extending screening to "distant relatives" (second, third, and fourth cousins and their offspring). At the present time, the MEDPED collaborators are setting an example of case detection through relative screening. Assistance for patients suspected or known to have FH (see criteria in Table 5–5), GRA, or Liddle's syndrome can be obtained by this toll-free number in the United States: 1-888-2Hi-CHOL.

MEDPED collaborators in 38 countries have collectively identified over 30,000 patients with FH, in part by contacting relatives of known FH cases. By educating patients and their personal physicians and by helping them get additional help from referral specialists, the MEDPED effort has made it possible for many FH patients to experience dramatic (40 to 50 percent) reductions in LDL-C levels. Annual follow-up contacts and involvement in FH support groups and lay organizations help address the most important challenge to

lifelong medication: *long-term compliance.* Because relatives in high-risk families have different health plans and HMOs and live in different states or even different countries, some recommend that MEDPED efforts be supported by national governments and even coordinated by the World Health Organization (WHO). These efforts should include coordinated relative tracing, registration of severe gene carriers, education of personal physicians, and long-term follow-up to prevent the discontinuing of lifesaving medications. The WHO has convened two meetings devoted to FH and the MEDPED concept and has published a report with practical recommendations for this approach.[69] This same approach could work for similar diseases as long as they meet these criteria:

1. A single dominant gene causes preventable serious illness.
2. Validated diagnostic tests are available (gene test or clinical test).
3. Some form of treatment or prevention is available and has been shown to be effective.

Several other single-gene disorders that fit these criteria are presented in Table 5–6.

The cost-effectiveness of drug therapy for FH has been rigorously analyzed and documented.[69,269] Daily treatment with a low dose of lovastatin was projected to save money as well as lives. Higher-dose therapy was associated with an acceptable cost per year of life saved in one conservative analysis,[269] and it was more cost-effective than secondary prevention in men from the 4S study.[69]

Although some social scientists have raised concerns that projects like MEDPED might cause psychological stress by contacting relatives to talk about their family history, MEDPED collaborators in several countries report a large preponderance of positive reactions from relatives contacted in FH families. The dramatic occurrence of very early heart attack deaths in FH families is usually well known to relatives. Whether they know their cholesterol levels or not, many relatives in FH pedigrees already worry, long before being contacted by MEDPED, about having an early heart attack death. Because of MEDPED, thousands of relatives have been screened and found to have normal cholesterol and reassured that their fear of early death from heart attack was not warranted. Others found to have very high cholesterol levels have learned something very few of them knew before MEDPED: their severely elevated cholesterol levels can be dramatically reduced and early heart attack deaths prevented. In a recent study of patient attitudes regarding diagnosis of FH, patients diagnosed with FH reported modest anxiety about high serum cholesterol, use of cholesterol-lowering drugs, and risk of heart disease. However over 80 percent agreed with the statement, "I'm satisfied to know that I have heterozygous FH; then I can do something about it." Over 80 percent strongly disagreed (79.3 percent) or partly disagreed (4.0 percent) with the statement, "I wish I didn't know that I have heterozygous FH." Nearly 90 percent believed that their family should be screened and that people should be told of disease risks and what they can do to reduce risk.[270] Not examined in this survey was the benefit of reassurance that can be given to unaffected relatives. Similar observations are likely to be found in the dominant hypertension families.

Gene Therapy

As we enter the twenty-first century, the promise of benefits from gene therapy for human disease is analogous to what the anticipated benefits of commercial aviation might have been shortly after the Wright brothers' first flight at Kitty Hawk. For atherosclerotic diseases, the first short flight was launched in 1992 for a person with homozygous FH, although with very limited success.[271] In contrast, the future promise of gene therapy is a permanent cure for 10 million FH heterozygotes. Ongoing drug costs, side effects, and compliance issues could be things of the past. As other genetic diseases are clearly defined, they too could yield to complete eradication by gene therapy.

Basic technical challenges of gene therapy include obtaining a gene sequence with beneficial effects when expressed in the appropriate tissue, attaching the therapeutic DNA to a vehicle like a virus, and delivering the DNA in large numbers to cells where its effect is needed. These are not trivial tasks, but solutions to technical challenges often require time

before ingenious minds can forge the path from first flight to jet flight. Ongoing gene therapy research suggests potentially promising results for upregulating nitric oxide production in endothelium,[272] decreasing cholesterol levels in Apo-E–deficient mice,[273] efficient gene transfer to the liver using Apo-E3 peptides,[274] and promotion of reverse cholesterol transport with Apo-A–I Milano.[275]

Gene therapy has potential beyond replacing defective genes. It can override the effects of existing genes. It can carry the benefits of antiatherogenic genes from naturally protected humans to others born without this good fortune. Some speculate that within a few decades, we may well be writing prescriptions for genes, and that high-risk genes that now cause tragedy in some families will be conquered, and protective genes that now prevent atherosclerosis in a few lucky families may be shared with all those who need them. The social and economic factors, as well as perfection of the technology, may be the rate-limiting steps in applying this new science to individuals.

Summary

A large proportion of cardiovascular disease can be attributed to inherited or familial predisposition. Over the past few decades, important methods of studying these issues have been developed, including family studies to quantify familial aggregation, quantitative methods to study phenotype transmission, and examination of specific genes through linkage analysis or association studies. Genetic disorders leading to lipid problems, essential hypertension, type 2 diabetes, and obesity have been best studied. In order to apply genetic principles clinically, it is important to understand practical differences between monogenic and polygenic factors, and the interaction between genes and the environment. For certain genetic disorders such as familial hypercholesterolemia, international efforts have been launched to identify and treat cases worldwide. Finally, the refinement of techniques for, and application of, gene therapy holds potential promise for the treatment of certain genetic disorders and improved prevention of cardiovascular diseases, as we begin the twenty-first century.

APPENDIX 5–1 A QUESTIONNAIRE FOR OBTAINING A DETAILED LIPID FAMILY HISTORY[*]

Medical Family History   *This section is important. Please complete it as accurately as possible*

List all relatives, not just those with problems. Please make an effort to obtain as much information as possible. **Give approximate age for first occurrence or diagnosis for each disease or problem listed.** See the example provided. **You may need to call your relatives for missing information. Circle either Bro / Sis, Son / Dau, A / U for gender.**

BLOOD LEVELS: List the worst levels known - highest serum cholesterol, triglycerides. Approximate levels may be listed. Phone calls may be necessary to verify.

RELATIONSHIP	First Name	Living (L) or Dead (D)	Age (now or at death)	CAUSE OF DEATH IF DECEASED	AGE OF FIRST OCCURRENCE						CIGARETTES (Current (F)ormer (N)ever	WEIGHT (A)verage (O)verweight 50+ lbs	Total Cholesterol	Triglycerides	HDL Cholesterol
					HEART ATTACK	CORONARY BYPASS SURGERY	CORONARY ANGIOPLASTY (PTCA)	STROKE	HIGH BLOOD PRESSURE (treated)	DIABETES					
Example	John	D	70	Heart Attack	50	52			40		C	A	255	140	35
You															
Father															
Mother															
Bro / Sis															
Bro / Sis															
Bro / Sis															
Bro / Sis															
Bro / Sis															
Spouse															
Son / Dau															
Son / Dau															
Son / Dau															
Son / Dau															
Pat GF															
Pat GM															
Pat A / U															
Pat A / U															
Pat A / U															
Pat A / U															
Pat A / U															
Mat GF															
Mat GM															
Mat A / U															
Mat A / U															
Mat A / U															
Mat A / U															
Mat A / U															

[*]It may often take about 6 months of writing letters and making phone calls to collect all of this information from the relatives listed. Once collected, this information usually leads to a specific diagnosis and also identifies affected relatives needing treatment.

Key: Pat = paternal, Mat = maternal, GF = grandfather, GM = grandmother, A = aunt, U = uncle.

Source: Reproduced with permission from Cardiovascular Genetics Research, University of Utah, Salt Lake City, UT.

References

1. Mitchell BD, Dyke B: Use of genetic epidemiological methods to study complex genetic diseases. *Nutr Metab Cardiovasc Dis* 1997; 7:467–479.

2. Kee F, Tiret L, Robo JY, et al: Reliability of reported family history of myocardial infarction. *BMJ* 1993; 307:1528–1530.

3. Hopkins PN, Williams RR, Hunt SC: Magnified risks from cigarette smoking for coronary prone families in Utah. *West J Med* 1984; 141:196–202.

4. Hopkins PN, Williams RR, Kuida H, et al: Family history as an independent risk factor for incident coronary artery disease in a high-risk cohort in Utah. *Am J Cardiol* 1988; 62:703–707.

5. Hopkins PN, Williams RR: Human genetics and coronary heart disease: a public health perspective. *Annu Rev Nutr* 1989; 9:303–345.

6. Ciruzzi M, Schargrodsky H, Rozlosnik J, et al: Frequency of family history of acute myocardial infarction in patients with acute myocardial infarction. *Am J Cardiol* 1997; 80:122–127.

7. Friedlander Y, Siscovick DS, Weinmann S, et al: Family history as a risk factor for primary cardiac arrest. *Circulation* 1998; 97:155–160.

8. Marenberg ME, Risch N, Berkman LF, et al: Genetic susceptibility to death from coronary heart disease in a study of twins. *N Engl J Med* 1994; 330:1041–1046.

9. Hunt SC, Williams RR, Barlow GK: A comparison of positive family history definitions for defining risk of future disease. *J Chronic Dis* 1986; 39:809–821.

10. Hunt SC, Hasstedt SJ, Kuida H, et al: Genetic heritability and common environmental components of resting and stressed blood pressures, lipids, and body mass index in Utah pedigrees and twins. *Am J Epidemiol* 1989; 129:625–638.

11. Williams RR, Hasstedt SJ, Hunt SC, et al: Genetic traits related to hypertension and electrolyte metabolism. *Hypertension* 1991; 17(suppl I):I-69–I-73.

12. Hasstedt SJ, Wu LL, Ash KO, et al: Hypertension and sodium-lithium countertransport in Utah pedigrees: evidence for major-locus inheritance. *Am J Hum Genet* 1988; 43:14–22.

13. Hunt SC, Stephenson SH, Hopkins PN, et al: A prospective study of sodium-lithium countertransport and hypertension in Utah. *Hypertension* 1991; 17:1–7.

14. Berry TD, Hasstedt SJ, Hunt SC, et al: A gene for high urinary kallikrein may protect against hypertension in Utah kindreds. *Hypertension* 1989; 13:3–8.

15. Hunt SC, Hasstedt SJ, Wu LL, Williams RR: A gene-environment interaction between inferred kallikrein genotype and potassium. *Hypertension* 1993; 22:161–168.

16. Schumacher MC, Hasstedt SJ, Hunt SC, et al: Major gene effect for insulin levels in familial NIDDM pedigrees. *Diabetes* 1992; 41:416–423.

17. Hasstedt SJ, Ramirez ME, Hiroshi K, Williams RR: Recessive inheritance of a relative fat pattern. *Am J Hum Genet* 1989; 45:917–928.

18. Hasstedt SJ, Hunt SC, Wu LL, Williams RR: Evidence for multiple genes determining sodium transport. *Genet Epidemiol* 1994; 11:553–568.

19. Pritchard JK, Rosenberg NA: Use of unlinked genetic markers to detect population stratification in association studies. *Am J Hum Genet* 1999; 65:220–228.

20. Williams RR, Hasstedt SJ, Wilson DE, et al: Evidence that men with familial hypercholesterolemia can avoid early coronary death: an analysis of 77 gene carriers in four Utah pedigrees. *JAMA* 1986; 255:219–224.

21. Saarinen K, Swan H, Kainulainen K, et al: Molecular genetics of the long QT syndrome: two novel mutations of the KVLQT1 gene and phenotypic expression of the mutant gene in a large kindred. *Hum Mutat* 1998; 11:158–165.

22. Persu A, Barbry P, Bassilana F, et al: Genetic analysis of the beta subunit of the epithelial Na^+ channel in essential hypertension. *Hypertension* 1998; 32:129–137.

23. Lifton RP, Hunt SC, Williams RR, et al: Exclusion of the Na^+-H^+ antiporter as a candidate gene in human essential hypertension. *Hypertension* 1991; 17:8–14.

24. Jeunemaitre X, Lifton RP, Hunt SC, et al: Absence of linkage between the angiotensin converting enzyme and human essential hypertension. *Nature Genet* 1992; 1:72–75.

25. Jeunemaitre X, Charru A, Rigat B, et al: Sib pair linkage analysis of renin gene haplotypes in human essential hypertension. *Hum Genet* 88:301–306, 1992.

26. Hunt SC, Williams CS, Sharma AM, et al: Lack of linkage between the endothelial nitric oxide synthase gene and hypertension. *J Hum Hypertens* 1996; 10:27–30.

27. Haddad L, Day INM, Hunt S, et al: Evidence for a third genetic locus causing familial hypercholesterolaemia: a non-LDLR, non-ApoB kindred. *J Lipid Res* 1999; 40:1113–1122.

28. Varret M, Rabes JP, Saint-Jore B, et al: A third major locus for autosomal dominant hypercholesterolemia maps to 1p34.1-p32. *Am J Hum Genet* 1999; 64:1378–1387.

29. Hopkins PN, Wu LL, Williams RR: Dyslipidemias, in Noe DA, Rock RC (eds): *Laboratory Medicine: The Selection and Interpretation of Clinical Laboratory Studies.* Baltimore, Williams & Wilkins, 1994:476–511.

30. Wetterau JR, Aggerbeck LP, Bouma M-E, et al: Absence of microsomal triglyceride transfer protein in individuals with abetalipoproteinemia. *Science* 1992; 258:999–1001.

31. Wetterau JR, Gregg RE, Harrity TW, et al: An MTP inhibitor that normalizes atherogenic lipoprotein levels in WHHL rabbits. *Science* 1998; 282:751–754.

32. Wu J, Kim J, Li Q, Kwok PY, et al: Known mutations of apoB account for only a small minority of hypobetalipoproteinemia. *J Lipid Res* 1999; 40:955–959.

33. Hardman DA, Pullinger CR, Hamilton RL, et al: Molecular and metabolic basis for the metabolic disorder nor-

motriglyceridemic abetalipoproteinemia. *J Clin Invest* 1991; 88:1722–1729.

34. Pullinger CR, Hillas E, Hardman DA, et al: Two apolipo-protein B gene defects in a kindred with hypo-betalipoproteinemia, one of which results in a truncated variant, apoB-61, in VLDL and LDL. *J Lipid Res* 1992; 33:699–710.

35. Brunzell JD: Familial lipoprotein lipase deficiency and other causes of chylomicronemia syndrome. In: Scriver CR, Beaudet AL, Sly WS, Valle D (eds): *The Metabolic and Molecular Bases of Inherited Disease.* New York, McGraw-Hill, 1995:1913–1932.

36. Gianturco SH, Ramprasad MP, Song R, et al: Apolipo-protein B-48 or its apolipoprotein B-100 equivalent mediates the binding of triglyceride-rich lipoproteins to their unique human monocyte-macrophage receptor. *Arterioscler Thromb Vasc Biol* 1998; 18:968–976.

37. Nordestgaard BG, Zilversmit DB: Large lipoproteins are excluded from the arterial wall in diabetic cholesterol-fed rabbits. *J Lipid Res* 1988; 29:1491–1500.

38. Greenberg BH, Blackwelder WC, Levy RI: Primary type V hyperlipoproteinemia: a descriptive study in 32 families. *Ann Intern Med* 1977; 87:526–534.

39. Malekzadeh S, Dressler FA, Hoeg JM, et al: Left atrial endocardial lipid deposits and absent to minimal arterial lipid deposits in familial hyperchylomicronemia. *Am J Cardiol* 1991; 67:1431–1434.

40. Minnich A, Kessling A, Roy M, et al: Prevalence of alleles encoding defective lipoprotein lipase in hyper-triglyceridemic patients of French Canadian descent. *J Lipid Res* 1995; 36:117–124.

41. Li WW, Dammerman MM, Smith JD, et al: Common genetic variation in the promoter of the human apo CIII gene abolishes regulation by insulin and may contribute to hypertriglyceridemia. *J Clin Invest* 1995; 96:2601–2605.

42. Helio T, Palotie A, Sane T, et al: No evidence for linkage between familial hypertriglyceridemia and apolipoprotein B, apolipoprotein C-III or lipoprotein lipase genes. *Hum Genet* 1994; 94:271–278.

43. Santamarina-Fojo S, Dugi KA: Structure, function and role of lipoprotein lipase in lipoprotein metabolism. *Curr Opin Lipidol* 1994; 5:117–125.

44. Wilson DE, Emi M, Iverius PH, et al: Phenotypic expression of heterozygous lipoprotein lipase deficiency in the extended pedigree of a proband homozygous for a missense mutation. *J Clin Invest* 1990; 86:735–750.

45. Thorn JA, Chamberlain JC, Alcolado JC, et al: Lipoprotein and hepatic lipase gene variants in coronary atherosclerosis. *Atherosclerosis* 1990; 85:55–60.

46. Jukema JW, van Boven AJ, Groenemeijer B, et al: The Asp9 Asn mutation in the lipoprotein lipase gene is associated with increased progression of coronary atherosclerosis. *Circulation* 1996; 94:1913–1918.

47. Nordestgaard BG, Abildgaard S, Wittrup HH, et al: Heterozygous lipoprotein lipase deficiency: frequency in the general population, effect on plasma lipid levels, and risk of ischemic heart disease. *Circulation* 1997; 96:1737–1744.

48. Wittekoek ME, Pimstone SN, Reymer PWA, et al: A common mutation in the lipoprotein lipase gene (N291S) alters the lipoprotein phenotype and risk for cardiovascular disease in patients with familial hypercholesterolemia. *Circulation* 1998; 97:729–735.

49. Hunt SC, Province MA, Atwood LD, et al: No linkage of the lipoprotein lipase locus to hypertension in Caucasians. J Hypertens 1999; 17:39–43.

50. Fredrickson DS, Morganroth J, Levy RI: Type III hyperlipoproteinemia: an analysis of two contemporary definitions. *Ann Intern Med* 1975; 82:150–157.

51. Morganroth J, Levy RI, Fredrickson DS: The biochemical, clinical, and genetic features of type III hyperlipoproteinemia. *Ann Intern Med* 1975; 82:158–174.

52. LaRosa JC, Chambless LE, Criqui MH, et al: Patterns of dyslipoproteinemia in selected North American populations: the Lipid Research Clinics Program Prevalence Study. *Circulation* 1986; 73:1–12.

53. Goldstein J, Hazzard W, Schrott H: Hyperlipidemia in coronary heart disease: I. Lipid levels in 500 survivors of myocardial infarction. *J Clin Invest* 1973; 52:1533–1543.

54. Goldstein J, Schrott H, Hazzard W: Hyperlipidemia in coronary heart disease: II. Genetic analysis of lipid levels in 176 families and delineation of a new inherited disorder, combined hyperlipidemia. *J Clin Invest* 1973; 52:1544–1568.

55. Williams RR, Hopkins PN, Hunt SC, et al: Population-based frequency of dyslipidemia syndromes in coronary prone families in Utah. *Arch Intern Med* 1990; 150:582–588.

56. Hopkins PN, Wu LL, Williams RR, et al: Type III hyperlipidemia and lipoprotein remnants in early onset familial coronary artery disease. *Circulation* 1998; 98 (suppl I):I-791.

57. Mahley RW, Rall SC: Type III hyperlipoproteinemia (dysbetalipoproteinemia): the role of apolipoprotein E in normal and abnormal lipoprotein metabolism. In: Scriver CR, Beaudet AL, Sly WS, Valle D (eds): *The metabolic basis of inherited disease.* New York, McGraw Hill, 1989:1195–1213.

58. Hopkins PN, Wu LL, Schumacher MC, et al: Type III dyslipoproteinemia in patients heterozygous for familial hypercholesterolemia and apolipoprotein E2: evidence for a gene-gene interaction. *Arterioscler Thromb* 1991; 11:1137–1146.

59. Nakajima K, Saito T, Tamura A, et al: A new approach for the detection of type III hyperlipoproteinemia by RLP-cholesterol assay. *J Atheroscler Thromb* 1994; 1:30–36.

60. Mahley RW, Rall SC: Type III hyperlipoproteinemia (dysbetalipoproteinemia): the role of apolipoprotein E in normal and abnormal lipoprotein metabolism. In: Scriver

CR, Beaudet AL, Sly WS, Valle D (eds): *The Metabolic and Molecular Bases of Inherited Disease*. New York, McGraw-Hill, 1995:1953–1980.

61. Emi M, Hegele RM, Hopkins PN, et al: Effects of three genetic loci in a pedigree with multiple lipoprotein phenotypes. *Arteriosclerosis* 1991; 11:1349–1355.

62. Goldstein JL, Brown MS: Lipoprotein metabolism in the macrophage: implications for cholesterol deposition in atherosclerosis. *Annu Rev Biochem* 1983; 52:223–261.

63. Connelly PW, Maguire GF, Lee M, Little JA: Plasma lipoproteins in familial hepatic lipase deficiency. *Arteriosclerosis* 1990; 10:40–48.

64. Carlson LA, Holmquist L, Nilsson-Ehle P: Deficiency of hepatic lipase activity in post-heparin plasma in familial hypertriglyceridemia. *Acta Med Scand* 1986; 219:435–447.

65. Auwerx JH, Babirak SP, Hokanson JE, et al: Coexistence of abnormalities of hepatic lipase and lipoprotein lipase in a large family. *Am J Hum Genet* 1990; 46:470–477.

66. Demant T, Carlson LA, Holmquist L, et al: Lipoprotein metabolism in hepatic lipase deficiency: studies on the turnover of apolipoprotein B and on the effect of hepatic lipase on high density lipoprotein. *J Lipid Res* 1988; 29:1603–1611.

67. Hobbs HH, Russel DW, Brown MS, Goldstein JL: The LDL receptor locus in familial hypercholesterolemia: mutational analysis of a membrane protein. *Annu Rev Genet* 1990; 24:133–170.

68. Goldstein JL, Hobbs HH, Brown MS: Familial hyper-cholesterolemia. In: Scriver CR, Beaudet AL, Sly WS, Valle D (eds): *The Metabolic and Molecular Bases of Inherited Disease*. New York, McGraw-Hill, 1995:1981–2030.

69. World Health Organization Familial Hypercholesterolemia Consultation Group: *Familial Hypercholesterolemia: Report of a WHO Consultation*. Paris, World Health Organization, 1998.

70. Stone N, Levy R, Fredrickson D, Verter J: Coronary artery disease in 116 kindred with familial type II hyperlipoproteinemia. *Circulation* 1974; 49:476–488.

71. Mabuchi H, Miyamoto S, Ueda K, et al: Causes of death in patients with familial hypercholesterolemia. *Atherosclerosis* 1986; 61:1–6.

72. Kane JP, Malloy MJ, Ports TA, et al: Regression of coronary atherosclerosis during treatment of familial hypercholesterolemia with combined drug regimens. *JAMA* 1990; 264:3007–3012.

73. Thompson GR, Maher VMG, Matthews S, et al: Familial Hypercholesterolaemia Regression Study: a randomised trial of low-density-lipoprotein apheresis. *Lancet* 1995; 345:811–816.

74. Heiberg A, Slack J: Family similarities in the age at coronary death in familial hypercholesterolaemia. *BMJ* 1977; 2:493–495.

75. Innerarity TL, Weisgraber KH, Arnold KS, et al: Familial defective apolipoprotein B-100: low density lipoproteins with abnormal receptor binding. *Proc Natl Acad Sci USA* 1987; 84:6919–6923.

76. Innerarity TL, Mahley RW, Weisgraber KH, et al: Familial defective apolipoprotein B-100: a mutation of apolipoprotein B that causes hypercholesterolemia. *J Lipid Res* 1990; 31:1337–1349.

77. Ludwig EH, Hopkins PN, Allen A, et al: Association of genetic variations in apolipoprotein B with hypercholesterolemia, coronary artery disease, and receptor binding of low density lipoproteins. *J Lipid Res* 1997; 38:1361–1373.

78. Boren J, Lee I, Zhu W, et al: Identification of the low density lipoprotein receptor-binding site in apolipoprotein B100 and the modulation of its binding activity by the carboxyl terminus in familial defective apo-B100. *J Clin Invest* 1998; 101:1084–1093.

79. Boren J, Olin K, Lee I, et al: Identification of the principal proteoglycan-binding site in LDL. A single-point mutation in apo-B100 severely affects proteoglycan interaction without affecting LDL receptor binding. *J Clin Invest* 1998; 101:2658–2664.

80. Brugger D, Schuster H, Zollner N: Familial hypercholesterolemia and familial defective apolipoprotein B-100: comparison of the phenotypic expression in 116 cases. *Eur J Med Res* 1996; 1:383–386.

81. Funke H: Genetic determinants of high density lipoprotein levels. *Curr Opin Lipidol* 1997; 8:189–196.

82. Rader DJ, Ikewaki K, Duverger N, et al: Very low high-density lipoproteins without coronary atherosclerosis. *Lancet* 1993; 342:1455–1458.

83. Heimberg M, Van Harken DR, Brown TO: Hepatic lipid metabolism in experimental diabetes: II. Incorporation of [I-14C]palmitate into lipids of the liver and of the d less than 1.020 perfusate lipoproteins. *Biochim Biophys Acta* 1967; 137:435–445.

84. Nestel PJ, Poyser A: Changes in cholesterol synthesis and excretion when cholesterol intake is increased. *Atherosclerosis* 1979; 34:193–196.

85. Fielding PE, Fielding CJ, Havel RJ: Cholesterol net transport, esterification, and transfer in human hyperlipidemic plasma. *J Clin Invest* 1983; 71:449–460.

86. Inazu A, Brown ML, Hesler CB, et al: Increased high-density lipoprotein levels caused by a common cholesteryl-ester transfer protein gene mutation. *N Engl J Med* 1990; 323:1234–1238.

87. Inazu A, Jiang XC, Haraki T, et al: Genetic cholesteryl ester transfer protein deficiency caused by two prevalent mutations as a major determinant of increased levels of high density lipoprotein cholesterol. *J Clin Invest* 1994; 94:1872–1882.

88. Zhong S, Sharp DS, Grove JS, et al: Increased coronary heart disease in Japanese-American men with mutation in the cholesteryl ester transfer protein gene despite increased HDL levels. *J Clin Invest* 1996; 97:2917–2923.

89. Boerwinkle E, Leffert CC, Lin J, et al: Apolipoprotein (a) gene accounts for greater than 90% of the variation in

plasma lipoprotein (a) concentrations. *J Clin Invest* 1992; 90:52–60.

90. Stein JH, Rosenson RS: Lipoprotein Lp(a) excess and coronary heart disease. *Arch Intern Med* 1997; 157:1170–1176.

91. Espeland MA, Marcovina SM, Miller V, et al for the PEPI Investigators. Effect of postmenopausal hormone therapy on lipoprotein(a) concentration. *Circulation* 1998; 97:979–986.

92. Hopkins PN, Wu LL, Hunt SC, et al: Lipoprotein(a) interactions with lipid and non-lipid risk factors in early familial coronary artery disease. *Arterioscler Thromb Vasc Biol* 1997; 17:2783–2792.

93. Hopkins PN, Hunt SC, Schreiner PJ, et al: Lipoprotein(a) interactions with lipid and non-lipid risk factors in patients with early onset coronary artery disease: results from the NHLBI Family Heart Study. *Atherosclerosis* 1998; 141:333–345.

94. Seed M, Hoppichler F, Reaveley D, et al: Relation of serum lipoprotein (a) concentration and apolipoprotein (a) phenotype to coronary heart disease in patients with familial hypercholesterolemia. *N Engl J Med* 1990; 322:1494–1499.

95. Maher VMG, Kitano Y, Neuwirth C, et al: Lp(a) and coronary atherosclerosis in familial hypercholesterolaemia. *Arterioscler Thromb* 1991; 11:1520.

96. Ridker PM, Hennekens CH, Stampfer MJ: A prospective study of lipoprotein(a) and the risk of myocardial infarction. *JAMA* 1993; 270:2195–2199.

97. Maher VMG, Brown BG, Marcovina SM, et al: Effects of lowering elevated LDL cholesterol on the cardiovascular risk of lipoprotein(a). *JAMA* 1995; 274:1771–1774.

98. Maher MG, Brown B: Lipoprotein (a) and coronary heart disease. *Curr Opin Lipidol* 1995; 6:229–235.

99. Armstrong VW, Cremer P, Eberle E, et al: The association between serum Lp(a) concentrations and angiographically assessed coronary atherosclerosis: dependence on serum LDL levels. *Atherosclerosis* 1986; 62:249–257.

100. Cambillau M, Simon A, Amar J, et al: Serum Lp(a) as a discriminant marker of early atherosclerotic plaque at three extracoronary sites in hypercholesterolemic men: the PCVMETRA Group. *Arterioscler Thromb* 1992; 12:1346–1352.

101. Solymoss BC, Marcil M, Wesolowska E, et al: Relation of coronary artery disease in women <60 years of age to the combined elevation of serum lipoprotein (a) and total cholesterol to high-density cholesterol ratio. *Am J Cardiol* 1993; 72:1215–1219.

102. Williams RR, Hunt SC, Hopkins PN, et al: Genetic basis of familial dyslipidemia and hypertension: 15-year results from Utah. *Am J Hypertens* 1993; 6:319S–327S.

103. Genest JJ, Martin-Munley SS, McNamara JR, et al: Familial lipoprotein disorders in patients with premature coronary artery disease. *Circulation* 1992; 85:2025–2033.

104. Genest JJ, McNamara JR, Salem DN, Schaefer EJ: Prevalence of risk factors in men with premature coronary artery disease. *Am J Cardiol* 1991; 67:1185–1189.

105. Hazzard W, Goldstein J, Schrott H: Hyperlipidemia in coronary heart disease: III. Evaluation of lipoprotein phenotypes of 156 genetically defined survivors of myocardial infarction. *J Clin Invest* 1973; 52:1569–1577.

106. Kesaniemi YA, Grundy SM: Significance of low density lipoprotein production in the regulation of plasma cholesterol level in man. *J Clin Invest* 1982; 70:13–22.

107. Turner PR, Konarska R, Revill J, et al: Metabolic study of variation in plasma cholesterol level in normal men. *Lancet* 1984; 2:663–665.

108. Grundy SM, Vega GL, Bilheimer DW: Kinetic mechanisms determining variability in low density lipoprotein levels and rise with age. *Arteriosclerosis* 1985; 5:623–630.

109. Davignon J, Gregg RE, Sing CF: Apolipoprotein E polymorphism and atherosclerosis. *Arteriosclerosis* 1988; 8:1–21.

110. Lefevre M, Ginsberg HN, Kris-Etherton PM, et al: ApoE genotype does not predict lipid response to changes in dietary saturated fatty acids in a heterogeneous normolipidemic population: the DELTA Research Group—Dietary Effects on Lipoproteins and Thrombogenic Activity. *Arterioscler Thromb Vasc Biol* 1997; 17:2914–2923.

111. Aouizerat BE, Allayee H, Bodnar J, et al: Novel genes for familial combined hyperlipidemia. *Curr Opin Lipidol* 1999; 10:113–122.

112. Cortner JA, Coates PM, Liacouras CA, Jarvik GP: Familial combined hyperlipidemia in children: clinical expression, metabolic defects, and management. *J Pediatr* 1993; 123:177–184.

113. Sane T, Nikkila EA: Very low density lipoprotein triglyceride metabolism in relatives of hypertriglyceridemic probands. *Arteriosclerosis* 1988; 8:217–226.

114. Aguilar-Salinas CA, Hugh P, Barrett R, et al: A familial combined hyperlipidemic kindred with impaired apolipoprotein B catabolism: kinetics of apolipoprotein B during placebo and pravastatin therapy. *Arterioscler Thromb Vasc Biol* 1997; 17:72–82.

115. Babirak SP, Iverius PH, Fujimoto WY, Brunzell JD: Detection and characterization of the heterozygote state for lipoprotein lipase deficiency. *Arteriosclerosis* 1989; 9:326–334.

116. Beisiegel U, Weber W, Bengtsson-Olivecrona G: Lipoprotein lipase enhances the binding of chylomicrons to low density lipoprotein receptor-related protein. *Proc Natl Acad Sci USA* 1991; 88:8342–8346.

117. Williams KJ, Petrie KA, Brocia RW, Swenson TL: Lipoprotein lipase modulates net secretory output of apolipoprotein B in vitro: a possible pathophysiologic explanation for familial combined hyperlipidemia. *J Clin Invest* 1991; 88:1300–1306.

118. Sniderman A, Vu H, Cianflone K: Effect of moderate hypertriglyceridemia on the relation of plasma total and LDL apo B levels. *Atherosclerosis* 1991; 89:109–116.

119. Sniderman A, Teng B, Genest J, et al: Familial aggregation and early expression of hyperapobetalipoproteinemia. *Am J Cardiol* 1985; 55:291–295.

120. Austin MA, Breslow JL, Hennekens CH, et al: Low-density lipoprotein subclass patterns and risk of myocardial infarction. *JAMA* 1988; 260:1917–1921.

121. Austin MA, King MC, Vranizan KM, Krauss RM: Atherogenic lipoprotein phenotype: a proposed genetic marker for coronary heart disease risk. *Circulation* 1990; 82:495–506.

122. Griffin BA, Freeman DJ, Tait GW, et al: Role of plasma triglyceride in the regulation of plasma low density lipoprotein (LDL) subfractions: relative contribution of small, dense LDL to coronary heart disease risk. *Atherosclerosis* 1994; 106:241–253.

123. Gardner CD, Fortmann SP, Krauss RM: Association of small low-density lipoprotein particles with the incidence of coronary artery disease in men and women. *JAMA* 1996; 276:875–881.

124. Stampfer MJ, Krauss RM, Ma J, et al: A prospective study of triglyceride level, low-density lipoprotein particle diameter, and risk of myocardial infarction. *JAMA* 1996; 276:882–888.

125. Lamarche B, Tchernof A, Moorjani S, et al: Small, dense low-density lipoprotein particles as a predictor of the risk of ischemic heart disease in men: prospective results from the Québec Cardiovascular Study. *Circulation* 1997; 95:69–75.

126. Lamarche B, Tchernof A, Mauriege P, et al: Fasting insulin and apolipoprotein B levels and low-density lipoprotein particle size as risk factors for ischemic heart disease. *JAMA* 1998; 279:1955–1961.

127. Tribble DL, Krauss RM, Lansberg MG, et al: Greater oxidative susceptibility of the surface monolayer in small dense LDL may contribute to differences in copper induced oxidation among LDL density subfractions. *J Lipid Res* 1995; 36:662–671.

128. Superko HR: What can we learn about dense low density lipoprotein and lipoprotein particles from clinical trials? *Curr Opin Lipidol* 1996; 7:363–368.

129. Williams RR, Hunt SC, Hopkins PN, et al: Familial dyslipidemic hypertension: evidence from 58 Utah families for a syndrome present in approximately 12% of patients with essential hypertension. *JAMA* 1988; 259:3579–3586.

130. Hunt SC, Wu LL, Hopkins PN, et al: Apolipoprotein, low density lipoprotein subfraction, and insulin associations with familial combined hyperlipidemia: study of Utah patients with familial dyslipidemic hypertension. *Arteriosclerosis* 1989; 9:335–344.

131. Hopkins PN, Hunt SC, Wu LL, et al: Hypertension, dyslipidemia, and insulin resistance: links in a chain or spokes on a wheel? *Curr Opin Lipidol* 1996; 7:241–253.

132. Kaplan NM: The deadly quartet: upper-body obesity, glucose intolerance, hypertriglyceridemia, and hypertension. *Arch Intern Med* 1989; 149:1514–1520.

133. Hall JE, Brands MW, Zappe DH, Alonso Galicia M: Insulin resistance, hyperinsulinemia, and hypertension: causes, consequences, or merely correlations? *Proc Soc Exp Biol Med* 1995; 208:317–329.

134. Hong Y, Pedersen NL, Brismar K, de Faire U: Genetic and environmental architecture of the features of the insulin-resistance syndrome. *Am J Hum Genet* 1997; 60:143–152.

135. Selby JV, Newman B, Quiroga J, et al: Concordance for dyslipidemic hypertension in male twins. *JAMA* 1991; 265:2079–2084.

136. Williams RR, Hunt SC, Wu LL, et al: Dyslipidemic hypertension in families with hypertension, non-insulin-dependent diabetes mellitus, and coronary heart disease. *Atheroscler Rev* 1991; 22:107–111.

137. Lifton RP, Dluhy RG, Powers M, et al: A chimaeric 11β-hydroxylase/aldosterone synthase gene causes glucocorticoid-remediable aldosteronism and human hypertension. *Nature* 1992; 355:262–265.

138. Shimkets RA, Warnock DG, Bositis CM, et al: Liddle's syndrome: heritable human hypertension caused by mutations in the β subunit of the epithelial sodium channel. *Cell* 1994; 79:407–414.

139. Scheinman SJ, Guay-Woodford LM, Thakker RV, Warnock DG: Genetic disorders of renal electrolyte transport. *N Engl J Med* 1999; 340:1177–1187.

140. Garrison RJ, Kannel WB, Stokes J, Castelli WP: Incidence and precursors of hypertension in young adults: the Framingham Offspring Study. *Prev Med* 1987; 16:235–251.

141. INTERSALT Cooperative Research Group. INTERSALT: an international study of electrolyte excretion and blood pressure: results for 24 hour urinary sodium and potassium excretion. *BMJ* 1988; 297:319–328.

142. Law MR, Frost CD, Wald NJ: By how much does dietary salt reduction lower blood pressure? I. Analysis of observational data among populations. *BMJ* 1991; 302:811–815.

143. Frost CD, Law MR, Wald NJ. By how much does dietary salt reduction lower blood pressure? II. Analysis of observational data within populations. *BMJ* 1991; 302:815–818.

144. Law MR, Frost CD, Wald NJ: By how much does dietary salt reduction lower blood pressure? III. Analysis of data from trials of salt reduction. *BMJ* 1991; 302:819–824.

145. Cutler JA, Follmann D, Allender PS: Randomized trials of sodium reduction: an overview. *Am J Clin Nutr* 1997; 65 (suppl):643S–651S.

146. Working Group on Primary Prevention of Hypertension: National High Blood Pressure Education Program Working Group report on primary prevention of hypertension. *Arch Intern Med* 1993; 153:186–208.

147. Joint National Committee on Prevention, Detection, Evaluation, and Treatment of High Blood Pressure: The

sixth report of the Joint National Committee on Prevention, Detection, Evaluation, and Treatment of High Blood Pressure. *Arch Intern Med* 1997; 157:2413–2446.

148. Guyton AC, Hall JE, Coleman TG, Manning RD, Norman RA: The dominant role of the kidney in long-term arterial pressure regulation in normal and hypertensive states. In: Laragh JH, Brenner BM (eds): Hypertension: pathophysiology, diagnosis, and management. New York, Raven Press, 1995:1311–1326.

149. Ward R: Familial aggregation and genetic epidemiology of blood pressure. In: Laragh JH, Brenner BM (eds): Hypertension: pathophysiology, diagnosis, and management. New York: Raven Press, 1995:67–88.

150. Hamilton M, Pickering GW, Roberts JA, Sowry GSC: The aetiology of essential hypertension: 1. The arterial pressure in the general population. *Clin Sci* 1954; 13:11–35.

151. Hamilton M, Pickering GW, Roberts JA, Sowry GSC: The aetiology of essential hypertension: 2. Scores for arterial blood pressures adjusted for differences in age and sex. *Clin Sci* 1954; 13:37–49.

152. Hamilton M, Pickering GW, Roberts JAF, Sowry GSC: The aetiology of essential hypertension: 4. The role of inheritance. *Clin Sci* 1954; 13:273–304.

153. Rapp JP: The search for the genetic basis of blood pressure variation in rats. In: Laragh JH, Brenner BM (eds): Hypertension: pathophysiology, diagnosis, and management. New York, Raven Press, 1995:1289–1300.

154. Jeunemaitre X, Soubrier P, Kotelevtsev YV, et al: Molecular basis of human hypertension: role of angiotensinogen. *Cell* 1992; 71:169–180.

155. Caulfield M, Lavender P, Farrall M, et al: Linkage of the angiotensinogen gene to essential hypertension. *N Engl J Med* 1994; 330:1629–1633.

156. Caulfield M, Lavender P, Newell-Price J, et al: Linkage of the angiotensinogen gene locus to human essential hypertension in African Caribbeans. *J Clin Invest* 1995; 96:687–692.

157. Caulfield M, Lavender P, Newell-Price J, et al: Angiotensinogen in human essential hypertension. *Hypertension* 1996; 28:1123–1125.

158. Hunt SC, Hopkins PN, Williams RR: Hypertension: genetics and mechanisms. In: Fuster V, Ross R, Topol EJ (eds): *Atherosclerosis and Coronary Artery Disease.* Philadelphia, Lippincott-Raven, 1996:209–235.

159. Johnson AG, Simons LA, Friedlander Y, et al: M235ØT polymorphism of the angiotensinogen gene predicts hypertension in the elderly. *J Hypertens* 1996; 14:1061–1065.

160. Inoue I, Nakajima T, Williams CS, et al: A nucleotide substitution in the promoter of human angiotensinogen is associated with essential hypertension and affects basal transcription in vitro. *J Clin Invest* 1997; 99:1786–1797.

161. Rotimi C, Cooper R, Ogunbiyi O, et al: Hypertension, serum angiotensinogen, and molecular variants of the angiotensinogen gene among Nigerians. *Circulation* 1997; 95:2348–2350.

162. Bloem LJ, Foroud TM, Ambrosius WT, et al: Association of the angiotensinogen gene to serum angiotensinogen in blacks and whites. *Hypertension* 1997; 29:1078–1082.

163. Hegele RA, Harris SB, Hanley AJG, et al: Angiotensinogen gene variation associated with variation in blood pressure in aboriginal Canadians. *Hypertension* 1997; 29:1073–1077.

164. Schunkert H, Hense H-W, Gimenez-Roqueplo A, et al: The angiotensinogen T235 variant and the use of antihypertensive drugs in a population-based cohort. *Hypertension* 1997; 29:628–633.

165. Borecki IB, Province MA, Ludwig EH, et al: Associations of candidate loci angiotensinogen and angiotensin-converting enzyme with severe hypertension: the NHLBI Family Heart Study. *Ann Epidemiol* 1997; 7:13–21.

166. Kunz R, Kreutz R, Beige J, et al: Association between the angiotensinogen 235T-variant and essential hypertension in whites: a systematic review and methodological appraisal. *Hypertension* 1997; 30:1331–1337.

167. Brand E, Chatelain N, Keavney B, et al: Evaluation of the angiotensinogen locus in human essential hypertension: a European study. *Hypertension* 1998; 31:725–729.

168. Cooper R, Rotimi C, Ogunbiyi O, Ward R: Angiotensinogen genotype, serum level and hypertension in blacks (abstr). *Am J Hypertens* 1997; 10:33A.

169. Pratt JH, Ambrosius WT, Tewksbury DA, et al: Serum angiotensinogen concentration in relation to gonadal hormones, body size, and genotype in growing young people. *Hypertension* 1998; 32:875–879.

170. Walker WG, Whelton PK, Saito H, et al: Relation between blood pressure and renin, renin substrate, angiotensin II, aldosterone and urinary sodium and potassium in 574 ambulatory subjects. *Hypertension* 1979; 1:287–291.

171. Hopkins PN, Lifton RP, Hollenberg NK, et al: Blunted renal vascular response to angiotensin II is associated with a common variant of the angiotensinogen gene and obesity. *J Hypertens* 1996; 14:199–207.

172. The Trials of Hypertension Prevention Collaborative Research Group: Effects of weight loss and sodium reduction intervention on blood pressure and hypertension incidence in overweight people with high-normal blood pressure: the Trials of Hypertension Prevention, Phase II. *Arch Intern Med* 1997; 157:657–667.

173. Hunt SC, Cook NR, Oberman A, et al: Angiotensinogen genotype, sodium reduction, weight loss, and prevention of hypertension: Trials of Hypertension Prevention, Phase II. *Hypertension* 1998; 32:393–401.

174. Hunt SC, Geleijnse JM, Wu LL, et al: Enhanced blood pressure response to mild sodium reduction in subjects with the 235T variant of the angiotensinogen gene. *Am J Hypertens* 1999; 12:460–466.

175. Cusi D, Barlassina C, Azzani T, et al: Polymorphisms of α-adducin and salt sensitivity in patients with essential hypertension. *Lancet* 1997; 349:1353–1357.

176. Tripodi G, Valtorta F, Torielli L, et al: Hypertension-associated point mutations in the adducin alpha and beta subunits affect actin cytoskeleton and ion transport. *J Clin Invest* 1996; 97:2815–2822.

177. Manunta P, Cusi D, Barlassina C, et al: Alpha-adducin polymorphisms and renal sodium handling in essential hypertensive patients. *Kidney Int* 1998; 53:1471–1478.

178. Tamaki S, Iwai N, Tsujita Y, et al: Polymorphism of alpha-adducin in Japanese patients with essential hypertension. *Hypertens Res* 1998; 21:29–32.

179. Kamitani A, Wong ZY, Fraser R, et al: Human alpha-adducin gene, blood pressure, and sodium metabolism. *Hypertension* 1998; 32:138–143.

180. Kato N, Sugiyama T, Nabika T, et al: Lack of association between the alpha-adducin locus and essential hypertension in the Japanese population. *Hypertension* 1998; 31:730–733.

181. Wang WY, Adams DJ, Glenn CL, Morris BJ: The Gly460Trp variant of alpha-adducin is not associated with hypertension in white Anglo-Australians. *Am J Hypertens* 1999; 12:632–636.

182. Ishikawa K, Katsuya T, Sato N, et al: No association between alpha-adducin 460 polymorphism and essential hypertension in a Japanese population. *Am J Hypertens* 1998; 11:502–506.

183. Hopkins PN, Williams RR: Identification and relative weight of cardiovascular risk factors. *Cardiol Clin* 1986; 4:3–31.

184. Haffner SM, Stern MP, Hazuda HP, et al: Cardiovascular risk factors in confirmed prediabetic individuals: does the clock for coronary heart disease start ticking before the onset of clinical diabetes? *JAMA* 1990; 263:2893–2898.

185. Morwessel NJ: The genetic basis of diabetes mellitus. *AACN Clin Issues* 1998; 9:539–554.

186. Ghosh S, Schork NJ: Genetic analysis of NIDDM: the study of quantitative traits. *Diabetes* 1996; 45:1–14.

187. Ravussin E, Valencia ME, Esparza J, et al: Effects of a traditional lifestyle on obesity in Pima Indians. *Diabetes Care* 1994; 17:1067–1074.

188. Pratley RE: Gene-environment interactions in the pathogenesis of type 2 diabetes mellitus: lessons learned from the Pima Indians. *Proc Nutr Soc* 1998; 57:175–181.

189. Knowler W, Bennett P, Ballintine E: Increased incidence of retinopathy in diabetics with elevated blood pressure: a six-year follow-up study in Pima Indians. *N Engl J Med* 1980; 302:645–650.

190. Neel JV: Diabetes mellitus: a "thrifty" genotype rendered detrimental by "progress"? *Am J Hum Genet* 1962; 14:353–362.

191. Ferrannini E: Insulin resistance versus insulin deficiency in non-insulin-dependent diabetes mellitus: problems and prospects. *Endocrinol Rev* 1998; 19:477–490.

192. DeFronzo RA, Ferrannini E: Insulin resistance: a multi-faceted syndrome responsible for NIDDM, obesity, hypertension, dyslipidemia, and atherosclerotic cardiovascular disease. *Diabetes Care* 1991; 14:173–194.

193. Pimenta W, Korytkowski M, Mitrakou A, et al: Pancreatic beta cell dysfunction as the primary genetic lesion in NIDDM. Evidence from studies in normal glucose tolerant individuals with a first degree NIDDM relative. *JAMA* 1995; 273:1855–1861.

194. Polonsky KS, Sturis J, Bell GI: Non-insulin-dependent diabetes mellitus—a genetically programmed failure of the beta cell to compensate for insulin resistance. *N Engl J Med* 1996; 334:777–783.

195. Walston J, Silver K, Bogardus C, et al: Time of onset of non-insulin-dependent diabetes mellitus and genetic variation in the β_3-adrenergic-receptor gene. *N Engl J Med* 1995; 333:343–347.

196. Sakane N, Yoshida T, Umekawa T, et al: Beta 3-adrenergic-receptor polymorphism: a genetic marker for visceral fat obesity and the insulin resistance syndrome. *Diabetologia* 1997; 40:200–204.

197. Yamada K, Ishiyama-Shigemoto S, Ichikawa F, et al: Polymorphism in the 5′-leader cistron of the beta2-adrenergic receptor gene associated with obesity and type 2 diabetes. *J Clin Endocrinol Metab* 1999; 84:1754–1757.

198. Schalin-Jäntti C, Nikula-Ijäs P, Huang X, et al: Polymorphism of the glycogen synthase gene in hypertensive and normotensive subjects. *Hypertension* 1996; 27:67–71.

199. Seldin MF, Mott D, Bhat D, et al: Glycogen synthase: a putative locus for diet-induced hyperglycemia. *J Clin Invest* 1994; 94:269–276.

200. Groop LC, Kankuri M, Schalin-Jäntti C, et al: Association between polymorphism of the glycogen synthase gene and non-insulin-dependent diabetes mellitus. *N Engl J Med* 1993; 328:10–14.

201. Hani EH, Clement K, Velho G, et al: Genetic studies of the sulfonylurea receptor gene locus in NIDDM and in morbid obesity among French Caucasians. *Diabetes* 1997; 46:688–694.

202. Fleury C, Neverova M, Collins S, et al: Uncoupling protein-2: a novel gene linked to obesity and hyperinsulinemia. *Nature Genet* 1997; 15:269–272.

203. Elbein SC, Leppert M, Hasstedt S: Uncoupling protein 2 region on chromosome 11q13 is not linked to markers of obesity in familial type 2 diabetes. *Diabetes* 1997; 46:2105–2107.

204. Urhammer SA, Dalgaard LT, Sorensen TI, et al: Mutational analysis of the coding region of the uncoupling protein 2 gene in obese NIDDM patients: impact of a common amino acid polymorphism on juvenile and maturity onset forms of obesity and insulin resistance. *Diabetologia* 1997; 40:1227–1230.

205. Shiinoki T, Suehiro T, Ikeda Y, et al: Screening for variants of the uncoupling protein 2 gene in Japanese patients with non-insulin-dependent diabetes mellitus. *Metabolism* 1999; 48:581–584.

206. Cassell PG, Neverova M, Janmohamed S, et al: An uncoupling protein 2 gene variant is associated with a raised body mass index but not type II diabetes. *Diabetologia* 1999; 42:688–692.

207. Pedersen O: Genetics of insulin resistance. *Exp Clin Endocrinol Diabetes* 1999; 107:113–118.

208. Hansen L, Fjordvang H, Rasmussen SK, et al: Mutational analysis of the coding regions of the genes encoding protein kinase B-alpha and -beta, phosphoinositide-dependent protein kinase-1, phosphatase targeting to glycogen, protein phosphatase inhibitor-1, and glycogenin: lessons from a search for genetic variability of the insulin-stimulated glycogen synthesis pathway of skeletal muscle in NIDDM patients. *Diabetes* 1999; 48:403–407.

209. Taylor SI, Moller DE: Mutations of the insulin receptor gene. In: Moller DE (ed): Insulin resistance. Chichester, England, Wiley, 1993:83–121.

210. Kahn CR, Vicent D, Doria A: Genetics of non-insulin-dependent (type II) diabetes mellitus. *Annu Rev Med* 1996; 47:509–531.

211. Kan M, Kanai F, Iida M, et al: Frequency of mutations of insulin receptor gene in Japanese patients with NIDDM. *Diabetes* 1995; 44:1081–1086.

212. Velho G, Froguel P, Clement K, et al: Primary pancreatic beta-cell secretory defect caused by mutations in glucokinase gene in kindreds of maturity onset diabetes of the young. *Lancet* 1992; 340:444–448.

213. Vaxillaire M, Rouard M, Yamagata K, et al: Identification of nine novel mutations in the hepatocyte nuclear factor 1 alpha gene associated with maturity-onset diabetes of the young (MODY3). *Hum Mol Genet* 1997; 6:583–586.

214. Velho G, Froguel P: Genetic determinants of non-insulin-dependent diabetes mellitus: strategies and recent results. *Diabetes Metab* 1997; 23:7–17.

215. Aitman TJ, Todd JA: Molecular genetics of diabetes mellitus. *Baillieres Clin Endocrinol Metab* 1995; 9: 631–656.

216. Zouali H, Vaxillaire M, Lesage S, et al: Linkage analysis and molecular scanning of glucokinase gene in NIDDM families. *Diabetes* 1993; 42:1238–1245.

217. Elbein SC, Chiu KC, Hoffman MD, et al: Linkage analysis of 19 candidate regions for insulin resistance in familial NIDDM. *Diabetes* 1995; 44:1259–1265.

218. Vionnet N, Hani EH, Lesage S, et al: Genetics of NIDDM in France: studies with 19 candidate genes in affected sib pairs. *Diabetes* 1997; 46:1062–1068.

219. Lesage S, Zouali H, Vionnet N, et al: Genetic analyses of glucose transporter genes in French non-insulin-dependent diabetic families. *Diabetes Metab* 1997; 23:137–142.

220. Lepretre F, Vionnet N, Budhan S, et al: Genetic studies of polymorphisms in ten non-insulin-dependent diabetes mellitus candidate genes in Tamil Indians from Pondichery. *Diabetes Metab* 1998; 24:244–250.

221. Hanson RL, Elston RC, Pettitt DJ, et al: Segregation analysis of non-insulin-dependent diabetes mellitus in Pima Indians: evidence for a major-gene effect. *Am J Hum Genet* 1995; 57:160–170.

222. Permutt MA, Chiu K, Ferrer J, et al: Genetics of type II diabetes. *Recent Prog Horm Res* 1998; 53:201–216.

223. Hanis CL, Boerwinkle E, Chakraborty R, et al: A genome-wide search for human non-insulin-dependent (type 2) diabetes genes reveals a major susceptibility locus on chromosome 2. *Nature Genet* 1996; 13:161.

224. Elbein SC, Hoffman MD, Teng K, et al: A genome-wide search for type 2 diabetes susceptibility genes in Utah Caucasians. *Diabetes* 1999; 48:1175–1182.

225. Pratley RE, Thompson DB, Prochazka M, et al: An autosomal genomic scan for loci linked to prediabetic phenotypes in Pima Indians. *J Clin Invest* 1998; 101:1757–1764.

226. Bouchard C: Current understanding of the etiology of obesity: genetic and nongenetic factors. *Am J Clin Nutr* 1991; 53:1561S–1565S.

227. Rice T, Sjostrom CD, Perusse L, et al: Segregation analysis of body mass index in a large sample selected for obesity: the Swedish Obese Subjects study. *Obes Res* 1999; 7:246–255.

228. Pietilainen KH, Kaprio J, Rissanen A, et al: Distribution and heritability of BMI in Finnish adolescents aged 16y and 17y: a study of 4884 twins and 2509 singletons. *Int J Obes Relat Metab Disord* 1999; 23:107–115.

229. Stunkard AJ, Sorensen TIA, Hanis G, et al: An adoption study of human obesity. *N Engl J Med* 1986; 314:193–198.

230. Bouchard C, Tremblay A, Despres JP, et al: The response to long-term overfeeding in identical twins. *N Engl J Med* 1990; 322:1477–1482.

231. Bouchard C, Perusse L, Leblanc C, et al: Inheritance of the amount and distribution of human body fat. *Int J Obes* 1988; 12:205–215.

232. Borecki IB, Rice T, Pérusse L, et al: Major gene influence on the propensity to store fat in trunk versus extremity depots: evidence from the Québec Family Study. *Obes Res* 1995; 3:1–8.

233. Burns TL, Donohoue PA, Leibel R: Identification of obesity genes using sib-pair linkage analysis: the Muscatine Study. *Circulation* 1995; 91:929.

234. Hegele Ra, Brunt J, Connelly PW: Genetic variation on chromosome 1 associated with variation in body fat distribution in men. *Circulation* 1995; 92:1089–1093.

235. Andersson L, Haley CS, Ellegren H, et al: Genetic mapping of quantitative trait loci for growth and fatness in pigs. *Science* 1994; 263:1771–1774.

236. Widén E, Lehto M, Kanninea T, et al: Association of a polymorphism in the β_3-adrenergic-receptor gene with features of the insulin resistance syndrome in Finns. *N Engl J Med* 1995; 333:348–351.

237. Perusse L, Chagnon YC, Weisnagel J, Bouchard C: The human obesity gene map: the 1998 update. *Obes Res* 1999; 7:111–129.

238. Lee JH, Reed DR, Li WD, et al: Genome scan for human obesity and linkage to markers in 20q13. *Am J Hum Genet* 1999; 64:196–209.

239. Comuzzie AG, Hixson JE, Almasy L, et al: A major quantitative trait locus determining serum leptin levels and fat mass is located on human chromosome 2. *Nature Genet* 1997; 15:273–276.

240. Norman RA, Thompson DB, Foroud T, et al: Genomewide search for genes influencing percent body fat in Pima Indians: suggestive linkage at chromosome 11q21-q22. *Am J Hum Genet* 1997; 60:166–173.

241. Chagnon YC, Chung WK, Perusse L, et al: Linkages and associations between the leptin receptor (LEPR) gene and human body composition in the Quebec Family Study. *Int J Obes Relat Metab Disord* 1999; 23:278–286.

242. McCully KS: Homocysteine and vascular disease. *Nature Med* 1996; 2:386–389.

243. Wu LL, Wu J, Hunt SC, et al: Plasma homocyst(e)ine as a risk factor for early familial coronary artery disease. *Clin Chem* 1994; 40:552–561.

244. Hopkins PN, Wu LL, Wu J, et al: Higher plasma homocyst(e)ine and increased susceptibility to adverse effects of low folate in early familial coronary artery disease. *Arterioscler Thromb Vasc Biol* 1995; 15:1314–1329.

245. Graham IM, Daly LE, Refsum HM, et al: Plasma homocysteine as a risk factor for vascular disease: the European Concerted Action Project. *JAMA* 1997; 277:1775–1781.

246. den Heijer M, Brouwer IA, Bos GMJ, et al: Vitamin supplementation reduces blood homocysteine levels: a controlled trial in patients with venous thrombosis and healthy volunteers. *Arterioscler Thromb Vasc Biol* 1998; 18:356–361.

247. Christensen B, Frosst P, Lussier-Cacan S, et al: Correlation of a common mutation in the methylenetetrahydrofolate reductase gene with plasma homocysteine in patients with premature coronary artery disease. *Arterioscler Thromb Vasc Biol* 1997; 17:569–573.

248. Gudnason V, Stansbie D, Scott J, et al on behalf of the EARS group: C677T (thermolabile alanine/valine) polymorphism in methylenetetrahydrofolate reductase (MTHFR): its frequency and impact on plasma homocysteine concentration in different European populations. *Atherosclerosis* 1998; 136:347–354.

249. Adams M, Smith PD, Martin D, et al: Genetic analysis of thermolabile methylenetetrahydrofolate reductase as a risk factor for myocardial infarction. *Q J Med* 1996; 89:437–444.

250. Morita H, Taguchi J-i, Kurihara H, et al: Genetic polymorphism of 5,10-methylenetetrahydrofolate reductase (MTHFR) as a risk factor for coronary artery disease. *Circulation* 1997; 95:2032–2036.

251. Kluijtmans LAJ, Kastelein JJP, Lindemans J, et al: Thermolabile methylenetetrahydrofolate reductase in coronary artery disease. *Circulation* 1997; 96:2573–2577.

252. Clarke R, Daly L, Robinson K, et al: Hyperhomocysteinemia: an independent risk factor for vascular disease. *N Engl J Med* 1991; 324:1149–1155.

253. Kluijtmans LA, Boers GH, Kraus JP, et al: The molecular basis of cystathionine beta-synthase deficiency in Dutch patients with homocystinuria: effect of CBS genotype on biochemical and clinical phenotype and on response to treatment. *Am J Hum Genet* 1999; 65:59–67.

254. de Jong SC, Stehouwer CDA, Mackaay AJC, et al: High prevalence of hyperhomocysteinemia and asymptomatic vascular disease in siblings of young patients with vascular disease and hyperhomocysteinemia. *Arterioscler Thromb Vasc Biol* 1997; 17:2655–2662.

255. Williams RR, Hopkins PN, Wu LL, Hunt SC: Guidelines for managing severe familial lipid disorders. *Primary Cardiol* 1995; 21:47–53.

256. Williams RR, Hunt SC, Schumacher MC, et al: Diagnosing heterozygous familial hypercholesterolemia using new practical criteria validated by molecular genetics. *Am J Cardiol* 1993; 72:171–176.

257. Neumann HP, Eng C, Mulligan LM, et al: Consequences of direct genetic testing for germline mutations in the clinical management of families with multiple endocrine neoplasia, type II. *JAMA* 1995; 274:1149–1151.

258. Jacques PF, Bostom AG, Williams RR, et al: Relation between folate status, a common mutation in methylenetetrahydrofolate reductase, and plasma homocysteine concentrations. *Circulation* 1996; 93:7–9.

259. Folsom AR, Nieto FJ, McGovern PG, et al: Prospective study of coronary heart disease incidence in relation to fasting total homocysteine, related genetic polymorphisms, and B vitamins: the Atherosclerosis Risk in Communities (ARIC) study (in process citation). *Circulation* 1998; 98:204–210.

260. Davis TA, Anderson EC, Ginsburg AV, Goldberg AP: Weight loss improves lipoprotein lipid profiles in patients with hypercholesterolemia. *J Lab Clin Med* 1985; 106:447–454.

261. Katzel LI, Bleecker ER, Rogus EM, Goldberg AP: Sequential effects of aerobic exercise training and weight loss on risk factors for coronary disease in healthy, obese middle-aged and older men. *Metabolism* 1997; 46:1441–1447.

262. Wood PD, Stefanick ML, Dreon DM, et al: Changes in plasma lipids and lipoproteins in overweight men during weight loss through dieting as compared with exercise. *N Engl J Med* 1988; 319:1173–1179.

263. Wood PD, Stefanick ML, Williams PT, Haskell WL: The effects on plasma lipoproteins of a prudent weight-reducing diet, with or without exercise, in overweight men and women. *N Engl J Med* 1991; 325:461–466.

264. King AC, Haskell WL, Young DR, et al: Long-term effects of varying intensities and formats of physical activity on participation rates, fitness, and lipoproteins in men and women aged 50 to 65 years. *Circulation* 1995; 91:2596–2604.

265. Barnard RJ: Effects of life-style modification on serum lipids. *Arch Intern Med* 1991; 151:1389–1394.

266. Ornish D, Brown SE, Scherwitz LW, et al: Can lifestyle changes reverse coronary heart disease? The Lifestyle Heart Trial. *Lancet* 1990; 336:129–133.

267. Mouratidis B, Vaughan-Neil EF, Gilday DL, et al: Detection of silent coronary artery disease in adolescents and young adults with familial hypercholesterolemia by single-photon emission computed tomography thallium-201 scanning. *Am J Cardiol* 1992; 70:1109–1112.

268. Williams RR, Schumacher MC, Barlow GK, et al: Documented need for more effective diagnosis and treatment of familial hypercholesterolemia according to data from 502 heterozygotes in Utah. *Am J Cardiol* 1993; 72:18D–24D.

269. Goldman L, Goldman PA, Williams LW, Weinstein MC: Cost effectiveness considerations in the treatment of heterozygous familial hypercholesterolemia with medications. *Am J Cardiol* 1993; 72:75D–79D.

270. Andersen LK, Jensen HK, Juul S, Faergeman O: Patients' attitudes toward detection of heterozygous familial hypercholesterolemia. *Arch Intern Med* 1997; 157:553–560.

271. Grossman M, Raper SE, Kozarsky K, et al: Successful ex vivo gene therapy directed to liver in a patient with familial hypercholesterolaemia. *Nature Genet* 1994; 6:335–341.

272. Kullow IJ, Mozes G, Schwartz RS, et al: Adventitial gene transfer of recombinant endothelial nitric oxide synthase to rabbit carotid arteries alters vascular reactivity. *Circulation* 1997; 96:2254–2261.

273. Fazio VM, Rinaldi M, Ciafre SA, et al: Functional chronic correction of dyslipidemia in apo E deficient mice by direct intramuscular injection of naked plasmid DNA. *66th Congress of the European Atherosclerosis Society, Florence, Italy.* Milan, Italy, Giovanni Lorenzini Medical Foundation, 1996:28.

274. Gottschalk S, Sparrow JT, Hauer J, et al: A novel DNA-peptide complex for efficient gene transfer and expression in mammalian cells. *Gene Ther* 1996; 3:48–57.

275. Chiesa G, Stoltzfus LJ, Michelagnoli S, et al: Elevated triglycerides and low HDL cholesterol in transgenic mice expressing human apolipoprotein A-I (Milano). *Atherosclerosis* 1998; 136:139–146.

CHAPTER 6

Hypertension: Epidemiology and Contemporary Management Strategies

Jackson T. Wright, Jr.
Victoria C. Hammonds

Hypertension is undisputedly a major risk factor for cardiovascular disease (CVD), the most common cause of morbidity and mortality in the industrialized world. However, its impact is not uniform, and some patient populations have a greater burden of complications. In addition, certain concomitant diseases and the presence of other risk factors may also alter the risk profile in the hypertensive patient. This chapter reviews the cardiovascular risk of hypertension and its management and considers these issues in selected special populations including the elderly, minority groups, the hypertensive with other risk factors, and patients with selected target organ damage.

Association between Blood Pressure and Cardiovascular Risk

Blood pressure correlates highly with cardiovascular risk. This correlation has been demonstrated in multiple epidemiologic studies, and reduction in CVD risk has been documented in numerous primary prevention therapeutic trials.[1-3] The Seven Countries Study[1] demonstrated a direct relation of systolic and diastolic blood pressures within 16 communities to coronary death rates. These data showed a doubling in risk for every increment of 10 mmHg in the population's median systolic blood pressure. Within in-

dividuals, further evidence of a direct relation of increasing systolic and diastolic blood pressure levels with the subsequent incidence of coronary heart disease (CHD) mortality over 11.6 years of follow-up is documented in men initially free of CHD screened for the Multiple Risk Factor Intervention Trial (Figs. 6–1 and 6–2).[2] The pooling of results from nine prospective observational studies including 418,343 persons initially free of CHD shows the increase in risk for CHD mortality to begin at levels of diastolic blood pressure between 73 and 78 mmHg and to increase more than fivefold between levels of 73 and 105 mmHg.[4]

Hypertension is a leading cause of ischemic coronary and cerebrovascular disease, the second leading cause of end-stage renal disease, and the leading cause of congestive heart failure and hemorrhagic stroke in the United States. Treatment of hypertension has contributed to the reduction of CHD and stroke mortality over the past 20 years.[3]

However, despite the huge burden of disease attributable to hypertension, the level of awareness, treatment and control of this disorder remains a national tragedy (Table 6–1). Furthermore, at the current rate, it appears that blood pressure control rates in the United States will fall well below the 50 to 55 percent levels established as national goals for the years 2000 and 2010. As discussed below, the magnitude of the problem in selected populations is even more challenging.

FIGURE 6–1 Baseline systolic blood pressure and adjusted coronary heart disease death rates for men screened for the Multiple Risk Factor Intervention Trial. Rate per 10,000 person-years adjusted by direct method of age, race, serum cholesterol, cigarettes per day, use of medication for diabetes, and income (average follow-up, 11.6 years). Relative risk (RR) adjusted by proportional hazards regression for age, race, serum cholesterol, cigarettes per day, use of medication for diabetes, and income. $p = .05$ for 118 to 120 mmHg and $p = .001$ for all higher deciles. (Adapted from Stamler et al.,[2] with permission.)

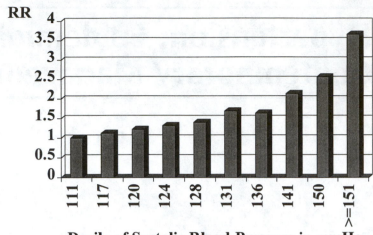

Decile of Systolic Blood Pressure in mmHg (Upper Cutpoint)

FIGURE 6–2 Baseline diastolic blood pressure and adjusted coronary heart disease death rates for men screened for the Multiple Risk Factor Intervention Trial. Rate per 10,000 person-years adjusted by direct method of age, race, serum cholesterol, cigarettes per day, use of medication for diabetes, and income (average follow-up, 11.6 years). Relative risk (RR) adjusted by proportional hazards regression for age, race, serum cholesterol, cigarettes per day, use of medication for diabetes, and income. $p = .01$ for 79 to 80 mmHg and $p = .001$ for all higher deciles. (Adapted from Stamler et al.,[2] with permission.)

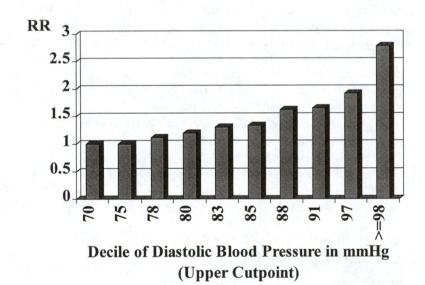

Decile of Diastolic Blood Pressure in mmHg (Upper Cutpoint)

Blood Pressure Measurement and Risk Assessment

Assessment and monitoring blood pressure–related risk in individual patients require the routine use of standardized measurement techniques.[3,5–7] Blood pressures should be measured by determining the average of at least two seated blood pressures taken 2 min apart after the patient has rested quietly for at least 5 min in the chair in which the blood pressures are to be measured.[6] When the blood pressure is measured, the arm should be supported at heart level, the back supported, the legs uncrossed, and feet resting firmly on the floor rather than dangling. Blood pressures obtained with the patient on the examining table or shortly after entering the examin-

TABLE 6–1 Hypertension Awareness, Treatment, and Control Rates in the United States*

	NHANES[†] II	NHANES III (Phase 1) (1988–1991)	NHANES III (Phase 2) (1991–1994)
Hypertensives aware	51	73	68
Hypertensives under treatment	31	55	53
Hypertensives controlled (BP <140/90 mmHg)	10	29	27

*Percentage of adults aged 18–74 with SBP ≥ 140 mmHg or DBP ≥ 90 mmHg or taking antihypertensive medications.
†National Health and Nutrition Examination Survey.
Sources: From JNC VI[3] and Burt et al.,[54] with permission.

ing room, even after a long wait in the waiting room, can be significantly misleading. An essential step in measuring blood pressure is the use of an appropriately sized cuff fitted to a recently calibrated sphygmomanometer (if mercury devices are not available).

Hypertension has been defined by multiple consensus panels as a mean systolic blood pressure (SBP) greater than or equal to 140 mmHg and/or mean diastolic blood pressure (DBP) greater than or equal to 90 mmHg on two or more occasions in patients not taking antihypertensive medication (Table 6–2). Normal blood pressure is defined as below 130/85 mmHg, though a blood pressure below 120/80 mmHg is associated with the lowest cardiovascular risk and is thus considered to be the optimum blood pressure. Additionally, data are accumulating correlating blood pressures obtained by 24-h ambulatory blood pressure monitoring (ABPM) with the presence of target organ damage (Table 6–3).[8–12] Individuals with mean 24-h readings below 130/80 mmHg, mean sleep readings below 120/75 mmHg, and a 10 to 20 percent decrease in blood pressures during sleep are unlikely to have evidence of blood pressure–related target organ damage. However, there are still few data relating the prognostic value of 24-h ABPM to clinical events. Additionally, since serial 24-h ABPM measurements are currently financially and logistically impractical, they have utility in identifying low-risk individuals but are not yet useful in guiding therapy in those under treatment.

There is general agreement that decisions relating blood pressure level and treatment intensity should be determined by risk stratification.[3,13–15] Hypertensives at greatest risk for complications or who already have evidence of CVD should receive the earliest and most aggressive treatment (Table 6–4). Risk factors associated with increased CVD risk in hypertensives include age above 60 years, diabetes mellitus, smoking, dyslipidemia, family history of premature CVD, and male gender or postmenopausal status in women. Hypertensives

TABLE 6–2 Classification of Blood Pressure for Adults 18 ≥ Years*

Category	Systolic Blood Pressure, mmHg		Diastolic Blood Pressure, mmHg
Optimal	<120	and	<80
Normal	<130	and	<85
High normal	130–139	or	85–89
Hypertension	≥140	or	≥90
Stage 1	140–159	or	≥90–99
Stage 2	160–179	or	100–109
Stage 3	≥180	or	≥110

*JNC-VI classification of blood pressure based upon office readings with the patient seated.
Source: From JNC VI,[3] with permission.

TABLE 6–3 Normal Blood Pressure Defined by 24-h Ambulatory Blood Pressure Monitor

	Systolic/Diastolic, mmHg
Mean 24-h BP	<130/80
Awake mean BP	<135/85
Sleep mean BP	<120/75
Nocturnal BP decline	10–20%

Sources: From JNC VI,[3] Pickering,[11] and Appel and Stason.[12]

with preexisting coronary artery disease (myocardial infarction, angina, previous revascularization) and other target organ damage—left ventricular hypertrophy (LVH), heart failure, stroke or transient ischemic attacks (TIAs), nephropathy, retinopathy, or peripheral vascular disease—are at highest risk for CVD complications and benefit from the most aggressive treatment. Therefore, in addition to focusing on evaluating for secondary causes of hypertension, the clinician should undertake an aggressive search for these risk factors and the presence of target organ damage.

Appendix 6–1 includes a quick reference guide to JNC VI recommendations for blood pressure measurement, primary prevention, goals, treatment, and adherence.[3]

Management of Hypertension to Prevent Cardiovascular Disease

Treatment Goals

The primary focus of treatment in the hypertensive patient is to lower blood pressure to the recommended blood pressure goal using whatever agents are necessary to achieve this. Accumulating evidence is beginning to suggest that cardiovascular benefit is achieved with blood pressure lowering regardless of the treatment regimen selected.[16–20] Although some agents may offer proven or theoretical additional advantages in patients with specific clinical conditions,

TABLE 6–4 Risk Stratification and Indication for Antihypertensive Treatment*

Blood Pressure Stages, mmHg	Risk Group A, without Risk Factors, TOD, or CCD	Risk Group B Nondiabetics with ≥ or at least 1 Risk Factor, without TOD or CCD	Risk Group C, Diabetics and Hypertensives with TOD and/or CCD
High-normal (130–139/85–89)	Lifestyle modification	Lifestyle modification	Drug therapy and simultaneous lifestyle modification for risk group C with CHF, renal insufficiency, and/or diabetes only
Stage 1 (140–159/90–99)	Drug therapy after 12 months of lifestyle modification if goal BP not reached	Drug therapy after 6 months of lifestyle modification if goal BP not reached	Drug therapy and simultaneous lifestyle modification
Stage 2 (≥160/≥100)	Drug therapy and simultaneous lifestyle modification	Drug therapy and simultaneous lifestyle modification	Drug therapy and simultaneous lifestyle modification

*Graded intervention strategies for the management of elevated blood pressure based upon the presence of target organ damage (TOD), clinical cardiovascular disease (CCD), and risk factors.

Sources: From JNC VI[3] and the National High Blood Pressure Education Working Group,[142] with permission.

these advantages are maximized only if blood pressure control is also achieved. Lowering SBP to less than 140 mmHg and DBP to less than 90 mmHg is therefore uniformly recommended as the minimal goal for all hypertensives.[3,13–15,21–23] In patients with diabetes, renal insufficiency, or heart failure, blood pressure control to less than 130/85 mmHg (and to less than 125/75 in the hypertensive with renal insufficiency and proteinuria) is the recommended treatment goal.[3]

Lifestyle modification is the first therapeutic modality utilized for the management of hypertension. The benefit of lifestyle modification in reducing hypertension-related complications has not been established by prospective long-term clinical trials. However, there is general consensus that it should be utilized alone as initial therapy in low- to moderate-risk hypertensives and as concomitant therapy in all hypertensives on drug therapy (Table 6–4). In addition to its potential to lower blood pressure, lifestyle modification also contributes to improved overall cardiovascular health. Furthermore, recent data suggest that its greatest utility may be in the primary prevention of hypertension and potential reduction of population-based risk.[24–28]

The antihypertensive drug regimen should include agents proven efficacious by clinical outcome trial data unless they are contraindicated or not tolerated. However, the overriding focus should be to prescribe whatever agents are necessary to achieve the blood pressure goal in conjunction with lifestyle modifications. Even when a specific drug class is indicated for its particular non–blood pressure lowering attributes, achieving the therapeutic goal blood pressure remains critical for maximal target-organ protection and overall risk reduction. It is a tragedy that in the United States only about one-quarter of all hypertensives and fewer than half of all drug-treated hypertensives are controlled to less than 140/90 mmHg.[3]

Lifestyle Modification in the Treatment of Hypertension

Two recent studies have regenerated enthusiasm about lifestyle modification in the management of mild hypertension and high-normal blood pressure. The Treatment of Mild Hypertension Study (TOMHS), utilizing an intensive lifestyle intervention program, reported an 8- to 9-mmHg reduction in both systolic and diastolic blood pressures. Additional reductions in blood pressure and reduction in cardiovascular events were noted in this trial with the addition of drug therapy.[29] In the Dietary Approach to Stop Hypertension (DASH) study, hypertensive patients following a diet that was rich in fruits, vegetables, and low-fat dairy products (Table 6–5) had a mean reduction in blood pressure of 11 mmHg systolic and 5 mmHg diastolic below that seen with the traditional U.S. diet.[25] This effect on blood pressure in DASH was noted even without calorie or salt restriction. Specific lifestyle modification strategies have been recommended by the Joint National Committee on Prevention, Evaluation, and Treatment of High Blood Pressure (JNC VI) (Table 6–6).[3]

Excess body weight, especially with abdominal obesity, has been associated with an increased risk for high blood pressure and adverse effects on other CVD risk factors. In the Trials of Hypertension Prevention (TOHP),[24] the Trial of Nonpharmacologic Interventions in the Elderly (TONE),[27] and other studies, an 8- to 10-lb reduction in weight produced a 3- to 4-mm Hg lowering of systolic blood pressure in overweight hypertensives. In the TOMHS trial, weight reduction incremented the blood pressure–lowering effect of antihypertensive drug therapy.[29] Regular aerobic physical activity is recommended to lower blood pressure as well as to enhance weight loss and improve overall cardiovascular health.[30–32] Brisk walking for 30 to 45 min most days of the week is often sufficient to meet these goals.[33] Obviously, high-risk patients should have a thorough evaluation of their cardiovascular status, including stress testing, before initiating a more aggressive exercise program.

Restriction of sodium intake to 2.4 g/day or less is recommended in hypertensive patients by nearly all consensus panels. These recommendations are based on extensive data from epidemiologic studies and clinical trials. Several population-based studies have shown significant correlations between the levels of salt intake and blood pressure. One of the

TABLE 6–5 The DASH Diet*

Food Group	Daily Servings	Serving Sizes	Examples and Notes	Significance to the DASH Diet Pattern
Grains and grain products	7–8	1 slice bread 1/2 c (0.12 L) dry cereal 1/2 c (0.12 L) cooked rice, pasta, or cereal	Whole wheat bread, English muffin, pita bread, bagel, cereals, grits, oatmeal	Major sources of energy and fiber
Vegetables	4–5	1 c (0.24 L) raw leafy vegetable 1/2 c (0.12 L) cooked vegetable 6 oz (180 mL) vegetable juice	Tomatoes, potatoes, carrots, peas, squash, broccoli, turnip greens, collards, kale, spinach, artichokes, beans, sweet potatoes	Rich sources of potassium, magnesium, and fiber
Fruits	4–5	6 oz (180 mL) fruit juice 1 medium fruit 1/4 c (0.06 L) dried fruit 1/2 c (0.12 L) fresh, frozen, or canned fruit	Apricots, bananas, dates, grapes, oranges, orange juice, grapefruit, grapefruit juice, mangoes, melons, peaches, pineapples, prunes, raisins, strawberries, tangerines	Important sources of potassium, magnesium, and fiber
Low-fat or nonfat dairy foods	2–3	8 oz (240 mL) milk 1 c (0.24 L) yogurt 1.5 oz (45 g) cheese	Skim or 1% milk, skim or low-fat buttermilk, nonfat or low-fat yogurt, part-skim mozzarella cheese, nonfat cheese	Major sources of calcium and protein
Meats, poultry, and fish	≤2	3 oz (84 g) cooked meats, poultry, or fish	Select only lean meats; trim away visible fats; broil, roast, or boil, instead of frying; remove skin from poultry	Rich sources of protein and magnesium
Nuts, seeds, and legumes	4–5/wk	1.5 oz (42 g) or 1/3 c (0.08 L) nuts 0.5 oz (14 g) or 2 tbsp (3 mL) seeds 1/2 c (0.12 L) cooked legumes	Almonds, filberts, mixed nuts, peanuts, walnuts, sunflower seeds, kidney beans, lentils	Rich sources of energy, magnesium, potassium, protein, and fiber

*DASH's final results appear in *N Engl J Med* 1997; 366:1117–1124. The results show that the DASH "combination diet" lowered blood pressure and, so, may help prevent and control high blood pressure. The "combination diet" is rich in fruits, vegetables, and low-fat dairy foods, and low in saturated and total fat. It also is low in cholesterol; high in dietary fiber, potassium, calcium, and magnesium; and moderately high in protein. The DASH eating plan shown above is based on 2000 calories a day (8400 J/d). Depending on energy needs, the number of daily servings in a food group may vary from those listed.

Source: Adapted from JNC VI,[3] with permission.

TABLE 6–6 Lifestyle Modification Strategies in the Management of Hypertension

1. Encourage weight loss to achieve desirable body weight

2. Increase aerobic physical activity (30–45 min most days of the week)

3. Reduce sodium intake to no more than 100 mmol per day

4. Maintain adequate dietary intake of potassium, calcium, and magnesium; reduce dietary intake of saturated fat and cholesterol

5. Limit alcohol intake to <1 oz (30 mL) ethanol per day

6. Cessation of smoking

Source: Adapted from JNC VI,[3] with permission.

largest studies demonstrating the association, the Intersalt Study, was conducted in 52 centers around the world and involved more than 10,000 patients.[34] Other clinical trials have also shown that restriction of sodium intake lowers blood pressure. A meta-analysis of 17 such trials reported a mean reduction of 6 mmHg systolic and 2 mmHg diastolic blood pressure associated with a reduction in urinary sodium excretion by 95 mmol/day.[35] Furthermore, the blood pressure reduction possible with universal reduction in sodium intake by 50 mmol/day has been estimated to result in a potential 22 percent reduction in the 500,000 incident cases of strokes and a potential 16 percent reduction in the 1.5 million incident cases of coronary artery disease.[36] Large subgroups of the general population are reported to be most sensitive to the blood pressure effects of changes in dietary salt intake. They include African Americans, the elderly, diabetics, the obese, those with renal impairment, and the vast majority of hypertensives.[37] In addition to a direct effect on blood pressure, sodium restriction augments the response to other antihypertensives and reduces potassium loss in patients on diuretics.[3]

A few observational studies have recently questioned the safety of restricting dietary sodium intake. In one, Alderman et al. reported an increased incidence of myocardial infarctions in a workplace survey of hypertensive patients with urinary sodium excretion in the lowest quartile.[38] An analysis of the NHANES I (National Health and Nutrition Examination Survey) database by this author reached similar conclusions.[39] However, both studies have significant methodologic limitations, including use of a single baseline sodium determination (one consisting of a single 24-h dietary recall) and then attempting to correlate this value with clinical events occurring decades later. There are no prospective studies available to support these observations. Therefore, given the overwhelming data supporting the benefits of sodium restriction, at this time there is little reason to abandon current recommendations about reducing salt intake.

Adequate intake of both potassium (50 to 90 mmol/day) and calcium (800 to 1200 mg/day) is recommended for patients with hypertension.[3] A pooled analysis of 33 randomized controlled studies reported a reduction of more than 3 mmHg in systolic blood pressure with potassium supplementation.[40] An inverse relationship between dietary calcium intake and blood pressure has also been reported.[41] In addition, calcium supplements have been reported to lower blood pressure.[42] However, the blood pressure reduction associated with increased calcium intake is minimal. Therefore, while hypertensive patients are advised to maintain adequate dietary intake of potassium except for that contained in low-fat diary products, calcium supplements are not routinely recommended for blood pressure lowering at this time.[3] Although potassium supplements may be required in hypokalemic patients, most patients should be able to obtain an adequate intake of potassium through diet, primarily from fruits and vegetables. A diet low in saturated fat and smoking cessation are important adjunctive measures in improving the overall cardiovascular health of hypertensive patients.

Excessive alcohol intake also has a deleterious effect on blood pressure, and abrupt withdrawal from heavy alcohol consumption can significantly elevate blood pressure. In the Multiple Risk Factor Intervention Trial (MRFIT), increasing levels of alcohol intake were associated with increased blood pressure.[43] Excessive alcohol ingestion is also associated with the development of resistant hypertension.

Therefore, estimation of alcohol intake is recommended as a routine part of the evaluation of hypertensive patients, and all consensus panels recommend counseling of hypertensives to limit their ethanol intake to no more than 1 oz/day.[3]

In addition to using lifestyle modification strategies to treat hypertension, the primary prevention of hypertension may be their greatest benefit. The rationale for primary prevention efforts to prevent the development of hypertension, in addition to blood pressure control efforts focused on the detection and treatment of preexisting hypertension, are well known.[28] This is reinforced by the low blood pressure control rates[14,28,44] observed in the most hypertensive populations, the many hypertensives who are unaware that they even have the disease, and the significant cost (financial and potential risk of adverse drug reaction) of identifying and treating hypertensives. Thus, population-based approaches, especially those efforts directed at high-risk individuals, are clearly indicated. In order to facilitate population-based programs directed at maximizing the life-style changes recommended, significant changes in public policy directed at public educational campaigns, food industry practices, and reimbursement for preventive care will be necessary.

Principles of Antihypertensive Drug Selection

Although therapeutic aims focus on achieving a goal blood pressure, the primary purpose of antihypertensive therapy is to prevent the complications of elevated blood pressure. Thus, agents that have been shown to reduce CVD outcomes as well as to lower blood pressure are preferred for initial drug selection over those shown only to lower blood pressure. However, while much of the attention has been directed at the initial drug selection, most patients require a multiple drug regimen to achieve blood pressure goals, especially those patients whose blood pressure goal is lower than the usual 140/90 mmHg.[45,46] The general algorithm for drug treatment of hypertension, as recommended by the JNC VI is shown in Fig. 6–3.[3] Guidelines for improving patient adherence to antihypertensive therapy appear in Table 6–7.[3]

Table 6–8 shows the choices of initial pharmacologic therapy for uncomplicated patients, and for those with specific comorbidities. Thiazide diuretics and beta blockers have been studied in multiple well-designed clinical outcome trials documenting their efficacy in reducing CVD events, as shown in a recent meta-analysis (Fig. 6–4).[47] In patients without specific indications for other agents, they are uniformly recommended for initial therapy. Recently, the results of a prospective placebo-controlled clinical trial that evaluated nitrendipine, the long-acting dihydropyridine calcium channel blocker as initial therapy in older hypertensives with isolated systolic hypertension were released.[18] This trial was stopped prematurely by the trial's data safety and monitoring board when the active therapy group had significantly

TABLE 6–7 General Guidelines to Improve Patient Adherence to Antihypertensive Therapy

Be aware of signs of patient nonadherence to antihypertensive therapy.

Establish the goal of therapy: to reduce blood pressure to nonhypertensive levels with minimal or no adverse events.

Educate patients about the disease and involve them and their families in its treatment. Have them measure blood pressure at home.

Maintain contact with patients; consider telecommunication.

Keep care inexpensive and simple.

Encourage lifestyle modifications.

Integrate pill-taking into routine activities of daily living.

Prescribe medications according to pharmacologic principles, favoring long-acting formulations.

Be willing to stop unsuccessful therapy and try a different approach.

Anticipate adverse events and adjust therapy to prevent, minimize, or ameliorate side effects.

Continue to add effective and tolerated drugs, stepwise, in sufficient doses to achieve the goal of therapy.

Encourage a positive attitude about achieving therapeutic goals.

Consider using nurse case management.

Source: Adapted from JNC VI,[3] with permission.

FIGURE 6–3 Algorithm for the treatment of hypertension. ACE, angiotensin-converting enzyme; ISA, intrinsic sympathomimetic activity. (From JNC VI,[3] with permission.)

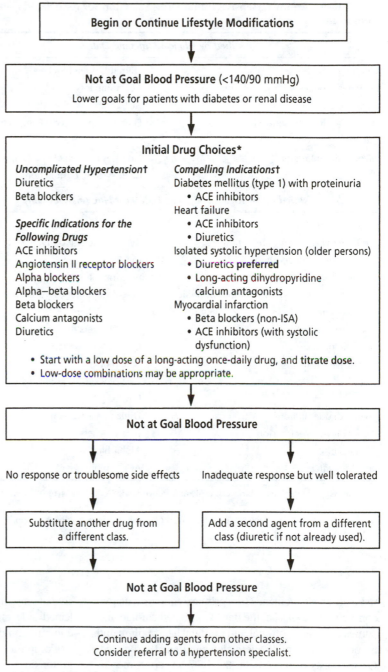

Begin or Continue Lifestyle Modifications

Not at Goal Blood Pressure (<140/90 mmHg)
Lower goals for patients with diabetes or renal disease

Initial Drug Choices*

Uncomplicated Hypertension†
Diuretics
Beta blockers

Specific Indications for the Following Drugs
ACE inhibitors
Angiotensin II receptor blockers
Alpha blockers
Alpha–beta blockers
Beta blockers
Calcium antagonists
Diuretics

Compelling Indications†
Diabetes mellitus (type 1) with proteinuria
• ACE inhibitors
Heart failure
• ACE inhibitors
• Diuretics
Isolated systolic hypertension (older persons)
• Diuretics **preferred**
• Long-acting dihydropyridine calcium antagonists
Myocardial infarction
• Beta blockers (non-ISA)
• ACE inhibitors (with systolic dysfunction)

• Start with a low dose of a long-acting once-daily drug, and **titrate dose**.
• Low-dose combinations may be appropriate.

Not at Goal Blood Pressure

No response or troublesome side effects

Inadequate response but well tolerated

Substitute another drug from a different class.

Add a second agent from a different class (diuretic if not already used).

Not at Goal Blood Pressure

Continue adding agents from other classes.
Consider referral to a hypertension specialist.

* Unless contraindicated.
† Based on randomized controlled trials.

TABLE 6–8 Antihypertensive Initial Drug Selection for Associated Comorbidities

Justified by Clinical Outcome Data	
Uncomplicated	Diuretics, beta blockers
Diabetes mellitus with proteinuria	ACE inhibitors
Heart failure	ACE inhibitors, diuretics
Isolated systolic hypertension	Diuretics (preferred), Long-acting DHP
CaCBs	
Myocardial infarction	Non-ISA beta blockers, ACE inhibitors (with systolic dysfunction)

Justified by Surrogate Endpoints Data/Post Hoc Analyses Only	
Angina	Beta blockers, CaCBs
Atrial tachycardia and fibrillation	Beta blockers, Non-DHP CaCBs
Cyclosporine-induced hypertension	CaCBs
Diabetes mellitus (type 2) with proteinuria	ACE inhibitors
Diabetes mellitus (type 2) without proteinuria	Low-dose diuretics, ACE inhibitors
Dyslipidemia	Alpha blockers
Essential tremor	Beta blockers (nonselective)
Heart failure	Carvedilol, losartan
Hyperthyroidism	Beta blockers
Migraine	Beta blockers (nonselective), Non-DHP CaCBs
Myocardial infarction	Diltiazem, verapamil
Preoperative hypertension	Beta blockers
Prostatism	Alpha blockers
Renal insufficiency	ACE inhibitors

Key: CaCBs, calcium channel blockers; DHP, dihydropyridine; ISA, intrinsic sympathomimetic activity.

Sources: From JNC VI[3] and the National High Blood Pressure Education Working Group,[142] with permission.

reduced stroke incidence (the primary endpoint) on two consecutive "looks" at the data. Combined cardiac outcomes consisting of fatal and nonfatal heart failure and myocardial infarction were also significantly reduced. On the basis of these data, the JNC VI report recommended long-acting dihydropyridine calcium channel blockers as alternatives to thiazide diuretics for patients with isolated systolic hypertension.[3] Appendix 6–2 provides a listing of currently marketed antihyperten-

sive agents, including their usual dose range and selected side effects. Appendix 6–3 provides a list of combination drugs for hypertension.

Comparative clinical outcome trials with angiotensin-converting enzyme (ACE) inhibitors, angiotensin-receptor blockers, and alpha blockers are not yet available. The results of one open-label trial, the Captopril Primary Prevention (CAPPP) Trial, were recently reported showing no advantage of this

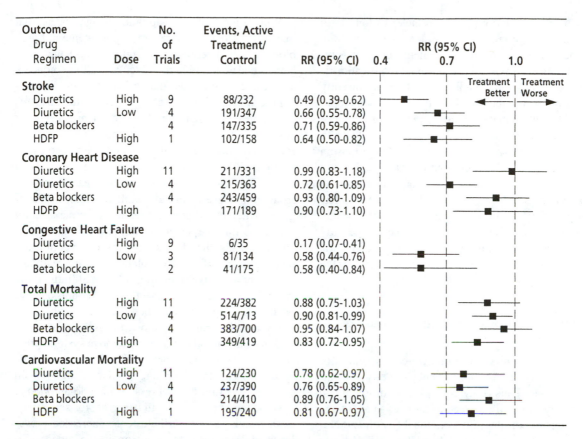

Outcome Drug Regimen	Dose	No. of Trials	Events, Active Treatment/ Control	RR (95% CI)
Stroke				
Diuretics	High	9	88/232	0.49 (0.39-0.62)
Diuretics	Low	4	191/347	0.66 (0.55-0.78)
Beta blockers		4	147/335	0.71 (0.59-0.86)
HDFP	High	1	102/158	0.64 (0.50-0.82)
Coronary Heart Disease				
Diuretics	High	11	211/331	0.99 (0.83-1.18)
Diuretics	Low	4	215/363	0.72 (0.61-0.85)
Beta blockers		4	243/459	0.93 (0.80-1.09)
HDFP	High	1	171/189	0.90 (0.73-1.10)
Congestive Heart Failure				
Diuretics	High	9	6/35	0.17 (0.07-0.41)
Diuretics	Low	3	81/134	0.58 (0.44-0.76)
Beta blockers		2	41/175	0.58 (0.40-0.84)
Total Mortality				
Diuretics	High	11	224/382	0.88 (0.75-1.03)
Diuretics	Low	4	514/713	0.90 (0.81-0.99)
Beta blockers		4	383/700	0.95 (0.84-1.07)
HDFP	High	1	349/419	0.83 (0.72-0.95)
Cardiovascular Mortality				
Diuretics	High	11	124/230	0.78 (0.62-0.97)
Diuretics	Low	4	237/390	0.76 (0.65-0.89)
Beta blockers		4	214/410	0.89 (0.76-1.05)
HDFP	High	1	195/240	0.81 (0.67-0.97)

FIGURE 6–4   Meta-analysis of randomized placebo-controlled clinical trials in hypertension according to first-line treatment strategy. Shown are the number of trials with the indicated endpoint of interest. For these comparisons, the numbers of participants randomized to active treatment and placebo, respectively, were 7768 and 12,075 for high-dose diuretic therapy and 6736 and 12,147 for beta-blocker therapy. Because the Medical Research Council trials included two active arms, the placebo group is included twice in these totals (for diuretic comparison and for beta-blocker comparison). The total numbers of participants randomized to active and control therapy were 24,294 and 23,926, respectively. RR, relative risk; CI, confidence interval; HDFP, Hypertension Detection and Follow-up Program. (Data from Psaty et al.,[47] with permission. Copyright 1997, American Medical Association.)

ACE inhibitor over a diuretic/beta blocker–based regimen with respect to clinical outcomes. The diuretic/beta blocker–based regimen was actually better in preventing strokes, but captopril showed an advantage in preventing diabetes.[48] More definitive trials are now in progress.[49] By the end of the year 2003, clinical endpoint data from more than 36 trials on over 195,000 patients and almost 900,000 patient/years will be available. The results of these trials and a planned prospective meta-analysis should provide the comparative data to define the role of specific drug classes more precisely.

One major challenge in achieving blood pressure goals is maintaining patients on the therapeutic regimen. Patients need to remain convinced of the importance of adhering to therapy and may require assistance in overcoming the obstacles to long-term adherence. A program of constant communication, patient education and reinforcement, problem solving, attention to regimen cost, and simplification is essential to maximizing adherence. There is currently greater interest in the use of fixed combination preparations for the management of hypertension. The last two updates to the JNC reports and the World Health Organization/International Society of Hypertension have acknowledged that combining antihypertensives with different mechanisms of action may allow use of both agents at lower doses and with greater tolerability.[3,14,50,51] Additionally, fixed combinations may also allow simplification of the regimen, especially in hypertensives requiring multiple drugs, and some combinations can be used with little increase over the cost of the agents prescribed separately.[52]

Recommendations for Blood Pressure Management in Selected Populations

Older hypertensives   The clinical consequences of hypertension increase in frequency directly with increasing age. Thus, they occur most commonly in the elderly, currently defined as those 65 years of age and older. According to the National Health and Nutrition Examination Survey III (NHANES III), the prevalence of hypertension in persons aged 65 to 74 was 63 percent.[53] The greatest prevalence was seen in African Americans at 72 percent, followed by Mexican Americans (55 percent) and non-Hispanic whites (53 percent). By the year 2000, it is estimated that there will be approximately 35 million Americans above 65 years of age, and the number will double by the year 2050.[54] Thus, with the financial cost of cardiovascular disease–related morbidity and mortality (i.e., heart disease and stroke) currently estimated to be more than $269 billion dollars annually,[55] the effective management of hypertension in this population is clearly of major public health concern. Current estimates indicate that only 15 percent of elderly hypertensives are adequately treated versus the population average of 27 percent.[56] Thus, those hypertensives at highest risk and likely to derive the greatest benefit from therapy are least likely to be treated to recommended blood pressure goals.

With aging, pathophysiologic changes occur that may affect blood pressure and its management. Large blood vessels become more rigid because the numbers of elastic fibers in the vascular wall are reduced. This elevates total vascular resistance, thus increasing the workload of the left ventricle. Clinically, this condition is associated with a greater prevalence of isolated systolic hypertension and, in its extreme form, may contribute to the pseudohypertension seen in some elderly patients. Pseudohypertension or a falsely elevated sphygmomanometer reading results from an increase in vascular wall stiffness. It is suggested when blood pressure readings are persistently elevated with no evidence of target organ damage or when patients manifest symptoms of hypertension that are not confirmed by blood pressure readings. The Osler maneuver identifies a physical finding that is reportedly helpful in detecting this condition.[57] A positive finding is noted when the radial or brachial artery remains palpable (though pulseless) after inflation of the blood pressure cuff above systolic pressure. However, two recent reports have questioned the specificity of this finding.[58,59] Other age-related changes affecting blood pressure include autonomic dysfunction and a decline in baroreceptor sensitivity. Both factors may contribute to an increased prevalence of orthostatic hypotension in the elderly. Finally, reduced renal function may make the elderly more salt-sensitive, and reduced hepatic function may augment the action of agents utilizing this method of elimination (e.g., calcium channel blockers).[60]

Hypertension in the elderly can be divided into three subtypes: (1) isolated systolic hypertension, (2) isolated diastolic hypertension, and (3) combined systolic and diastolic hypertension. In general, average DBP increases with age until the sixth decade of life and then begins to decline, while average SBP continues to increase with age, and isolated systolic hypertension is the most common form of hypertension in those over age 60.[61] More recently, pulse pressure, has been shown to be an important predictor of risk for CHD events in middle-aged and older individuals.[62]

Isolated systolic hypertension is defined by an SBP equal to or greater than 140 mmHg and a DBP equal to or less than 90 mmHg.[3] It is seldom seen before age 45 and begins to increase in prevalence in those over age 55. The prevalence increases in both sexes with aging but the condition is 60 to 100 percent more prevalent in females.[63] Although isolated systolic hypertension is most commonly associated with decreased elasticity of large blood vessels due to arteriosclerosis, other etiologies—including aortic insufficiency, Paget's disease, coarctation of the aorta, arteriovenous malformation, and severe anemia—may also be responsible.[64]

The evaluation and diagnosis of hypertension in the elderly are similar to those in other adult populations. However, because of the higher risk of postural hypotension in the elderly, blood pressure readings should be taken in both sitting and standing positions. The history should also look for clues that might suggest a secondary cause of hypertension. Although not common, most secondary causes of hypertension increase with increasing age and should be considered in cases where the onset of hypertension is sudden or previously good blood pressure control becomes difficult to maintain. In this population, one of the most common reversible secondary causes results from renovascular disease. Primary aldosteronism should be considered when hypokalemia is noted. Other secondary causes found in the elderly include pheochromocytoma, sleep apnea, hyperparathyroidism, and Cushing's syndrome.

Multiple studies support the benefits of antihypertensive therapy for reducing cardiovascular risk in older hypertensives. Individuals at highest risk experience the greatest benefit of antihypertensive drug therapy.[10] Thus, the elderly are one of the subgroups that show the greatest absolute risk reduction. The Systolic Hypertension in the Elderly (SHEP) trial compared the outcomes of patients 60 years of age or older with isolated systolic hypertension who were randomly assigned to treatment with either placebo or a diuretic/beta blocker–based regimen. The study reported a 36 percent reduction in stroke, a 27 percent reduction in CHD, a 55 percent decrease in CHF, and a decrease in cardiovascular mortality of 32 percent among those randomized to active treatment (Table 6–9).[65] Similar results were noted in another trial utilizing a long-acting dihydropyridine calcium channel blocker–based regimen.[18] The Swedish Trial

TABLE 6–9 Percent Reduction (Treated/Controls) in Events in Clinical Trials on the Elderly with Isolated Systolic Hypertension

Trial	Age Range	Stroke	CHD	CHF	All CVD
SHEP[65] (n = 4736)	60–96	36*	27*	55*	32*
SYST-EUR**[18]† (n = 4695)	60–100	42*	30	29	31*

Key: CHD, coronary heart disease; CHF, congestive heart failure; CVD, cardiovascular disease.

*$p < .05$.

†Trial discontinued early by its data safety and monitoring board.

Source: From the National High Blood Pressure Education Program Working Group,[142] with permission.

in Old Patients with Hypertension (STOP) reported a 47 percent decrease in stroke and a 43 percent reduction in all-cause mortality with active treatment of hypertensives aged 70 to 84.[66] The Medical Research Council in the Elderly trial included 4396 patients 65 to 74 years of age and compared diuretic versus beta blocker versus placebo treatment groups.[67] The combined actively treated patient groups demonstrated a 25 percent reduction in stroke and a 17 percent reduction in all cardiovascular events. The diuretic-based but not the beta blocker–based regimen reduced CHD events. Based on these and other data, the recommendation for all hypertensives, especially the elderly, is to lower SBP to less than 140 mmHg and DBP to less than 90 mmHg. In older hypertensives with isolated systolic hypertension and a markedly elevated SBP, an initial goal to reduce SBP below 160 mmHg may be considered.[53]

Concerns have been raised about limiting the level to which diastolic blood pressure should be lowered in the older hypertensive patient. Some have suggested a "J curve" relationship between diastolic blood pressure and cardiac morbidity/mortality, where lowering the DBP below a critical point may no longer be beneficial and potentially harmful (especially in patients with preexisting CHD).[68] This concept has been refuted by the trials of patients with isolated systolic hypertension that showed no increase in CVD event rate when mean DBP was lowered from 85 to 67 mmHg.[18,65] It was also most recently evaluated in the Hypertension Optimal Treatment (HOT) study, which studied 19,193 hypertensives from 26 countries between the ages of 50 and 80 years with DBPs between 110 and 115 mmHg.[20] The results confirmed the benefits of reduction of SBP to less than 140 mmHg and DBP to less than 85 mmHg. The lowest risk for major cardiovascular events was achieved at a diastolic blood pressure of 82.6 mmHg and a mean systolic blood pressure of 138.5 mmHg. Although the number of patients achieving DBP of less than 80 mmHg was too small to evaluate benefit of the lower DBP, SBP as low as 120 mmHg and DBP as low as 70 mmHg did not appear to cause significant additional risk, even in patients with CHD.

As with all segments of the population with hypertension, nonpharmacologic treatment and lifestyle modifications should be part of all therapeutic interventions. The efficacy of nondrug therapy has been clearly established, even in older populations.[27,62] Pharmacologic therapies are initiated based on blood pressure classifications, other CVD risk factors, and the extent of target organ damage as outlined in the JNC VI (Table 6–4). Special considerations must be made when choosing a drug regimen for older patients. Frequency in dosing, existence of other comorbid disease states, side-effect profiles, and drug-drug interactions must be considered. In general, all drug therapies should be initiated at low doses and doses titrated deliberately to lower blood pressure to goal levels, though more slowly.

Thiazide diuretics are the initial drugs of choice for most older hypertensives. They have been well studied as initial therapy for combined systolic/diastolic hypertension as well as for isolated systolic hypertension in the elderly. Numerous clinical trials have clearly documented a decrease in cardiovascular-related morbidity and mortality with their use.[3] In addition to their efficacy in lowering blood pressure and CVD risk, diuretics are also easily affordable—a significant factor for this group of patients with often limited financial resources. A functional disadvantage of diuretics may relate to an increased incidence of urinary incontinence in the elderly, which may reduce compliance. The lower doses used in the elderly (25 mg/day or less) reduces the occurrence of significant adverse metabolic side effects (e.g., hypokalemia, hyperglycemia, and dyslipidemia). The publication of the results of the Sys-Eur Trial using long acting dihydropyridine calcium channel blockers has led to the recommendation of these agents as an alternative to initial therapy with thiazide diuretics for patients with isolated systolic hypertension.[3,18]

Beta blockers have also been shown in clinical outcome trials to reduce hypertension-related cardiovascular morbidity and mortality. However, in older hypertensives, therapy initiated with beta blockers has proven to be less effective at reducing CHD events than antihypertensive therapy initiated with thiazide diuretics.[67] Nonetheless, beta blockers are drugs of choice in all hypertensives, including the elderly, who have had a myocardial infarction and/or symptoms of angina pectoris. Beta blockers should be used cautiously in those taking nondihydropyridine calcium channel blockers because of their additive potential to depress atrioventricular node conduction and heart rate. Additionally, because of a higher expected prevalence of occult CHD in older patients, discontinuation of these drugs should be accomplished by tapering rather than by abrupt withdrawal.[3]

ACE inhibitors should be considered in older hypertensives with heart failure secondary to left ventricular systolic dysfunction and in those with diabetes mellitus. Alpha blockers may be useful in older hypertensives with specific comorbid diseases such as dyslipidemia and those with symptomatic prostatic hypertrophy. However, they should be used cautiously because of their tendency to exacerbate orthostatic hypotension, dizziness, and syncope.

Minorities The prevalence of hypertension in the United States remains highest among African Americans as compared with non-Hispanic whites and Mexican Americans. Although increasing data suggest that the prevalence and severity of hypertension are less marked in Mexican Americans, hypertension control rates are also less and CVD rates are at least as high in this subgroup. In African

Americans, the added excess prevalence of diabetes mellitus, other cardiovascular risk factors (cigarette smoking, obesity, lipid disorders, and LVH), in addition to the greater severity of hypertension make the need for aggressive blood pressure control even more critical. The excess blood pressure–related end-organ damage observed in this population leads to an excess hypertension-related morbidity and mortality.[69] Hypertension in African Americans is associated with a 320 percent higher rate of end-stage renal disease, an 80 percent higher rate of stroke, and a 50 percent higher incidence of CHD mortality than in other U.S. populations.[70–72] It is noteworthy that several major clinical trials have now documented that rational antihypertensive therapy can achieve excellent levels of blood pressure control even in the most difficult to manage African-American patient.[73–75]

A review of the proposed mechanisms and pathophysiologic characteristics responsible for the observed racial/ethnic differences in blood pressure–related manifestations is beyond the scope of this text. However, significant racial/ethnic diversity exists in the pathophysiology of essential hypertension, supporting the notion that this condition is a complex disorder of polygenetic and environmental factors.[76] Compared with whites, African Americans are more likely to have volume-dependent, salt-sensitive hypertension associated with low levels of plasma renin activity.[77–79] Several population-based studies have shown a positive correlation between high intracellular sodium (Na) levels and hypertension prevalence among African Americans.[76] Moreover, intracellular sodium levels are consistently higher among them than among whites. An elevated intracellular sodium level has been proposed to trigger a cascade of compensatory pathophysiologic changes leading to elevated intracellular calcium and enhanced vascular reactivity.[80]

Diuretics have been shown to decrease hypertensive morbidity and mortality in both African Americans and in whites.[73] Moreover, diuretics reduce LVH, which has a higher prevalence among African Americans and contributes to excess cardiovascular mortality.[81] In a Veterans Administration Cooperative Studies Group trial, monotherapy with the non-dihydropyridine calcium channel blocker diltiazem was also effective in lowering blood pressure as compared with captopril, atenolol, clonidine, prazosin, hydrochlorothiazide, or placebo.[82] However, in this as well as other trial populations, though specifically selected for a long-term monotherapy trial, no more than 64 percent of participants achieved DBP goal with any one agent. African-American hypertensives have consistently been shown to respond less well to beta blockers, ACE inhibitors, and angiotensin receptor blockers than to other classes of antihypertensive agents. For this reason, these agents are often underutilized in African-American hypertensives even when they are indicated for other conditions (e.g. CHD, heart failure).[3,83] Substantial evidence is now available to document that when these drugs are combined with a diuretic, African Americans respond as well to them as do other racial/ethnic groups.[84–86]

After lifestyle modification, antihypertensive drug therapy initiated with diuretics is recommended for African Americans with uncomplicated essential hypertension, with other agents added to decrease systolic and diastolic blood pressure to less than 140/90.[3] The high risk of complications, the proven efficacy of these agents in reducing blood pressure as well as CVD outcomes in this population, and their ability to augment the antihypertensive efficacy of other agents are among the reasons for this recommendation. Given the greater severity of hypertension in African Americans, there is a greater likelihood that more than one antihypertensive agent will be needed to achieve optimal blood pressure control. African Americans may often require three to four drugs to reach this goal.[74] The importance of achieving recommended blood pressure goals in African-American hypertensives cannot be overstated.[3]

Effect of Concomitant Diseases on Hypertension Management

The coexistence of other clinical conditions may affect the choice of antihypertensive therapy. JNC VI and other consensus documents list several concomitant diseases and subgroups of patients that may affect the management of hypertension (Table 6–8).

Diabetes mellitus The hypertensive with diabetes is at particularly high risk of CVD, and these two disorders commonly occur together.[87] Hypertension occurs twice as often in diabetics as in nondiabetics. Diabetes and glucose intolerance occur in over one-third of hypertensives, and the incidence and prevalence of diabetes is rapidly increasing in this country and worldwide. An estimated 35 to 75 percent of diabetic complications can be related to hypertension.[88] Atherogenic complications, including CHD, as well as cerebrovascular, peripheral vascular, and renovascular disease are all increased in diabetic hypertensives as compared with those who have one or none of these disorders.

The evaluation of the hypertensive diabetic is similar to that of other hypertensives. The higher risk associated this combination is further increased by the presence of other CVD risk factors that often accompany both disorders, including hyperlipidemia and unhealthy lifestyles (e.g., obesity, physical inactivity, smoking). These should be identified and every attempt made to correct them. Careful attention to how blood pressure is measured is especially important in the diabetic hypertensive. Because blood pressure is more variable in diabetics, more readings are required to obtain accurate mean readings. In addition, orthostatic hypotension is more common, making standing readings essential at all clinic visits. Secondary causes of hypertension associated with diabetes and hypertension include renovascular hypertension, Cushing's syndrome, pheochromocytoma, and primary aldosteronism. The fundoscopic examination and the evaluation of all large arteries and pulses for bruits are important on physical examination.

Therapy is directed at aggressive treatment of both diseases to their respective (HbA$_{1c}$ and blood pressure) goals.[3] In the United States, while there are no clinical outcome data documenting the benefit of this lower goal, the consensus is that antihypertensive drug therapy and goals of blood pressure treatment should be directed at maintaining blood pressure below 130/85 mmHg in the hypertensive with diabetes rather than the usual goal of less than 140/90 mmHg. In the Hypertension Optimal Treatment (HOT) trial,

diabetics randomized to the lower blood pressure goal (diastolic blood pressure below 80 mmHg) had a significantly lower (by 51 percent) CVD event rate than those randomized to the DBP goal of less than 90 mmHg.[20] However, the blood pressure that was actually achieved in the diabetics randomized to these two arms was not provided, and the achieved blood pressure in the majority of trial participants was higher than the goal to which they were randomized. Thus, the blood pressure–producing optimal risk reduction for the diabetics in this trial has not yet been reported.

In the hypertensive with type 1 diabetes and proteinuria, the data support the inclusion of an ACE inhibitor in the antihypertensive regimen (or an angiotensin receptor blocker in the ACE inhibitor–intolerant patient).[3,13,14,21–23] The primary goal is to prevent diabetic end-stage renal disease, the most frequent life-threatening complication in the type 1 diabetic. The data are less compelling regarding initial drug selection in the hypertensive with type 2 diabetes, especially in older type 2 diabetics without proteinuria where the major morbidity and mortality are related to cardiovascular events.[89]

In addition to their potential to produce adverse effects on blood lipids, potassium, and/or glucose, high-dose diuretics and nonselective beta blockers have been reported to also increase insulin resistance.[90,91] This has resulted in their association with worsening the adverse metabolic profile of the insulin-resistance syndrome. However, reduction of cardiovascular events (including coronary events) has been reported to be even greater in diabetic than in nondiabetic hypertensives using diuretic/sympatholytic–based antihypertensive regimens.[17,92,93] Definitive clinical outcome data from studies specifically designed to compare the effect of other agents—including ACE inhibitors, angiotensin receptor blockers, alpha blockers, or calcium channel blockers—with diuretic/sympatholytic–based regimens on cardiovascular event rate are not yet available.

The results of two recently completed small trials comparing the effect of dihydropyridine calcium channel blockers and ACE inhibitors in hypertensive diabetics have been published. They suggest a greater reduction of cardiovascular events (mostly CHD) in those receiving an ACE inhibitor than in those taking the dihydropyridine calcium channel blocker.[94,95] However, in addition to their small size (only about 200 in each of the treatment groups) and one having an open-label design, neither of these trials was designed to evaluate cardiovascular endpoints as a primary objective. Additionally, since the comparison was between two agents whose effect on CVD outcomes were unknown, it is unclear whether the difference in the endpoints was due to an increase or lack of decrease in events in the calcium-channel-blocker arms or to a comparatively greater reduction in events in the ACE-inhibitor arms. On the other hand, post hoc analysis of data from two other trials[18,20] reported a greater reduction of CVD events with a dihydropyridine calcium channel blocker–based regimen in the diabetic versus the entire cohort.

A post hoc analysis of another trial has been presented but not published and suggests a favorable comparison between an ACE inhibitor–based compared to a beta blocker/diuretic–based regimen in diabetics.[48] However, the recently reported United Kingdom Prospective Diabetes Study Group trial comparing blood pressure lowering with an ACE inhibitor–based regimen to one containing a beta blocker confirmed the benefit of blood pressure lowering with these agents but reported no difference in either microvascular (e.g., nephropathy, retinopathy) or macrovascular (e.g., CVD, stroke) event rate in comparing the two drug treatment arms. However, there were more reported side effects as well as a greater weight gain in the beta-blocker group.[96,97] Several larger trials specifically designed to evaluate CVD events in diabetic hypertensives are ongoing. The results of the largest trial, the Antihypertensive and Lipid-Lowering Treatment to Prevent Heart Attack trial (ALLHAT), comparing a thiazide diuretic to a dihydropyridine calcium channel blocker, an ACE inhibitor, and an alpha blocker, and including approximately 15,000 hypertensive diabetics, should be available by 2003.[98]

Thus, until more definitive data are available, current recommendations for the hypertensive diabetic are to aggressively reduce blood pressure to achieve the blood pressure goal. It is clearly reasonable to accomplish this with a regimen that includes an ACE inhibitor, especially in a patient with diabetic nephropathy.[3,13,14,22] Although clinical outcomes data are not yet available for the angiotensin receptor blockers, their related mechanism of action makes their selection for diabetics intolerant to ACE inhibitors a reasonable recommendation until the results of ongoing clinical trials with these agents are available.[3] Since significant reduction of cardiovascular outcomes including CHD has been documented with a low-dose diuretic-based antihypertensive therapy, this represents a reasonable alternative or additional agent to use to achieve the target blood pressure.[17,94,95] The role of calcium channel blockers in this population (except when needed for blood pressure control) remains to be established. As in all high-risk populations, the importance of achieving the blood pressure goal regardless of agent(s) prescribed cannot be overemphasized.

Hyperlipidemia Hyperlipidemia and hypertension commonly occur concomitantly, and in combination their associated risk is more than additive.[99] Lifestyle modification is the first approach to the treatment of both conditions. Thus, recommended management mandates even greater emphasis on control of obesity, reduction of cholesterol and saturated fat intake, and increased physical activity. If lifestyle modifications are insufficient, drug therapy for either or both risk factors must be added. The goal of therapy is to attain both the recommended low-density lipoprotein (LDL) cholesterol and blood pressure goals.

Although several classes of antihypertensives may alter plasma lipids and lipoproteins, the clinical significance of these drug-induced changes on CVD risk has never been examined in a clinical outcome trial. Thiazide and loop diuretics can cause small though usually transient elevations in total cholesterol, triglycerides, and LDL cholesterol.[100–106] The absence of a long-term adverse effect of thiazide diuretics on cholesterol levels compared with placebo and the other classes of antihypertensives has been confirmed in two recent long-term comparative trials.[29,83] Beta blockers can increase levels of plasma triglycerides and reduce high-density lipoprotein (HDL) cholesterol levels.[8,9] Labetalol, carvedilol, and beta blockers with intrinsic sympathomimetic activity

(ISA) have little or no adverse effect on lipids. Interestingly, unlike agents of this class without ISA activity, ISA-active agents have not demonstrated cardioprotection after a myocardial infarction. The alpha$_1$-receptor blockers may produce modest decreases in serum cholesterol, especially in the very low density lipoprotein (VLDL) subfraction, and increase HDL.[100,107,108] Thus, these agents may offer an advantage in managing hypertensive patients with dyslipidemia, though clinical outcome data to document this are still pending. ALLHAT will be the first test of the benefit of an alpha blocker (doxazosin) in preventing CVD morbidity and mortality in hypertensives with and without hyperlipidemia.[98] ACE inhibitors, angiotensin-receptor blockers, calcium channel blockers, and the central adrenergic agonists only minimally affect serum lipids and lipoproteins.[100]

The lipid-altering effects of an antihypertensive agent should not take precedence over features normally considered in selecting therapy. In hypertensives with modest financial resources who require lipid-lowering drug therapy, the potential adverse effect of lower-cost diuretics and beta blockers on serum lipids prescribed with the more potent though more expensive lipid-lowering agents may be more rational than the selection of more expensive antihypertensive agents that have only marginal beneficial effects on blood lipids. A trial of antihypertensive agents with lipid-neutral or beneficial effects on plasma lipids may be considered in patients with only modest elevations of blood lipids in whom additional lipid-lowering therapy is being considered or in those who remain above goal even on maximal lipid-lowering therapy. The lipid-lowering arm of ALLHAT will provide important comparative clinical outcome data on the effect of lipid-lowering therapy with an HMG-CoA reductase inhibitor in hypertensives treated with classes of antihypertensive agents having varying beneficial and adverse effects on plasma lipids.[98]

Hypertension Management in Patients with Coexistent Target-Organ-Damage Heart Disease

In hypertensives with heart disease (i.e., LVH, CHF, and/or CHD), control of blood pressure is particu-

larly important. LVH is a major independent CVD risk factor. In hypertensives with LVH, the risk of a CVD event increases three- to fourfold.[109] Reduction of blood pressure with any of the available classes of antihypertensives (except monotherapy with hydralazine and minoxidil) or with lifestyle changes will reduce LV mass.[110–114] The mechanisms by which LVH increases cardiovascular events are not certain. Increased ventricular ectopy, predisposition to reentrant arrhythmias, and a lowered threshold for myocardial ischemia have been postulated.[115] Observational data suggest that regression of LVH reduces CVD risk.[113] However, a beneficial effect of regression of LVH by antihypertensive therapy on cardiovascular morbidity and mortality beyond that seen with blood pressure reduction needs to be conclusively demonstrated.[116,117] This is currently being prospectively evaluated in at least one long-term clinical outcome trial.[118]

The electrocardiogram (ECG) has a low sensitivity for detecting LVH but is highly specific in most populations. However, the significance of LVH determined by ECG in African Americans is unclear. Multiple studies have reported LVH determined by ECG to be more prevalent in African Americans than in white hypertensives.[119–124] However, several studies reported that the assessment of LVH by ECG in African Americans is significantly less accurate than in other populations.[119–121] Uncertainty also exists regarding the CVD risk associated with ECG-determined LVH in African American populations.[125–127] The reasons for the difference in accuracy of the ECG in identifying LVH in African American versus white populations are unclear.[128–130]

Although echocardiography is more sensitive and specific than the ECG in detecting LVH, its widespread use in hypertensives without other indications is not recommended except in untreated stage 1 hypertensives without cardiovascular risk factors or evidence of target organ damage. In this case, the presence of LVH on echocardiogram may increase the tendency to initiate more aggressive therapy earlier. Some have recommended greater use of a "limited" echocardiographic study in centers where such studies are available for reduced cost.[131]

Cardiac failure Hypertension is now the leading cause of CHF in the United States.[132] LVH with progressive ventricular dilatation, myocardial ischemia, and diastolic dysfunction are among the mechanisms responsible for the development of heart failure in hypertensive patients.[132] Multiple studies have shown that blood pressure control and ACE inhibitors used alone or in combination with digoxin and/or diuretics are effective in reducing morbidity and mortality in hypertensives with CHF.[3,14,15,22] ACE inhibitors are the agents of choice in patients with hypertension and systolic dysfunction leading to heart failure. Angiotensin II receptor antagonists and carvedilol, a combined alpha and beta blocker, also appear promising in preliminary studies of patients with congestive heart failure.[3,133,134] In hypertensives with heart failure, a normal or high ejection fraction suggests diastolic dysfunction; beta-adrenergic blockers and nondihydropyridine calcium channel blockers may be effective in this setting.[135]

Coronary artery disease Coronary artery disease (CAD) is both a common coexistent condition and a consequence of hypertension. Since beta-adrenergic blockers and calcium channel antagonists have antianginal properties in addition to their antihypertensive effects, they are preferred agents in patients with hypertension and CAD.[3,14,15,22] The Beta Blocker in Heart Attack Trial (BHAT) and other post–myocardial infarction trials of beta blockers have documented the efficacy of beta blockers without ISA in reducing mortality in nearly all patients with prior myocardial infarctions, even in some with relative contraindications.[136,137] Unless there are contraindications to their use, beta blockers are the drugs of choice in these patients. Similarly, patients who develop systolic dysfunction following a myocardial infarction benefit from the use of ACE inhibitors.[138]

Cerebrovascular disease Hypertension is a major risk factor for both hemorrhagic and atherosclerotic stroke. Normalization of blood pressure with diuretics, beta blockers, and long-acting dihydropyridine calcium channel blocker–based therapy has been shown to reduce stroke incidence in primary prevention trials.[3,18,20,65] However, there are few data on the effect of antihypertensive therapy in preventing recurrent stroke in patients with preexisting cerebrovascular disease. Thus, secondary prevention of recurrent stroke with antihypertensive therapy is still unproved, though data suggest that antihypertensive therapy protects against other CVD complications in this high-risk group.[139]

Renal disease Hypertension is the second leading cause of chronic renal disease in the United States and the leading cause in African Americans.[72] In patients with end-stage renal disease, CVD is the major cause of death, and all patients with renal dysfunction are considered to be in the "highest risk" group for CVD.[140] Elevated blood pressure in patients on hemodialysis is associated with increased CVD incidence. However, it is unclear what blood pressure represents optimal control, since there is also evidence of a "J" relationship. In this population, even the timing of blood pressure measurement to assess optimal blood pressure control (e.g., before or after dialysis, on days between dialysis) remains uncertain.[140,141] Most consensus panels recommend lowering blood pressure to less than 125/75 mmHg in patients with proteinuria above 1 g/day and would favor the inclusion of ACE inhibitors in the regimen. However, this regimen is intended to slow the progression of the renal disease,[3,142] since there are few data evaluating the benefit of antihypertensive therapy in preventing CVD in this population.[95,96,140]

Peripheral vascular disease The CVD risk in patients with peripheral vascular disease is similar to that of patients with CHD. There are limited data regarding the choice of antihypertensive therapy in patients with atherosclerotic peripheral vascular disease. Beta-adrenergic blockers, especially nonselective agents, may worsen intermittent claudication; on a theoretical basis, calcium channel antagonists and alpha blockers, because of their vasodilator properties, may be useful in this scenario.[3] Normalization of blood pressure as well as other risk factors is essential.

Conclusions

Hypertension is a very common and important risk factor for cardiovascular disease. There is an extensive database of experience on the most effective approaches to diagnose, evaluate, and treat the disorder. These approaches are also backed by substantial clinical outcome data documenting the benefit of these approaches in preventing its CVD complications. Current recommendations focus on identifying hypertensives at greatest risk for complications for earlier and more aggressive treatment. The results of ongoing clinical trials should clarify the role of specific classes of antihypertensives in various hypertensive subgroups. For now, while most recommendations recognize the benefit of using specific agents for special indications and subpopulations of hypertensives, all emphasize the need to lower blood pressure to achieve the blood pressure goals.

Furthermore, while enhanced efforts to treat and improve control in those already under treatment are needed, enhanced screening programs in high-risk populations are essential to identify the large numbers of hypertensives in those populations that have not yet been detected. Moreover, public health campaigns aimed at promoting preventive behaviors to prevent hypertension would have the most dramatic impact.

APPENDIX 6-1 QUICK REFERENCE GUIDE TO JNC VI RECOMMENDATIONS FOR BLOOD PRESSURE MEASUREMENT, PRIMARY PREVENTION, GOALS, TREATMENT, AND ADHERENCE

Blood Pressure Measurement

Patient should:
- Rest for 5 minutes before measurement.
- Refrain from smoking or ingesting caffeine for 30 minutes prior to measurement.
- Be seated with feet flat on floor, back and arm supported, arm at heart level.

Clinician should:
- Use the appropriate size cuff for the patient; the bladder should encircle at least 80 percent of the upper arm.
- Use calibrated or mercury manometer.
- Average two or more readings, separated by at least 2 minutes.

Primary Prevention

Encourage patients to make healthy lifestyle choices:
- Quit smoking to reduce cardiovascular risk.
- Lose weight, if needed.
- Restrict sodium intake to no more than 100 mmol per day.
- Limit alcohol intake to no more than 1–2 drinks per day.
- Get at least 30–45 minutes of aerobic activity on most days.
- Maintain adequate potassium intake—about 90 mmol per day.
- Maintain adequate intakes of calcium and magnesium for general health.

Goal

Set a clear goal of therapy based on patient's risk. Control blood pressure **to below:**
- 140/90 mmHg for patients with uncomplicated hypertension; set a lower goal for those with target organ damage or clinical cardiovascular disease.
- 130/85 mmHg for patients with diabetes.
- 125/75 mmHg for patients with renal insufficiency with proteinuria greater than 1 gram per 24 hours.

Treatment

Begin with lifestyle modifications (see Primary Prevention above) for all patients. Be supportive!
- Add pharmacologic therapy if blood pressure remains uncontrolled.
- Start with a diuretic or beta blocker unless there are compelling indications to use other agents. Use low dose and titrate upward. Consider low-dose combinations.
- If no response, try a drug from another class or add a second agent from a different class (diuretic if not already used).

Adherence

- Encourage lifestyle modifications. Be supportive!
- Educate patient and family about disease. Involve them in measurement and treatment.
- Maintain communications with patient.
- Discuss how to integrate treatment into daily activities.
- Keep care inexpensive and simple.
- Favor once-daily, long-acting formulations.
- Use combination tablets, when needed.
- Consider using generic formulas or larger tablets that can be divided. This may be less expensive.
- Be willing to stop unsuccessful therapy and try a different approach.
- Consider using nurse case management.

(continued)

- Determine blood pressure stage.
- Determine risk group by major risk and TOD/CCD.
- Determine treatment recommendations (by using the table below).
- Determine goal blood pressure.
- Refer to specific treatment recommendations.

Major Risk Factors
- Smoking factors
- Dyslipidemia
- Diabetes mellitus
- Age >60 years
- Gender:
  —Men
  —Postmenopausal women
- Family history:
  —Women < age 65
  —Men < age 55

TOD/CCD (Target Organ Damage/ Clinical Cardiovascular Disease
Heart diseases
- LVH
- Angina/prior MI
- Prior CABG
- Heart failure
Stroke or TIA
Nephropathy
Peripheral arterial disease
Hypertensive retinopathy

Blood pressure stages (mmHg)	Risk Group A No major risk factors No TOD/CCD	Risk Group B At least one major risk factor, not including diabetes No TOD/CCD	Risk Group C TOD/CCD and/or diabetes, with or without other risk factors
High-normal (130–139/85–89)	Lifestyle modification	Lifestyle modification	Drug therapy for those with heart failure, renal insufficiency or diabetes Lifestyle modification
Stage 1 (140–159/90–99)	Lifestyle modification (up to 12 months)	Lifestyle modification (up to 6 months) For patients with multiple risk factors, clinicians should consider drugs as initial therapy plus lifestyle modifications.	Drug therapy Lifestyle modification
Stages 2 and 3 (≥160/≥100)	Drug therapy Lifestyle modification	Drug therapy Lifestyle modification	Drug therapy Lifestyle modification

Example: A patient with diabetes and a blood pressure of 142/94 mmHg plus left ventricular hypertrophy should be classified as having stage 1 hypertension with target organ disease (left ventricular hypertrophy) and with another major risk factor (diabetes). This patient would be categorized as **Stage 1, Risk Group C,** and recommended for immediate initiation of pharmacologic treatment.

Goal Blood Pressure

<140/90 mmHg	Uncomplicated hypertension, Risk Group A, Risk Group B, Risk Group C except for the following:
<130/85 mmHg	Diabetes; renal failure; heart failure
<125/75 mmHg	Renal failure with proteinuria >1 gram/24 hours

Specific Treatment Recommendations

Lifestyle modification should be definitive therapy for some patients and adjunctive therapy for all patients recommended for pharmacologic therapy. Turn page over for a list of recommended lifestyle modifications.

Initial Drug Choices

- Start with a low dose of a long-acting once-daily drug, and **titrate dose**
- Low-dose combinations may be appropriate

Uncomplicated Hypertension	Compelling Indications		Specific Indications for the Following Drugs:
Diuretics Beta blockers	Diabetes type 1 (IDDM)	start with ACE inhibitor if proteinuria is present	(See Table 9 in JNC VI for specific indications)
	Heart failure	start with ACE inhibitor or diuretic	ACE inhibitors
	Myocardial infarction	beta blocker (non-ISA) after MI; ACE inhibitor for LV dysfunction after MI	Angiotensin II receptor blockers Alpha blockers Alpha–beta blockers
	Isolated systolic hypertension (older patients)	diuretics (preferred) or calcium antagonists (long-acting DHP)	Beta blockers Calcium antagonists Diuretics

Source: From the National Heart, Lung, and Blood Institute.

APPENDIX 6–2 ORAL HYPERTENSIVE DRUGS*

Drug	Trade Name	Usual Dose Range, Total mg/day* (Frequency per Day)	Selected Side Effects and Comments*
Diuretics (partial list)			Short-term: increases cholesterol and glucose levels; biochemical abnormalities: decreases potassium, sodium, and magnesium levels, increases uric acid and calcium levels; rare: blood dyscrasias, photosensitivity, pancreatitis, hyponatremia
Chlorthalidone (G)†	Hygroton	12.5–50 (1)	
Hydrochlorothiazide (G)	Hydrodiuril, Microzide, Esidrix	12.5–50 (1)	
Indapamide	Lozol	1.25–5 (1)	(Less or no hypercholesterolemia)
Metolazone	Mykrox	0.5–1.0 (1)	
	Zaroxolyn	2.5–10 (1)	
Loop diuretics			
Bumetanide (G)	Bumex	0.5–4 (2–3)	(Short duration of action, no hypercalcemia)
Ethacrynic acid	Edecrin	25–100 (2–3)	(Only nonsulfonamide diuretic, ototoxicity)
Furosemide (G)	Lasix	40–240 (2–3)	(Short duration of action, no hypercalcemia)
Torsemide	Demadex	5–100 (1–2)	
Potassium-sparing agents			Hyperkalemia
Amiloride hydro-chloride (G)	Midamore	5–10 (1)	
Spironolactone (G)	Aldactone	25–100 (1)	(Gynecomastia)
Triamterene (G)	Dyrenium	25–100 (1)	
Adrenergic inhibitors			
Peripheral agents			
Guanadrel	Hylorel	10–75 (2)	(Postural hypotension, diarrhea)
Guanethidine monosulfate	Ismelin	10–150 (1)	(Postural hypotension, diarrhea)
Reserpine (G)**	Serpasil	0.05–0.25 (1)	(Nasal congestion, sedation, depression, activation of peptic ulcer)
Central alpha-agonists			Sedation, dry mouth, bradycardia, withdrawal hypertension
Clonidine hydrochloride (G)	Catapres	0.2–1.2 (2–3)	(More withdrawal)
Guanabenz acetate (G)	Wytensin	8–32 (2)	
Guanfacine hydrochloride (G)	Tenex	1–3 (1)	(Less withdrawal)
Methyldopa (G)	Aldomet	500–3,000 (2)	(Hepatic and "autoimmune" disorders)

(continued)

Alpha blockers			Postural hypotension
Doxazosin mesylate	Cardura	1–16 (1)	
Prazosin hydrochloride (G)	Minipress	2–30 (2–3)	
Terazosin hydrochloride	Hytrin	1–20 (1)	
Beta blockers			Bronchospasm, bradycardia, heart failure, may mask insulin-induced hypoglycemia; less serious: impaired peripheral circulation, insomnia, fatigue, decreased exercise tolerance, hypertriglyceridemia (except agents with intrinsic sympathomimetic activity)
Acebutolol§‡	Sectral	200–800 (1)	
Atenolol (G)§	Tenormin	25–100 (1–2)	
Betaxolol§	Kerlone	5–20 (1)	
Bisoprolol fumarate§	Zebeta	2.5–10 (1)	
Carteolol hydrochloride‡	Cartrol	2.5–10 (1)	
Metoprolol tartrate (G)§	Lopressor	50–300 (2)	
Metoprolol succinate§	Toprol-XL	50–300 (1)	
Nadolol (G)	Corgard	40–320 (1)	
Penbutolol sulfate‡	Levatol	10–20 (1)	
Pindolol (G)‡	Visken	10–60 (2)	
Propranolol hydrochloride (G)	Inderal / Inderal LA	40–480 (1) / 40–480 (2)	
Timolol maleate (G)	Blocadren	20–60 (2)	
Combined alpha and beta blockers			Postural hypotension, bronchospasm
Carvedilol	Coreg	12.5–50 (2)	
Labetalol hydrochloride (G)	Normodyne, Trandate	200–1,200 (2)	
Direct vasodilators			Headaches, fluid retention, tachycardia
Hydralazine hydrochloride (G)	Apresoline	50–300 (2)	(Lupus syndrome)
Minoxidil (G)	Loniten	5–100 (1)	(Hirsutism)
Calcium antagonists			
Nondihydropyridines			Conduction defects, worsening of systolic dysfunction, gingival hyperplasia
Diltiazem hydrochloride	Cardizem SR / Cardizem CD, Dilacor XR, Tiazac	120–360 (2) / 120–360 (1)	(Nausea, headache)
Verapamil hydrochloride	Isoptin SR, Calan SR / Verelan, Covera HS	90–480 (2) / 120–480 (1)	(Constipation)
Dihydropyridines			Edema of the ankle, flushing, headache, gingival hypertrophy

(continued)

Amlodipine besylate	Norvasc	2.5–10 (1)
Felodipine	Plendil	2.5–20 (1)
Isradipine	DynaCirc	5–20 (2)
	DynaCirc CR	5–20 (1)
Nicardipine	Cardene SR	60–90 (2)
Nifedipine	Procardia XL, Adalat CC	30–120 (1)
Nisoldipine	Sular	20–60 (1)

ACE inhibitors

Common: cough; rare: angioedema, hyperkalemia, rash, loss of taste, leukopenia

Benazepril hydrochloride	Lotensin	5–40 (1–2)
Captopril (G)	Capoten	25–150 (2–3)
Enalapril maleate	Vasotec	5–40 (1–2)
Eosinopril sodium	Monopril	10–40 (1–2)
Lisinopril	Prinivil, Zestril	5–40 (1)
Moexipril	Univasc	7.5–15 (2)
Quinapril hydrochloride	Accupril	5–80 (1–2)
Ramipril	Altace	1.25–20 (1–2)
Trandolapril	Mavik	1–4 (1)

Angiotensin II receptor blockers

Angioedema (very rare), hyperkalemia

Losartan potassium	Cozaar	25–100 (1–2)
Valsartan	Diovan	80–320 (1)
Irbesartan	Avapro	150–300 (1)

*These dosages may vary from those listed in the *Physicians' Desk Reference* (52d edition), which may be consulted for additional information. The listing of side effects is not all-inclusive, and side effects are for the class of drugs except where noted for individual drugs (in parentheses); clinicians are urged to refer to the package insert for a more detailed listing.

†(G) indicates generc available.

‡Has intrinsic sympathomimetic activity.

§Cardioselective.

**Also acts centrally.

Source: Adapted from JNC VI,[3] with permission.

APPENDIX 6–3 COMBINATION DRUGS IN HYPERTENSION

Drug	Trade Name
Beta-adrenergic blockers and diuretics	
Atenolol, 50 or 100 mg/chlorthalidone, 25 mg	Tenoretic
Bisoprolol fumarate, 2.5 5, or 10 mg/hydrochlorothiazide, 6.25 mg	Ziac*
Metoprolol tartrate, 50 or 100 mg/hydrochlorothiazide, 25 or 50 mg	Lopressor HCT
Nadolol, 40 or 80 mg/bendroflumethiazide, 5 mg	Corzide
Propranolol hydrochloride, 40 or 80 mg/hydrochlorothiazide, 25 mg	Inderide
Propranolol hydrochloride (extended release), 80, 120, or 160 mg/hydrochlorothiazide, 50 mg	Inderide LA
Timolol maleate, 10 mg/hydrochlorothiazide, 25 mg	Timolide
ACE inhibitors and diuretics	
Benazepril hydrochloride, 5, 10, or 20 mg/hydrochlorothiazide, 6.25, 12.5, or 25 mg	Lotensin HCT
Captopril, 25 or 50 mg/hydrochlorothiazide, 15 or 25 mg	Capozide*
Enalapril maleate, 5 or 10 mg/hydrochlorothiazide, 12.5 or 25 mg	Vaseretic
Lisinopril, 10 or 20 mg/hydrochlorothiazide, 12.5 or 25 mg	Prinzide, Zestoretic
Angiotensin II receptor antagonists and diuretics	
Losartan potassium, 50 mg/hydrochlorothiazide, 12.5 mg	Hyzaar
Calcium antagonists and ACE inhibitors	
Amlodipine besylate, 2.5 or 5 mg/benazepril hydrochloride, 10 or 20 g	Lotrel
Diltiazem hydrochloride, 180 mg/enalapril maleate, 5 mg	Teczem
Verapamil hydrochloride (extended release), 180 or 240 mg/trandolapril, 1, 2, or 4 mg	Tarka
Felodipine, 5 mg/enalapril maleate, 5 mg	Lexxel
Other combinations	
Triamterene, 37.5, 50, or 75 mg/hydrochlorothiazide, 25 or 50 mg	Dyazide, Maxide
Spironolactone, 25 or 50 mg/hydrochlorothiazide, 25 or 50 mg	Aldactazide
Amiloride hydrochloride, 5 mg/hydrochlorothiazide, 50 mg	Moduretic
Guanethidine monosulfate, 10 mg/hydrochlorothiazide, 25 mg	Esimil
Hydralazine hydrochloride, 25, 50, or 100 mg/hydrochlorothiazide, 25 or 50 mg	Apresazide
Methyldopa, 250 or 500 mg/hydrochlorothiazide, 15, 25, 30, or 50 mg	Aldoril
Reserpine, 0.125 mg/hydrochlorothiazide, 25 or 50 mg	Hydropres
Clonidine hydrochloride, 0.1, 0.2, or 0.3 mg/chlorthalidone, 15 mg	Combipres
Methyldopa, 250 mg/chlorothiazide, 150 or 250 mg	Aldochlor
Reserpine, 0.125 or 0.25 mg/chlorthalidone, 25 or 50 mg	Demi-Regroton
Reserpine, 0.125 or 0.25 mg/chlorothiazide, 250 or 500 mg	Diupres
Prazosin hydrochloride, 1, 2, or 5 mg/polythiazide, 0.5 mg	Minizide

*Approved for initial therapy.
Source: Adapted from JNC VI,[3] with permission.

References

1. Keys A: *Seven Countries: A Multivariate Analysis of Death and Coronary Heart Disease.* Cambridge, MA, Harvard University Press, 1980.

2. Stamler J, Stamler R, Neaton JD: Blood pressure, systolic and diastolic, and cardiovascular risks: U.S. population data. *Arch Intern Med* 1993; 153:598–615.

3. Joint National Committee on Prevention, Detection, Evaluation, and Treatment of High Blood Pressure: The Sixth Report of the Joint National Committee on Prevention, Detection, Evaluation, and Treatment of High Blood Pressure. *Arch Intern Med* 1997; 157:2413–2446.

4. McMahon S, Peto R, Cutler J, et al: Blood pressure, stroke, and coronary heart disease: Part 1. Prolonged differences in blood pressure: prospective observational studies corrected for the regression dilution bias. *Lancet* 1990; 335:765–774.

5. Prisant LM, Alpert BS, Robbins CB, et al: American national standard for nonautomated sphygmomanometers: summary report. *Am J Hypertens* 1995; 8:210–213.

6. Perloff D, Grim C, Flack J, et al: *Special Report: Human Blood Pressure Determination by sphygmomanometry: AHA Medical/Scientific Statement.* Dallas, American Heart Association, 1998.

7. Perloff D, Grim C, Flack J, et al: Human blood pressure determination by sphygmomanometry. *Circulation* 1993; 88:2460–2467.

8. Lind L, Pollare T, Berne C, et al: Long-term metabolic effects of antihypertensive drugs. *Am Heart J* 1993; 128:1177–1183.

9. Rabkin SW: Mechanisms of action of adrenergic receptor-blockers on lipids during antihypertensive drug treatment. *J Clin Pharmacol* 1993; 33:286–291.

10. Lever AF, Ramsay LE: Treatment of hypertension in the elderly. *J Hypertens* 1995; 13:571–579.

11. Pickering T, for an American Society of Hypertension ad hoc panel: Recommendations for the use of home (self) and ambulatory blood pressure monitoring. *Am J Hypertens* 1995; 9:1–11.

12. Appel LJ, Stason WB: Ambulatory blood pressure monitoring and blood pressure self-measurement in the diagnosis and management of hypertension. *Ann Intern Med* 1993; 118:867–882.

13. Alderman MH, Cushman WC, Hill MN, et al: International roundtable discussion of national guidelines for the detection, evaluation, and treatment of hypertension. *Am J Hypertens* 1993; 6:974–981.

14. Chalmers J, Zanchetti A: The 1996 report of a World Health Organization Expert Committee on Hypertension Control. *J Hypertens* 1996; 14:929–933.

15. The Core Services Committee: *Guidelines for the Management of Mildly Raised Blood Pressure in New Zealand, 1–22. 1995.* Wellington, NZ, Core Service Committee, 1995.

16. Lewis EJ, Hunsicker LG, Bain RP, et al: The effect of angiotensin-converting-enzyme inhibition on diabetic nephropathy. *N Engl J Med* 1993; 329:1456–1462.

17. Curb JD, Pressel SL, Cutler JA, et al: Effect of diuretic-based antihypertensive treatment on cardiovascular disease risk in older diabetic patients with isolated systolic hypertension. *JAMA* 1996; 278:40–43.

18. Staessen JA, Fagard R, Thijs L, et al: Randomised double-blind comparison of placebo and active treatment for older patients with isolated systolic hypertension. *Lancet* 1997; 350:757–764.

19. Parving HH, Smidt UM, Hommel E, et al: Effect of antihypertensive treatment on kidney function in diabetic nephropathy. *Am J Kidney Dis* 1993; 22:188–195.

20. Hansson L, Zanchetti A, Carruthers SG, et al: Effects of intensive blood pressure lowering and low dose aspirin in patients with hypertension: principal results of the Hypertension Optimal Treatment (HOT) randomized trial. *Lancet* 1998; 351:1755–1762.

21. Haynes RB, Lacourciere Y, Rabkin SW, et al: Diagnosis of hypertension in adults. *Can Med Assoc J* 1993; 149:409–418.

22. Ogilvie RI, Burgess ED, Cusson JR, et al: Pharmacologic treatment of essential hypertension. *Can Med Assoc J* 1993; 149:575–584.

23. Peters TJ, Fahey TP: What constitutes controlled hypertension? Patient based comparison of hypertension guidelines. *BMJ* 1996; 313:93–96.

24. Trials of Hypertension Prevention Collaborative Research Group: The effects nonpharmacologic interventions on blood pressure of persons with high normal levels: results of the Trials of Hypertension Prevention, Phase I. *JAMA* 1992; 267:1213–1220.

25. Appel LJ, Moore TJ, Obarzanek E, et al: A clinical trial of the effects of dietary patterns on blood pressure. *N Engl J Med* 1997; 336:1117–1124.

26. Trials of Hypertension Prevention Collaborative Group: Effects of weight loss and sodium reduction intervention on blood pressure and hypertension incidence in overweight people with high-normal blood pressure: the Trials of Hypertension Prevention, Phase II. *Arch Intern Med* 1997; 157:657–667.

27. Whelton PK, Appel LJ, Eilspeland MA, et al: Sodium and reduction of weight in the treatment of hypertension in older persons: a randomized controlled trial of nonpharmacologic in the elderly (TONE). *JAMA* 1998; 279:839–846.

28. National High Blood Pressure Education Program: National High Blood Pressure Education Program Working Group report on primary prevention of hypertension. *Arch Intern Med* 1993; 153:186–208.

29. Neaton JD, Grimm RH, Prineas RJ, et al: Treatment of Mild Hypertension Study: final results. *JAMA* 1993; 270:713–724.

30. Paffenbarger RS, Jr., Hyde RT, Wing AL, et al: The association of changes in physical-activity level and other lifestyle characteristics with mortality among men. *N Engl J Med* 1993; 328:538–545.

31. Kokkinos PF, Narayan P, Colleran JA, et al: Effects of regular exercise on blood pressure and left ventricular hypertrophy in African-American men with severe hypertension. *N Engl J Med* 1995; 333:1462–1467.

32. Blair SN, Goodyear NN, Gibbons LW, et al: Physical fitness and incidence of hypertension in healthy normotensive men and women. *JAMA* 1984; 252:487–490.

33. U.S. Department of Health and Human Services: Physical Activity and Health: A report of the Surgeon General, Washington, DC, 1996.

34. Stamler J, Elliott P, Kesteloot H, et al: Inverse relation of dietary protein markers with blood pressure: findings for 10,020 men and women in the INTER-SALT study. *Circulation* 1996; 94:1629–1634.

35. Midgley JP, Matthew AG, Greenwood CMT, et al: Effect of reduced dietary sodium on blood pressure: a meta-analysis of randomized controlled trials. *JAMA* 1996; 275:1590–1597.

36. Law MR, Frost ED, Wald NJI: Analysis of data from trials of salt reduction. *BMJ* 1991; 302:819–824.

37. Weinberger MH: Salt sensitivity of blood pressure in humans. *Hypertension* 1996; 27:481–490.

38. Alderman MH, Madhavan S, Cohen H, et al: Low urinary sodium is associated with greater risk of myocardial infarction among treated hypertensive men. *Hypertension* 1995; 25:1144–1152.

39. Alderman MH, Cohen H, Madhavan S: Dietary sodium intake and mortality: The National Health and Nutrition Examination Survey (NHANES 1). *Lancet* 1998; 351: 781–785.

40. Whelton PK, He J, Cutler JA, et al: Effects of oral potassium on blood pressure: meta-analysis of randomized controlled clinical trials. *JAMA* 1997; 277:1624–1632.

41. Cappuccio FP, Elliott P, Allender PS, et al: Epidemiologic association between dietary calcium intake and blood pressure: a meta-analysis of published data. *Am J Epidemiol* 1995; 142:935–945.

42. Allender PS, Cutler JA, Follmann D, et al: Dietary calcium and blood pressure: a meta-analysis of randomized clinical trials. *Ann Intern Med* 1996; 124:825–831.

43. Stamler J, Caggiula AW, Grandits GA: Relation of body mass and alcohol, nutrient, fiber and caffeine intakes to blood pressure in the special intervention and usual care groups in the Multiple Risk Factor Intervention Trial. *Am J Clin Nutr* 1997; 65:338S-365S.

44. Chockalingham A, Abbott D, Bass M, et al: Recommendations of the Canadian Consensus Conference on Non-pharmacological Approaches to the Management of High Blood Pressure. *Can Med Assoc J* 1990; 142:1397–1409.

45. Materson BJ, Reda DJ, Cushman WC, et al: Single-drug therapy for hypertension in men: a comparison of six antihypertensive agents with placebo. *N Engl J Med* 1993; 328:914–921.

46. Veterans Administration Cooperative Study Group on Antihypertensive Agents: Comparison of propranolol and hydrochlorothiazide for the initial treatment of hypertension: II. Results of long-term therapy. *JAMA* 1982; 248: 2004–2011.

47. Psaty BM, Smith NL, Siscovick DS, et al: Health outcomes associated with antihypertensive therapies used as first-line agent: a systematic review and meta-analysis. *JAMA* 1997; 277:739–745.

48. Hansson L, Lindholm LH, Niskanen L, et al, for the Captopril Prevention Project (CAPPP) study group: Effect of angiotensin-converting-enzyme inhibition compared with conventional therapy on cardiovascular morbidity and mortality in hypertension: the Captopril Prevention Project (CAPPP) randomized trial. *Lancet* 1999; 353:611–616.

49. World Health Organization—International Society of Hypertension Blood Pressure Lowering Treatment Trialists' Collaboration: Protocol for prospective collaborative overviews of major randomized trials of blood pressure lowering treatments. *J Hypertens* 1998; 16:127–137.

50. Guidelines Subcommittee: 1993 guidelines for the management of mild hypertension: memorandum from a WHO/ISH meeting. *J Hypertens* 1993; 11:905–918.

51. Joint National Committee on Prevention, Detection, Evaluation, and Treatment of High Blood Pressure: The fifth report of the Joint National Committee on Detection, Evaluation, and Treatment of High Blood Pressure (JNC V). *Arch Intern Med* 1993; 153:154–183.

52. Wright JT Jr: Use of combination antihypertensive therapy in the black hypertensive. *Ethn Dis* 1997; 2:172–174.

53. National High Blood Pressure Education Program Working Group: National High Blood Pressure Education Program Working Group Report on hypertension in the elderly. *Hypertension* 1994; 23:275–285.

54. Burt VL, Cutler JA, Higgins M, et al: Trends in the prevalence, awareness, treatment, and control of hypertension in the adult U.S. population. *Hypertension* 1995; 26:60–69.

55. National Heart Lung and Blood Institute: *Fact Book Fiscal Yr 1996*. Bethesda, MD, U.S. Department of Health and Human Services, National Institutes of Health, 1997.

56. Schappert SM: National ambulatory medical care survey from vital and health statistics for the Centers for Disease Control and Prevention. National Center for Health Statistics. *Adv Data* 1993; 230:1–20.

57. Messerli FH, Ventura HO, Amodeal C: Osler's maneuver and pseudohypertension. *N Engl J Med* 1985; 312:1548–1551.

58. Wright JC, Looney SW: Prevalence of positive Osler's maneuver in 3387 persons screened for the Systolic

Hypertension in the Elderly Program (SHEP) (see comments). *J Hum Hypertens* 1997; 11:285–289.

59. Belmin J, Visintin JM, Salvatore R, et al: Osler's maneuver: absence of usefulness for the detection of pseudohypertension in an elderly population. *Am J Med* 1995; 98:42–49.

60. Flack J, Wright JT Jr: Optimal utilization of calcium channel blockers in African-American and other special hypertensive populations. *Urban Cardiol* 1998; 5:1–13.

61. Sagie A, Larson MG, Levy D: The natural history of borderline isolated systolic hypertension. *N Engl J Med* 1993; 329:1912–1917.

62. Franklin SS, Khan SA, Wong ND, et al: Is pulse pressure useful in predicting risk for coronary heart disease? The Framingham Heart Study. *Circulation* 1999; 100:354–360.

63. Gifford RW Jr: Geriatric hypertension: chairman's comments on the NIH working report. *Geriatrics* 1987; 42:45–50.

64. Brest AN: Should systolic hypertension be treated? in Corday E (ed): *Controversies in Cardiology*. Philadelphia, Davis, 1978:217–220.

65. SHEP Cooperative Research Group: Prevention of stroke by antihypertensive drug treatment in older persons with isolated systolic hypertension: final results of the Systolic Hypertension in the Elderly Program (SHEP). *JAMA* 1991; 265:3255–3264.

66. Dahlof B, Linholm LH, Hansson L, et al: Morbidity and mortality in the Swedish trial in older patients with hypertension. *Lancet* 1991; 339:1281–1285.

67. MRC Working Party: Medical Research Council Trial of treatment of hypertension in older adults. *BMJ* 1992; 304:405–412.

68. Farnett L, Mulcrow CD, Linn WD, et al: The J-curve phenomena and the treatment of hypertension: is there a point beyond which pressure reduction is dangerous? *JAMA* 1991; 265:489–495.

69. Douglas JG: Hypertension and diabetes in blacks. *Diabetes Care* 1990; 14:1191S–1195S.

70. Singh GK, Kochanek KD, MacDorman MF: Advance report of final mortality statistics 1994. *Mon Vital Stat Rep* 1996; 45:1–76.

71. Lewis CE, Raczynski JM, Oberman A, et al: Risk factors and the natural history of coronary heart disease in blacks, in Saunders E (ed): *Cardiovascular Diseases in Blacks*. Philadelphia, Davis, 1991:29–45.

72. Klag MJ, Whelton PK, Randall BL, et al: End-stage renal disease in African-American and white men: 16-year MRFIT findings. *JAMA* 1997; 277:1293–1298.

73. Hypertension Detection and Follow-up Program Cooperative Group: Five-year findings of the Hypertension Detection and Follow-up Program: II. Mortality by race, sex, and age. *JAMA* 1979; 242:3572–3577.

74. Wright JT Jr, Bakris GL, Douglas M, et al: Baseline and achieved blood pressure in the African American Study

of Kidney Disease and Hypertension (AASK). *Ethn Dis* 1997; 7:S1.

75. Cushman WC, Black HR, Probstfield JL, et al: Blood pressure control in the Antihypertensive and Lipid Lowering Treatment to Prevent Heart Attack Trial (ALLHAT) (abstr). *Am J Hypertens* 1998; 11:17A.

76. Douglas JG, Thibonnier M, Wright JT: Essential hypertension: racial/ethnic differences in pathophysiology. *J Assoc Acad Minority Physicians* 1996; 7:16–21.

77. Sullivan JM, Prewitt RL, Ratts TE: Sodium sensitivity in normotensive and borderline and hypertensive humans. *Am J Med Sci* 1998; 295:370–377.

78. Weinberger M, Miller JZ, Luft FC, et al: Definitions and characteristics of sodium sensitivity and blood pressure resistance. *Hypertension* 1998; 8:II-127–II-134.

79. Rahman M, Douglas JG, Wright JT: Pathophysiology and treatment implications of hypertension in the African-American population. *Endocrinol Metab Clin North Am* 1997; 26:125–144.

80. Douglas, JG, Wright, JT: *Blacks and Hypertension: Current Concepts*. Kalamazoo, MI, Upjohn, 1998.

81. Liao Y, Cooper RS, McGee DL, et al: The relative effects of left ventricular hypertrophy, coronary artery disease and ventricular dysfunction on survival among black adults. *JAMA* 1995; 277:739–745.

82. Masterson BJ, Reda DJ, Cushman WC, et al: Single drug therapy for hypertension in men: a comparison of six antihypertensive agents with placebo: the Department of Veterans Affairs Cooperative Study Group on anti-hypertensive agents. *N Engl J Med* 1993; 328:914–921.

83. Prisant LM, Mensah GA: Use of beta-adrenergic receptor-blockers in blacks. *J Clin Pharmacol* 1996; 36:867–873.

84. Wright JT: Use of combination antihypertensive therapy in the black hypertensive. *Ethn Dis* 1997; 7:172–174.

85. Sica DA: Fixed-dose combination antihypertensive drugs: do they have a role in rational therapy? *Drugs* 1994; 48:16–24.

86. Saunders E, Neutel J: A new antihypertensive strategy for black patients: low-dose multimechanism therapy? *J Natl Med Assoc.* 1994; 88:171–175.

87. The National High Blood Pressure Working Group: National High Blood Pressure Education Program Working Group on Hypertension in Diabetes. *Hypertension* 1994; 23:145–158.

88. Bild, D, Teutsch SM: The control of hypertension in persons with diabetes: a public health approach. *Public Health Rep* 1987; 102:522–529.

89. Moss SE, Klein BE: Cause-specific mortality in a population-based study of diabetes. *Am J Public Health* 1991; 81:1158–1162.

90. Jacob S, Rett K, Henriksen EJ: Antihypertensive therapy and insulin sensitivity: do we have to redefine the role of beta-blocking agents? *Am J Hypertens* 1998; 11:1258–1265.

91. DeFronzo RA, Ferrannini E: Insulin resistance: a multi-faceted syndrome responsible for NIDDM, obesity, hypertension, dyslipidemia. *Diabetes Care* 1991; 14:173–177.

92. The Hypertension Detection and Follow-up Program Cooperative Research Group: Mortality findings for stepped-care and referred-care participants in the Hypertension Detection and Follow-up Program, stratified by other risk factors. *Prev Med* 1985; 14:312–335.

93. Amery A, Brixko P, Cohen H, et al: Mortality and morbidity results from the European Working Party on High Blood Pressure in the Elderly Trial. *Lancet* 1985; 1:1349–1354.

94. Estacio RO, Jeffers BW, Hiatt WR, et al: The effect of nisoldipine as compared with enalapril on cardiovascular outcomes in patients with non-insulin-dependent diabetes and hypertension. *N Engl J Med* 1998; 338:645–652.

95. Tatti P, Pahor M, Byington RP, et al: Outcome results of the fosinopril versus amlodipine cardiovascular events randomized trial (FACET) in patients with hypertension and NIDDM. *Diabetes Care* 1998; 21:597.

96. UK Prospective Diabetes Study Group: Efficacy of atenolol and captopril in reducing risk of macrovascular and microvascular complications in type 2 diabetes: UKPDS 39. *BMJ* 1998; 317:713–720.

97. UK Prospective Diabetes Study Group: Tight blood pressure control and risk of macrovascular and microvascular complications in type 2 diabetes: UKPDS 38. *BMJ* 1998; 317:703–713.

98. Davis BR, Cutler JA, Gordon DJ, et al: Rationale and design for the Antihypertensive and Lipid Lowering Treatment to Prevent Heart Attack Trial (ALLHAT). *Am J Hypertens* 1996; 9:342–360.

99. National Cholesterol Education Program Working Group: Working Group on Management of Patients with Hypertension and High Blood Cholesterol: report on the management of hypertension and high blood cholesterol. *Arch Intern Med* 1991; 114:224–237.

100. Kasiske BL, Ma JZ, Kalil RSN, et al: Effects of antihypertensive therapy on serum lipids. *Ann Intern Med* 1995; 122:133–141.

101. Lehtonen A, Gordin A: A metabolic parameter after changing from hydrochlorothiazide on the plasma levels of triglycerides, total cholesterol and HDL cholesterol in patients with essential hypertension. *Eur J Clin Pharmacol* 1984; 27:153–157.

102. Chrysant SG, Neller GK, Dillard B, et al: Effects of diuretics on lipid metabolism in patients with essential hypertension. *Angiology* 1976; 27:707–711.

103. van Brummelen P, Geveres Leuvn JA, van Gen CM: Influence of hydrochlorothiazide on the plasma levels of triglycerides, total cholesterol and HDL cholesterol in patients with essential hypertension. *Curr Med Res Opin* 1979; 6:24–29.

104. Glueck Z, Weidmann P, Mordasini R, et al: Increased serum low-density lipoprotein cholesterol in men treated short-term with diuretic chlorthalidone. *Metab Clin Exp* 1980; 29:240–245.

105. Williams WR, Schneider KA, Borhani NO, et al: The relationship between diuretics and serum cholesterol in hypertension detection follow-up participants. *Am J Prev Med* 1986; 2:248–255.

106. Ames RP, Hill P: Increase in serum lipids during treatment of hypertension with chlorthalidone. *Lancet* 1976; 1:721–723.

107. Andersson P, Lithell H: Metabolic effects of doxazosin and enalapril in hypertriglyceridemic hypertensive men. Relationship to changes in skeletal muscle blood flow. *Am J Hypertens* 1996; 9(4pt.1):323–333.

108. Pool JL: Effects of doxazosin on serum lipids: a review of the clinical data and molecular basis for altered lipid metabolism. *Am Heart J* 1991; 121:251–259.

109. Levy D, Garrison RH, Savage DD: Prognostic implications of echocardiographically determined left ventricular mass in the Framingham Heart Study. *N Engl J Med* 1990; 322:1561–1566.

110. Gibson RS, Boden WE: Calcium channel antagonists: friend or foe in postinfarction patients? *Am J Hypertens* 1996; 9:172S–176S.

111. Koren MJ, Devereux RB, Casale PN, et al: Relation of left ventricular mass and geometry to morbidity and mortality in uncomplicated essential hypertension. *Ann Intern Med* 1991; 114:345–352.

112. Liao Y, Cooper RS, McGee DL, et al: The relative effects of left ventricular hypertrophy, coronary artery disease, and ventricular dysfunction on survival among black adults. *JAMA* 1995; 273:1592–1597.

113. Devereux RB: Do antihypertensive drugs differ in their ability to regress left ventricular hypertrophy? *Circulation* 1997; 95:1983–1985.

114. Gottdiener JS, Reda DJ, Massie BM, et al: Effect of single-drug therapy on reduction of left ventricular mass in mild to moderate hypertension: comparison of six antihypertensive agents; the Department of Veterans Affairs Cooperative Study Group on Antihypertensive Agents. *Circulation* 1997; 1994:1786–1793.

115. Frohlich ED: Pathophysiology of systemic arterial hypertension. In: Schlant RC, Alexander RW (eds): *Hurst's The Heart,* 8th ed. New York, McGraw-Hill, 1994: 1391–1401.

116. Levy D, Salomon M, D'Agostino RB, et al: Prognostic implications of baseline electrocardiographic features and their serial changes in subjects with left ventricular hypertrophy. *Circulation* 1994; 90:1786–1793.

117. Devereux RB, Agabiti-Rosei E, Dahlof B, et al: Regression of left ventricular hypertrophy as a surrogate endpoint for morbid events in hypertension treatment trials. *J Hypertens* 1996; 14 (suppl):S95-S102.

118. Dahlof B, Devereux RB, de Faire U, et al: The Losartan Intervention For Endpoint Reduction (LIFE) in Hypertension Study: rationale, design, and methods: The LIFE Study Group. *Am J Hypertens* 1997; 10:705–713.

‎

119. Gottdiener JS, Reda DJ, Materson BJ, et al: Importance of obesity, race and age to the cardiac structural and functional effects of hypertension. *J Am Coll Cardiol* 1994; 24:1492–1498.

120. Lee DK, Marantz PR, Devereux RB, et al: Left ventricular hypertrophy in black and white hypertensives: standard electrocardiographic criteria overestimate racial differences in prevalence. *JAMA* 1992; 267:3294–3299.

121. Crow RS, Prineas RJ, Rautaharju P, et al: Relation between electrocardiography and echocardiography for left ventricular mass in mild systemic hypertension (results from Treatment of Mild Hypertension Study). *Am J Cardiol* 1995; 75:1233–1238.

122. Savage DD, Henry WL, Mitchell JR, et al: Echocardiographic comparison of black and white hypertensive subjects. *J Natl Med Assoc* 1979; 71:709–712.

123. Dunn FG, Oigman W, Sungaard-Riise K, et al: Racial differences in cardiac adaptation to essential hypertension determined by echocardiographic indexes. *J Am Coll Cardiol* 1983; 1:1348–1351.

124. Hammond IW, Alderman MH, Devereux RB, et al: Contrast in cardiac anatomy and function between black and white patients with hypertension. *J Natl Med Assoc* 1984; 76:247–255.

125. Tyroler HA: Overview of risk factors for coronary heart disease in black populations. *Am Heart J* 1984; 108:658–660.

126. Rautaharju PM, LaCroiz AZ, Savage DD, et al: Electrocardiographic estimate of left ventricular mass versus radiographic cardiac size and disease mortality in the epidemiologic follow-up study of First National Health and Nutritional Examination Survey. *Am J Cardiol* 1988; 62:59–66.

127. Bartel A, Heyden S, Tyroler HA, et al: Electrocardiographic predictors of coronary heart disease. *Arch Intern Med* 1971; 128:929–937.

128. Horton J, Sherber HS, Lakatta EG: Distance correction for precordial electrocardiographic voltage in estimating left ventricular mass: an echocardiographic study. *Circulation* 1977; 55:509–512.

129. Watkins L: Impact of interracial comparisons of inappropriate criteria for cardiac enlargement in blacks. *Hypertension* 1985; 7:1031–1033.

130. Feldman T, Barow KM, Neuman A, et al: Relation of electrocardiographic R-wave amplitude to changes in left ventricular chamber size and position in normal subjects. *Am J Cardiol* 1985; 55:1168–1174.

131. Sheps SG, Frohlich ED: Limited echocardiography for hypertensive left ventricular hypertrophy. *Hypertension* 1997; 29:560–563.

132. Vasan RS, Levy D: The role of hypertension in the pathogenesis of heart failure: a clinical mechanistic overview. *Arch Intern Med* 1996; 156:1789–1796.

133. Australia/New Zealand Heart Failure Research Collaborative Group: Randomized, placebo-controlled trial of carvedilol in patients with congestive heart failure due to ischaemic heart disease. *Lancet* 1997; 349:375–380.

134. Pitt B, Segal R, Martinez FA, et al: Randomized trial of losartan versus captopril in patients over 65 with heart failure (Evaluation of Losartan in the Elderly Study, ELITE). *N Engl J Med* 1997; 349:747–752.

135. Gaasch WH: Diagnosis and treatment of heart failure based on left ventricular systolic and diastolic dysfunction. *JAMA* 1994; 271:1276–1280.

136. Frishman WH, Furberg CD, Friedewald WT: Beta-adrenergic blockade for survivors of acute myocardial infarction. *N Engl J Med* 1984; 310:830–837.

137. Gottlieb SS, McCarter RJ, Vogel RA: Effect of beta-blockade on mortality among high-risk and low-risk patients after myocardial infarction. *N Engl J Med* 1998; 339:489–497.

138. Hennekens CH, Albert CM, Godfried SL, et al: Adjunctive drug therapy of acute myocardial infarction—evidence from clinical trials. *N Engl J Med* 1996; 335:1660–1667.

139. Hypertension-Stroke Collaborative Study Group: Effect of cintihypertensive treatment on stroke recurrence. *JAMA* 1974; 229:409–418.

140. Levey AS, Beto JA, Coronado BE, et al: Controlling the epidemic of cardiovascular disease on chronic renal disease: What do we know? What do we need to know? Where do we go from here? The National Kidney Foundation Task Force on Cardiovascular Disease. *Am J Kidney Dis* 1998; 32:853–906.

141. Wright JTJ, Douglas JG, Rahman M: Guidelines for the prevention of cardiovascular disease in hypertensive patients with normal renal function. *Am J Kidney Dis* 1998; 32(suppl 2):S1–S15.

142. National High Blood Pressure Education Program Working Group: 1995 Update of the working group reports on chronic renal failure and renovascular hypertension. *Arch Intern Med* 1996; 156:1938–1947.

CHAPTER 7

Cholesterol and Lipids

Nathan D. Wong
Moti L. Kashyap

The importance of elevated total and low-density-lipoprotein cholesterol (LDL-C) in the etiology of coronary heart disease (CHD) and the value of their reduction in the primary and secondary prevention of CHD are well recognized.[1,2] In addition, high-density lipoproteins (HDL) have been linked to protection for CHD.[3,4] Evidence indicates that HDL-cholesterol (HDL-C) participates in the process of reverse cholesterol transport, whereby excess cholesterol is removed from tissues,[5] and may also inhibit atherogenesis.[6,7] The raising of HDL-C levels has also been shown to protect against initial coronary events[8] and documented to be of benefit in the secondary prevention of CHD.[9]

Despite lower rates of CHD events and mortality among those receiving lipid-regulating therapy, many individuals who receive effective treatment still suffer events. This has, in part, led to increasing efforts to understand more detailed aspects of lipids, including the atherogenic lipoprotein phenotype (ALP), characterized by small-sized and highly dense LDL, lipoprotein(a), and subfractions of HDL.

Important challenges we face include (1) adequate identification of the many individuals in need of treatment, both among those with and without coronary artery disease; (2) more effectively treating the many persons with preexisting coronary artery disease who are either not on lipid-regulating treatment or are inadequately treated; and (3) adequately treating other high-risk patient populations, such as diabetics, hypertensives, and the elderly, who would clearly benefit from lipid management. Although there have been major accomplishments in detection of dyslipidemia and treatment with newer therapies

over the past 15 years, many patients clinically indicated for treatment still remain inadequately controlled.

Epidemiologic Perspective

Total and Low-Density-Lipoprotein Cholesterol

A direct relation between levels of total or LDL-C with the risk of CHD has been demonstrated by numerous studies, both across and within populations. The Seven Countries Study showed that, among populations with higher mean levels of total cholesterol, rates of CHD were also higher (Fig. 7–1).[10] Migration studies in Japanese showed mean total cholesterol levels and corresponding rates of CHD to be lowest in their native country (181 mg/dL and 25.4 per 1000, respectively), intermediate among those living in Hawaii (218 mg/dL and 34.7 per 1000, respectively), and highest among Japanese living in San Francisco (228 mg/dL and 44.6 per 1000, respectively).[11] Within a large sample of middle-aged men, a curvilinear relation of total cholesterol to CHD risk was demonstrated by the Multiple Risk Factor Intervention Trial (MRFIT) (Fig. 7–2)[12] and in both men and women by the Framingham Heart Study.[3] Similar relationships are also seen among those with elevated levels of LDL-C.[13] In contrast, the U.S. Pooling Project showed the lowest rate of coronary events to be in the second rather than the first quintile of cholesterol levels.[14] In addition, the relation of total cholesterol to CHD risk is amplified as a function of the number of other risk factors

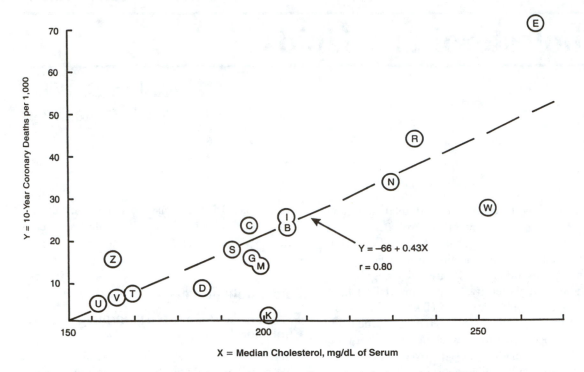

FIGURE 7–1   Ten-year coronary death rates and median serum cholesterol level. B, Belgrade; C, Crevalcore; D, Dalmatia; E, East Finland; G, Corfu; I, Italian railroad; K, Crete; M, Montegiorgio; N, Zutphen; R, American railroad; S, Slavonia; T, Tanushimaru; U, Ushibuka; V, Velika Krsna; W, West Finland; Z, Zrenjanin. (From Keys,[10] with permission. Copyright 1980 by the President and Fellows of Harvard College.)

present, as demonstrated by the Framingham Heart Study (Fig. 7–3).[15] Among persons with a prior history of myocardial infarction, an elevated total cholesterol following recovery remains a significant independent risk factor for reinfarction, death from CHD, and total mortality.[16]

Falling cholesterol levels are associated with future total mortality, possibly being a consequence of certain diseases, such as cancers, predisposing to death.[17] In the Honolulu Heart Study,[18] men with low total cholesterol levels were more likely to have had preexisting adverse health characteristics, such as a higher prevalence of current smoking, heavy drinking, and certain gastrointestinal conditions, and those with the lowest levels of total cholesterol were at a significantly higher risk for hemorrhagic stroke,

cancer, and all-cause mortality. Falling levels of total cholesterol over a 6-year period were also associated with a subsequent increase in the risk of all-cause mortality.[19,20]

High-Density-Lipoprotein Cholesterol

HDL-C plays a role in reverse cholesterol transport, protecting against CHD. HDLs also have antioxidant and profibrinolytic properties and transport important apolipoproteins mediating triglyceride metabolism.[21] An inverse relation of HDL-C to CHD risk is well documented.[20,22] From a 12-year follow-up of individuals 50 to 79 years of age in the Framingham Heart Study, both men and women in the first through third quartiles of HDL-C were at substan-

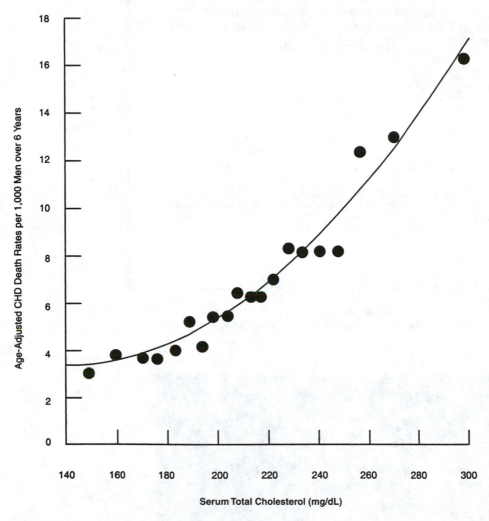

FIGURE 7–2 Total cholesterol and coronary heart disease incidence among MRFIT screenees. (From Stamler et al.,[12] with permission.)

tially higher risk of incident myocardial infarction than those in the highest quartile (Figs. 7–4 and 7–5).[22] Even for those with levels of total cholesterol less than 200 mg/dL, risk for myocardial infarction was high when HDL-C was low. For men (Fig. 7–4) and particularly for women (Fig. 7–5), CHD risk was lower among those in the highest quartile of HDL-C, even if total cholesterol levels were

elevated. Additional evidence from the placebo group of the Helsinki Heart Study showed the LDL-C/HDL-C ratio to be the single best predictor of cardiac events.[8] When this ratio exceeded 5.0 in combination with triglycerides of 200 mg/dL or higher, there was nearly a fourfold higher risk of new coronary events versus those with lower LDL-C/HDL-C ratios and triglycerides.

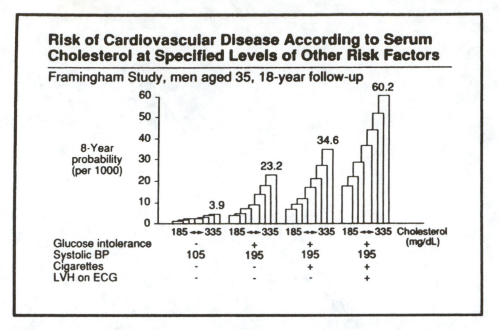

FIGURE 7–3 Impact of multiple risk factors on relation of total cholesterol to coronary heart disease risk: Framingham Heart Study. (From Kannel et al.,[15] with permission.)

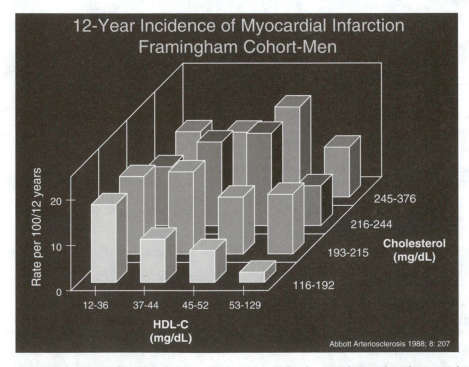

FIGURE 7–4 Twelve-year incidence of myocardial infarction by total and HDL-C levels: Framingham cohort, men. (Adapted from Abbott et al.,[22] with permission.)

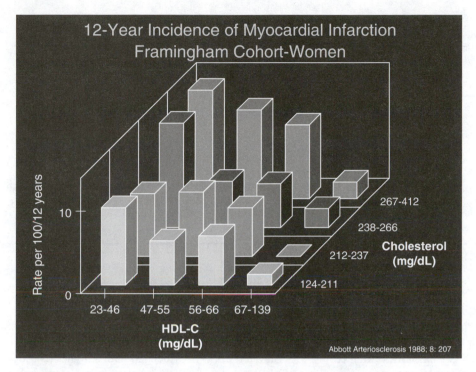

FIGURE 7–5 Coronary heart disease incidence by total and HDL-C levels: Framingham cohort, women. (Adapted from Abbott et al.,[22] with permission.)

Population Levels of Total Cholesterol, LDL Cholesterol, and HDL Cholesterol

The National Health and Nutrition Examination Survey III (NHANES III)[23] provides data on the distribution (prevalence of high-risk levels and percentile levels) by age, gender, and ethnicity of total cholesterol, LDL-C, and HDL-C levels among a large population sample of individuals aged 20 and above. These data on the prevalence of borderline and elevated total and LDL-C and low HDL-C are shown in Table 7–1.

Triglycerides

The relation of triglyceride levels to risk for CHD has been controversial. Although triglycerides were associated with an increased risk of CHD among women aged 50 to 69 in the Framingham Heart Study and men aged 53 to 74 in the Copenhagen Male

Study,[24,25] the Lipid Research Clinics Follow-up study showed no independent relation of triglycerides with CHD mortality except among subjects with lower HDL-C and higher LDL-C as well as in younger subjects.[26] More recently, Gaziano et al., in a case-control study, showed a significant relation of fasting triglycerides to risk of myocardial infarction even after adjusting for HDL-C and other risk factors [relative risk (RR) in the highest versus lowest quartile 2.7; 95 percent confidence interval (CI) 1.4 to 5.5]. The ratio of triglycerides to HDL-C was also strongly associated with risk of myocardial infarction.[27] Further, a large meta-analysis of population-based prospective studies showed a direct relation of triglycerides (per mmol/L or 88.5 mg/dL) and CHD incidence (RR = 1.14; 95 percent CI, 1.05 to 1.28 for men and RR = 1.37; 95 percent CI, 1.13 to 1.66 for women), independent of HDL-C and other risk factors.[28]

TABLE 7–1 Proportion (%) of Adults Aged 20 to 74 with Borderline and Elevated Total and LDL Cholesterol and Low HDL Cholesterol by Ethnicity and Gender

	Total Sample		Non-Hispanic White		Non-Hispanic Black		Mexican-American	
	M	F	M	F	M	F	M	F
Total cholesterol								
200–239 mg/dL	32.5	29.5	32.8	29.6	31.5	31.2	33.0	30.3
240 mg/dL or higher	18.9	20.2	18.8	20.1	16.9	20.1	20.5	19.0
LDL cholesterol								
130–159 mg/dL	27.0	24.7	27.3	24.2	26.6	24.6	22.7	25.1
160 mg/dL or higher	21.1	17.7	22.0	18.7	17.2	16.9	16.2	13.2
HDL cholesterol								
less than 35 mg/dL	16.3	5.7	17.8	6.2	9.3	3.3	15.2	5.5

Source: NHANES III (1988–1991).[23]

In light of the existing evidence, triglycerides should be measured in the evaluation of patients at risk for CHD as part of a fasting lipid profile.[24] Measurement of triglycerides is especially warranted in diabetics or those with glucose intolerance, insulin resistance, obesity, or low HDL-C. From this, the additional risk from elevated triglycerides can be better evaluated along with knowledge about levels of the other lipoprotein fractions.

Apolipoproteins and Lipoprotein(a)

There exist limited prospective data relating apolipoproteins AI and B to CHD risk. The Quebec Cardiovascular Study reported, among 2155 men aged 45 to 76, a direct relation of plasma apolipoprotein B (Apo-B) concentrations with onset of ischemic heart disease over the next 5 years (RR = 1.4; 95 percent CI, 1.2 to 1.7) independent of other risk factors. A weaker, inverse association of Apo-AI with ischemic heart disease (RR = 0.85; 95 percent CI, 0.7 to 1.0) did not persist after adjustment for risk factors.[29]

Lipoprotein(a) [Lp(a)] excess has been identified as a powerful risk factor for developing CHD (Table 7–2) and is also elevated in those with premature CHD.[30] Lp(a) can contribute to atherosclerosis by

impairing fibrinolysis, increasing lipid deposition in the arterial wall, and increasing oxidation of LDL-C.

Elevated Lp(a) is associated with a higher risk for cerebrovascular disease, peripheral arterial disease, myocardial infarction, restenosis after angioplasty, and failure of coronary artery bypass grafts.[31] In Swedish middle-aged asymptomatic men, elevated Lp(a) was also associated with subsequent myocardial infarction,[32] and the Lipid Research Clinics also reported a relation of Lp(a) to CHD.[33] Further, the Framingham Heart Study has reported, among 2191 men aged 20 to 54 at baseline with a median follow-up of 15.4 years, elevated Lp(a) (as indicated by sinking pre–beta lipoprotein bands) to be associated with a twofold greater risk (adjusted for other risk factors) of premature CHD.[34] A 12-year follow-up of 3103 women in the Framingham Heart Study similarly showed that those with this marker for Lp(a) were at a significantly increased risk of myocardial infarction, intermittent claudication, cerebrovascular disease, and total coronary and cardiovascular events (RR = 1.61; 95 percent CI, 1.13 to 2.29 for CHD events).[35]

But neither the Helsinki Heart Study[36] nor the Physician's Health Study[37] showed Lp(a) to be a significant risk factor. A recently reported community-

TABLE 7–2 Observational Studies of the Relation of Lipoprotein(a) and Coronary Heart Disease

Reference	Study Population	Result
Rosengren et al., 1990[32]	135 men aged 50, nested case-control, 6-year follow-up	RR* = 3.3 (p = .02) unadjusted; p = .01 risk factor–adjusted
Ridker et al., 1993[37]	592 male physicians, nested case-control, 5-year follow-up	RR = 0.83 (1.36–1.89), fifth vs first quintile, age, risk factor–adjusted
Schaefer et al., 1994[33]	623 men aged 35–39, nested case-control, 7–10 year follow-up	RR = 2.08 (1.19–3.63), fifth vs first quintile, age, risk factor–adjusted
Bostom et al., 1994[35]	3101 women, prospective, 12-year follow-up	RR = 2.37 (1.48–3.81) (MI) RR = 1.61 (1.13–2.29) (CAD) RR = 1.44 (1.09–1.91) (CVD); age, risk factor–adjusted
Bostom et al., 1996[34]	2191 men aged 20–54, prospective, CAD age <55, 15-year follow-up	RR = 1.9 (1.2–2.9); age, risk factor–adjusted
Nguyen et al., 1997[38]	9936 men and women, 14-year follow-up, CAD	RR = 1.9 (1.3–2.9) (women) RR = 1.6 (1.0–2.5) (men)
Cantin et al., 1998[41]	2156 men aged 47–76, 5-year follow-up, CAD	RR = 1.16 (0.83–1.85) Lp(a) >33 mg/dL vs <11 mg/dL

*RR, relative risk, with 95% confidence interval in parentheses; CAD, coronary artery disease; MI, myocardial infarction; CVD, cardiovascular disease.

based cohort of 9936 men and women, disease-free at baseline, who were followed up for 14 years for the development of cardiovascular endpoints, showed an increased level of Lp(a) to be associated with a 1.9-fold increased risk of CHD events in women and a 1.6-fold increased risk in men but no consistent relationship to cerebrovascular events.[38]

Most recently, the Scandinavian Simvastatin Survival Study showed Lp(a) levels to be significantly higher in those sustaining major coronary events than in subjects without such events. This study also showed a significant relation of Lp(a) levels to total mortality.[39] In patients undergoing coronary angiography, Lp(a) levels are also higher in patients with higher numbers of blocked coronary vessels as well as degree and extent of blockages.[40] Finally, in the Quebec Cardiovascular Study, Lp(a) was not an independent risk factor for ischemic heart disease but instead amplified the risks associated with elevated total and LDL-C and Apo-B and retarded the protective effect associated with elevated HDL-C.[41]

Atherogenic Lipoprotein Phenotype and Other Inherited Lipid Disorders

Of increasing interest is the possible relation of small LDL-C particle size, also referred to as the atherogenic lipoprotein phenotype (ALP), to an increased risk of CHD. ALP consists of a major peak of small, dense LDL-C particles (denoted phenotype B), distinct from predominantly large, buoyant LDL-C particles (denoted phenotype A). The LDL pattern B trait is associated with a tendency toward elevated levels of triglycerides, very low-density lipoprotein (VLDL) and intermediate-density lipoprotein, and reduced levels of HDL-C; however, it can occur even when levels of these lipoproteins are normal.[42]

Several observational studies have described a relation of small, dense LDL-C to risk for CHD (Table 7–3). Austin et al. showed small, dense LDL-C to be associated with a threefold greater odds of myocardial infarction (MI) from a case-control study; however, risk was attenuated after adjustment for other lipid fractions.[43] The Physicians' Health Survey also confirmed this threefold increased risk for CHD associated with pattern B individuals,[44] which persisted after adjustment for total and HDL-C and Apo-B. Also, the Stanford Five Cities project showed, among 248 individuals, LDL size to be significantly smaller among CHD cases compared with controls, independent of HDL-C, non-HDL-C, triglycerides, body-mass index, and smoking. Small LDL-C was found in about 50 percent of cases, and there was a graded relation between LDL-C size and odds of CHD.[45] Others have also shown that while triglycerides, LDL-C, and/or Apo-B were associated with progression of angiographic disease in 335 men and women enrolled in a quantitative angiographic follow-up study, triglyceride-rich lipoproteins, which included cholesterol in intermediate-density lipoproteins, were directly related to lesion progression.[46]

Moreover, the Familial Atherosclerosis Treatment Study (FATS)[47] showed changes in standard lipid variables to explain about 30 percent of the variance in atherosclerosis regression, including 18 percent explained by LDL-C alone. But when LDL-C density was added into the equation, 59 percent of the variance was explained, most of which (48 percent) was contributed by change in LDL-C density, followed (in decreasing order of contribution) by LDL-C, hepatic lipase, and Lp(a). Finally, a nested case-control study was based on 2103 men in the Quebec Cardiovascular Study followed for 5 years. During that time, 114 developed ischemic heart disease, and those in the first tertile of LDL peak particle diameter were shown to have a 3.6-fold increased risk (95 percent CI, 1.5 to 8.8) of ischemic heart disease, which remained largely unaffected after adjustment for other lipid variables.[48]

Apo-E is the most common gene affecting LDL-C levels and includes as its major isoforms, E2, E3, and E4. LDL-C catabolism is greater in those with the less common E2 isoform compared to the most common E3 isoform. The E4 isoform is associated with a reduced catabolism of LDL and with suppression

TABLE 7–3   Studies of the Relation of the Atherogenic Lipoprotein Phenotype (Small, Dense LDL-C) with Coronary Heart Disease

Reference	Study Population	Result
Austin[43]	109 cases and 121 controls; MI hospital admissions	OR = 3.0 (1.7–5.3) (adjusted for age, sex, BMI) OR = 1.5 (0.7–3.3) (adjusted for above and other lipid fractions)
Krauss[44]	Physicians' Health Survey	Threefold CAD risk associated with pattern B, independent of total and HDL-C and Apo-B
Gardner[45]	248 individuals, nested case-control within Stanford Five Cities Study	LDL-C size significantly smaller in cases, independent of other factors; also graded odds of CAD with LDL-C size
Phillips[46]	335 men and women with CAD; angiographic follow-up	Triglyceride-rich lipoproteins directly related to lesion progression
Zambon[47]	Nested case-control within Familial Atherosclerosis Treatment Study (FATS)	LDL-C size most important indicator of CAD progression, explained 48% of variance in model including other lipids
Lamarche[48]	Nested case-control within Quebec Cardiovascular Study; 114 cases, 5-year follow-up	RR = 3.6 (1.5–8.8) first vs third tertile of LDL particle diameter

Key: MI, myocardial infarction; CAD, coronary artery disease; OR, odds ratio; HDL-C, high-density-lipoprotein cholesterol; Apo-B, apolipoprotein B; LDL-C, low-density-lipoprotein cholesterol; RR, relative risk, with 95% confidence interval in parentheses; BMI, body mass index.

of LDL-C receptors. There is also evidence of an increased risk of MI associated with the E4 allele.[49]

Clinical Trial Evidence for Lipid Intervention

Primary Prevention Studies

Numerous primary prevention studies document the importance of cholesterol lowering in patients without previous CHD (Table 7–4).[50] Among contemporary trials, the Lipid Research Clinics Coronary Primary Prevention Trial (LRC-CPPT) enrolled approximately 3800 men between the ages of 35 and 59 with elevated total and LDL-C and no evidence of prior CHD.[51] In those randomized to cholestyramine versus placebo, after 7 years of follow-up, there was an unequivocal reduction in the incidence of the primary endpoint of fatal plus nonfatal myocardial infarction. There was a 20 percent reduction in LDL-C, and a corresponding 19 percent reduction in coronary events. No significant reduction in coronary or total mortality, however, was realized.

The Helsinki Heart Study reported that among more than 4000 middle-aged men without prior evidence of CHD who were randomized to gemfibrozil (as compared with placebo), there was a highly significant reduction of 34 percent in the incidence of coronary events.[52] A subanalysis showed that elevation in HDL-C was independently associated with reduction in risk,[8] supporting the importance not only of reducing LDL-C but also of raising HDL-C in efforts to prevent CHD.

More recently, the West of Scotland Coronary Prevention Study reported results on 6595 men aged 45 to 64 years with hypercholesterolemia assigned to pravastatin or placebo, with a mean follow-up of 4.9 years.[53] Nonfatal MI or CHD death, the primary endpoint, was reduced significantly by 31 percent in the pravastatin treated group. The divergence of the curves related to event rates began after 6 months of therapy and became highly significant by the end of the study. The incidence of coronary angiography, coronary angioplasty, and coronary artery bypass surgery was also significantly reduced. Total mortality was also reduced by 22 percent ($p = .05$). More recently reported analyses have shown this mortality advantage to widen to a 26 percent reduction ($p = .01$) by 6 months after completion of the study but to weaken to 17 percent after 1 year, suggesting the importance of continuing therapy.[54] In addition, no further benefit was obtained beyond the second quintile of LDL-C lowering (where a 45 percent risk reduction was observed with mean LDL-C reduction of 24 percent) in risk factor–adjusted analyses.[55]

TABLE 7–4 Primary Prevention Studies of Lipid Modification

Trial	Therapy	LDL-C, Treatment Group			Percent Risk Reduction	
		n	Δ%	Achieved	CAD Events	Total Mortality
WHO[128]	Clofibrate	10,627	−9 (TC)*	224 mg/dL†	20	−30
LRC-CPPT[51]	Cholestyramine	3806	−20	175 mg/dL	19	7
Helsinki[52]	Gemfibrozil	4081	−10‡	174 mg/dL	34	−6
WOSCOPS[53]	Pravastatin	6595	−26	142 mg/dL	31¶	22§
AFCAPS/TexCAPS[56]	Lovastatin	6605	−25	115 mg/dL	37¶	−4

*Total cholesterol.
†Estimated based on baseline of 249 mg/dL.
‡Also accompanied by a 43% reduction in triglycerides and an increase of 10% in HDL-C.
§$p = .05$
¶$p < .001$

The Air Force/Texas Coronary Atherosclerosis Prevention Study (AFCAPS/TexCAPS) provides further evidence for the role of lipid lowering in primary prevention among men and women with average cholesterol levels similar in distribution to the national population based on NHANES III data.[56] In this study, 5608 men and 997 women were enrolled, with average total and LDL-cholesterol levels (mean 221 and 150 mg/dL, respectively) and below average HDL-cholesterol levels (mean 36 mg/dL in men and 40 mg/dL in women), and were randomized to lovastatin or placebo. After a mean follow-up of 5.2 years, there was a 37 percent reduction in major coronary events (fatal or nonfatal MI, unstable angina, or sudden cardiac death), a 33 percent reduction in new revascularization, and a 25 percent reduction in total cardiovascular events.

Secondary Prevention Studies

A number of clinical trials in persons with preexisting CHD demonstrate the efficacy of lipid intervention in reducing subsequent coronary events and total mortality (Table 7–5). The Coronary Drug Project, published in 1975, compared the efficacy of niacin, clofibrate, and other medications in reducing coronary events in men 30 to 64 years old with a history of MI. After 5 years of treatment, niacin was associated with a 27 percent reduction in the incidence of definite nonfatal myocardial infarction, but there was little effect on total mortality.[57] A 15-year follow-up of this cohort,[58] however, yielded a significant 11 percent lower total mortality rate in those originally randomized to niacin, despite the fact that many patients were off therapy for 9 years and other confounding variables were not controlled for. No significant differences in mortality were observed in the clofibrate- or dextrothyrozine-treated groups as compared with those on placebo. Other smaller secondary prevention studies examining the effect of clofibrate[59] or combined clofibrate and niacin[60] have also shown treatment benefits.

Although not involving pharmacologic therapy, the Program on the Surgical Control of the Hyperlipidemias (POSCH) study showed that regression of atherosclerosis and significant reductions in morbidity and mortality from CHD as well as total mortality could be obtained from total and LDL-C reduc-

TABLE 7–5 Secondary Prevention Studies of Lipid Modification

Trial	Therapy	n	LDL-C Δ%	LDL-C Achieved	Percent Risk Reduction[‡] CHD Events	Percent Risk Reduction[‡] Total Mortality
CDP[57*]	Niacin	3908	−10 (TC)	—	27	11[¶]
	Clofibrate	3892	−5 (TC)	—	4.7	−1
	Dextrothyroxine	3872	−10 (TC)	—	−13	−22
POSCH[61]	Partial ileal bypass	838	−38	103 mg/dL	35[§]	22
4S[62]	Simvastatin	4444	−34	121 mg/dL	42[¶]	30[¶]
CARE[2]	Pravastatin	4159	−28	100 mg/dL	24[§]	9
LIPID[64]	Pravastatin	9014	−25	113 mg/dL	24[¶]	22[¶]
HIT[9]	Gemfibrozil	2531	3.6[†]	—	22	10

Key: LDL-C, low-density-lipoprotein cholesterol; CHD, coronary heart disease; TC, total cholesterol. Negative (−) sign indicates increase in risk.

[*]Lipid changes available only for total cholesterol; CHD events based on 5-year follow-up, total mortality based on 15-year follow-up.

[†]Accompanied by a 7.5 percent increase in HDL-C and a 24.5 percent decrease in triglycerides.

[‡]$p < .05$

[§]$p < .01$

[¶]$p < .001$

tion effected by partial ileal bypass of patients with significant hypercholesterolemia.[61]

The Scandinavian Simvastatin Survival Study (4S) showed lipid lowering in patients with preexisting CHD not only to prevent subsequent coronary events but also to reduce total mortality and stroke.[62] In the 4444 men and women aged 35 to 70 with a history of MI or angina pectoris randomized to simvastatin or placebo for a mean follow-up of 5.4 years, the primary endpoint of total mortality was reduced significantly by 30 percent in the treatment group versus those on placebo. The secondary endpoint of all coronary events was reduced by 42 percent. Total mortality was also significantly lower in those under age 60 (RR = 0.63), as well as age 60 and over (RR = 0.73); coronary events were also lower in these age groups (RRs of 0.61 and 0.71, respectively). Both men and women had a similar reduction in the risk for all coronary events as well. Rates for revascularizations and cardiovascular disease events and mortality were also significantly lower in the treated group. A later report included published data in the subgroup of 202 diabetic patients; coronary events were reduced significantly by 55 percent in these individuals, and there was a nonsignificant (RR = 0.57, p = .09) reduction in total mortality.[63]

The Cholesterol and Recurrent Events (CARE) study reported data from 5 years of treatment with pravastatin or placebo in 4159 men and women who had sustained a previous MI but who had a total cholesterol of less than 6.2 mmol/L (240 mg/dL) and mean LDL-C averaging 3.6 mmol/L (139 mg/dL).[2] The incidence of fatal coronary events or nonfatal MI was reduced significantly by 24 percent. There were also significant reductions in coronary bypass surgery (26 percent), coronary angioplasty (23 percent), and stroke (31 percent). Coronary event rates were decreased more in women (46 percent) than men (20 percent), and the benefit extended to the elderly (27 percent in those aged 60 and over, versus 20 percent in those under age 60), hypertensives (23 percent versus 24 percent in nonhypertensives), smokers (33 percent in current smokers, compared with 22 percent in others), and diabetics (25 percent versus 23 percent in nondiabetics). No significant difference in total mortality was observed in the treatment versus placebo group (9 percent reduction, p = .37); however, there was an unexpected increased risk of breast cancer in the treatment group, which could not be explained but is thus far inconsistent with results from any other trial. The results of CARE extend the importance of cholesterol lowering in the vast majority of patients with MI who do not have substantially elevated LDL-C levels.

The recently reported Long-Term Intervention with Pravastatin in Ischemic Disease (LIPID) study[64] investigated whether cholesterol reduction with pravastatin reduces CHD mortality in patients with a previous MI or unstable angina who had cholesterol levels between 155 and 271 mg/dL. Among the 9014 patients aged 31 to 75 years randomized to pravastatin 40 mg daily or placebo and followed for an average of 6 years, the primary endpoint of CHD mortality was reduced by 24 percent. Consistent with the results of the 4S study, a 23 percent reduction in total mortality was also achieved. Significant reductions in MI, revascularizations, and cardiovascular deaths were also reported. There was also a significant 20 percent reduction in the risk of stroke.

The efficacy of increasing HDL-C on reducing recurrent coronary events was recently examined in the HDL Intervention Trial (HIT). Subjects also had normal LDL-C ($\leq$140 mg/dL) but low HDL-C ($\leq$40 mg/dL) and were randomized to gemfibrozil or placebo.[65] Mean baseline HDL-C was 32 mg/dL; LDL-C, 111 mg/dL; and triglycerides, 161 mg/dL. After a median follow-up of 5.1 years, there was a 22 percent reduced risk of CHD death or nonfatal MI (p < .01) among those treated versus those on placebo, suggesting the value of increasing HDL-C in secondary prevention.[9]

Atherosclerosis Regression Studies

Although both primary and secondary event studies focusing on coronary event reduction have documented the efficacy of lipid lowering, a series of coronary angiographic follow-up studies have also been published, extending the importance of lipid intervention on retarding the progression and/or stimulating regression of coronary atherosclerosis (Table 7–6). A number of these studies show that, despite fairly modest angiographic changes, event rates are

TABLE 7–6 Arteriographic "Regression" Studies of Lipid Modification

Trial	Therapy	n, Treatment/ Control[*]	LDL-C, Treatment Group Δ%	LDL-C, Treatment Group Achieved	Outcomes, Treatment/Control, Percent of Patients[*] Progression	Outcomes, Treatment/Control, Percent of Patients[*] Regression
NHLBI[68]	Cholestyramine	59/57	−26	178 mg/dL	32/49	7/7
CLAS[67]	Colestipol + niacin	80/82	−38	105 mg/dL	9/61	16/2
FATS[70]	Colestipol + niacin	36/46	−32	129 mg/dL	25/46	39/11
	Lovastatin + colestipol	38/46	−46	107 mg/dL	21/46	32/11
Hahmann et al.[79]	Fenofibrate	21/21	−20	—	10/—	11/—
SCOR[129]	Colestipol, niacin, lovastatin	40/32	−28	172 mg/dL	20/41	33/13
SCRIP[80]	Colestipol, niacin, gemfibrozil, lovastatin, probucol	119/127	−23	121 mg/dL	50/50	20/10
STARS[69]	Cholestyramine	24/24	−33	136 mg/dL	4/38	21/4
STARS[69]	Diet	26/24	−16	164 mg/dL	15/38	31/4
MARS[73]	Lovastatin	114/106	−45	86 mg/dL	29/40	23/13
CCAIT[74]	Lovastatin	165/166	−30	120 mg/dL	33/50	10/7
MAAS[77]	Simvastatin	178/167	−31	117 mg/dL	23/32	19/12
REGRESS[75]	Pravastatin	314/327	−25	125 mg/dL	45/55	17/9
HARP[81]	Multiple agents	40/39	−39	85 mg/dL	35/38	10/13
POSCH[61]	Partial ileal bypass	333/301	−42	104 mg/dL	38/65	13/5
POST-CABG[84]	Multiple agents	628/628	−38	93–97 mg/dL	27/39	5/4
Lifestyle[71]	Diet, other	22/19	−36	95 mg/dL	14/32	41/32
Heidelberg[130]	Diet, exercise	40/52	−9	149 mg/dL	20/42	30/4
LOCAT[82]	Gemfibrozil	395	−12	131 mg/dL	4 (2%)	23 (14%)

[*]Data presented according to treatment/control group status.

Source: Modified from Rossouw,[66] with permission.

reduced substantially, suggesting that the effect of pharmacologic therapy on CHD risk reduction may be multifactorial and not limited to changes in arterial lumen diameter (see section below on Mechanisms of Event Reduction).[66]

In the Cholesterol Lowering Atherosclerosis Study,[67] patients with coronary artery bypass surgery were recruited and treated with a combination of colestipol and niacin and compared with a placebo group. Coronary angiograms were performed at baseline and again 2 years later, with qualitative,

blinded readings by a panel of angiographers. Of treated patients, 16 percent showed regression of atherosclerosis, compared with only 2 percent in the placebo group. Earlier angiographic trials involving therapy with cholestyramine showed that atherosclerotic progression could be retarded, but the drug was not powerful enough to effect significant changes in regression.[68,69]

The Familial Atherosclerosis Treatment Study (FATS)[70] involved two different treatment arms, one with combined niacin and colestipol treatment and a second with combined lovastatin and colestipol treatment; these were compared to a conventionally treated diet arm where cholesterol-lowering treatment was allowed if cholesterol levels exceeded the 90th percentile during follow-up. Both percentage stenosis and minimum lumen diameter decreased in those on active treatment, indicating regression of atherosclerosis, compared with significant progression in the conventionally treated arms. More than one-third of treated patients showed regression of atherosclerosis, compared with about one-tenth of control group patients.

The Lifestyle Heart Trial[71] was unique in being able to demonstrate regression of atherosclerosis as a result of a stringent nonpharmacologic lifestyle regimen that included a vegetarian low-fat diet (under 10 percent of calories in fat) and less than 5 mg intake of cholesterol daily, along with smoking cessation, stress management, and increased physical activity. A total of 41 patients completed the study, including 22 in the intervention and 19 in the control group. Although substantial reductions in total and LDL-C were obtained, triglycerides increased and HDL-C was reduced in the treatment group relative to the control group. Remarkably, 81 percent of patients in the treated group showed regression of atherosclerosis (and a 91 percent reduction in the frequency of angina). A recent follow-up report from this study showed continued improvements among the intervention group as determined by those completing the 5-year follow-up angiogram who maintained comprehensive lifestyle changes.[72]

Other studies have also demonstrated that HMG-CoA reductase monotherapy with lovastatin,[73,74] pravastatin,[75,76] or simvastatin[77] retarded the angiographic progression of atherosclerosis, as evidenced by less reduction in minimum lumen diameter in the intervention versus the control group. One of these studies, the Canadian Coronary Atherosclerosis Intervention Trial (CCAIT),[78] showed the rate of atherosclerosis progression to be significantly reduced among the subgroup of women as well (28 percent of treated versus 59 percent of placebo patients). Another study showed regression of atherosclerosis among those with lower total and LDL-C levels as obtained by therapy with a fibric acid derivative.[79]

The Stanford Coronary Risk Intervention Project (SCRIP) used a diet and exercise regimen to effectively modify lipid levels as well as lipid-lowering medications in many patients during the course of the study (90 percent of those in the risk reduction and 23 percent of those in the usual-care group were on lipid-lowering medications by the end of the study). This study showed less progression of atherosclerosis (small reduction in minimum lumen diameter) and fewer cardiac events in the risk-reduction group.[80] However, clinical events were not reduced consistently in all these studies, and a fairly large sample size was required in two of them. In one study, aggressive lipid management with multiple therapies did not induce regression or reduce progression of atherosclerosis in individuals with normal cholesterol levels.[81] A review of many angiographic trials of lipid lowering showed regression to be more common in trials where baseline mean LDL-C exceeded 170 mg/dL as compared with those where LDL-C was 170 mg/dL or lower at baseline.[66]

Atherosclerosis can also be retarded by interventions other than those designed to reduce LDL-C. The Lopid Coronary Angiography Trial (LOCAT) involved 372 patients randomized to gemfibrozil or placebo who received two angiograms separated by an average of 32 months and who had low HDL-C as their principal lipid abnormality. Progression of native coronary atherosclerosis was significantly retarded in the treatment group (-0.04 mm) as compared with the placebo group (-0.09 mm) ($p < .01$), and new lesions in the graft vessels were more common in the placebo group (14 percent) than in the gemfibrozil group (2 percent) ($p < .01$).[82] The results of this trial provide some support for the use of fibrates to treat CHD patients who have normal cholesterol levels but low HDL-C as well for as the role of several possible mechanisms (e.g., reducing VLDL-C, altering LDL-C size and density, and effecting reverse cholesterol transport) in retarding atherosclerosis.[83]

More recently, the issue of how low an LDL-C is required to retard progression of angiographic disease was examined. Among 1351 individuals who had undergone coronary artery bypass surgery, those

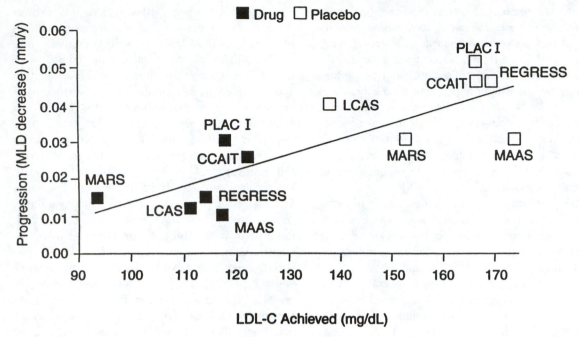

FIGURE 7–6 Relation of on-treatment LDL-C achieved to degree of atherosclerosis progression (decrease in minimum lumen diameter in millimeters per year) ($r^2 = .71$, $p = .0005$ from a weighted regression analysis of angiographic statin trials of at least 100 patients each). CCAIT, Canadian Coronary Atherosclerosis Intervention Trial; LCAS, Lipoprotein and Coronary Atherosclerosis Study; MAAS, Multicentre Anti-Atheroma Study; MARS, Monitored Atherosclerosis Regression Study; PLAC I, Pravastatin Limitation of Atherosclerosis in the Coronary Arteries; REGRESS, Regression Growth Evaluation Statin Study. (From Ballantyne,[85] with permission.)

who received aggressive treatment with lovastatin (and cholestyramine if needed) to maintain an LDL-C between 93 and 97 mg/dL were less likely to show progression of atherosclerosis (27 percent of grafts) compared with those who achieved only moderate lowering of LDL-C to 132 to 136 mg/dL (39 percent).[84] Data from most of the recent atherosclerosis regression trials involving measurement of minimum lumen diameter show less progression of atherosclerosis the lower the LDL-C achieved (Fig. 7–6).[85]

In many clinical trials, the reduction in cardiovascular disease (CVD) events appears to be beyond what would be expected based on changes in arterial lumen diameter from angiographic trials. An ef-

fect of lipid-lowering therapy on plaque stabilization is hypothesized as one mechanism for the prevention of clinical events. Other agents recommended for secondary prevention—e.g., antiplatelet agents such as aspirin and beta blockers—might explain the magnitude of risk reductions achievable with the addition of cholesterol-lowering agents.[86]

Relation of Baseline LDL-C and Extent of LDL-C Lowering to Coronary Event Risk

Coronary event reduction may also depend on the level of baseline LDL-C. The AFCAPS/TexCAPS study[56] showed event risk to be similar regardless of baseline LDL-C tertile; those in the lowest tertile

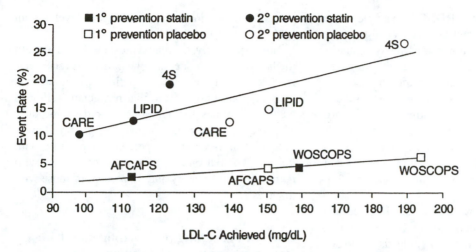

FIGURE 7–7 Relation of LDL-C achieved to coronary heart disease risk reduction from primary and secondary prevention studies involving statins. 4S, Scandinavian Simvastatin Survival Study; AFCAPS, Air Force/Texas Coronary Atherosclerosis Prevention Study; CARE, Cholesterol and Recurrent Events Trial; LIPID, Long-Term Intervention with Pravastatin in Ischaemic Disease Study; WOSCOPS, West of Scotland Coronary Prevention Study. (From Ballantyne,[87] with permission.)

(91 to 142 mg/dL) sustained a 34 percent reduction as compared with a reduction of 41 percent in the highest tertile (157 to 236 mg/dL). The West of Scotland Coronary Primary Prevention Study (WOSCOPS)[51] had much higher baseline LDL-C levels and showed greater efficacy among those with LDL-C levels below 189 mg/dL (37 percent risk reduction) as compared with 189 mg/dL or greater (27 percent risk reduction).

There is generally an incremental value of achieving low LDL-C levels on treatment both in primary and secondary prevention. From the major primary and secondary prevention studies, the lower the LDL-C achieved, the lower the coronary event rates (Fig. 7–7).[87] In secondary prevention, there are data to suggest that treatment may be of reduced or little benefit for those with baseline LDL-C levels below approximately 130 mg/dL. Among participants in the Cholesterol and Recurrent Events (CARE) study,[2] there was no benefit of treatment for those with baseline LDL-C levels below 125 mg/dL. The recently published Long-Term Intervention with Pravastatin in Ischemic Heart Disease (LIPID) study[64] corrobo-

rates these findings, as a nonsignificant 16 percent risk reduction was noted for those with LDL-C levels below 135 mg/dL, versus significant reductions in risk of 26 percent and 30 percent for those with baseline LDL-C levels of 135 to 173 mg/dL and 174 mg/dL or higher, respectively.

Mechanisms of Event Reduction

Ongoing investigations have tried to answer the question of potential mechanisms of action for the clinical benefit of lipid lowering. The first hypothesis is based on the theory that it is the small rather than large plaques that result in rupture and thrombosis, leading to the acute, serious, and eventually fatal complications of atherosclerosis. Small plaques have fresh lipid deposits in them; it has been hypothesized that sharp reductions in atherogenic LDL reduce the influx and increase the efflux of freshly deposited cholesterol, resulting in stabilization of these plaques and prevention of rupture and thrombosis.

The second theory is that lipid reduction restores the abnormal endothelial function that is often observed in patients with CHD. For example, when acetylcholine is introduced via catheter in the coronary arteries in normal subjects, coronary dilatation occurs. On the other hand, in patients with severe coronary atherosclerosis, vasoconstriction results instead. This paradoxical vasoconstriction is thought to be due to an inability of the atherosclerotic coronary artery to produce nitric oxide, considered to be a mediator for the vasodilatation.[88] Lipid reduction restores the ability of the endothelium to produce nitric oxide, thereby resulting in normalization of endothelial function.

The fact that lipid-lowering medications, particularly HMG-CoA reductase inhibitors, cause relatively modest angiographic changes leads one to postulate that nonlipid mechanisms could be involved. Possible beneficial effects on endothelial function, inflammatory responses, plaque stability, and thrombus formation have been proposed, and experimental studies have suggested that stability may be achieved through a reduction in macrophages and cholesterol ester content and an increase in volume of collagen and smooth muscle cells. Also, inhibition of platelet aggregation and maintenance of a favorable balance between prothrombotic and fibrinolytic mechanisms may also be involved.[89]

Screening and Evaluation of Dyslipidemia

Although there have been substantial increases in awareness of elevated cholesterol as well as increased treatment compliance during the past two decades, recent national surveys suggest substantial improvement is still needed.[90] Other data suggest that rates of lipid profile screening and treatment among persons with known CHD vary widely by physician.[91] A recent study showed that less than half of the patients who met National Cholesterol Education Program (NCEP) criteria for initiation of therapy actually received it, and among those given medications, only one-third achieved acceptable LDL-C reductions within a year.[92] In a large sample of postmenopausal women with heart disease, only 47 percent were taking lipid-lowering medication and 91

percent did not meet the NCEP goal level for an LDL-C of less than 100 mg/dL.[93]

Not surprisingly, the blame must be shared by both the health care provider and the patient. A recent retrospective chart review[94] of patients admitted to a coronary care unit showed that physicians followed NCEP guidelines for obtaining a lipid profile only 50 percent of the time. Moreover, a lipid profile was obtained (at best) in 74 percent of patients with known CHD but only in 56 percent of patients with a known family history and 37 percent of those with diabetes.

Current Screening and Management Recommendations in Adults

The National Cholesterol Education Program[1] and American Heart Association[95] recommend an initial measurement of serum total and HDL-C in all adults aged 20 and over as an initial screening for primary prevention (Fig. 7–8). If these lipids are normal (total cholesterol <200 mg/dL *and* HDL-C ≥35 mg/dL) and the individual is healthy, a repeat screening is recommended every 5 years. If either total cholesterol is 240 mg/dL or greater *or* HDL-C is less than 35 mg/dL (regardless of level of total cholesterol), a full fasting lipid profile should be obtained, from which LDL-C is determined and used as the criterion for treatment. For those with borderline-high blood cholesterol, if HDL-C is equal to or greater than 35 mg/dL *and* fewer than two other CHD risk factors (Fig. 7–8) are present, reevaluation within 2 years and lifestyle modification are recommended. For those with evidence of CHD, a full fasting lipid profile is essential for appropriate evaluation.

Generally, the average of two or more fasting measurements of LDL-C, which can be made over consecutive days, provides the most accurate baseline for the purposes of determining appropriateness for initiating pharmacologic therapy.[95] Although studies have shown that fasting lipoprotein measurements made immediately upon admission for an acute coronary event reasonably estimate baseline levels, total cholesterol and LDL-C can subsequently fall below baseline following the event. It may be necessary to

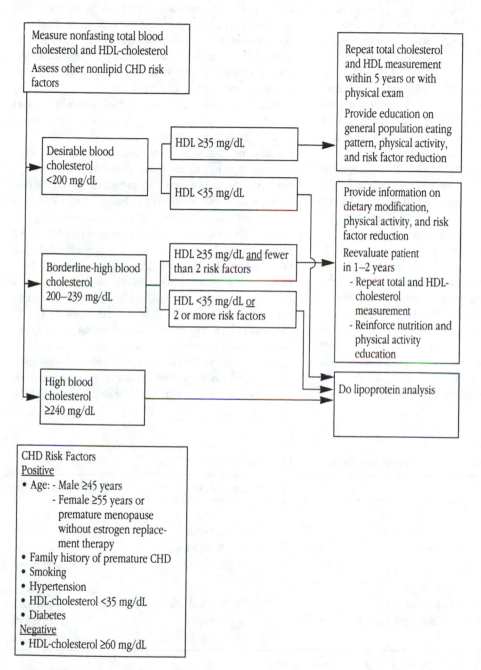

FIGURE 7–8 Primary prevention in adults without evidence of CHD: initial classification based on total cholesterol and HDL-C. (From the National Cholesterol Education Program, 1993.[1])

wait several weeks or longer in order to obtain accurate baseline measures.[96] But one has to weigh this against the possibility of not getting a measurement at all once the patient leaves the hospital. In primary prevention, guidelines suggesting limiting lipid screening only to men aged 35 to 65 and women aged 45 to 65 and using only a measure of total cholesterol were recently proposed by the American College of Physicians[97]; however, these recommendations have been criticized by other experts.[98]

The Adult Treatment Plan (ATP) II guidelines of the National Cholesterol Education Program[1] base initiation and treatment goals for dietary and pharmacologic therapy on LDL-C levels, number of preexisting CHD risk factors, and whether or not the patient has prior coronary artery disease (Table 7–7). Specifically, an LDL-C target value of 2.6 mM/L (100 mg/dL) or below is recommended for patients with preexisting evidence of atherosclerotic cardiovascular disease. Patients with other risk factors are treated to achieve LDL-C levels below 130 mg/dL (if two or more risk factors are present) or 160 mg/dL (if fewer than two risk factors are present). In addition, secondary lipid goals of an HDL-C above 35 mg/dL (and ideally higher) and triglycerides under 200 mg/dL are recommended both in primary and secondary prevention.[95,99] The American Diabetes Association has recently recommended treatment to lower LDL-C to less than 100 mg/dL in all diabetics who have at least one additional coronary risk factor or preexisting CHD.[100]

Many patients with elevated cholesterol and CHD are patients who are at very high risk and are not treated for this condition. In one study,[101] only 16.7 percent of patients were treated before cardiac catheterization, although the diagnoses of both hypercholesterolemia and the presence of CHD had been established. What was frustrating was that 1 to 2 years following cardiac catheterization (among patients with CHD), only 36 percent of patients were being treated; of those treated, fewer were treated to target goal. Thus, we are treating only a small proportion of patients who need medical management for dyslipidemia. As staffing to provide adequate screening and identification is limited, many health care providers and even pharmaceutical companies are placing increasing attention on efforts to adequately identify and control dyslipidemia among patients with existing coronary artery disease (secondary prevention). It is among these individuals that the

TABLE 7–7   Treatment Decisions Based on LDL-C

	Initiation Level	LDL-C Goal
Dietary therapy		
Without CHD and fewer than two risk factors	>160 mg/dL	<160 mg/dL
Without CHD and with two or more risk factors	>130 mg/dL	<130 mg/dL
With CHD	>100 mg/dL	<100 mg/dL
Drug therapy		
Without CHD and fewer than two risk factors	>190 mg/dL[*]	<160 mg/dL
Without CHD and with two or more risk factors	>160 mg/dL	<130 mg/dL
With CHD	>130 mg/dL[†]	<100 mg/dL

Key: LDL-C, low-density-lipoprotein cholesterol; CHD, coronary heart disease.

[*]In men under 35 years of age and premenopausal women with LDL-C levels 190 to 219 mg/dL, drug therapy should be delayed except in high-risk patients such as those with diabetes.

[†]In CHD patients with LDL-C levels 100 to 129 mg/dL, the physician should exercise clinical judgment in deciding whether to initiate drug treatment.

Source: From the National Cholesterol Education Program.[1]

magnitude of risk reduction and cost-benefit of lipid-lowering therapy can be most convincingly demonstrated.[98]

Dietary Management of Dyslipidemia

The initial treatment for hypercholesterolemia is, of course, diet and other nonpharmacologic measures, including physical activity. These interventions are considered in greater depth in other chapters of this book specifically dealing with nutrition (Chap. 13), physical activity (Chap. 12), and behavioral management (Chap. 14). Basic nutritional principles are based on the American Heart Association and National Cholesterol Education Program Step 1 and 2 Diets. The Step 1 Diet can lower LDL-C by 7 to 9 percent, while the Step 2 Diet lowers LDL-C by 10 to 20 percent; lower-fat diets can provide 20 to 25 percent LDL-C reductions.[102] The Step 1 Diet is recommended for all healthy Americans over the age of 2 years and calls for less than 10 percent of calories in saturated fat, a cholesterol content of less than 300 mg daily, and no more than 30 percent of total calories from fat.

Among patients with coronary disease or those with multiple risk factors who are at highest risk, it is recommended that the Step 2 Diet be prescribed as soon as possible. This diet has less than 7 percent of total caloric intake from saturated fat, with the rest from monounsaturated fatty acids and up to 10 percent from polyunsaturated fatty acids, with no more than 30 percent of total calories from fat. The cholesterol intake should be reduced to less than 200 mg per day. It is emphasized that the patient should engage in sufficient exercise and the total caloric content should be designed to maintain a desirable body weight. Very low fat diets can sometimes reduce HDL-C as well as apolipoprotein A levels; there is controversy as to whether this may be harmful.[103]

Once it is decided that the patient is exhibiting maximum compliance to diet therapy, usually within 3 to 6 months, drugs should be considered if LDL-C levels remain above NCEP-specified initiation levels for pharmacologic intervention (see Table 7–7). Also, many Americans may be unable to achieve maximum lipid-lowering potential from lifestyle and will thus require pharmacologic therapy.[102] There is an increasing consensus, however, on beginning drug therapy concurrently with diet in the treatment of individuals whose LDL-C is at 130 mg/dL or greater and among patients with preexisting coronary artery disease, since maximal dietary therapy will usually reduce LDL-C levels by no more than 15 to 25 mg/dL.[96]

Pharmacologic Management of Dyslipidemia

Major Classes of Medications

The drugs that are available for lipid lowering are the bile acid sequestrants, nicotinic acid (niacin), fibric acid derivatives, and HMG-CoA reductase inhibitors. Other measures that may be effective are estrogen replacement therapy (for modest elevations in LDL-C and low HDL-C) and the use of fish oils (for elevated triglycerides). For this reason, they are traditionally recommended as first-line agents for the control of dyslipidemia. Selection of the appropriate agent depends on the lipid disorder, including the extent of LDL-C elevation, whether triglycerides are elevated or HDL-C decreased, the presence of other known risk factors,[1] known tolerability to previously used agents, and medical history. The following is a discussion of the individual agents followed by a discussion on drug selection in practice.

Bile acid sequestrants Bile acid–binding resins, which include cholestyramine and colestipol, primarily lower LDL-C (up to 25 percent reduction with maximal dosages of 25 to 30 g per day), do not affect HDL-C significantly, but may increase triglycerides in some patients. These agents are resins that prevent reabsorption of bile salts. This results in increased conversion of hepatocellular cholesterol to bile acids. Decreased hepatocellular cholesterol content results in upregulation of LDL-C receptors and increased clearance of circulating LDL-C particles.

Gastrointestinal discomfort, including constipation and bloating as well as heartburn, are the most common side effects.[103] In order to minimize the likelihood of side effects, the intiation dosage should be small. This dosage is gradually increased over several weeks, and a stool softner or psyllium may be included. One suggested regimen is to start with one dose (4 g of cholestyramine or 5 g of colestipol) at mealtime for 2 weeks and to increase this by a dose every 2 weeks (given subsequently twice daily) until a dosage of 16 or 20 g of cholestyramine or colestipol, respectively, is reached. In the few patients who can tolerate this dosage well, an increase by an additional two doses can be considered.

The resin is supplied as a powder, which is suspended in a (4- to 12-oz) glass of water. The suspension should stand for at least 5 min in order to improve its palatability and decrease the side effect of gagging experienced by some patients. To prevent constipation, it is preferable to precede resin administration with 1 to 2 tsp of psyllium powder given for 3 to 5 days. Psyllium itself is a mild bile acid–binding agent and may lower LDL-C by approximately 5 percent.[104] If constipation remains a problem, a stool softener (e.g., sodium docusate) may be added in appropriate patients to improve compliance. Bile acid resins also bind certain commonly used medications. These include digoxin, beta-adrenergic blockers, thyroid extracts, etc. Therefore, resins should be taken at least 1 h after or 4 h before other oral medications.

Niacin Among lipid-regulating agents, niacin is unique in that it is the only agent that favorably affects all major lipoprotein subfractions, resulting in a 20 to 30 percent reduction in LDL-C, increases in HDL-C of 15 to 30 percent, and even greater reductions in triglycerides (20 to 50 percent). It also lowers Lp(a) by as much as 30 to 40 percent and may convert individuals from the "small, dense" LDL-C pattern B to a larger, more buoyant pattern A.[49] Recent studies indicate that niacin also increases lipoprotein A-I (LpA-I), a subfraction of HDL that is considered to be antiatherogenic, versus lipoprotein A-II, which is not.[21] Older studies indicated that niacin decreased free fatty acid mobilization by inhibition of adipose tissue lipolysis;[105] however, more recent studies have focused on its mechanism in raising HDL and lowering Apo-B–containing lipoproteins. In culturated human hepatocytes (Hep G_2) cells, niacin decreases the uptake of Apo A-I.[106] Thus, the in vivo catabolism of the major protein of HDL (Apo A-I) is retarded, a finding that is consistent with previous turnover studies indicating an effect in delaying catabolism.[107] Because hepatic removal of cholesteryl ester is not affected,[106] more efficient reverse cholesterol transport would result. Niacin also inhibits hepatic synthesis of triglycerides, which results in acceleration of intracellular degradation of Apo-B prior to its secretion, thereby lowering triglyceride-rich very low density lipoproteins (VLDL), which are precursors of low-density lipoproteins.

Niacin is frequently not recommended in diabetics because it may stimulate hyperglycemia; however, with the advent of powerful glycemic control agents, this may be less of a concern given its powerful effects on all three lipids that frequently require control in diabetics. It is also contraindicated in patients with a history of gout or active peptic ulcer disease and hepatic dysfunction.

Whereas hepatotoxicity can occur with sustained-release preparations and flushing is the most common side effect, particularly for immediate-release preparations, newer, extended-release preparations[108,109] may prove more tolerable than immediate or older sustained-release preparations. Other side effects include dry skin, itching, gastritis, hepatitis, increased uric acid levels, and hyperglycemia. Tips for improving tolerability include starting at a low dosage and gradually increasing the dosage over several weeks to a maximum in the range of 1 to 3 g per day as necessary and tolerated. Enteric-coated aspirin minimizes flushing and can be given once daily. A newer, extended-release preparation of niacin (Niaspan) is dispensed as a convenient starter pack. Liver enzyme elevations often accompany use of higher dosages. They should be monitored and niacin dosage reduced or withdrawn if enzyme levels exceed three times the upper limit of normal.

Fibric acid derivatives The fibric acid derivatives, or "fibrates" (gemfibrozil and fenofibrate are available in the United States), lower triglycerides by 30 percent or more and raise HDL-C by up to 15 percent, with greater changes for both lipids in patients with severe hypertriglyceridemia. They also lower LDL-C modestly, usually about 10 percent from use of gemfibrozil, somewhat greater from fenofibrate. In hypertriglyceridemic patients, however, LDL-C levels may increase. Fibrates lower triglycerides by stimulating lipoprotein lipase.[110] Cell culture studies indicate that gemfibrozil stabilizes Apo-AI messenger RNA and fenofibrate activates the peroxisome proliferator–activated receptor.[21] Gallstone disease, dyspepsia, abdominal pain, and rashes are the most common side effects.

Hepatoxicity may occur, but the incidence (less than 2 percent) is low. The drug should be withdrawn if this occurs. The dose of gemfibrozil is 600 mg given twice a day orally half an hour before meals. Fenofibrate comes in a micronized form (67 mg per capsule), and the usual dose is two to three capsules daily.

HMG-CoA reductase inhibitors HMG-CoA reductase inhibitors ("statins") have come into wide use in the United States only within the last decade, during which six such agents have been marketed, each varying in cost and effectiveness in lowering LDL-C. These include lovastatin, pravastatin, simvastatin, fluvastatin, atorvastatin, and cerivastatin. The statins inhibit hydroxymethyl-coenzyme A (HMG-CoA), a key enzyme in cholesterol biosynthesis. In the liver, statins lower free cholesterol concentration, which results in upregulation of LDL-C receptors. LDL-C particles are cleared more rapidly, resulting in lower LDL-C concentrations. Hepatotoxicity, myopathy, and teratogenicity are the adverse events of greatest concern, but they generally affect a small (less than 1 to 2 percent) number of patients and are dose-related; dyspepsia and abdominal discomfort are more common and may occur in up to 5 percent of patients.

At higher dosages of atorvastatin[111] and simvastatin,[112] a 40 to 60 percent reduction in LDL-C can be expected. There is generally less than a 10 percent reduction in triglycerides and less than a 10 percent increase in HDL-C associated with use of the HMG-CoA reductase inhibitors at lower dosages, although higher recommended dosages of simvastatin and atorvastatin have shown reductions in triglyc-

erides by as much as 30 percent. The comparative efficacy of other statins in development or recently marketed (such as cerivastatin) is being evaluated. Short-term studies report greater LDL-C lowering efficacy, at a given dose, with atorvastatin as compared with simvastatin, as well as a greater proportion of patients reaching LDL-C target goal at a given dosage of atorvastatin.[113] The vast majority of patients can generally reach target NCEP LDL-C goals at higher dosages. The quantity and strength of the research evidence supporting the efficacy of each statin in primary and/or secondary prevention studies varies dramatically from one drug to the other; lovastatin, pravastatin, and simvastatin have the strongest data to support treatment benefits in primary and secondary prevention of coronary events as well as studies showing substantial reductions in total mortality (see above, under "Clinical Trial Evidence for Lipid Intervention"). Although the HMG-CoA reductase inhibitors generally provide the greatest LDL-C reduction with the best tolerability, it should be realized that maximal CHD risk reduction may not necessarily require LDL-C reduction beyond that provided by modest dosages of most formulations.[55] Yet this question remains open for investigation, as the lowest LDL-C level beyond which no further benefit is achieved is unclear.

Estrogen replacement therapy Estrogen replacement therapy can be used in postmenopausal women and generally results in lowering of LDL-C and raising of HDL-C by approximately 10 percent each. The use of progestin in combination with estrogen for women with an intact uterus often blunts some of the beneficial lipid effects obtained from estrogens alone.[114] Observational studies, however, suggest significant reductions in CHD risk associated both with estrogen used alone[115,116] and estrogens in combination with progestin.[116] The true risk-benefit of estrogen replacement therapy in patients without known coronary artery disease must await the results of the Women's Health Initiative.[117] However, one large trial [Heart and Estrogen/Progestin Replacement Study (HERS)] in postmenopausal women with known coronary artery disease reported no overall benefit on preventing future cardiovascular outcomes over a 4-year follow-up period[118] despite a 14 percent reduction in LDL-C levels and an 8 percent increase in HDL-C levels during the first year. A trend toward improving benefit was noted after a worse prognosis in the initial year of HERS, presumably resulting partly from the increasing antiatherogenic benefit conferred over time by the lipid changes.

Estrogens appear to increase the production of HDL as assessed by human turnover studies of HDL apoproteins.[119] Recent hepatocyte culture studies indicate that estradiol stimulates the production of HDL subfraction LP-AI particles, but not LP-AI + AII, by increasing the mRNA transcription rate of Apo-AI but not Apo-AII.[120]

Fish oils Fish oils contain omega-3 fatty acids, which also lower triglycerides. In total dosages of 3 to 6 g per day, triglyceride lowering can be achieved, but HDL-C levels are largely unaffected. Several fish-oil preparations are sold over the counter and are useful in treating severe hypertriglyceridemia (in addition to a very low fat diet) where pancreatitis is a potential risk.

Clinical Approach and Principles of Drug Selection

The selection of these agents should be highly individualized, although general guidelines can be formulated. Once the decision to initiate drug therapy is made, the choice of agent depends on two major considerations: first, the nature of the lipid disorder, and second, the assessment of risk (for atherosclerotic CVD and pancreatitis). These must be considered and the lipid goal established using NCEP recommendations as a guide. In the vast majority of patients, the lipid disorder falls into one of four patterns as shown in Table 7–8. Secondary causes (especially diabetes mellitus, hypothyroidism, and nephrotic syndrome) should be ruled out and treated optimally when present.

TABLE 7–8 Overview of Pharmacologic Treatment of Common Lipid Disorders

Lipid Pattern			
↑ LDL-C	↑ LDL-C and TG	↑ TG	↓ HDL-C (Normal LDL-C and TG)
IIA*	IIB	IV/V	—
Monotherapy			
1. Statin	1. Niacin	1. Niacin	1. Niacin
2. Resin	2. Statin	2. Fibrate	2. Fibrate
3. Niacin	3. Fibrate	3. Fish oil	3. Estrogen[†]
	4. Resin		4. Ethanol[‡]
Combinations			
1. Statin + resin	1. Niacin + statin	1. Niacin + fibrate	1. Niacin + fibrate
2. Niacin + resin	2. Niacin + resin	2. Add fish oil	2. Niacin + estrogen
	3. Statin + fibrate		3. Fibrate + estrogen
	4. Resin + fibrate		

Key: LDL-C, low-density-lipoprotein cholesterol; TG, triglycerides; HDL-C, high-density-lipoprotein cholesterol.
*Phenotype (Frederickson classification).
[†]In postmenopausal women.

Elevated LDL-C levels When the principal lipid disorder involves elevated LDL-C levels (i.e., above the NCEP threshold for pharmacologic intervention), the use of a statin should be considered first. In patients with established CHD and those with type 2 diabetes mellitus, this level is 130 mg/dL (goal < 100 mg/dL). Among those with two or more risk factors, the initiation level is 160 mg/dL and the goal below 130 mg/dL; in those with less than two risk factors, the initiation level is 190 mg/dL and the goal below 160 mg/dL. If the goal is not achieved with the highest dose of a potent statin, combined therapy is indicated. Bile acid–binding resins should be added next, to the highest tolerated dose, because they act synergistically. If the patient is unable to tolerate resins, niacin should be considered. An extended-release niacin (Niaspan), recently approved by the Food and Drug Administration, should be considered, as this agent is conveniently taken once nightly with the statins. Compliance is better with this formulation, which has lower side effects than immediate-release niacin, but more experience is needed to confirm initial reports of lower side effects and hepatotoxicity.[108,109]

Hypertriglyceridemia When hypertriglyceridemia is the main presenting feature and the LDL-C levels are on target for a given patient, the initial drug of choice is either niacin or a fibrate (or a combination of the two). In patients with diabetes mellitus, a fibrate should be considered initially; in nondiabetics with low HDL-C levels, niacin may be considered first-line therapy because of its greater potency as compared with fibrates. In patients with severe hypertriglyceridemia (with fasting chylomicronemia), the addition of fish-oil capsules to a fibrate or niacin should be considered, especially in patients with a history of pancreatitis.

In patients with combined hyperlipidemia (i.e., elevated LDL-C and triglycerides), niacin often can correct these lipid problems. Statins lower LDL-C with moderate effects on triglycerides and HDL-C. Fibrates lower triglycerides but have a neutral or moderate effect on LDL-C. Niacin also lowers small, dense LDL and Lp(a) levels, which statins do not generally affect. For these reasons, niacin should be considered first-line therapy, especially with the advent of newer extended-release preparations given once nightly. However, if the patient is unable to tolerate niacin or has contraindications, statins would be the next choice if the LDL-C elevation is a greater problem than the triglyceride elevations. If hypertriglyceridemia is the dominant problem, fibrates may be chosen. Combination therapy is indicated when monotherapy fails to meet goals. The use of a statin with niacin is very effective in lowering LDL-C to aggressive goals in high-risk patients. This combination also raises low HDL-C, which often accompanies this lipid disorder. The risk of myositis is increased but still remains uncommon. The exact incidence of myositis from this combination is unclear; large clinical trials are needed and are under way to answer this question. Resins can be used instead of statins, but compliance may be a problem in some patients. The addition of fibrates is indicated in patients with hypertriglyceridemia as a predominant problem.

Therapy for increasing HDL-C levels Although LDL-C reduction remains the primary goal of therapy, as recommended by the National Cholesterol Education Program, emerging data are establishing the rationale for raising HDL-C levels as an important therapeutic goal, particularly in patients with preexisting CHD.[65] Lifestyle alterations, including smoking cessation, weight loss, exercise, and optimal control of diabetes remain the first step in efforts to increase HDL-C.[21] Although alcohol use in moderation may also raise HDL-C levels, it cannot be advocated for use by the general public because of its potential for abuse; its use by selected individuals at high risk needs to be a decision made with the health care provider, and only after considering potential risks.[21,121]

When low HDL-C is the primary abnormality, the use of drugs has been controversial. However, recent results of the HDL Intervention Trial (HIT) in veterans[9] have provided a more firm rationale for pharmacologic treatment. A low HDL-C is the primary abnormality in 20 to 25 percent of patients with CHD. In such patients, gemfibrozil should be considered for initial use. If more aggressive increases in HDL-C are desired, niacin or a combination of niacin and gemfibrozil should be considered. The rationale for this combination is that whereas gemfibrozil increases Apo-AI production, niacin decreases its catabolism. Thus, these mechanisms of action are complementary and yield the greatest rise in HDL-C.[21] In postmenopausal women, estrogens should be considered in addition to or combination with fibrates or niacin.

Other Considerations

The above approach is usually successful in achieving lipid goals in the vast majority of patients. Patients with rare dyslipidemias (e.g., type I hypertriglyceridemia) and those with severe lipid level elevations in spite of maximal drug therapy should be referred to a specialized lipid center. In some high-risk patients (e.g., with CHD and LDL-C levels over 200 mg/dL persisting in spite of drug treatment), LDL-apheresis must be considered. The Food and Drug Administration has recently approved the use of this procedure, in which the patients' blood plasma is processed through a column that specifically removes Apo-B–containing lipoproteins. This procedure is performed twice a month and requires trained personnel.

Cost-Effectiveness of Lipid-Lowering

The cost-effectiveness of lipid-lowering therapy depends not only on the actual cost of the medication used for a given patient or in a given institution but also the risk status of the patient. The cost to produce health benefits (increased longevity and improved quality of life) will generally be lowest in groups with the highest near-term risk for CHD, such as those with preexisting CHD.[1] Next in cost are those with multiple risk factors or severely high cholesterol levels who have a fairly high risk of developing clinical events. Least cost-effective are those who have only moderate elevations of blood cholesterol without other risk factors.

In the 4S study, among high-risk men and women with preexisting CHD, the cost per year of life gained depended on the age, gender, and baseline lipid levels; it ranged from $3800 for 70-year-old men with a mean cholesterol of 309 mg/dL to $27,400 for 35-year-old women with a mean cholesterol of 213 mg/dL.[122] Other models creating estimates for primary prevention of CHD have estimated costs per year of life saved in the range of $19,000 to $56,000, depending on dosage and formulation of medication (HMG-CoA reductase inhibitor in all cases). The cost per life-year saved was about three times greater among women than men at age 40, twice as great at age 60, and 1.3 times greater at age 70 as compared with age 40.[123,124] A recent survey found that although cardiologists tended to recommend pharmacologic treatment in situations where published studies suggested it to be more cost-effective, treatment in the primary prevention setting tended to be more aggressive than would be recommended on the basis of cost-effectiveness analyses.[125] Others have calculated cost-effectiveness based on populationwide approaches to reduce cholesterol levels in the U.S. adult population, estimating cost per year of life saved ($3200) to be similar to that of many medical interventions.[126]

Conclusion

There are considerable data showing that the lowering of atherogenic lipoproteins (especially LDL-C) can reduce cardiovascular morbidity and mortality (including all-cause mortality) and effect some degree of regression of atherosclerosis and stabilization of atherosclerotic plaque. There is also mounting evidence regarding the increasing role that HDL-C and certain lipoprotein subspecies, such as small, dense LDL-C and Lp(a), may play in the atherosclerotic process. Effective and tolerable pharmacologic agents exist for ameliorating these lipid risk factors.

Significant progress has been made in reducing the prevalence of dyslipidemia, increasing professional and public cholesterol awareness, and reducing dietary fat intake, which together have been associated with a continuing decline in CHD mortality. Significant challenges remain, however. Dyslipidemia—in particular elevated total and LDL-C as well as low HDL-C—still remains undertreated, particularly among those with known CHD.[127]

It remains important to identify patients at risk for CHD, based on lipid levels and accompanying risk factors, and to use appropriate lifestyle measures combined with pharmacologic agents when needed to maximize the potential for prevention of CHD.

References

1. Expert Panel on Detection, Evaluation, and Treatment of High Blood Cholesterol in Adults. Summary of the Second Report of the National Cholesterol Education Program (NCEP) Expert Panel on Detection, Evaluation, and Treatment of High Blood Cholesterol in Adults (Adult Treatment Panel II). *JAMA* 1993; 269:3015–3023.

2. Sacks FM, Pfeffer MA, Moye LA, et al: The effect of pravastatin on coronary events after myocardial infarction in patients with average cholesterol levels. *N Engl J Med* 1996; 335:1001–1009.

3. Kannel WB, Castelli WP, Gordon T: Cholesterol in the prediction of atherosclerotic disease: new perspective based on the Framingham Heart Study. *Ann Intern Med* 1979; 90:85–91.

4. Gordon T, Castelli WP, Hjortland MC, et al: High density lipoprotein as a protective factor against heart disease: the Framingham Heart Study. *Am J Med* 1977; 62:707–714.

5. Kashyap ML: Basic considerations in the reversal of atherosclerosis—significance of high-density lipoproteins in stimulating reverse cholesterol transport. *Am J Cardiol* 1989; 63:56H–59H.

6. Rubin EM, Krauss RM, Spangler EA, et al: Inhibition of early atherogenesis in transgenic mice by human apolipoprotein AI. *Nature* 1991; 353:265–267.

7. Badimon JJ, Badimon L, Fuster V: Regression of atherosclerotic lesions by high-density lipoprotein fraction in the cholesterol-fed rabbit. *J Clin Invest* 1990; 85:1234–1241.

8. Manninen V, Tenkanen L, Koskinen P, et al: Joint effects of serum triglyceride and LDL-cholesterol and HDL-cholesterol concentrations on coronary heart disease risk in the Helsinki Heart Study: implications for treatment. *Circulation* 1992; 85:37–45.

9. Bloomfield-Rubins H, Robins SJ, Collins D for the Department of Veterans Affairs HIT Study Group: Gemfibrozil for the secondary prevention of coronary heart disease in men with low levels of high-density lipoprotein cholesterol. *N Engl J Med* 1999; 341:410–418.

10. Keys A: *Seven Countries: A Multivariate Analysis of Death and Coronary Heart Disease.* Cambridge, MA, Harvard University Press, 1980.

11. Robertson TL, Kato H, Rhoads GG, et al: Epidemiologic studies of coronary heart disease and stroke in Japanese men living in Japan, Hawaii and California: incidence of myocardial infarction and death from coronary heart disease. *Am J Cardiol* 1977; 39:239–243.

12. Stamler J, Wentworth D, Neaton JD: Is the relationship between serum cholesterol and risk of premature death from coronary heart disease continuous and graded? Findings in 356,333 primary screenees of the Multiple Risk Factor Intervention Trial (MRFIT). *JAMA* 1986; 256:2823–2828.

13. Kannel WB, Castelli WP, Gordon T, McNamara PM: Serum cholesterol, lipoproteins, and the risk of coronary heart disease: the Framingham study.

14. The Pooling Project Research Group: Relationship of blood pressure, serum cholesterol, smoking habit, relative weight and ECG abnormalities to incidence of major coronary events: final report of the Pooling Project. *J Chronic Dis* 1978; 31:201–306.

15. Kannel WB: High-density lipoproteins: epidemiologic profile and risks of coronary artery disease. *Am J Cardiol* 1983; 52:9B–12B.

16. Wong ND, Wilson PWF, Kannel WB: Serum cholesterol as a prognostic factor after myocardial infarction: the Framingham study. *Ann Intern Med* 1991; 115:687–693.

17. Anderson KM, Castelli WP, Levy D: Cholesterol and mortality: 30 years of follow-up from the Framingham study. *JAMA* 1987; 257:2176–2180.

18. Iribarren C, Reed DM, Chen R, et al: Low serum cholesterol and mortality: which is the cause and which is the effect? *Circulation* 1995; 92:2396–2403.

19. Iribarren C, Reed DM, Burchfiel CM, Dwyer JH: Serum total cholesterol and mortality: confounding factors and risk modification in Japanese-American men. *JAMA* 1995; 273:1926–1932.

20. Abbott RD, Yano K, Hakim AA, et al: Changes in total and high-density lipoprotein cholesterol over 10- and 20-year periods (the Honolulu Heart Program). *Am J Cardiol* 1998; 82:172–178.

21. Kashyap ML: Mechanistic studies of high-density lipoproteins. *Am J Cardiol* 1998; 82:42U–48U.

22. Abbott RD, Wilson PWF, Kannel WB, Castelli WP: High density lipoprotein cholesterol, total cholesterol screening, and myocardial infarction: the Framingham study. *Arteriosclerosis* 1988; 8:207–211.

23. Third Report on Nutrition Monitoring in the United States: Volume I. Washington, DC, U.S. Government Printing Office, 1995.

24. Gotto AM: Triglyceride as a risk factor for coronary artery disease. *Am J Cardiol* 1998; 82(suppl 9A):22Q–25Q.

25. Jeppesen J, Hein HO, Suadicani P, Gyntelberg F: Triglyceride concentration and ischemic heart disease: an eight-year follow-up in the Copenhagen Male Study. *Circulation* 1998; 97:1029–1036.

26. Criqui MH, Heiss G, Cohn R, et al: Plasma triglyceride level and mortality from coronary heart disease. *N Engl J Med* 1993; 328:1220–1225.

27. Gaziano JM, Hennekens CH, O'Donnell CJ, et al: Fasting triglycerides, high-density lipoprotein, and risk of myocardial infarction. *Circulation* 1997; 96:2520–2525.

28. Hokanson JE, Austin MA: Plasma triglyceride level is a risk factor in cardiovascular disease independent of high-density lipoprotein cholesterol level: a meta-analysis of population-based prospective studies. *J Cardiovasc Risk* 1996; 3:213–219.

29. Lamarche B, Moorjani S, Lupien PJ, et al: Apolipoprotein AI and B levels and the risk of ischemic heart disease during a five-year follow-up of men in the Quebec Cardiovascular Study. *Circulation* 1996; 94:273–278.

30. Stein JH, Rosenson RS: Lipoprotein lp(a) excess and coronary heart disease. *Arch Intern Med* 1997; 157:1170–1176.

31. Seed M: Lipoprotein (a)—its role in cardiovascular disease. In: Betteridge DJ (ed): *Lipids: Current Perspectives,* vol 1, *Lipids and Lipoproteins.* London, Martin Dunitz, 1996.

32. Rosengren A, Wilhelmsen L, Eriksson E, et al: Lipoprotein(a) and coronary heart disease risk: a prospective case-control study in a general population sample of middle-aged men. *BMJ* 1990; 301:1248–1251.

33. Schaefer EJ, Lamon-Fava S, Janner J, et al: Lipoprotein(a) levels and risk of coronary heart disease in men: the Lipid Research Clinics Primary Prevention Trial. *JAMA* 1994; 271:999–1003.

34. Bostom AG, Cupples LA, Jenner JL, et al: Elevated plasma lipoprotein(a) and coronary heart disease in men aged 55 years and younger: a prospective study. *JAMA* 1996; 276:544–548.

35. Bostom AG, Gagnon DR, Cupples LA, et al: A prospective investigation of elevated lp(a) detected by electrophoresis and cardiovascular disease in women: the Framingham Heart Study. *Circulation* 1994; 90:1688–1695.

36. Jauhiainen M, Koskinen P, Ehnholm C, et al: Lipoprotein(a) and coronary heart disease risk: a nested case-control study of the Helsinki Heart Study participants. *Atherosclerosis* 1991; 89:59–67.

37. Ridker RM, Hennekens CH, Stampfer MJ: A prospective study of lipoprotein(a) and risk of myocardial infarction. *JAMA* 1993; 270:2195–2199.

38. Nguyen TT, Ellefson RD, Hodge DO, et al: Predictive value of electrophoretically detected lipoprotein(a) for coronary heart disease and cerebrovascular disease in a community-based cohort of 9,936 men and women. *Circulation* 1997; 96:1390–1397.

39. Berg K, Dahlen G, Christophersen B, et al: Lp(a) lipoprotein level predicts survival and major coronary events in the Scandinavian Simvastatin Survival Study. *Clin Genet* 1997; 52:254–561.

40. Budde T, Fechtrup C, Bosenberg E, et al: Plasma lp(a) levels correlate with the number, severity, and length-extension of coronary lesions in male patients undergoing coronary arteriography for clinically suspected coronary atherosclerosis. *Arterioscler Thromb* 1994; 14:1730–1736.

41. Cantin B, Gagnon F, Moorjani S, et al: Lipoprotein(a) is an independent risk factor for ischemic heart disease in man? The Quebec Cardiovascular Study. *J Am Coll Cardiol* 1998; 31:519–525.

42. Krauss RM: Heterogeneity of plasma low-density lipoproteins and atherosclerosis risk. *Curr Opin Lipidol* 1994; 5:339–349.

43. Austin MA, Breslow JL, Hennekens CH, et al: Low-density lipoprotein subclass patterns and risk of myocardial infarction. *JAMA* 1988; 260:1917–1921.

44. Krauss RM, Stampfer MJ, Blanche PJ, et al: Particle diameter and risk of myocardial infarction. *Circulation* 1994; 90:I-460.

45 Gardner CD, Fortmann SP, Krauss RM: Small low-density lipoprotein particles are associated with the incidence of coronary artery disease in men and women. *JAMA* 1996; 276:875–881.

46. Phillips NR, Waters D, Havel RJ: Plasma lipoproteins and progression of coronary artery disease evaluated by angiography and clinical events. *Circulation* 1993; 88:2762–2770.

47. Zambon A, Brown BG, Hokansen JE, Brunzell JD: Hepatic lipase changes predict coronary artery disease regression progression in the Familial Atherosclerosis Treatment Study (abstr). *Circulation* 1996; 94:I-539.

48. Lamarche B, Tchernof A, Moorjani S, et al: Small, dense low-density lipoprotein particles as a predictor of the risk of ischemic heart disease in men: prospective results from the Quebec Cardiovascular Study. *Circulation* 1997; 95:69–75.

49. Superko HR: New aspects of risk factors for the development of atherosclerosis, including small low-density lipoprotein, homocysteine, and lipoprotein(a). *Curr Opin Cardiol* 1995; 10:347–354.

50. Holme I: Cholesterol reduction and its impact on coronary artery disease and total mortality. *Am J Cardiol* 1995; 76:10C–17C.

51. Lipid Research Clinics Program: The Lipid Research Clinics Coronary Primary Prevention Trial Results: I. reduction in incidence of coronary heart disease. *JAMA* 1984; 251:351–364.

52. Frick MH, Elo O, Kaapa K, et al: Helsinki Heart Study: primary-prevention trial with gemfibrozil in middle-aged men with dyslipidemia: safety of treatment, changes in risk factors, and incidence of coronary heart disease. *N Engl J Med* 1987; 317:1237–1245.

53. Shepherd J, Cobbe SM, Ford I, et al: Prevention of coronary heart disease with pravastatin in men with hyper-

cholesterolemia: West of Scotland Coronary Prevention Study Group. *N Engl J Med* 1995; 333:1301–1307.

54. Ford I for the WOSCOPS Study Group: A follow-up report on mortality in the West of Scotland Coronary Prevention Study (WOSCOPS). 11th International Symposium on Atherosclerosis, Paris, October 1997. Abstract P-145.

55. West of Scotland Coronary Prevention Study Group: Influence of pravastatin and plasma lipids on clinical events in the West of Scotland Coronary Prevention Study (WOSCOPS). *Circulation* 1998; 97:1440–1445.

56. Downs JR, Clearfield M, Weis S, et al. for the AFCAPS/TexCAPS Research Group: Primary prevention of acute coronary events with lovastatin in men and women with average cholesterol levels. *JAMA* 1998; 279:1615–1622.

57. The Coronary Drug Project Research Group: Clofibrate and niacin in coronary heart disease. *JAMA* 1975; 231:360–381.

58. Canner PL, Berge KG, Wenger NK, et al: Fifteen-year mortality in Coronary Drug Project patients: long-term benefit with niacin. *J Am Coll Cardiol* 1986; 8:1245–1255.

59. Research Committee of the Scottish Society of Physicians: Ischaemic heart disease: a secondary prevention trial using clofibrate. *BMJ* 1971; 4:775–784.

60. Carlson LA, Rosenhamer G: Reduction of mortality in the Stockholm Ischaemic Heart Disease Secondary Prevention Study by combined treatment with clofibrate and nicotonic acid. *Acta Med Scand* 1988; 223:405–418.

61. Buchwald H, Varco RL, Matts JP, et al and the POSCH group: Report of the program on the Surgical Control of the Hyperlipidemias (POSCH): effect of partial ileal bypass surgery on mortality and morbidity from coronary heart disease in patients with hypercholesterolemia. *N Engl J Med* 1990; 323:946–955.

62. Scandinavian Simvastatin Survival Study Group: Randomized trial of cholesterol lowering in 4444 patients with coronary heart disease: the Scandinavian Simvastatin Survival Study (4S). *Lancet* 1994; 344:1383–1389.

63. Pyorala K, Pedersen TR, Kjekshus J, et al: Cholesterol lowering with simvastatin improves prognosis of diabetic patients with coronary heart disease: a subgroup analysis of the Scandinavian Simvastatin Survival Study (4S). *Diabetes Care* 1997; 20:614–620.

64. The Long-Term Intervention with Pravastatin in Ischaemic Disease (LIPID) Study Group: Prevention of cardiovascular events and death with pravastatin in patients with coronary heart disease and a broad range of initial cholesterol levels. *N Engl J Med* 1998; 339:1349–1357.

65. Bloomfield-Rubins H, Robins SJ, Iwane MK, et al for the Department of Veterans Affairs HIT Study Group: Rationale and design of the Department of Veterans Affairs high-density lipoprotein cholesterol intervention trial (HIT) for secondary prevention of coronary artery disease in men with low high-density lipoprotein cholesterol and desirable low-density lipoprotein cholesterol. *Am J Cardiol* 1993; 71:45–52.

66. Rossouw JE: Lipid-lowering interventions in angiographic trials. *Am J Cardiol* 1995; 76:86C–92C.

67. Blankenhorn DH, Nessim SA, Johnson RL, et al: Beneficial effects of combined colestipol-niacin therapy on coronary atherosclerosis and coronary venous bypass grafts. *JAMA* 1987; 257:3233–3240.

68. Brenskie JF, Levy RI, Kelsey SF, et al: Effects of therapy with cholestyramine on progression of coronary arteriosclerosis: results of the NHLBI Type II Coronary Intervention Study. *Circulation* 1984; 69:313–324.

69. Watts GF, Lewis B, Brunt JNH: Effects on coronary artery disease of a lipid-lowering diet, or diet, plus cholestyramine, in the St. Thomas Atherosclerosis Regression Study (STARS). *Lancet* 1992; 339:563–569.

70. Brown BG, Albers JJ, Fisher LD: Regression of coronary artery disease as a result of intensive lipid-lowering therapy in men with high levels of apolipoprotein B. *N Engl J Med* 1990; 323:1289–1298.

71. Ornish D, Brown SE, Scherwitz LW, et al: Can lifestyle changes reverse coronary heart disease? The Lifestyle Heart Trial. *Lancet* 1990; 336:129–133.

72. Ornish D, Scherwitz LW, Billings JH, et al: Intensive lifestyle changes for reversal of coronary heart disease. *JAMA* 1998; 280:2001–2007.

73. Blankenhorn DH, Azen SP, Kramsch DM, et al: The Monitored Atherosclerosis Regression Study (MARS): coronary angiographic changes with lovastatin therapy. *Ann Intern Med* 1993; 119:969–976.

74. Waters D, Higginson L, Gladstone P, et al: Effect of monotherapy with an HMG-CoA reductase inhibitor on the progression of coronary atherosclerosis as assessed by serial quantitative arteriography: the Canadian Coronary Atherosclerosis Intervention Trial. *Circulation* 1994; 89:959–968.

75. Jukema JW, Bruschke AVG, Van Boven AJ, et al: Effects of lipid lowering by pravastatin on progression and regression of coronary artery disease in symptomatic men with normal to moderately elevated serum cholesterol levels: the Regression Growth Evaluation Statin Study (REGRESS). *Circulation* 1995; 91:2528–2540.

76. Pitt B, Mancini GBJ, Ellis SG, et al for the PLAC I Investigators: Pravastatin Limitation of Atherosclerosis in the Coronary Arteries (PLAC I): reduction in atherosclerosis progression and clinical events. *J Am Coll Cardiol* 1995; 26:1133–1139.

77. MAAS Investigators: Effect of simvastatin on coronary atheroma in the multicentre anti-atheroma study (MAAS). *Lancet* 1994; 344:633–638.

78. Waters D, Hinninson L, Gladstone P, et al: Effects of cholesterol-lowering on the progression of coronary ath-

erosclerosis in women: a Canadian Coronary Atherosclerosis Intervention Trial (CCAIT) substudy. *Circulation* 1995; 92:2404–2410.

79. Hahmann HW, Bunte T, Hellwig N, et al: Progression and regression of mild coronary arterial narrowings by quantitative angiography after fenofibrate therapy. *Am J Cardiol* 1991; 67:957–961.

80. Haskell WL, Alderman EL, Fair JM, et al: Effects of intensive multiple risk factor reduction on coronary atherosclerosis and clinical cardiac events in men and women with coronary artery disease: the Stanford Coronary Risk Intervention Project (SCRIP). *Circulation* 1994; 89:975–990.

81. Sacks FM, Pasternak RC, Gibson CM, et al: Effect on coronary atherosclerosis of decrease in plasma cholesterol concentrations in normocholesterolaemic patients. *Lancet* 1994; 344:1182–1186.

82. Frick MH, Syvanne M, Nieminen MS, et al: Prevention of the angiographic progression of coronary and vein-graft atherosclerosis by gemfibrozil after coronary bypass surgery in men with low levels of HDL-cholesterol: Lopid Coronary Angiography Trial (LOCAT) Study Group. *Circulation* 1997; 96:2137–2143.

83. Havel RJ: Benefits of fibrate drugs in coronary heart disease patients with normal cholesterol levels. *Circulation* 1997; 96:2113–2114.

84. The Post Coronary Artery Bypass Graft Trial Investigators: The effect of aggressive lowering of low-density lipoprotein cholesterol levels and low-dose anticoagulation on obstructive changes in saphenous vein coronary-artery bypass grafts. *JAMA* 1997; 336:153–161.

85. Ballantyne CM, Herd JA, Dunn JK, et al: Effects of lipid lowering therapy on progression of coronary and carotid artery disease. *Curr Opin Lipidol* 1997; 8:354–361.

86. Yusuf S, Lessem J, Jha P, Lonn E: Primary and secondary prevention of myocardial infarction and strokes: an update of randomly allocated controlled trials. *J Hypertens* 1993; 11(suppl 4):S61–S73.

87. Ballantyne CM: Low-density lipoproteins and risk for coronary artery disease. *Am J Cardiol* 1998; 82(suppl 9A):3Q–12Q.

88. Pearson TA, Marx HJ: The rapid reduction in cardiac events with lipid-lowering therapy: mechanisms and implications. *Am J Cardiol* 1993; 72:1072–1073.

89. Rosenson RS, Tangney CC: Antiatherothrombotic properties of statins: implications for cardiovascular event reduction. *JAMA* 1998; 279:1643–1650.

90. Stafford RS, Blumenthal D, Pasternak RC: Variations in cholesterol management practices by U.S. physicians. *J Am Coll Cardiol* 1997; 29:139–146.

91. Harnick DJ, Cohen JL, Schechter CB, et al: Effects of practice setting on quality of lipid-lowering management in patients with coronary artery disease. *Am J Cardiol* 1998; 81:1416–1420.

92. Danias PG, O'Mahony S, Radford M, et al: Serum cholesterol levels are underevaluated and undertreated. *Am J Cardiol* 1998: 81:1353–1355.

93. Schrott HG, Bittner V, Vittinghoff E, et al: Adherence to National Cholesterol Education Program treatment goals in postmenopausal women with heart disease: the Heart and Estrogen/Progestin Replacement Study (HERS). *JAMA* 1997; 277:1281–1286.

94. Frolkis JP, Zyzanski SJ, Schwartz JM, Suhan PS: Physician noncompliance with the 1993 National Cholesterol Education Program (NCEP-ATPII) guidelines. *Circulation* 1998; 98:851–855.

95. Grundy SM, Balady GJ, Criqui MH, et al: AHA Science Advisory: guide to primary prevention of cardiovascular diseases. *Circulation* 1997; 95:2329–2331.

96. Grundy SM, Balady GJ, Criqui MH, et al: When to start cholesterol-lowering therapy in patients with coronary heart disease: a statement for healthcare professionals from the American Heart Association Task Force on Risk Reduction. *Circulation* 1997; 95:1683–1685.

97. American College of Physicians guidelines for using serum cholesterol, high-density lipoprotein cholesterol, and triglycerides as screening tests for the prevention of coronary heart disease in adults. *Ann Intern Med* 1996; 124:515–517.

98. Task Force on Risk Reduction, American Heart Association: Cholesterol screening in asymptomatic adults: no cause to change. *Circulation* 1996; 93:1067–1068.

99. Smith SC, Blair SN, Criqui MH, et al: Preventing heart attack and death in patients with coronary disease. *Circulation* 1995; 92:204.

100. American Diabetes Association: Consensus statement: detection and management of lipid disorders in diabetes. *Diabetes Care* 1996; 19(suppl 1):S96–S102.

101. Cohen MV, Byrne MJ, Levine B, et al: Low rate of treatment of hypercholesterolemia by cardiologists in patients with suspected and proven coronary artery disease. *Circulation* 1991; 83:1294–1304.

102. Stone NH, Nicolosi RJ, Kris-Etherton P, et al: Summary of the scientific conference on the efficacy of hypocholesterolemia dietary interventions. *Circulation* 1996; 94:3388–3391.

103. Wong ND, Kashyap ML: Dyslipidemia in the elderly: prevalence and implications for clinical management in the prevention of coronary artery disease. *Cardiol Elderly* 1994; 2:348–354.

104. Sprecher DL, Harris BV, Goldberg AC, et al: Efficacy of psyllium in reducing serum cholesterol levels in hypercholesterolemic patients on high- or low-fat diets. *Ann Intern Med* 1993; 119(7 pt 1):545–554.

105. Carlson LA: Studies on the effect of nicotinic acid on catecholamide stimulated lipolysis in adipose tissue in vitro. *Acta Med Scand* 1963; 173:719–722.

106. Jin FY, Kamanna VS, Kashyap ML: Niacin decreases removal of high density lipoprotein apolipoprotein A-I but

not cholesterol ester by Hep G₂ cells: implications for reverse cholesterol transport. *Arterioscler Thromb Vasc Biol* 1997; 17:2020–2028.

107. Shepherd J, Packard CJ, Patsch JR, et al: Effect of nicotinic acid therapy on plasma high-density lipoprotein subfraction distribution and composition and on apolipoprotein A metabolism. *J Clin Invest* 1979; 63:858–867.

108. Knopp RH, Alagona P, Davidson M, et al: Equivalent efficacy of a time-release form of niacin (Niaspan) given once-a-night versus plain niacin in the management of hyperlipidemia. *Metabolism* 1998; 47:1097–1104.

109. Morgan JM, Capuzzi DM, Guyton JR: A new extended-release niacin (Niaspan): efficacy, tolerability, and safety in hypercholesterolemic patients. *Am J Cardiol* 1998; 82(12A):29V–34V.

110. Saku K, Gartside PS, Hynd BA, Kashyap ML: Mechanism of action of gemfibrozil on lipoprotein metabolism. *J Clin Invest* 1995; 75:1702–1712.

111. Nawrocki JW, Weiss SR, Davidson MH, et al: Reduction in LDL cholesterol of 25% to 60% in patients with primary hypercholesterolemia by atorvastatin, a new HMG-CoA reductase inhibitor. *Arterioscl Thromb Vasc Biol* 1995; 15:678–682.

112. Stein EA, Davidson MH, Dobs AS, et al: Efficacy and safety of simvastatin 90 mg/day in hypercholesterolemic patients. *Am J Cardiol* 1998; 82:311–316.

113. Dart A, Jerums G, Nicholson G, et al: A multicenter, double-blind, one-year study comparing safety and efficacy of atorvastatin versus simvastatin in patients with hypercholesterolemia. *Am J Cardiol* 1997; 80:39–44.

114. Writing Group for the PEPI Trial: Effects of estrogen or estrogen/progestin regimens on heart disease risk factors in postmenopausal women. *JAMA* 1995; 273:199–208.

115. Bush TL, Barrett-Connor E, Cowan LD, et al: Cardiovascular mortality and noncontraceptive use of estrogen in women: results of the Lipid Research Clinics Program Follow-up Study. *Circulation* 1987; 75:1102–1109.

116. Grodstein F, Stampfer MH, Manson JE, et al: Postmenopausal estrogen and progestin use and the risk of cardiovascular disease. *N Engl J Med* 1996; 335:453–461.

117. The Women's Health Initiative Study Group: Design of the Women's Health Initiative clinical trial and observational study. *Control Clin Trials* 1998; 19:61–109.

118. Hulley S, Grady D, Bush T, et al: Randomized trial of estrogen plus progestin for secondary prevention of coronary heart disease in postmenopausal women. *JAMA* 1998: 280:605–613.

119. Sacks FM, Walsh BW: Sex hormones and lipoprotein metabolism. *Curr Opin Lipidol* 1994; 5:236–240.

120. Jin FY, Kamanna VS, Kashyap ML: Estradiol stimulates apolipoprotein A-I but not A-II containing particle synthesis and scretion by stimulating mRNA transcription rate in Hep G2 cells. *Arterioscler Thromb Vasc Biol* 1998; 18:999–1006.

121. Pearson TA: Alcohol and heart disease: AHA medical/scientific statement. *Circulation* 1996; 94:3023–3025.

122. Johannesson M, Jonsson B, Kjekshus J, et al: Cost-effectiveness of simvastatin treatment to lower cholesterol levels in patients with coronary heart disease. *N Engl J Med* 1997; 336:332–336.

123. Martens LL, Guibert R: Cost-effectiveness analysis of lipid-modifying therapy in Canada: comparison of HMG-CoA reductase inhibitors in the primary prevention of coronary heart disease. *Clin Therapeut* 1994; 16:1052–1062.

124. Thorvik E, Aursnes I, Kristiansen IS, Waller HT: Cost-effectiveness of cholesterol-lowering drugs: a review of the evidence. *Wiener Klin Wochensch* 1996; 108:234–243.

125. Gaspoz JM, Kennedy JW, Orav EJ, Goldman L: Cost-effectiveness of prescription recommendations for cholesterol-lowering drugs: a survey of a representative sample of cardiologists. *J Am Coll Cardiol* 1996; 27:1232–1237.

126. Tosteson ANA, Weinstein MC, Hunink MGM: Cost-effectiveness of populationwide educational approaches to reduce serum cholesterol levels. *Circulation* 1997; 95:24–30.

127. Cleeman JI, Lenfant C: The National Cholesterol Education Program: progress and prospects. *JAMA* 1998; 280:2099–2104.

128. Committee on Principal Investigation: A co-operative trial in the primary prevention of ischaemic heart disease using clofibrate. *Br Heart J* 1978; 40:1069–1118.

129. Kane JP, Malloy MJ, Ports TA, et al: Regression of coronary atherosclerosis during treatment of familial hypercholesterolemia with combined drug regimens. *JAMA* 1990; 264:3007–3012.

130. Hambrecht R, Niebauer J, Marburger C, et al: Various intensities of leisure time physical activity in patients with coronary artery disease: effects on cardiorespiratory fitness and progression of coronary atherosclerotic lesions. *J Am Coll Cardiol* 1993; 22:468–477.

CHAPTER 8

Diabetes

Jennifer Kaseta
James R. Sowers

Diabetes mellitus is known to be a risk factor for cardiovascular disease (CVD). It causes both macrovascular and microvascular disease, leading to cardiovascular complications. The macrovascular complications include coronary heart disease (CHD), stroke, and peripheral vascular disease, while microvascular complications present as diabetic nephropathy, retinopathy, and cardiomyopathy.[1] CVD, including myocardial infarction and stroke, is the leading cause of death among diabetic persons.[1,2] Several studies have shown that diabetes mellitus is an independent risk factor for CVD.[3–5]

Epidemiology

Population- and occupation-based cohort studies generally show type 2 diabetes mellitus to confer about a twofold greater risk for CHD in men but a threefold greater risk in women. Reported national incidence rates (per 1000 person-years) for CHD range from 4.1 in nondiabetic versus 10.5 in diabetic women aged 40 to 77 years to 10.2 in nondiabetic versus 28.4 in diabetic men.[5] Multiple studies have also described important risk factors for cardiovascular disease (CVD) in diabetics to include hypertension, hyperlipidemia, hyperinsulinemia, advancing age, cigarette smoking, obesity, physical inactivity, and microalbuminuria.[2–8]

In the Framingham study,[3] the presence of diabetes doubled the age-adjusted risk of CVD in men and tripled it in women. Myocardial infarction, angina, and sudden death were two times higher in the diabetic as compared with the nondiabetic. Subjects with diabetes in all age groups had a significantly higher rate of cardiac failure as compared with the nondiabetic subjects. This difference was more pronounced in the oldest age groups (65 to 75 years). Diabetes continued to be a major independent cardiovascular risk factor when all other risk factors for CVD were adjusted for.

Within the Multiple Risk Factor Intervention Trial (MRFIT),[4] more than 5000 diabetics were followed for 12 years and compared with over 350,000 nondiabetics. The risk of cardiovascular death at the 12-year follow-up was approximately three times higher in diabetic males as compared with their nondiabetic controls, regardless of age, ethnic group, serum cholesterol, systolic blood pressure, or tobacco use. When patients had optimal control of systolic blood pressure (<120 mmHg) and serum cholesterol (<200 mg/dL), and were nonsmokers, the relative risk (RR) of cardiovascular death was 5.1 times higher in the diabetic than in the nondiabetic. The MRFIT study confirmed that diabetes is a strong independent risk factor for cardiovascular mortality, above the risk incurred from hypercholesterolemia, systolic hypertension, and cigarette use. It also confirmed that hypercholesterolemia, systolic blood pressure, and cigarette smoking were significant independent predictors of mortality in men with and without diabetes. The presence of one or more of these risk factors had a greater impact on increasing CVD risk in diabetics than in nondiabetics (Fig. 8–1).

Among over 115,000 female nurses aged 30 to 55 years at baseline, those with, versus those without, an onset of diabetes prior to age 30 had an age-adjusted risk ratio for CHD of 12.2, versus 6.7 among

FIGURE 8-1 Age-adjusted CVD death rates by presence of number of risk factors for men screened for MRFIT, with and without diabetes at baseline. Risk factors include serum cholesterol ≥200 mg/dL, cigarette smoking (any), and systolic blood pressure ≥120 mmHg. (Adapted from Stamler et al.[4])

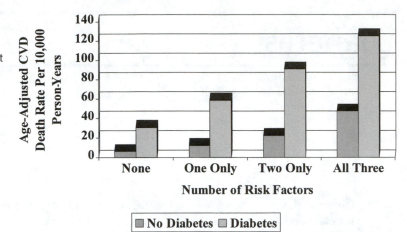

those having diabetes at age 30 or greater. After adjustment for other risk factors, this risk remained significant but was attenuated (RR = 3.1).[7]

Diabetes mellitus and hypertension are interrelated diseases. Hypertension in type 2 diabetics is associated with an increased risk of macrovascular as well as microvascular complications.[9,10] The United Kingdom Prospective Diabetes Study (UKPDS) Group documented an increased risk of stroke over an 8-year observational period in diabetic persons with associated hypertension or elevated levels of systolic blood pressure[11] and also showed that blood pressure lowering reduced the incidence of macrovascular and microvascular complications in type 2 diabetics.[12] Tight control of blood pressure with either an angiotensin-converting enzyme (ACE) inhibitor or a beta blocker resulted in a reduced risk of both macrovascular and microvascular complications in hypertensive patients with type 2 diabetes.[11-13] The risk of any diabetes-related endpoints was reduced by 24 percent, strokes were reduced by 44 percent, and microvascular endpoints by 37 percent.[12] The Hypertension Optimal Treatment Trial provides additional support for aggressive treatment of hypertension in diabetics.[14] The most aggressively treated subjects had a 30 percent reduction in stroke as compared with the least aggressively treated group, although this difference was not statistically significant owing to the small cohort of diabetics and short duration of follow-up.

Type 2 diabetes mellitus is the most prevalent form of diabetes. It is characterized by insulin resistance and decreased insulin production by pancreatic beta cells. Both obesity and physical inactivity predispose individuals to type 2 diabetes mellitus, and both contribute to insulin resistance.[15] Insulin resistance is associated with other cardiovascular risk factors—dyslipidemia, hypertension, and prothrombotic factors.[15] This association underscores the importance of metabolic abnormalities in CVD among diabetics.

Pathophysiology

Many factors contribute to the increased incidence of CVD among diabetics. These include microalbuminuria, lipoprotein and coagulation abnormalities, hypertension, hyperinsulinemia, endothelial dysfunction, increased oxidative stress,[16] and abnormalities of platelet function and coagulation[17] (Tables 8-1 to 8-3).

Microalbuminuria

Microalbuminuria, indicated by an albumin excretion rate of (0.03 to 0.3 g/dL), has been shown to be a risk factor for cardiovascular mortality in type 2 diabetes mellitus. It has also been associated with adverse cardiovascular events in type 1 diabetics.[18-20] The exact

TABLE 8–1 Lipids, Coagulation and Fibrinolytic Abnormalities in Diabetes

Elevated plasma levels of VLDL, LDL, and Lp(a)

Decreased plasma HDL cholesterol

Increased small dense LDL cholesterol products

Decreased lipoprotein lipase activity

Elevated plasma levels of factor VII and VIII

Increased levels of fibrinogen and PAI-1

Elevated thrombin-antithrombin complexes

Decreased levels of antithrombin II, protein C, and protein S

Decreased plasminogen activators and fibrinolytic activity

Increased endothelial expression of adhesion molecules

Increased adhesion of platelets and leukocytes to the endothelium

Key: VLDL, very low density lipoprotein; LDL, low-density lipoprotein; Lp(a), lipoprotein(a); HDL, high-density lipoprotein; PAI-1, plasminogen activator inhibitor-1.

TABLE 8–2 Abnormalities of Platelet Function in Diabetes

Increased platelet adhesiveness

Increased platelet aggregation

Decreased platelet survival

Increased platelet generation of vasoconstrictor prostanoids

Reduced platelet generation of prostacyclin and other vasodilator prostanoids

Altered platelet divalent cation homeostasis—i.e., decreased $[Mg^{2+}]_i$ and increased $[Ca^{2+}]_i$

Increased nonenzymatic glycosylation of platelet proteins

Decreased platelet polyphosphoinositide content

Decreased platelet production of nitric oxide

Increased platelet myosin light chain phosphorylation

Increased platelet adhesion to endothelium

TABLE 8–3 Alterations in Vascular Endothelium Associated with Diabetes

Elevated plasma levels of von Willebrand factor

Elevated expression, synthesis, and plasma levels of endothelin-1

Diminished prostacyclin release

Decreased release of endothelium-derived relaxing factor Nitric oxide (NO) and reduced responsiveness to NO

Impaired fibrinolytic activity

Increased endothelial cell surface thrombomodulin

Increased endothelial cell procoagulant activity

Impaired plasmin degradation of glycosylated fibrin

Increased levels of advanced glycosylated end products

Increased superoxide anion generation and NO destruction

Increased expression of adhesion molecules

betic first-degree relatives of patients with type 2 diabetes often have microalbuminuria associated with insulin resistance. This suggests that microalbuminuria in nondiabetic individuals may foreshadow the onset of type 2 diabetes mellitus.[5]

Lipoprotein Abnormalities

Although many diabetics do have elevated levels of total and low-density lipoprotein cholesterol (LDL-C), hypertriglyceridemia and/or low levels of high-density lipoprotein cholesterol (HDL-C), are the most commonly occurring lipid abnormalities in diabetics. For any lipoprotein level, diabetics have a greater coronary risk than do nondiabetics. Among the 5163 men in the MRFIT study who reported taking medication for diabetes, those with a total cholesterol of 260 mg/dL and higher were at more than twice the risk of cardiovascular death over 12 years than those with levels under 180 mg/dL. In contrast, triglycerides, but not total cholesterol, were associated with the presence of ischemic heart disease.[4] The few data regarding the predictive value of lipoprotein levels in diabetics derive from a registry study of 1059 Finnish diabetics receiving drug reimbursement who were followed for 7 years for

mechanism is unknown. It is thought that albuminuria may be the result of generalized endothelial dysfunction that enhances the penetration of atherogenic lipoproteins in the arterial wall.[19] Microalbuminuria has been associated with several cardiovascular risk factors including hyperinsulinemia, insulin resistance, central obesity, and dyslipidemia.[15] Nondia-

CHD events.[21] Compared with those with HDL-C of 35 mg/dL or higher, those with an HDL-C below 35 mg/dL were at a twofold greater risk of coronary events, as were those with triglycerides of 400 mg/dL or greater, compared with less than 200 mg/dL. Those with levels of LDL-C of 160 mg/dL or greater also were at greater risk.

The characteristics of lipoproteins may also differ between diabetics and nondiabetics. Oxidation of lipoproteins is enhanced in the presence of hyperglycemia and hypertriglyceridemia.[20] Triglycerides are elevated in the diabetic secondary to a decrease in lipoprotein lipase activity.[17] Oxidized lipoproteins are cytotoxic to vascular endothelial and smooth muscle cells and probably contribute to atherogenesis.[16] There is increased glycation of apoB in the hyperglycemic state.[14] This results in impaired recognition of LDL by hepatocyte receptors and an increase in LDL half-life. The glycation of HDL increases the clearance of HDL and decreases its half-life. The net result is an increase in plasma very low density lipoprotein (VLDL), LDL, and lipoprotein(a) and a decrease in plasma HDL.[22] Lipoprotein(a) is a modified form of LDL that can bind to endothelium and components of the extracellular matrix.[23] This results in localized cholesterol accumulation. In several large prospective studies, lipoprotein(a) has been shown to be a powerful predictor of premature atherosclerotic vascular disease.[24–26] Its structure is similar to that of plasminogen; it interferes with fibrinolysis and accentuates thrombosis by competing with plasminogen for binding sites. Several other mechanisms have been elucidated in the diabetic milieu that skew the coagulation cascade in favor of thrombosis. Finally, a small, dense LDL particle size (phenotype B) appears to be an important risk factor for the development of type 2 diabetes, possibly mediated through its association with insulin resistance.[27]

Coagulation Abnormalities

Diabetic individuals are prone to thrombosis, in part through disruptions in platelet function (Table 8–2) and the vascular endothelium (Table 8–3).[28]

Diabetics have higher levels of plasminogen activator inhibitor-1 (PAI-1)[29] than nondiabetics. Elevated levels of PAI-1, which inhibit fibrinolysis, have been associated with hyperinsulinemia and hypertriglyceridemia;[30] they are also found in diabetic survivors of myocardial infarction.[31] This increase in PAI-1 may predispose individuals to recurrent myocardial infarction or abrupt closure of a lesion previously opened by angioplasty.[14] Fibrinolytic activity is also decreased. There are decreased levels of antithrombin III, protein C, and protein S,[22] which predispose these patients to thrombosis. The procoagulant state associated with diabetes can also be attributed to higher-than-normal levels of coagulation factors. Plasma levels of von Willebrand factor are elevated, especially in association with endothelial cell injury, microvascular and macrovascular damage, and poor diabetic control. High concentrations of factor VIII with hyperglycemia accelerate the rate of thrombin formation, which may contribute to occlusive vascular disease. Fibrinogen, factor VII, and thrombin-antithrombin complexes have been noted to be higher in diabetics. This prolongs the survival of provisional clots on injured endothelium. Increased concentrations of thrombin-antithrombin complexes result in increased clot generation.

Platelet adhesion and aggregation is enhanced in diabetics, further contributing to a procoagulant milieu.[32] Studies have suggested that the release of the contents of the alpha granules (thromboglobulin and platelet factor 4) is increased in platelets of diabetic individuals.[33] Platelets of diabetics also appear to have decreased levels of platelet-derived growth factor (PDGF) and serotonin, suggesting increased release. Nitric oxide (NO) is produced by platelets[34] as well as other tissues and inhibits platelet aggregation and adhesion to endothelial cells.[15,31,32,34] In diabetes mellitus, there is reduced production and increased destruction of NO.[1,35] This results in increased platelet aggregation. Other platelet abnormalities in diabetics include decreased platelet survival, increased platelet generation of vasoconstrictor prostanoids, reduced platelet generation of prostacyclin and other vasodilator prostanoids, and increased glycosylation of platelet proteins.[1,32]

Endothelial Cell Dysfunction

Abnormalities in the vascular endothelium are also associated with diabetes mellitus[1,35] (Table 8–3). Endothelial cell lipoprotein lipase activity is decreased. This impairs conversion of VLDL to LDL, which, in turn, is injurious to the endothelial cells. Hyperglycemia alters endothelial matrix production, which is thought to lead to basement membrane thickening. It also increases endothelial cell collagen and fibronectin synthesis while delaying endothelial cell replication and cell death by enhancing both oxidation and glycation. Hypercholesterolemia, frequently a disease of the diabetic, impairs endothelium-dependent relaxation. There is decreased release of endothelium-derived relaxing factor (NO)[35,36] and reduced responsiveness to NO, as previously discussed with regard to platelets. In addition, there is impaired degradation of glycosylated fibrin, increased concentrations of glycated end products and elevated expression, synthesis, and plasma concentrations of endothelin-1.

Insulin Resistance

Hyperinsulinemia, or insulin resistance, has traditionally been considered to be an important risk factor for diabetes as well as for CVD in diabetics.[6] Hyperinsulinemia is frequently associated with dyslipidemia and central obesity as well as hypertension.[37,38] In fact, among Framingham offspring subjects (mean age 54 years), approximately one-fourth—now middle-aged adults—were found to have this "central metabolic syndrome" characterized by hyperinsulinemia, dyslipidemia, and obesity.[38] More recent studies in adults with type 2 diabetes or impaired glucose tolerance do not consistently show a relation of endogenous insulin to heart disease.[39] However, among those without diabetes at baseline, a recent meta-analysis involving data from 12 population-based or nested case-control studies showed an overall weak positive association of nonfasting insulin levels and cardiovascular disease incidence [RR of 1.18 with 95 percent confidence intervals (CI) 1.08–1.29].[40] A recent 22-year follow-up from the study of Helsinki policemen showed a significant positive association for a major coronary event in the highest quintile versus the lower four quintiles of insulin response to an oral glucose tolerance test (area under the curve) with relative risks ranging from 1.32 (22-year follow-up) to 2.36 (5-year follow-up) after adjustment for other risk factors.[41] Hyperinsulinemia may increase cardiovascular risk through its promotion of hypertension, possibly a result of chronic enhancement of sympathetic nervous system activity, thus increasing renal tubular sodium reabsorption, modulating cation transport, or inducing vascular smooth muscle cell hypertrophy.[37] Low HDL cholesterol, also a risk factor for CHD, is promoted by insulin resistance through diminished activity of lipoprotein lipase, which may result in excessive transfer of triglycerides from chylomicrons and VLDL particles in exchange for cholesterol esters from HDL particles, thus reducing HDL cholesterol levels.[42]

Prevention and Management

Lifestyle Modification

Obesity and physical inactivity can predispose one to type 2 diabetes mellitus and cardiovascular disease.[43,44] The incidence of type 2 diabetes mellitus increases when obesity is severe. The National Institutes of Health Obesity Education Intiative[45] defines overweight as a body mass index (BMI) of 25 to 29.9 kg/m^2 and obesity as a BMI of greater than 30 kg/m^2. Upper-body obesity (central, android) is usually an indicator of insulin resistance. The waist-to-hip ratio and the waist circumference can be used to assess upper-body obesity. A waist-to-hip ratio greater than 0.9 in men or 0.8 in women indicates upper-body obesity and represents predominant upper-body fat distribution.[38,39] A waist circumference greater than 40 in (102 cm) in men or 36 in (88 cm) in women is indicative of abdominal obesity.

Approximately 50 percent of adult Americans are overweight, with nearly half of these classified as obese.[45] Obesity contributes to hyperlipidemia, low HDL cholesterol, hypertension, insulin resistance, and a prothrombotic state. Obesity acts as a risk factor for both diabetes and CVD by enhancing the metabolic milieu created by the other risk factors of diabetes mellitus and CVD. Regular exercise reduces insulin resistance and a sedentary lifestyle increases it. As with obesity, physical inactivity contributes to the metabolic abnormalities that precede the onset of hyperglycemia and subsequent cardiovascular disease. There is indirect evidence indicating that decreased physical activity results in an increased risk for type 2 diabetes mellitus, and less active population groups have an increased prevalence of type 2 diabetes. This prevalence increases as physical activity decreases. Physical activity increases insulin sensitivity. Endurance exercise causes weight loss and improves glucose tolerance.

Given the above information, lifestyle modifications are recommended as initial therapy for the prevention and management of diabetes mellitus. These include weight loss if the individual has exceeded the recommendations of the National Institutes of Health Obesity Education Initiative,[45] adhering to American Diabetes Association (ADA) recommendations on medical nutrition therapy,[46] increasing physical activity, and smoking cessation.

The focus of medical nutrition therapy in type 2 diabetes should be on achieving glucose, lipid, and blood pressure goals. Therapy should be individualized, giving consideration to usual eating habits and other lifestyle factors. Weight loss, when needed, as well as hypocaloric diets can improve glycemic control and may have the potential for long-term metabolic control. The recommended proportion of calories from fat depends on desired glucose, lipid, and weight goals. For those with normal lipid levels at desirable weight, the general goal of 30 percent or less calories from total fat, less than 10 percent calories from saturated fat, and under 300 mg/day of dietary cholesterol can be implemented. Less saturated fat and cholesterol, as from a step 2 diet (<7 percent of calories from saturated fat and <200 mg of dietary cholesterol), can be recommended for those with elevated LDL cholesterol levels. In general, 10 to 20 percent of calories should come from protein, which would leave the remaining 50 to 60 percent from carbohydrates, given the goal of 30 percent or less calories from fat. Although a commonly held belief has been that simple sugars should be avoided

and complex carbohydrates emphasized, there is limited scientific evidence to support this. There is no reason to avoid consumption of fruits and vegetables, in which fructose occurs naturally. Intake of 20 to 35 g/day of dietary fiber is also recommended, as is reduction of sodium intake to no more than 2400 mg/day and less than 2000 mg/day in those with hypertension and nephropathy. Recommendations regarding alcohol use are generally the same for diabetics as for the general public, but reduction or abstention may be advisable in those diabetics with other problems such as pancreatitis, dyslipidemia, or neuropathy as well as those being treated with insulin or sulfonylureas.[46] A nutrition guide for people with diabetes published by the ADA appears in Appendix 8–1.

Some type of regular exercise is likely to be beneficial in most diabetics. For those patients over age 35 and those who have had diabetes for more than 10 years, a complete physical exam and exercise stress test should be performed prior to the onset of an exercise program. It is well established that sudden exercise in sedentary individuals, including nondiabetics, can precipitate myocardial infarction.[47,48] Patients will be more compliant with activities that they enjoy, and regular encouragement and suggestions should be offered.[49,50] A reasonable initial exercise program should include 10 min of warmup and stretching, followed by 20 min of aerobic activity (walking, biking, swimming, etc.). This should be done at regular intervals (at least three times a week). The duration and intensity of the exercise program should be increased gradually. Although aerobic exercise is preferred, this may be limited by existing microvascular complications. Patients with proliferative retinopathy should avoid intense isometric exercise (weight lifting), as it can cause an increase in blood pressure and, in turn, intraocular bleeding. Patients with significant neuropathy should avoid traumatic weight-bearing activities (long distance running, prolonged downhill skiing). These have the potential to precipitate stress fractures in the foot and ankle and to cause pressure ulcers on the feet. A list of frequently asked questions about exercise and diabetes, as well as answers to these questions appears in Appendix 8–2.

Nonpharmacologic therapy in diabetic hypertensive patients may be beneficial for mild hypertension and may be used in combination with pharmacologic therapy to attain adequate blood pressure control. The ADA diet has been reported to lower blood pressure in diabetic patients. Moderate salt restriction can reduce systolic blood pressure. Weight reduction reduces blood pressure. For every 10 lb in weight reduction, systolic and diastolic blood pressures can be expected to decrease by 10 and 5 mmHg, respectively.[51,52]

Cigarette smoking is an independent risk factor for all-cause mortality, largely due to CVD. Smoking is associated with increased plasma total cholesterol and VLDL, a reduction in HDL, and a greater degree of insulin resistance.[53] In addition, smokers have worse glycemic control than do nonsmokers.[54,55] In type 1 diabetics, smoking is independently associated with an increase in urinary albumin excretion and nonproliferative retinopathy.[56] The degree of albuminuria approaches that of the non-smoking diabetic when smoking is discontinued.[55,56] A meta-analysis of several cardiovascular risk reduction trials has shown that smoking cessation had a much greater benefit on survival than most other nonpharmacologic interventions.[57] Smoking cessation is one of the most important lifestyle modifications one can make that will decrease cardiovascular morbidity and mortality.[52,58]

Management of Hypertension

The goal in treatment of hypertension in individuals with diabetes mellitus is a blood pressure less than 130/85 mmHg.[59] This is lower than the recommendation for those without diabetes (less than 140/80 mmHg) because of the increased risk of cardiovascular disease in diabetics (Figs. 8–2 and 8–3). Angiotensin-converting enzyme (ACE) inhibitors, calcium channel blockers, alpha blockers or low-dose thiazide diuretics can be used alone or in combination with lifestyle modifications. Reduction in blood pressure is the goal of antihypertensive therapy and is more important than the antihypertensive agent chosen. The UKPDS studies[11–13] and others have shown benefit with therapy using different classes of antihypertensives, including diuretics, ACE inhibitors, beta blockers, and calcium channel blockers.

ACE inhibitors are recommended as first-line therapy for the hypertensive diabetic[60] regardless of the presence or absence of proteinuria. They have no adverse effects on lipid levels or glycemic control[59] and have been shown to slow the progression of diabetic nephropathy.[60,61] Adverse effects of ACE inhibitors include acceleration of renal insufficiency in patients with bilateral renal artery stenosis, angioedema, and cough. When diabetics are intolerant to ACE inhibitors, angiotensin II receptor blockers may be considered; however, their long-term efficacy in preventing diabetic nephropathy, while promising, remains to be established.

Thiazide diuretics have been shown to reduce cardiovascular morbidity and mortality in large population-based trials. The diabetic hypertensive patient is generally volume-expanded; thus, diuretics are often needed for adequate blood pressure control. Disadvantages of thiazides include short-term dyslipidemia, altered carbohydrate metabolism, hypokalemia, hypomagnesemia, and hyperuricemia. These side effects are minimal if the patient receives a low dose (i.e., 25 mg or less of hydrochlorothiazide or chlorthalidone). When used in combination with ACE inhibitors, diuretics often have a synergistic effect in blood pressure lowering and the metabolic adverse effects of diuretics are minimized.[59–63]

Calcium channel blockers, alpha blockers, and beta blockers are not recommended as first-line therapy in the treatment of the hypertensive diabetic individual. Calcium channel blockers, however, may be beneficial in the treatment of microalbuminuria. Beta blockers may have adverse effects on glucose and lipid metabolism. They can blunt the catecholamine-mediated symptoms of hypoglycemia and prolong the recovery from hypoglycemia. Beta blockers can also decrease peripheral blood flow and worsen claudication and vasospasm in patients with an already compromised peripheral vasculature. Alpha blockers may cause or exacerbate sexual dysfunction.

Management of Dyslipidemia

Given the lipid abnormalities associated with diabetes mellitus, optimal lipid levels in diabetics correspond

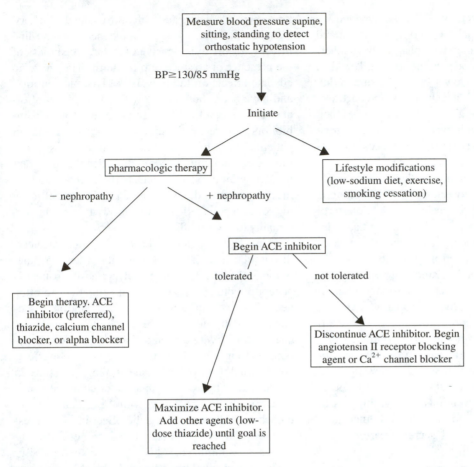

FIGURE 8–2 JNC VI recommendations for the treatment of hypertension in diabetics. (Adapted from the Sixth Report of the Joint National Committee on Detection, Evaluation, and Treatment of High Blood Pressure.[59])

to an LDL-C of less than or equal to 100 mg/dL, an HDL-C of over 45 mg/dL, and triglycerides below 200 mg/dL (Table 8–4).[64] Consideration should be given to obtaining a fasting lipid profile annually in adult patients and beginning at age 2 in children with diabetes.

In adults, the primary goal of a reduction of LDL-C can usually be achieved with a low-fat diet, achievement of ideal body weight, and, if necessary, pharmacologic therapy. If the baseline LDL-C is

equal to or less than 100 mg/dL, cholesterol-lowering agents are not required; if the baseline LDL exceeds 100 mg/dL, dietary therapy is initially recommended, after which, if it persists at or above 130 mg/dL, cholesterol-lowering medication should be initiated (Table 8–5).[64] A goal to reduce the LDL-C to below 130 mg/dL is generally recommended; however, some authorities do recommend reductions to below 100 mg/dL in diabetics who have at least one of the following other coronary risk factors:

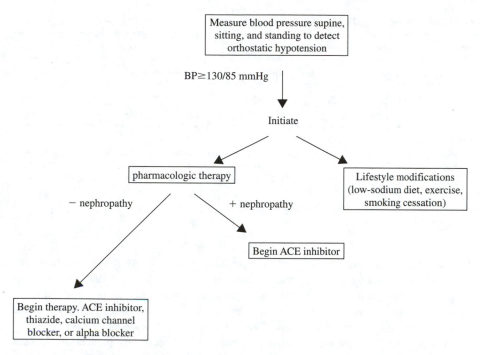

FIGURE 8–3   ADA recommendations for the treatment of hypertension in diabetics. (Adapted from the American Diabetes Association.)

HDL-C < 35 mg/dL, hypertension, smoking, family history of cardiovascular disease, or microalbuminuria or proteinuria. Among diabetics with preexisting CHD, peripheral vascular disease, or cerebrovascular disease, pharmacologic therapy should be initiated if the LDL-C persists above 100 mg/dL after lifestyle changes and glucose-lowering therapy have been utilized (Table 8–5). The favored drugs for treatment of hyperlipidemia in diabetics are the HMG-CoA reductase inhibitors ("statins"), recommended in part due to existing clinical trial data from the Scandinavian Simvastatin Survival Study documenting their efficacy in reducing coronary heart disease events, as shown in subgroup analysis in diabetics.[65] Bile-acid sequestrants (resins) and nicotinic acid are also effective, but they are less potent and are not as well tolerated. In addition, bile-acid sequestrants may raise triglyceride levels and niacin can exacerbate hyperinsulinemia and hyperglycemia.

Secondary goals of lipid therapy in diabetics are to reduce serum triglycerides and raise HDL cholesterol. The first-line of therapy to attain these goals is for the patient to achieve desired body weight and

TABLE 8–4   Category of Risk Based on Lipoprotein Levels in Adult Diabetics

Risk	LDL Cholesterol	HDL Cholesterol	Triglycerides
Higher	≥130 mg/dL	<35 mg/dL	≥400 mg/dL
Borderline	100–129 mg/dL	35–45 mg/dL	200–399 mg/dL
Lower	<100 mg/dL	>45 mg/dL	<200 mg/dL

Key: LDL, low-density lipoprotein; HDL, high-density lipoprotein.
Source: Adapted from the American Diabetes Association,[64] with permission.

TABLE 8–5 Treatment Decisions Based on LDL Cholesterol Level in Adults

	Medical Nutrition Therapy		Drug Therapy	
	Initiation Level	Goal	Initiation Level	Goal
With CHD, PVD, or CVD	>100 mg/dL	≤100 mg/dL	>100 mg/dL	≤100 mg/dL
Without CHD, PVD, or CVD	>100 mg/dL	≤100 mg/dL	≥130 mg/dL	<130 mg/dL*

Key: CHD, coronary heart disease; CVD, cardiovascular disease; PVD, peripheral vascular disease.

*For diabetic patients with one or more CHD risk factors—such as low HDL (<35 mg/dL), hypertension, smoking, family history of CVD, or microalbuminuria or proteinuria—some authorities recommend an LDL goal of <100 mg/dL. Caveats: (1) Medical nutrition therapy should be attempted before starting pharmacologic therapy. (2) Since diabetic men and women are considered to have equal CHD risk, age and sex are not considered "risk factors."

Source: Adapted from the American Diabetes Association,[64] with permission.

to increase physical activity. Smoking cessation will also aid in lowering triglycerides and raising HDL cholesterol. The goal for triglycerides is less than 200 mg/dL, or less than 150 mg/dL if macrovascular disease is present. While glucose-lowering agents do lower triglyceride levels, a fibrate may be added if elevated triglycerides persist and hypertriglyceridemia is the principal lipid abnormality. In cases where elevated LDL-C was the principal problem and a statin was prescribed as the initial agent, a fibrate may be added to provide additional triglyceride lowering beyond the modest reductions in triglycerides possible from high dosages of statins. The down side to this approach is that fibrates and statins in combination place the patient at an increased risk for myopathy. Nicotinic acid can be used as an alternative to fibrates, but unfortunately nicotinic acid increases insulin resistance and enhances hyperglycemia and has normally been contraindicated in diabetic patients. In some well-controlled diabetics, however, nicotinic acid may be a suitable choice, especially if hypertriglyceridemia and/or low HDL-C are the principal lipid abnormalities.

Aspirin Therapy

Diabetic individuals have enhanced platelet aggregation and adhesion.[66] Thromboxane, a potent vasoconstrictor and platelet-aggregating agent, is increased in patients with type 2 diabetes and cardiovascular disease.[66,67] Aspirin inhibits throm-

boxane synthesis by acetylating platelet cyclooxygenase. It has been used as both a primary and secondary intervention in nondiabetic and diabetic individuals to prevent cardiovascular disease.[68–70] The current guidelines for aspirin use provided by the ADA[71,72] include both primary and secondary prevention. Aspirin therapy is recommended as a secondary prevention strategy in diabetic individuals with large-vessel disease; this includes individuals with a history of myocardial infarction, vascular bypass procedures, or stroke or transient ischemic attacks, peripheral vascular disease, claudication, and/or angina. The ADA also recommends the consideration of aspirin therapy as a primary preventive strategy in high-risk individuals with type 1 or type 2 diabetes. This includes diabetics with one or more of the following characteristics: (1) tobacco use, (2) hypertension, (3) a family history of coronary heart disease, (4) obesity, (5) micro- or macroalbuminuria, and (6) dyslipidemia. The great majority of diabetics have at least one of these conditions that would warrant aspirin therapy. Aspirin therapy is not recommended to those individuals with an aspirin allergy, bleeding tendencies, anticoagulant therapy, recent gastrointestinal bleeding, and/or clinically active hepatic disease. The recommended dose is 81 to 325 mg of enteric-coated aspirin. Regular use of nonsteroidal anti-inflammatory drugs may increase the risk for developing chronic renal disease and impair blood pressure control in hypertensive patients. Low-dose aspirin is a weak inhibitor of prostaglandin synthesis and has no clinically significant effect on renal function or blood pressure control. Aspirin therapy is not associated with an increased risk or benefit in the progression of diabetic retinopathy and maculopathy.[72]

Pharmacologic Agents for Glycemic Control in Type 2 Diabetes Mellitus

The Diabetes Control and Complications Trial (DCCT)[73] showed the relationship of hyperglycemia to the development of microvascular disease and peripheral neuropathy. In patients with type 1 diabetes mellitus, improved glycemic control reduced both microvascular complications and peripheral neuropathy. There is evidence to support the same relationship between glycemic control and microvascular complications and peripheral neuropathy in type 2 diabetics.[74] Although no similar well-controlled prospective trial has been completed in type 2 diabetics, these results have been extrapolated to individuals with type 2 diabetes. The relationship between glycemic control and cardiovascular complications was not statistically significant in the DCCT. It is not known to what degree, if any, glycemic control will affect the progression of macrovascular disease in type 1 and type 2 diabetes. At least there does appear to be a strong relation of glycemic control to risk in nondiabetics, based on a recent report among more than 17,000 working nondiabetic men from three European cohorts. Over 20 years, those in the upper 2.5 percent of fasting glucose distributions (compared with the lower 80 percent) were at significantly greater risk of all-cause mortality (age-adjusted hazard ratio of 2.0, 95 percent confidence intervals 1.6 to 2.6) and cardiovascular death (hazard ratio 2.7, 95 percent confidence intervals 1.7 to 4.4).[75]

Based on the results of the DCCT and other similar studies, the ADA has recommended treatment goals for individuals with diabetes that emphasize glycemic control.[73] The initial treatment aimed at glycemic control in people with type 2 diabetes is a diet and exercise program. If progress toward glycemic control goals (e.g., $HbA_{1c} < 8$ percent) is not being met within a 3-month period, pharmacologic therapy is recommended after a diet and exercise program has been initiated.[74] Some patients may require initial therapy with medications at the time of diagnosis. These include individuals with symptoms of hyperglycemia, patients undergoing surgery, and those with ketosis.

Sulfonylureas are recommended as initial pharmacologic intervention in patients with type 2 diabetes because most of these are relatively insulin-deficient. An increase in endogenous insulin production is usually observed in patients taking sulfonylureas. After several years of sulfonylurea therapy, endogenous insulin secretion usually decreases and it is difficult to maintain near-normal glycemia. Biguanides have been used alone and in combination with sulfonylureas.[76] As with the sulfonureas, the effectiveness of therapy with biguanides slowly declines with time and other therapeutic interventions become necessary.

The thiazolidinediones (e.g., troglitazone) decrease hepatic gluconeogenesis and increase insulin-dependant glucose uptake in skeletal muscle. They require the presence of insulin for their action and can be used as monotherapy or in combination. Alpha-glucosidase inhibitors delay the hydrolysis of complex carbohydrates and thus slow absorption. These agents are useful in patients with postprandial hyperglycemia. As compared to sulfonylureas and biguanides, where there is usually a reduction in glycated hemoglobin of 1.5 to 2.0 percent,[77,78] the glycated hemoglobin from alpha-glucosidase therapy usually decreases by 0.5 to 1.0 percent.[78] As the effectiveness of oral agents decreases, insulin therapy is usually required to maintain glycemic control. The insulin regimen should be individualized to the patient.

Adverse events from sulfonylureas include hypoglycemia and weight gain. Biguanides are associated with lactic acidosis, especially in patients with renal disease and congestive heart failure, and are contraindicated in patients with renal insufficiency. The incidence of lactic acidosis with metformin is 0.03 per 1000 patient-years of use. Less concerning than lactic acidosis is gastrointestinal distress, most commonly diarrhea. Alpha-glucosidase inhibitors almost exclusively cause gastrointestinal side effects, most commonly flatulence and abdominal discomfort. This can be avoided by taking this medication with meals and by decreasing the amount of starch in the diet. Thiazolindinediones (troglitazone) have been associated with elevated serum transaminase levels as well as hepatic failure in patients taking this class of drug. It is currently not recommended to prescribe troglitazone to patients with serum transaminase levels of 1.5 times the upper limit of normal. Serum transaminase levels should be obtained at the initiation of troglitazone therapy, then monthly for 8 months, and then every 2 months for the remainder of the first year of therapy.

Summary

Macrovascular disease is the major cause of mortality in persons with type 2 diabetes mellitus. Many factors contribute to the high prevalence of macrovascular disease in persons with diabetes mellitus. Hypertension and dyslipidemia are two such factors. High blood pressure is about twice as frequent in persons with diabetes mellitus as those without. Information from death certificates indicates that hypertension was implicated in 4.4 percent of deaths coded to diabetes, and diabetes was involved in 10 percent of deaths coded to hypertension-related disease. Up to 75 percent of diabetes-related cardiovascular complications may be attributed to hypertension.[79] These observations have contributed to recommendations of more aggressive lowering of blood pressure (i.e., to less than 130/85 mmHg) in persons with coexistent diabetes and hypertension.

Diabetes is often accompanied by other metabolic abnormalities, including insulin resistance. These metabolic abnormalities of the coagulation-fibrinolytic system predispose to a procoagulant state. The nexus for all of these abnormalities may be central (visceral) obesity. The dyslipidemia accompanying hypertension frequently consists of low HDL cholesterol, elevated triglyceride levels, and an abnormal, more atherogenic LDL-cholesterol particle. Dyslipidemia interacts with associated hemodynamic (i.e., hypertension) and metabolic (i.e., increased platelet aggregation and PAI-1 levels) factors in a multiplicative manner, potentiating cardiovascular and renal disease. Accordingly, lipid therapy should be aggressive to attenuate these medical complications. The wide variety of lipid medications currently available, including many that are well toler-

ated and efficacious, leaves little excuse for not achieving adequate control of dyslipidemia in many persons with diabetes.

Despite the current recommendations regarding the goal of antihypertensive therapy in patients with diabetes mellitus, it is likely that in many medical care settings less than 10 percent of such persons are adequately controlled at blood pressure levels of less than 130/85 mmHg. Strategies for better control include combination therapy using several antihypertensive agents at relatively low doses that would result in synergism of their antihypertensive properties. It is also likely that less than 10 percent of diabetic persons have their LDL cholesterol lowered to less than 100 mg/dL, which is the goal for most of these patients.

Ideally, however, efforts aimed at preventing diabetes on a population level are essential if we are to reduce the population burden from this disease. Many risk factors for type 2 diabetes—such as obesity, physical inactivity, insulin resistance, and a high-fat diet—can largely be controlled. There exists the hypothesis that at least in some people, diabetes can be delayed if not prevented. While results of some behavioral and drug interventions are promising, further investigation is needed to determine the best approaches to preventing diabetes.[80]

APPENDIX 8–1 NUTRITION GUIDE FOR PEOPLE WITH DIABETES

Diabetes doesn't change the kinds of foods you eat. No matter what type of diabetes you have, the food choices you make are important. Smart food choices help keep your blood glucose level in good control. Poor food choices work against your efforts to stay healthy.

Your meal plan must match your unique needs. That's why there is no one diabetic diet. But the American Diabetes Association sets nutrition guidelines for people with diabetes to help with food choices. These guidelines are like a blueprint. When you work with a dietitian to create your meal plan, it's like turning that blueprint into a home. Just as you choose a certain roof material or paint color for your home, you can choose foods that suit your tastes. The most important guideline is that your meal plan needs to be individualized for you.

Your Food Plan

Diabetes doesn't change the kinds of foods you can eat. Basically, what's healthy for you is what's healthy for anyone who wants to eat well. Like everyone, you should focus on eating less fat, fewer sugary foods, and a variety of fresh fruits, vegetables, lean meats, and fish.

Your food plan should give you enough calories to stay at a healthy weight for you. This is a weight you can achieve and stay with and one that you and your doctor agree on. It may not be the ideal body weight found on the height/weight charts.

Your food choices can help you prevent or delay side effects of diabetes such as kidney disease, gastroparesis (slow stomach emptying), high blood pressure, and heart disease by helping you control blood glucose levels.

For people with type 1 diabetes: Food is one tool you can use to treat your diabetes. Your food plan should help you keep your blood glucose level as near to normal as possible. Plan your meals at consistent times so that you eat when your insulin is working the hardest. It's especially important for you to monitor your blood glucose levels. This will help you change your insulin dose to match the amount of food you usually eat.

Your meal plan should also help you prevent or treat very low blood glucose, even when you exercise. You also need food ideas for days when you're ill or don't eat normally. Even when you're sick, you still need to take insulin. A dietitian can help you plan ahead to avoid low blood glucose and teach you what and how much food to eat to treat a low blood glucose reaction.

Children and teens need a food plan that keeps them growing normally. Pregnant women, women who are planning to get pregnant, and women who are breast-feeding need to develop a food plan that will keep blood glucose under tight control. It's important for the health of mother and baby to have excellent blood glucose control from the first moment of pregnancy and while caring for an infant.

For people with type 2 diabetes: You seek several health goals—good control of your blood glucose levels, better blood fat levels, more normal blood pressure, and a healthy weight. You may be able to reach both of these goals with a healthy eating plan and regular exercise. If you also need insulin or diabetes pills, sticking with healthy food choices and portion sizes will help the medications work better.

Focus on cutting the fat in your diet, especially saturated fat and cholesterol. This objective works better than simply trying to lose weight. Space meals over the course of the day rather than eating a few large meals. Aim for a modest weight loss. For many people, losing only 10 to 20 pounds can mean improved blood glucose and blood fat levels and lower blood pressure.

The best way to lose weight is to eat fewer calories and increase your activity level. Minor changes can help. For example, cutting out 250 calories per day and walking briskly for 20 minutes three times a week may be all you need to do to control weight and blood glucose levels.

Source: From the American Diabetes Association, 1998, with permission.

Checking your blood glucose level at home is a great way to keep tabs on your progress.

Daily Guidelines

What are the basics of a nutritious diet for someone with diabetes? Nutrition means getting nutrients, protein, carbohydrates, fats, vitamins, and minerals from what you eat and drink. The amounts of carbohydrate, fat, and protein in your daily meal plan depend on your individual needs and tastes. They also depend on your overall health and your treatment goals (blood glucose, blood fat levels, and weight goals). Your nutrition needs change throughout life as your body changes. As your needs change, so should your food choices.

Protein: For most people, a healthy diet includes 10 to 20 percent of daily calories from protein (poultry, fish, dairy, and vegetable sources). If you have kidney disease, you and your doctor should talk about lowering your protein intake to around 10 percent of daily calories.

Fat: A healthy intake of fat is 30 percent or less of your daily calories. Less than 10 percent should come from saturated fats (fats that are solid at room temperature), and up to 10 percent should come from polyunsaturated fats (fats from fish and other seafood). Daily cholesterol intake should be 300 milligrams or less. Cholesterol is found in dairy products, eggs, and meats.

In general, Americans eat too much fat. To reduce our risk for heart disease, we all need to eat less saturated fat and cholesterol. Because having diabetes puts you at increased risk for heart disease, you have even more reason to watch your fat intake.

Carbohydrates: The rest of your daily calories will come from carbohydrates, which are found in fruits, vegetables, beans, dairy foods, and starchy foods such as breads.

Sugar is a type of carbohydrate. For the past 100 years, people with diabetes were told to avoid sugar. It was assumed that sugar, which quickly changes into glucose, would raise blood glucose levels more. But research has shown that this is not true.

Of course, there are still reasons why sugar is not a smart food choice. Your body depends on the nutrients supplied in the foods you eat. Sugary foods often contain empty calories that provide no nutrients. Your dietitian can help work foods with sugar into your meal plan. But sugary foods can't take the place of foods that supply vitamins and minerals. There is no reason to avoid table sugar in favor of other sweeteners, such as fructose (the sugar found in fruit), corn sweeteners, corn syrup, fruit juice or fruit juice concentrate, honey, molasses, dextrose, and maltose. On the other hand, there is no reason for people with diabetes to avoid foods that naturally contain sweeteners, such as fructose (fruits and vegetables) or lactose (dairy products).

Details: Unless you have special health concerns or problems, you can follow the same guidelines for eating fiber and sodium as the general public. If you eat a variety of healthful foods, you don't need to take extra vitamins and minerals.

Alcohol: The warnings the public hears about alcohol also apply to you. If you have well-controlled diabetes, you can work one or two drinks into your meal plan. Do not drink alcohol on an empty stomach. It can cause very low blood glucose. If you take insulin or diabetes pills, you need to know how alcohol affects your blood glucose level by testing during and after you drink.

Success with Food

You may have tried meal plans or diets only to fail time and again. You may have lost weight only to gain it back. Just the thought of changing your habits may seem overwhelming. The American Diabetes Association suggests that you think about food choices in a new way:

Don't try to do it alone. Working food choices into a diabetes treatment plan is a complex task. It takes teamwork. You want to wind up with a meal plan that fits you. Get the help of a registered dietitian and your doctor. A dietitian is a health-care professional with training and expertise in the field of food. The American Diabetes Association recommends that all adults with diabetes see a dietitian every 6 months to 1 year to help with meal plans. Look for one who has worked with many people with diabetes, because you want a dietitian who knows the current American Diabetes Association guidelines.

Look for the initials RD (registered dietitian), which indicate that the dietitian has passed a national credentialing exam. Many states also require dietitians to have a license, so you'll often see the initials LD (licensed dietitian). Good sources of recommendations are your primary care physician, area hospitals, the American Dietetic Association, and the American Diabetes Association (see below).

Dietitians teach you many useful skills, such as how to:

—Use Exchange Lists for Meal Planning, published by the American Diabetes Association and the American Dietetic Association.
—Count dietary carbohydrate and fat.
—Read food labels.
—Handle eating out in restaurants.
—Make healthy food choices when grocery shopping.

Dietitians help you discover a range of nutritional resources, including cookbooks and reference materials, so you can learn how to prepare healthy, delicious, and satisfying meals.

Start with what you are doing now. You and your dietitian should begin by looking at your current habits. This is called a nutrition assessment. Building on what you do now, you can come up with a plan that will help you meet your health goals. It should fit your food tastes, family or cultural customs, and lifestyle while it helps you meet your health goals.

You do not have to give up all your favorite foods. Make changes slowly.

For example, your goal might be to lose 10 pounds. You may be able to reach this goal by making some small changes:

—Cut down on portion size.
—Eat less fat.
—Eat more fresh fruits and vegetables.
—Walk briskly for 20 minutes three or four times a week.

Because there is no one diabetic diet, you have lots of food choices. As you change, your plan can change too.

Know your health goals. How does your meal plan help you meet these goals? By testing your blood glucose and having other regular health assessments, you get a picture of how your food plan is affecting your diabetes control. Talk to your doctor about how often you need to test your blood glucose at home. Keep track of your test results.

Staying healthy with diabetes will always be a challenge. When you work with your health care team on your meal plan, you are working on one of the most important tools for feeling your best. Although you need to follow a healthy eating plan, it's a blueprint that includes many choices. It's up to you to help shape a plan that you can live with.

APPENDIX 8–2 FREQUENTLY ASKED QUESTIONS: EXERCISE AND DIABETES

Why Is Exercise Important for People with Diabetes?

Exercise is beneficial to the health of people with both types of diabetes in two ways. First, exercise can take some glucose out of the blood to use for energy during and after exercise, which lowers blood glucose levels. Secondly, it helps delay or stop large blood vessel and heart (cardiovascular) disease. Cardiovascular disease is the leading killer of people with diabetes. All people with diabetes should exercise to counteract their increased risk of cardiovascular disease, to reach and maintain a healthy weight, and to enjoy themselves. An additional benefit for many people with diabetes is that exercise, plus other healthy lifestyle habits, can help them achieve good blood glucose control.

Getting Started

Q. How do I get started?

A. Your first steps toward a more active lifestyle should begin with a thorough medical examination. This is the only way to make sure your exercise program meets your individual needs. One exercise program does not fit all. Everyone is different, and your exercise plan needs to be based on your health and your body's needs. Working with your health care team will give you the confidence of knowing that you're doing all you can to avoid the pitfalls and reap only the benefits of exercise.

Q. I always put exercise off. How can I get going?

A. The first thing you should do is set some realistic goals for yourself. For example, this might be as simple as a walking program in which you walk around the block for 15 minutes a day. Then you should gradually build up your program and set new goals in order to stay motivated.

Q. Is it smart to exercise with someone else, or should I just do it alone?

A. Exercising with a partner is an excellent idea. When we exercise by ourselves we sometimes get discouraged and lose interest. However, an exercise buddy often provides the necessary encouragement and motivation to help us succeed.

Q. I've tried to exercise before and didn't stick with it. How can I keep from getting discouraged?

A. The following tips can help you stick with your exercise program:

1. Set a schedule and keep it. Make the commitment to exercise just as you would any other important appointment. Remember, habits are developed through practice.
2. Get a training partner. We all have days when we are easily tempted to skip our workout. Your partner and you can be strong for each other and strengthen your collective resolve. It also helps if you and your partner have similar goals so that you can exercise at the same level. A training partner who is aware of your diabetes can also keep your exercise sessions safer for you.
3. Cross-train. Doing the same thing every time you exercise can get boring. Many people alternate exercises daily. It's called cross-training. This is a method in which you alternate between forms of exercise to prevent putting a specific strain on a particular part of the body day after day. In other words, you might ride a bicycle one day, walk the next, and swim another day. It not only gives you variety in your routine but reduces the risk of injury by letting your body rest and repair between sessions using the same muscles.
4. Set goals. Setting specific goals for yourself and then evaluating how you are doing with your goals is a great way to keep on track. But goals can work against you, too. If you set a goal that is not quickly attainable, you might get discouraged when you don't see immediate progress.

Source: From the American Diabetes Association, 1998, with permission.

Be realistic in your goal-setting. Like Rome, your healthier body can't be built in a day.

5. Reward yourself. One good way to keep your motivation high is to reward yourself when you accomplish a goal. For example, decide that if you meet this month's goal, you will reward yourself with some new clothes, a compact disc, a new book—anything that will help keep you committed. Another hint: don't use food as a reward.

Q. Is it a good idea to drink fluids while I exercise?

A. Drinking fluids while exercising is a good idea. Actually you should try to drink something not only during the exercise but also before and after working out. This helps prevent dehydration and helps to replenish the fluids and nutrients your body loses during exercise. This is especially important for people with diabetes. Therefore during strenuous exercise, consider a high-glucose sports drink, which can help prevent your blood-sugar from going too low.

Q. I am elderly and it is rather hard for me to get around. Should I still try to exercise?

A. You should try to exercise regardless of your age. If it is difficult to get out, you can do various stretches in your home and even while sitting down. As our bodies age, warming up with stretching exercises becomes more and more important. You may find that after properly stretching, you can do more than you thought you could.

Q. I have both diabetes and arthritis. Can I still work out?

A. Yes, you can, but try two things to make exercising safer. One, make sure you stretch before all exercises, and, secondly, you should plan exercises which will strengthen your muscles and make you feel better.

Q. What is the best way to gain flexibility before I start working out?

A. The best way is to stretch as much as possible to decrease tension in your muscles. Flexibility can also help prevent injuries, so be sure to stretch plenty before you exercise.

Types of Exercise

Q. Is there a limit to types of exercise a person with diabetes can do?

A. There is no limit to what people with diabetes can do. Barring another medical condition, people with diabetes can do anything and everything. You can walk or bike, swim or hike for exercise. These are only examples and everyone is different, so be sure to ask your physician if you should have any limits in your exercise program.

Q. If I work out at the gym, what is the best machine I can use on a daily basis?

A. Stair-climbers and treadmills are excellent machines to use at the gym. They simulate walking and climbing, which can help burn fat, build endurance, and strengthen the cardiovascular system. Weight lifting can also provide a great workout. The important thing is to find something you enjoy and exercise safely.

Q. What is the best exercise to improve my blood sugar levels?

A. Walking seems to be an excellent exercise for a majority of people. Again, it is best to consult your physician to tailor an exercise program to fit your particular situation.

Q. As part of my workout, is it helpful to ride on a stationary bicycle?

A. Riding a stationary bicycle not only gives you a great aerobic workout, but it also strengthens your legs and helps build muscular endurance.

Diabetes, Exercise, and Weight Loss

Q. If I lower my blood sugar levels, is there a possibility that I could gain weight?

A. Yes, there is that possibility. To decrease your chances of gaining weight, begin to exercise more often and more intensely and reduce the amount of food that you eat. Consult your health professional to adjust your diet and exercise program accordingly.

Q. If I have diabetes, what is the most effective way to lose weight?

A. Regular exercise and good nutrition are the keys to weight loss. Regular exercise helps you lose weight by burning calories and increasing your metabolism. Eating well-balanced meals and controlling your caloric intake can also further your weight loss efforts.

Q. If I am planning on losing weight, why can't I just diet instead of exercising?

A. If you want to achieve permanent weight loss, most diets don't work by themselves. A diet that severely restricts calories is dangerous for anyone, especially for those of us with diabetes. Exercise, combined with your diet plan, helps maintain the weight loss and strengthens your body.

Exercise and Type 1 Diabetes

Q. My child has diabetes. Can she still play sports?

A. Yes, it is good to let children be competitive and show their interests. If they enjoy sports, tell them of professional athletes with diabetes such as NFL quarterback Wade Wilson or 1950s tennis star Bill Talbert. This can help show them that anything is possible and that if they pursue their dreams, anything can happen.

Q. How can I learn more about the effects on children with diabetes who play sports?

A. There are many ways. First, you should talk to your pediatrician and ask him/her what your child can and cannot do. Secondly, you could talk with another parent of a child with diabetes and find out which sport(s) their child plays. You can also find in-

formation in brochures from the International Diabetic Athletes' Association (IDAA).

Q. What can my child get out of playing sports if he or she has diabetes?

A. Playing sports can provide children many benefits. It gives them a chance to make new friends, develop physical confidence, and improve their self-esteem. As children with diabetes discover that they can play and be competitive with other children, it might improve their outlook for their future.

Q. I have type 1 diabetes. How is exercise different for me?

A. Exercise alone will not improve glucose control in type 1 diabetes. Increased exercise should help keep your weight under control with intensive management, but hypoglycemia is a very real risk. Adding exercise to your diabetes care plan will require the careful balance of food, insulin, and physical activity. You and your health care team should work together to find out what's best for you. There are strategies to get good blood glucose control and still let you lead an active life that promotes fitness.

Other Questions

Q. How can I be sure to avoid injury while exercising?

A. You can do two things to prevent injuries; one is to stretch before and after you exercise as a way to warm up and cool down. Secondly, you should gradually build up the intensity and duration of your exercise over many weeks or months to be sure that you do not overdo it early in your exercising.

Q. How can I prevent low blood sugar at night when I have exercised that day?

A. You need to balance your insulin, your food intake, and your exercise in order to have fewer low blood sugar episodes at night. You should work with your physician to maintain this balance.

Q. How can I find out how intense my workouts are?

A. To find out how intense your workouts are, you need to count your pulse. To count your pulse, place your first two fingers (not your thumb) over the radial artery, which is found in the top third of your other wrist on the thumb side, or over the carotid artery, which runs up the inside of your neck near the Adam's apple. Use light but firm pressure so that you can feel your pulse. Count the number of beats in 10 seconds quickly after you stop exercising. Otherwise your heart slows down too quickly to get an accurate number. Multiply that number by 6 to get the number of heartbeats per minute.

Q. Type 2 diabetes runs in my family. Does this mean I'm destined to develop diabetes?

A. No, exercise can help protect you from ever developing type 2 diabetes. Regular exercise fights insulin resistance and obesity, allowing people to avoid developing diabetes in the first place.

References

1. Sowers JR: Diabetes mellitus and cardiovascular disease in women. *Arch Intern Med* 1998; 158:617–621.
2. Muggeo M, Verlato G, Bonora E, et al: The Verona Diabetes Study: a population based survey on known diabetes mellitus prevalence and 5-year all cause mortality. *Diabetologia* 1995; 38:318–325.
3. Kannel WB, McGee DL: Diabetes and cardiovascular disease. The Framingham study. *JAMA* 1979; 241:2035–2038.
4. Stamler J, Vaccaro O, Neaton JD, Wentworth D and the Multiple Risk Factor Intervention Trail Group: Diabetes, other risk factors and 12 year cardiovascular mortality for men screened in the Multiple Risk Factor Intervention Trial. *Diabetes Care* 1993; 16:434–444.
5. Wingard DL, Barrett-Conner E: Heart disease and diabetes. In: *Diabetes in America,* 2nd ed. NIDDK,NIH pub. no. 95-1468. Bethesda, MD, National Institutes of Health, 1995.
6. Stout RW: Insulin and atheroma: 20-year perspective. *Diabetes Care* 1990; 13:631–654.
7. Manson JE, Colditz GA, Stampfer MJ, et al: A prospective study of maturity-onset diabetes mellitus and risk of coronary heart disease and stroke in women. *Arch Intern Med* 1991;151:1141–1147.
8. Raman M, Nesto RW: Heart disease in diabetes mellitus. *Endocrinol Metab Clin North Am* 1996; 25:425–438.
9. Ali SS, Sowers JR: Update on the management of hypertension; treatment of the elderly and diabetic hypertensives. Is the approach to management really different? *Cardiovasc Rev Rep* 1998;6:44–54.
10. The National High Blood Pressure Education Program Working Group: National High Blood Pressure Education Program Working Group report on hypertension in diabetes. *Hypertension* 1994; 23:145–158.
11. Davis TM, Millus H, Stratton IM, et al: Risk factors for stroke in type 2 diabetes mellitus: United Kingdom Prospective Diabetes Study (UKPDS) 29. *Arch Int Med* 1999; 159:1097–1103.
12. UKPDS Group: UK Prospective Diabetes Study 38: tight blood pressure control and risk of macrovascular and microvascular complications in type 2 diabetes. *BMJ* 1998; 317:703–713.
13. UKPDS Group: UK Prospective Diabetes Study 39: efficacy of atenolol and captopril in reducing risk of macrovascular and microvascular complications in type 2 diabetes. *BMJ* 1998; 317:713–720.
14. Hansson L, Zanchetti A, Carruthers SG, et al: For the HOT study group: effects of intensive blood-pressure lowering and low dose aspirin in patients with hypertension: principle results of the Hypertension Optimal Treatment (HOT) randomized trial. *Lancet* 1998; 351:1755–1762.
15. Hamaty M, Lamberti M, Sowers JR: Diabetic vascular disease and hypertension. *Curr Opin Cardiol* 1998; 13:298–303.
16. Sowers JR, Sowers PS, Peuler JD: Role of insulin resistance and hyperinsulinemia in the development of hypertension and atherosclerosis. *J Lab Clin Med* 1994; 123:647–652.
17. Guigliano D, Ceriello A, Paolisso G: Oxidative stress and diabetic complications. *Diabetes Care* 1996; 19:257–267.
18. Carmassi F, Morale M, Puccetti R, et al: Coagulation and fibrinolytic system impairment in insulin dependent diabetes mellitus. *Thromb Res* 1992; 67:643–654.
19. Kuusisto J, Mykkanen L, Pyorala K, et al: Hyperinsulinemia and microalbuminuria: a new risk indicator for coronary heart disease. *Circulation* 1995; 90:831.
20. Dinneen SF, Gerstein HC. The association of microalbuminuria and mortality in non-insulin-dependent diabetes mellitus: a systematic overview of the literature. *Arch Intern Med* 1997; 157:1413–1418.
21. Lehto S, Ronnemaa T, Haffner SM, et al: Dyslipidemia and hyperglycemia predict coronary heart disease events in middle-aged patients with NIDDM. *Diabetes* 1997; 48:1354–1359.
22. Lyons T: Lipoprotein glycation and its metabolic consequences. *Diabetes* 1992; 41(S2):67.
23. Chisolm G, Irwin K, Penn M: Lipoprotein oxidation and lipoprotein-induced cell injury in diabetes. *Diabetes* 1992; 41(S2):61.
24. Bostom AG, Cupples LA, Jenner JL, et al: Elevated

plasma lipoprotein (a) and coronary heart disease in men ages 55 years and younger: a prospective study. *JAMA* 1996; 276:544–548.

25. Schaefer EJ, Lamon-Fava S, Jenner JL, et al: Lipoprotein(a) levels and risk of coronary heart disease in men. *JAMA* 1994; 271:999–1003.

26. Bostom AG, Gagnon DR, Cupples LA, et al: A prospective investigation of elevated lipoprotein(a) detected by electrophoreseis and cardiovascular disease in women: the Framingham Heart Study. *Circulation* 1994; 90:1688–1695.

27. Austin MA, Mykkanen L, Kuusisto, et al: Prospective study of small LDLs as a risk factor for non-insulin dependent diabetes mellitus in elderly men and women. *Circulation* 1995; 92:1770–1778.

28. Ford I, Singh TP, Kitchen I, et al: Activation of coagulation in diabetes mellitus in relation to the presence of vascular complications. *Diabetes Med* 1991; 8:322–329.

29. Kwaan H: Changes in blood coagulation, platelet function and plasminogen-plasmin system in diabetes. *Diabetes* 1992; 41(S2):31.

30. Landin K, Tengborn L, Smith U: Elevated fibrinogen and plasminogen activator inhibitor (PAI-1) in hypertension is related to metabolic risk factors for cardiovascular disease. *J Intern Med* 1990; 227:273–278.

31. Gray R, Patterson D, Yudkin J: Plasminogen activator inhibitor activity in diabetic and nondiabetic survivors of myocardial infarction. *Atherothrombosis* 1993; 13:415.

32. Winocour P: Platelet abnormalities in diabetes mellitus. *Diabetes* 1992; 41(S2):26.

33. Davi G, Catalano I, Averna M, et al: Thromboxane biosynthesis and platelet function in type 2 diabetes mellitus. *N Eng J Med* 1990; 322:1769.

34. Mehta JL, Chen LY, Kone BC, et al: Identification of constitutive and inducible forms of nitric oxide synthase in human platelets. *J Lab Clin Med* 1995; 25:370–377.

35. Williams SB, Cusco JA, Roddy MA, et al: Impaired nitric oxide-mediated vasodilation in non-insulin dependent diabetes. *Circulation* 1994; 90:1–50.

36. Clarkson P, Celermajer DS, Donald AE, et al: Impaired vascular reactivity in insulin-dependent diabetes mellitus is related to disease duration and low-density lipopro-tein cholesterol levels. *J Am Coll Cardiol* 1996; 28:573–579.

37. Salone Jt, Lakka TA, Lakka H-M, et al: Hyperinsulinemia is associated with the incidence of hypertension and dyslipidemia in middle-aged men. *Diabetes* 1998; 47:270–275.

38. Meigs JB, D'Agostino RB Sr, Wilson PWF, et al: Risk variable clustering in the insulin resistance syndrome. *Diabetes* 1997; 46:1594–1600.

39. Wingard DL, Ferrara A, Barrett-Conner EL: Is insulin really a heart disease risk factor? *Diabetes Care* 1995; 18:1299–1304.

40. Ruige JB, Assendelft WJJ, Dekker JM, et al: Insulin and risk of cardiovascular disease: a meta-analysis. *Circulation* 1998; 97:996–1001.

41. Pyorala M, Miettinen H, Laakso M, Pyorala K: Hyperinsulinemia predicts coronary heart disease risk in healthy middle-aged men: the 22-year follow-up results of the Helsinki Policemen Study. *Circulation* 1998; 98:398–404.

42. Garg A: Insulin resistance in the pathogenesis of dyslipidemia. *Diabetes Care* 1996; 19:387–389.

43. Peiris AN, Sothmann MS, Hennes MI, et al: The relative contribution of obesity and body fat distribution to alterations in glucose and insulin homeostasis. *Am J Clin Nutr* 1989; 49:758–764.

44. Haffner SM, Stern MP, Hazuda HP, et al: Do upper body and centralized adiposity measure different aspects of regional body fat distribution? Relation to non-insulin-dependent diabetes mellitus, lipids, and lipoproteins. *Diabetes* 1987; 36:43–51.

45. National Institutes of Health: *Clinical Guidelines for the Identification, Evaluation, and Treatment of Overweight and Obesity in Adults.* Bethesda, MD: National Heart, Lung, and Blood Institute, 1998.

46. American Diabetes Association: Nutrition recommendation and principles for people with diabetes mellitus (position statement). *Diabetes Care* 1998; 21:S32–S35.

47. Mittleman MA, Maclure M, Tofler GH, et al: Triggering of acute myocardial infarction by heavy physical exertion-protection against trigger by regular exertion. *N Engl J Med* 1993; 329:1677.

48. Curfman, GD: Is exercise beneficial or hazardous to your heart? *N Engl J Med* 1993; 329:1730.

49. Calfas KJ, Long BJ, Sallis JF, et al: A controlled trial of physician counseling to promote the adoption of physical activity. *Prev Med* 1996; 25:225.

50. Long BJ, Calfas KJ, Wooten W, et al: A multi-site field test of the acceptability of Physical Activity Counseling in primary care: Project PACE. *Am J Prev Med* 1996; 12:73.

51. Sowers JR, Epstein M: Diabetes mellitus and hypertension: an update. *Hypertension* 1995; 26:869–879.

52. Sowers JR: Insulin and insulin-like growth factor in normal and pathological cardiovascular physiology. *Hypertension* 1997; 29:691–699.

53. Facchini FS, Hollenbeck CB, Jeppesen J, et al: Insulin resistance and cigarette smoking. *Lancet* 1992; 339:1128.

54. Lundman B, Asplund K, Norberg A: Smoking and metabolic control in patients with insulin-dependent diabetes mellitus. *J Intern Med* 1990; 227:101.

55. Chaturvedi N, Stephenson JM, Fuller JH, et al: The relationship between smoking and microvascular complication in the EURODIAB IDDM Complications Study. *Diabetes Care* 1995; 18:785.

56. Chase HP, Garg SK, Marshall G, et al: Cigarette smoking increases the risk of albuminuria among subjects with type 1 diabetes. *JAMA* 1991; 265:614.

57. Yudkin JS: How can we best prolong life? Benefits of coronary risk factor reduction in non-diabetic and diabetic subjects. *BMJ* 1993; 306:1313.

58. Ford ES, Malarcher AM, Herman WH, et al: Diabetes mel-

litus and cigarette smoking: findings from the 1989 National Health Interview Survey. *Diabetes Care* 1994; 17:688.

59. The Sixth Report of the Joint National Committee on Detection, Evaluation and Treatment of High Blood Pressure (JNC-VI). *Arch Intern Med* 1997; 157:2413–2446.

60. Lebovitz HE, Wiegmann TB, Cnaan A, et al: Renal protective effects of enalapril in hypertensive NIDDM: role of baseline albuminuria. *Kidney Int* 1994; 45:S150–S155.

61. Ravid M, Savin H, Jutrin I, et al: Long-term stabilizing effect of angiotensin-converting enzyme inhibition on plasma creatinine and on proteinuria in normotensive type II diabetic patients. *Ann Intern Med* 1993; 118:577–581.

62. Sowers JR, Lester MA: Diabetes and cardiovascular disease. *Diabetes Care* 1999; suppl 3: C14–20.

63. Sowers JR, Epstein M: Diabetes mellitus and associated hypertension, vascular disease, and nephropathy: an update. *Hypertension* 1995; 26:869–879.

64. American Diabetes Association: Management of dyslipidemia in adults with diabetes: position statement. *Diabetes Care* 1998; 21(suppl 1):S36–S39.

65. Pyorala K, Pedersen TR, Kjekshus J, et al: Cholesterol lowering with simvastatin improves prognosis of diabetic patients with coronary heart disease. *Diabetes Care* 1997; 20:614–620.

66. Sagel J, Colwell JA, Crook L, Laimins M: Increased platelet aggregation in early diabetes mellitus. *Ann Intern Med* 1975; 82:733–738.

67. Halushka PV, Rogers RC, Loadholt CB, et al: Increased platelet thromboxane synthesis in diabetes mellitus. *Ann Intern Med* 1981; 97:87–96.

68. Antiplatelet Trialists' Collaboration: Collaborative overview of randomized trials of antiplatelet therapy I: prevention of death, myocardial infarction, and stroke by prolonged antiplatelet therapy in various categories of patients. *BMJ* 1994; 308:71–72.

69. ETDRS Investigators: Aspirin effects on mortality and morbidity in patients with diabetes mellitus. *JAMA* 1992; 268:1292–1300.

70. Steering Committee of the Physicians' Health Study Research Group: Final report on the aspirin components of the ongoing Physicians' Health Study. *N Engl J Med* 1989; 321:129–135.

71. Colwell JA. Aspirin therapy in diabetes (technical review). *Diabetes Care* 1997; 20:1767–1771.

72. American Diabetes Association: Aspirin therapy in diabetes. *Diabetes Care* 1998; 21:(suppl):45–46.

73. DCCT Research Group: The effect of intensive diabetes treatment on the development and progression of long-term complications in insulin dependent diabetes mellitus. *N Engl J Med* 1983; 329:977–986.

74. The Pharmacological Treatment of Hyperglycemia in NIDDM: Consensus statement. *Diabetes Care* 1995; 18(suppl 7):1413–1418.

75. Balkau B, Shipley M, Jarrett RJ, et al: High blood glucose concentration is a risk factor for mortality middle-aged nondiabetic men. 20-year follow-up in the Whitehall Study, the Paris Prospective Study, and the Helsinki Policemen Study. *Diabetes Care* 1998; 21:360–367.

76. DeFronzo RA, Goodman AM: The multicenter metformin study group: efficacy of metformin in patients with non-insulin-dependent diabetes mellitus, *N Engl J Med* 1995; 333:541–549.

77. Hermann LS, Bitzen PO, Kjellstrom T, et al: Comparative efficacy of metformin and glibenclamide in patients with non-insulin-dependent diabetes mellitus. *Diabetes Metab* 1991; 17:201–208.

78. Chiasson JL, Josse RG, Hunt JA, et al: The efficacy of acarbose in treatment of patients with non-insulin-dependent diabetes mellitus: a multi-centered controlled clinical trial. *Ann Intern Med* 1994; 121:928–935.

79. Bild D, Teusch SM: The control of hypertension in persons with diabetes: a public health approach. *Public Health Rep* 1987; 102:522–529.

80. Knowler WC, Narayan KMV, Hanson RL, et al: Preventing non-insulin-dependent diabetes. *Diabetes* 1995; 44:483–488.

CHAPTER 9

Tobacco Use and Passive Smoking

Russell V. Luepker
Harry A. Lando

There are approximately 47 million adult smokers in the United States,[1] and it is estimated that 430,000 deaths annually are attributable to cigarette smoking (Fig. 9–1). These deaths are replenished by an estimated 3000 teenagers per day beginning the smoking habit. The economic costs are estimated to be $50 billion per year in medical expenses and $50 billion in indirect costs. The costs in lost health and in human suffering are incalculable.

The causal links between cigarette smoking and human disease are incontrovertible. Cigarettes are linked to many cancers and are the prime factor in lung cancer. Cigarettes are also linked to acute and chronic pulmonary diseases, including emphysema. Finally, tobacco smoking is among the three major

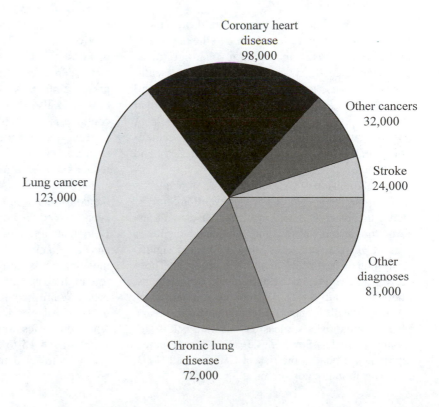

FIGURE 9–1 A total of 430,000 annual deaths were attributable to cigarette smoking in the United States, 1990–1994. (From the Centers for Disease Control and Prevention.[120])

Coronary heart
disease
98,000

Other cancers
32,000

Stroke
24,000

Other
diagnoses
81,000

Chronic lung
disease
72,000

Lung cancer
123,000

risk factors for cardiovascular disease (CVD). It is linked to sudden death, myocardial infarction, and stroke.[2] There is growing evidence that environmental tobacco smoke (ETS), which results in exposure of nonsmokers, poses health risks to that group. Lung cancer and respiratory tract infection among those exposed to ETS are well recognized.[3] More recent evidence suggests that ETS increases the risk of coronary heart disease (CHD).[4,5] These observations and others have resulted in a widespread call for prevention of tobacco uptake by teens, cessation among smoking adults, and restriction in the environment. This chapter discusses the epidemiologic evidence relating active and passive tobacco use to cardiovascular risk and the benefits of quitting. It also describes the trends in cigarette use. Finally, it discusses individual and population intervention strategies among youth and adults.

Effects of Cigarette Smoking on Cardiovascular Disease

There is a wealth of evidence over the past five decades linking cigarette smoking to the major cardiovascular diseases, including myocardial infarction, sudden death, stroke, and peripheral vascular disease.[2,6] These associations are found across all age, gender, and ethnic groups in the United States.[2] It is also apparent that the ill effects of smoking cut across national boundaries, as demonstrated in the Seven Countries Study of Keys and colleagues.[7]

The relationship of CHD mortality to smoking status from the 1959–1965 Cancer Prevention Study is shown in Fig. 9–2. CHD death increases with age for both men and women, with women having lower rates at all ages and ever smokers having significantly higher death rates than never smokers. Those differences are greatest in the younger age groups, where the relative risk of smoking approaches 8. However, the differences remain into the older years, where relative risks are less but absolute risk is significantly greater. Smoking cessation among adults significantly reduces the risk of CHD and all CVD, as shown in many populations.[8,9]

More recent data from the Multiple Risk Factor Intervention Trial (MRFIT) of 316,099 white men who were screened also confirms a graded relationship between number of cigarettes and CHD death.[10] The relative risk for 1 to 25 cigarettes per day is 2.1, rising to 2.9 for daily smoking consumption above 25 cigarettes per day. Similarly, the MRFIT Trial found that quitting smoking reduces CVD mortality.[11]

One of the most disturbing aspects of cigarette smoking is its strong association with sudden, unexpected death, particularly among younger individuals. Although sudden death is common among those with known CVD, Escobedo and Caspersen found that only smoking predicted sudden death in those thought to be disease-free.[12] Similarly, in both men and women, acute myocardial infarction in younger individuals (less than 50 years of age) is strongly associated with cigarette smoking.[13,14] The interaction of cigarette smoking with other known risk factors is well studied. Some suggest that the effect is additive, while others find a multiplicative effect. Cigarette smoking adds to the risk associated with lipids, obesity, diabetes mellitus, hypertension, oral contraceptive use, and electrocardiographic (ECG) abnormalities.[15-19] However, even without additional risk factors, smoking can increase the risk of CVD.[6] The presence of CHD, a strong risk factor for subsequent events, is also affected by smoking. Smokers who continue in the habit after an acute myocardial infarction have significantly higher rates of recurrent events and death.[20,21] Individuals who quit smoking reduce the risk of a subsequent event.[20]

The mechanisms by which cigarette smoking and the constituents in tobacco smoke affect CVD have been studied in both animal models and humans. Both acute and chronic mechanisms are postulated, and it is likely that both contribute. There is accumulating evidence that smoking plays an important role in the basic atherosclerotic process. This is elegantly confirmed in the Pathobiological Determinants of Atherosclerosis in Youth (PDAY) study,[22] where autopsies were performed on 1443 men and women aged 15 to 34 who died of external causes such as auto accidents. Smoking was associated with an excess of fatty streaks and raised lesions in the

FIGURE 9-2 Coronary Heart Disease Mortality. (From the U.S. Department of Health and Human Services.[6])

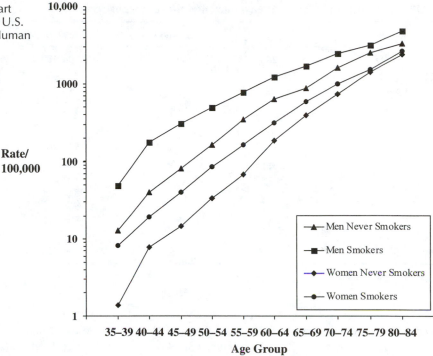

abdominal aorta in these otherwise healthy individuals.[22] Injury of the arterial endothelium is suggested by some as the mechanism for the atherosclerotic lesions.[23] Other mechanisms are also postulated.[24] The case for acute effects of smoking is supported by the known short-term vascular effects of nicotine and the rapid improvement in prognosis with smoking cessation. Postulated mechanisms for acute effects include alterations in clotting, including platelet adhesions, and acute coronary vasoconstriction due to nicotine.[25,26]

Environmental Tobacco Smoke

Recently, there has been increased emphasis on exposure to environmental tobacco smoke (ETS) among nonsmokers in the home, workplace, and public settings. This has become a more significant issue than individual smoking because it affects others who may not have a choice about being exposed to tobacco smoke. In the 1986 Surgeon General's Report, *The Health Consequences of Involuntary Smoking,* CVD is barely mentioned.[3] The report focuses principally on the cancer and respiratory disease effects of ETS. Recent increased research on ETS and CVD suggests a much larger problem.

A number of prospective epidemiologic studies have evaluated the role of ETS in CVD (Table 9–1). They are hampered by the difficulty of ascertaining the level of exposure and the potential for confounding by unmeasured or poorly measured risk factors for CVD. Some authors have suggested that cause and effect does not exist.[27] However, two recent metanalyses find the vast majority of studies to show a similar increased relative risk for both fatal and nonfatal CHD from ETS.[4,5] A follow-up of the American Cancer Society Cancer Prevention Study cohort from 1982 to 1989 found that male nonsmokers with smoking wives had a 1.2 relative risk, which was significant. Women living with smoking husbands had a relative risk of 1.1, which was not significant. There was no increase in risk for spouses of former smokers. This study was able to control

TABLE 9–1   Cohort Studies of Environmental Tobacco Smoke and Coronary Heart Disease

Source	Year	Location	Cases/Population	Adjusted RR (CI)
Hirayama[121]	1984	Japan	494/91,540	1.15 (0.93–1.42)
Garland[122]	1985	U.S.	19/695	2.7 (0.7–10.5)
Svendsen[123]	1987	U.S.	88/1245	2.2 (0.72–6.92)
Helsing[124]	1988	U.S.	1358/19,035	M 1.31 (1.05–1.64)
				F 1.24 (1.10–1.40)
Hole[125]	1989	U.K.	53/7987	2.01 (1.2–3.4)
Layard[126]	1995	U.S.	1389/2916	M 0.97 (0.73–1.28)
				F 0.99 (0.84–1.16)
Tunstall-Pedoe[127]	1995	U.K.	70/2278	2.7 (1.3–5.6)
Steenland et al.[5]	1996	U.S.	3819/309,599	M 1.22 (1.07–1.40)
				F 1.10 (0.96–1.27)
Kawachi et al.[28]	1997	U.S.	152/32,046	F 1.91 (1.11–3.28)

Key: RR, relative risk; CI, confidence interval.

for other CVD risk factors. A 10-year follow-up of 32,046 women ages 36 to 61 who had never smoked showed that those exposed to ETS had relative risks (RRs) for CHD (adjusted for other cardiovascular risk factors) of 1.58 [95 percent confidence interval (CI) = 0.93 to 2.68] in those with occasional exposure, and 1.91 (95 percent CI = 1.11 to 3.78) in those reporting regular exposure at work or home.[28]

The recently published analysis of the National Health and Nutrition Examination Survey (NHANES) attempted to answer the confounding question by comparing other risk measures, including classic risk factors and diet, in a large population sample. The investigators found few differences in cardiovascular risk factors between nonsmokers living in nonsmoking households and nonsmokers living in households with smokers.[29] They felt that confounding by unmeasured cardiovascular risk factors was unlikely.

Recently, a metanalysis incorporating more recent home-based studies along with workplace studies (total of 1699 cases) showed an overall increased risk associated with passive smoking (RR = 1.49, 95 percent CI = 1.29 to 1.72) and suggested similar relative risks for heart disease from work- versus home-based exposure.[30]

While the mechanism by which ETS affects individuals is still debated, considerable data are available on this issue. It is clear that mainstream smoke, that inhaled by the smoker, differs from sidestream smoke, which is released into the environment.[31] Sidestream smoke may be more toxic. It is apparent that nonsmokers who are exposed regularly to cigarette smoke develop a number of physiologic changes. Some authors suggest that nonsmokers are more sensitive to these changes than those regularly exposed.[32] These include the chronic effects of cigarette smoke, such as lower high-density-lipoprotein (HDL) cholesterol, as well as endothelial and platelet abnormalities.[30–32] It is also apparent that exposed nonsmokers have higher levels of carbon monoxide and lower exercise tolerance.[32]

These observations are all compatible with a pathologic effect in nonsmokers exposed to ETS. The effects on lung cancer and other respiratory diseases are already apparent.[24] Recent estimates suggest that 35,000 to 40,000 deaths per year from acute myocardial infarction are associated with environmental tobacco exposure. This effect is much larger than observed for lung cancer and suggests that attempts to reduce exposure of nonsmokers to tobacco smoke should be a high priority.[33]

Prevalence and Trends in Cigarette Smoking among Youth

Youth smoking issues are well described in the 1994 *Report of the Surgeon General.*[34] Most smokers begin this habit in their teenage years because of social pressure from the fact that friends, siblings, and parents smoke. Young people feel that smoking makes them look more adult and that it is associated with social success. It is related to independence and rebelliousness, common themes in the teenage years. The environment provides important support through advertising, which reinforces the "coolness" of smoking. The highly effective Joe Camel ads were clearly aimed at, and successful with, new-onset smokers.[35] The most vulnerable period is in the sixth through eighth grades (ages 12 to 14), when most smoking initiation occurs. There is little increase in regular use past age 18, although heavier use may occur then.

Early surveys of national trends showed a steady rise in cigarette smoking from 1968 to 1974.[36] During that time, smoking among teenage girls began to exceed that among boys. From 1975 to 1990, a national sample of high school seniors found a steady decline in smoking rates among this group. Importantly, the group of those who had never smoked was increasing. Female smoking exceeded that of males, but recently those differences have disappeared. There were also socioeconomic status differences, with college-bound seniors much less likely to smoke than those who did not plan to continue their studies.[37]

More recently, the favorable trends appear to have reversed. A recent survey by the Centers for Disease Control (CDC) compares 1991 with 1995 smoking rates for high school students. As shown in Fig. 9–3, cigarette smoking in the previous 30 days increased significantly between those two periods. There is also evidence from other data that cigarette smoking rates are no longer declining among youth.[37] In 1995, some 35 percent of high school students in the United States had smoked cigarettes in the previous month,[38] although there is great variability by state, ranging from a high of 43 percent in West Virginia to a low of 17 percent in Utah (Table 9–2). Moreover, a recent comparison of cigarette smoking prevalence between 1993 and 1997 among 116 nationally representative 4-year colleges showed a significant increase in current smoking (within the past 30 days) from 22.3 to 28.5 percent (a 27.8 percent increase).[39]

If the long-term health of the nation is to be improved, prevention of cigarette smoking initiation among youth is an essential element. After more than a decade of progress, there is now growing evidence that the trends are changing and that cigarette smoking is increasing among America's youth.

Prevalence and Trends among Adults

Cigarette consumption per capita for individuals aged 18 and older rose steadily from 1900 to the late 1960s. Since that time, it has steadily declined.[6] This has been the result of competing trends, including increased levels of smoking cessation and increasing recruitment of women smokers. There have also been early signs of a trend of increasing never smokers. The National Health Interview Survey (NHIS) found that 37.6 percent of adult men smoked in 1980 and 28.4 percent in 1990. Among women, the prevalence of current smoking was 29.3 percent in 1980 and 23.5 percent in 1990. These national rates confirm a declining number of adult smokers. But while rates nationally have further decreased since 1990, there still exists significant variation by region of the country.[38] In 1996, the percentage of adults who smoked ranged from a high of 31.7 percent in Kentucky to 15.8 percent in Utah, with most states reporting a prevalence under 25 percent (Table 9–3).

The Minnesota Heart Survey surveyed random samples of adults 25 to 74 years of age in the Minneapolis–St. Paul metropolitan area since 1980. Self-report of cigarette smoking has been validated by serum thiocyanate measures. As shown in Table 9–4, the never-smoked category has been grown substantially from 1980 to 1992 for both men and women. This, combined with former smokers, results in falling rates of cigarette smoking from 1980 to 1992.[40]

FIGURE 9–3 Cigarette smoking (one or more) at any time in the previous 30 days by grade in school—United States, 1991 and 1995. (From Everett et al.[128])

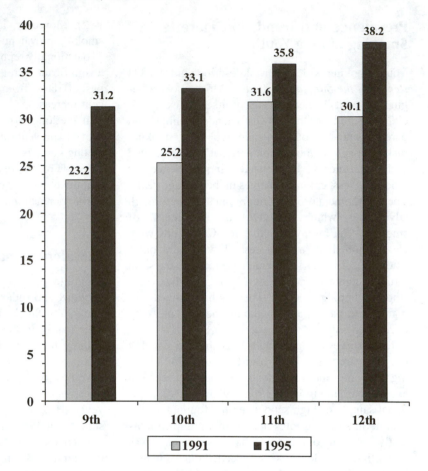

Although cigarette smoking among adults is declining, a substantial portion of the population is still addicted and the concerning trends among youth suggest that adult smoking may rise again.[37,40]

Prevention and Intervention among Youth

School-Based Prevention Programs

Much of the effort in preventing youth smoking has focused on the school setting. School-based prevention programs generally have been targeted at junior-high or middle-school children when the habit begins. Unfortunately, school-based programming alone may have limited impact in the absence of ac-

tive parental and community involvement.[34] At one time it was assumed that simply educating youths about the harmful effects of smoking would be sufficient to prevent them from initiating cigarette use.[41] However, it soon became apparent that such efforts alone were not sufficient to deter adolescents from beginning to smoke.

The social environment, including social influences within the environment, has been identified as a critical determinant of smoking onset. Rather than focusing on long-term disease risk, these interventions have stressed more immediate consequences of smoking, including negative social consequences. Adolescents are seen as often lacking in skills needed to resist peer pressure and other influences that promote smoking.[42] As described in the 1994 Surgeon

TABLE 9–2   Percentage of High School Students Who Reported Cigarette Smoking,* 1995

Rank	State	Percent	Rank	State	Percent
1.	West Virginia	43.0	17.	Massachusetts	35.7
2.	Missouri	39.8	18.	Tennessee[†]	35.3
3.	North Dakota	39.6	19.	Mississippi	35.0
4.	Wyoming	39.5	20.	Montana	34.8
5.	Michigan[†]	38.8	21.	Delaware[†]	34.5
6.	Ohio[†]	38.5	22.	Colorado	33.7
7.	South Dakota	38.0	23.	Nevada	32.9
8.	Maine	37.8	24.	South Carolina	32.6
9.	Vermont	37.7	25.	Hawaii	32.4
10.	Nebraska[†]	37.5	26.	North Carolina	31.3
11.	Arkansas	37.2	27.	Alabama	31.0
12.	Rhode Island[†]	37.1	28.	Georgia[†]	28.4
13.	Alaska	36.5	29.	Idaho[†]	27.1
14.	New Jersey	36.1	30.	California[†]	22.2
15.	New Hampshire	36.0	31.	District of Columbia[†]	22.0
16.	Illinois	35.7	32.	Utah	17.0

*Smoked cigarettes on 1 or more of the 30 days preceding the survey.

[†]Unweighted data. These surveys did not have an overall response rate of at least 60 percent and appropriate documentation. Thus, these data apply only to the students participating in the survey. 1995 data are not available for Arizona, Connecticut, Florida, Indiana, Iowa, Kansas, Kentucky, Louisiana, Maryland, Minnesota, New Mexico, New York, Oklahoma, Oregon, Pennsylvania, Texas, Virginia, Washington, and Wisconsin.

Source: Centers for Disease Control.[38]

General's report, the principal messages of skills-based interventions have focused on the negative, short-term social consequences of smoking, on the techniques of tobacco advertising that may be falsely appealing to adolescents, and on the socially salient advantages of being a nonsmoker.

Meta-analyses of school-based smoking prevention programs have indicated that these programs do have an impact in preventing smoking onset.[43–47] Furthermore, approaches through social influences appear to be the most effective types of school-based interventions. Based on the results of her metanalysis, Rooney concluded that the best results were obtained by social influence programs that (1) were delivered to sixth-grade students, (2) included booster sessions, (3) concentrated the program within a short time period, and (4) used an untrained peer to present the program.[46]

Glynn listed essential elements of effective smoking prevention programs based upon the consensus of a panel of experts.[48] These elements were summarized in the 1994 *Report of the Surgeon General*[34] as follows:

1. Classroom sessions should be delivered at least five times per year in each of two years in the sixth through eighth grades.
2. The program should emphasize the social factors that influence smoking onset, short-term consequences, and refusal skills.
3. The program should be incorporated into the existing school curricula.
4. The program should be introduced during the transition from elementary school to junior high or middle school (sixth or seventh grade).
5. Students should be involved in the presentation and delivery of the program.

TABLE 9–3 Percentage of Adults Who Reported Cigarette Smoking,* 1996†

Rank	State	Percent	Rank	State	Percent
1.	Kentucky	31.7	26.	Massachusetts	23.7
2.	Ohio	29.5	28.	New Jersey	23.6
3.	Indiana	28.8	28.	New York	23.6
4.	Nevada	28.1	28.	Oregon	23.6
5.	Missouri	28.0	28.	Washington	23.6
5.	Tennessee	28.0	32.	Colorado	23.5
7.	West Virginia	27.0	33.	Mississippi	23.1
8.	Arkansas	26.5	33.	Rhode Island	23.1
9.	Alaska	26.2	35.	Nebraska	23.0
10.	Maine	26.1	36.	Florida	22.9
11.	Louisiana	25.8	36.	Kansas	22.9
11.	Michigan	25.8	38.	New Mexico	22.8
13.	New Hampshire	25.7	38.	Texas	22.8
13.	North Carolina	25.7	40.	Alabama	22.6
15.	Pennsylvania	25.3	41.	Connecticut	22.2
16.	Wisconsin	25.2	42.	Montana	21.7
17.	Illinois	25.1	43.	South Dakota	21.5
18.	Iowa	24.6	44.	Idaho	21.3
18.	Oklahoma	24.6	45.	Minnesota	21.1
18.	Virginia	24.6	46.	District of Columbia	20.8
21.	South Carolina	24.4	46.	Maryland	20.8
22.	Delaware	24.3	48.	Georgia	19.9
22.	North Dakota	24.3	49.	California	18.7
24.	Vermont	24.2	50.	Hawaii‡	17.5
25.	Wyoming	24.0	51.	Utah	15.8
26.	Arizona	23.7			

**Ever smoked at least 100 cigarettes and now smoke every day or some days.
†All data are age-adjusted, 1970 total U.S. population.
‡Hawaii data are from 1995.
Source: CDC Behavioral Risk Factor Surveillance System (provisional data), Centers for Disease Control.[38]

6. Parental involvement should be encouraged.
7. Teachers should be adequately trained.
8. The program should be socially and culturally acceptable to each community.

Although some of these points might appear self-evident (e.g., adequate training of teachers, social and cultural acceptability of programs), they have often been overlooked in practice. Furthermore, in high-risk populations, including those of low socioeconomic status, many inner-city residents, and some ethnic minorities, considerable smoking onset already will have occurred by sixth grade. In these populations, it may be advisable to focus prevention efforts on younger children as well.

TABLE 9–4   Smoking Status 1980–1992

	1980–1982	1985–1987	1990–1992
Men			
Never	30.2%	34.5%	40.6%
Former	35.6%	35.9%	33.1%
Current	34.2%	29.6%	26.3%
Women			
Never	45.7%	46.9%	50.4%
Former	20.4%	25.3%	24.1%
Current	33.9%	27.8%	25.5%

Source: Adapted from Arnett et al.,[40] with permission.

Community-Based Prevention Programs

A few model prevention programs have actively involved parents and the larger community in addition to schools. One example is a project by Perry and colleagues in the context of the Minnesota Heart Health Program (MHHP),[49] a research and demonstration project designed to reduce cardiovascular disease at the community level.[50] Initiated in 1980, MHHP involved the entire population in three participating communities in the north central United States. These communities were exposed to a 5-year educational program that encouraged modifications in eating, exercise, and smoking.

Perry et al. hypothesized that school-based smoking prevention would be more effective in communities in which multiple complementary school and community programs were established.[49] Students participated in 5 years of school-based health education, including peer-led prevention, in a context in which adults were actively involved in community smoking-cessation programs and smoking restrictions were being considered both in schools and in the larger community. Results were very encouraging, with smoking prevalence significantly lower among students in the intervention community than among those in the control community. These differences persisted throughout junior and senior high school. At the end of the twelfth grade, students in the intervention community evidenced 40 percent lower smoking prevalence than did students in the comparison community: 14.6 percent of students were weekly smokers at the end of high school compared with 24.1 percent in the reference community.

State and Federal Prevention Initiatives

California, Massachusetts, and Arizona have operated comprehensive antitobacco programs funded by cigarette excise taxes. A major emphasis of these programs has been on preventing tobacco use in youth. Each of these initiatives has included aggressive and well-funded antitobacco media campaigns. The National Cancer Institute American Stop Smoking Intervention Study for Cancer Prevention (ASSIST) is the largest tobacco-control project undertaken in the United States. ASSIST is based upon a coalition model and is intended to demonstrate that a comprehensive, coordinated intervention can significantly reduce tobacco use. A major emphasis of ASSIST as well has been on primary prevention of tobacco use among children, adolescents, and young adults.

There have been few published evaluations of media campaigns targeted at youth initiation of smoking. Flynn et al. found that a combination of media intervention and school-based programming fared better than school-based intervention alone.[51] The media campaign included both radio and television spots that were broadcast as paid advertisements over local media. Reported smoking in the previous week was 35 percent less among youth in the school-and-media condition than in the school-only condition (12.8 versus 19.8 percent).

Prevention efforts should be considered within a broader context that also addresses policy issues and counteradvertising in addition to youth-focused prevention and cessation initiatives.[52] The tobacco industry spends approximately $5 billion each year on advertising and promotion in the United States, with these expenditures heavily targeted toward youth. A comprehensive public policy on tobacco should address tobacco advertising and promotion, access of minors to tobacco products, and tobacco excise taxes in addition to school-based and other community initiatives.

Restrictions on tobacco advertising targeted at youth, including use of cartoon imagery, may be effective in reducing the appeal of such advertising to youth. Restrictions on smoking in public places, including schools, and on tobacco availability to minors also may reduce smoking prevalence, although findings have been inconsistent.[52,53] All 50 states and the District of Columbia have adopted a minimum age of 18 for the purchase of tobacco, but these laws have not been widely enforced.

Increased taxation also may have an impact upon adolescent smoking. Adolescents appear to be at least as price sensitive, if not more so, as adults. The impact of significantly higher prices may be even greater in discouraging initiation than in reducing consumption among existing smokers. Furthermore, a substantial increase in excise taxes could not only be an important tool to discourage adolescent smoking but revenue from these taxes could be dedicated to comprehensive tobacco control programs that would further reduce youth onset of smoking.

Cessation

The vast majority of the work done with youth has focused upon prevention rather than cessation of smoking. Unfortunately, despite the best efforts at prevention, the annual number of adolescents who became daily smokers before the age of 18 years increased by 73 percent from 1988 (708,000) to 1996 (1.226 million). Among persons aged 12 to 17 years, the incidence of first use of cigarettes per 1000 potential new users has been rising continuously during the 1990s. If the rate of smoking initiation among young people had held constant since 1988, then 1.5 million fewer persons under the age of 18 years would have become daily smokers by 1996.[54] Clearly, prevention programs alone are not the sole answer to the problem of youth smoking.

Perhaps the most comprehensive and best designed study was the Project Towards No Tobacco Use.[55] This study was conducted in rural and suburban high schools in two states. The cessation component of this project was a group-based clinic. Students were randomly assigned to a clinic or to a wait list control. Clinics consisted of five sessions over

1 month, with an additional follow-up session held 3 months after the fifth session. Unfortunately, the clinics suffered high attrition, and results at the 3-month follow-up indicated no benefit of the clinic (6.8 percent chemically confirmed abstinence) over the wait list control (7.9 percent chemically confirmed abstinence). These results are especially discouraging because the investigators had previously undertaken extensive formative work, which included 31 focus groups with adolescents.

Hollis et al. reported a less intensive but well-designed intervention in the setting of a health maintenance organization (HMO).[56] Adolescents who indicated on a screening questionnaire as having smoked in the previous week were asked to participate in the study. Participants were randomly assigned to an intervention, consisting of either a 60-min office visit with a nurse practitioner or usual care. Intervention subjects who wished to quit smoking received a follow-up call 1 week later; additional calls were dependent on adolescents' continued interest in quitting. Those who quit smoking were eligible for a lottery with opportunities to win $100. One-year outcome data failed to indicate an intervention effect.

Many of the interventions that have been demonstrated to be effective in adults have not achieved comparable success in adolescent populations. Thus, although nicotine replacement has consistently led to good outcomes with adult smokers,[57] findings to date with adolescents have been disappointing. In a study by Smith et al., only 1 of 22 adolescent smokers aged 13 to 17 who received nicotine patch therapy was abstinent at 6-month follow-up.[58] In a second unpublished study with 101 adolescent smokers, 6-month abstinence was only 5 percent.

A more promising preliminary study was recently published by Colby and colleagues.[59] Intervention consisted of brief motivational interviewing for adolescent smokers (without follow-up) in a hospital emergency room. Motivational interviewing has been widely used with adults,[60] but there is very little published work with adolescents. Colby et al. randomly assigned 40 adolescents to either motivational interviewing or usual care. Three months after the intervention, 22 percent of the intervention group had quit smoking, compared with 10 percent in the control group. However, with only 40 adolescents, this difference was not significant. Motivational interviewing appears feasible with adolescents and, indeed, this client-centered method may be especially appropriate for adolescent smokers.

Lando and colleagues currently are undertaking a systems-based approach with adolescents in the context of dental practices within a large HMO. Adolescent smokers aged 14 to 17 years who have scheduled routine dental appointments are randomly assigned to either dental advice only or to dental advice plus face-to-face counseling and follow-up telephone support. The face-to-face counseling session and follow-up support emphasize motivational interviewing. The study is currently in progress, and no outcome data are available.

A recent review examined the literature on smoking cessation in adolescents.[61] The authors evaluated 17 cessation studies. Program content for these studies was derived from a wide range of theoretical perspectives. Most studies were conducted in school settings that reached less than half of the potential population of adolescent smokers. End-of-treatment quit rates reported in 12 of the 17 studies averaged 20.7 percent (range, 0 to 36 percent), while abstinence at follow-up declined to 13 percent. The most successful programs generally included some type of cognitive-behavioral intervention, such as instruction in coping skills and a focus on the immediate consequences of quitting.

Clearly more work is needed in this area. The vast majority of adolescents are not actively considering quitting. Most adolescents who smoke regularly believe it would be very difficult to quit,[62] but adolescents are unlikely to either enroll or remain in formal cessation programs.[34] Adolescents often have withdrawal symptoms, much like adults. Despite these withdrawal symptoms and the perceived difficulty of quitting, many adolescents view organized cessation programs as irrelevant largely on the grounds that they see no immediate need for assistance. The importance of effective cessation programs for adolescents is underscored, however, by the fact that more than 80 percent of those who smoked a half pack a day or more as high school

seniors were smoking 5 to 6 years later as young adults; over half of these smokers were consuming a pack or more a day at follow-up. Prevention and intervention programs among youth are summarized in Table 9–5.

Interventions among Adults

Interventions with adults have focused on cessation rather than prevention—for obvious reasons. There is, however, some initiation of smoking even in adulthood. A summary of adult smoking cessation strategies is found in Table 9–6. Adult initiation is relatively common in certain settings, as in the military. Thus, Klesges and his colleagues reported that 7 percent of never smokers who entered the Air Force and completed Basic Military Training were regular smokers 1 year later.[63] Ethnic differences have also been found in smoking initiation: African Americans tend to initiate later than European Americans.[64] In some other countries, initiation of smoking tends to occur considerably later than in the United States. In China, for example, one cohort study found the mean age for starting smoking to be 22 years.[65]

TABLE 9–5 Prevention and Intervention Strategies in Youth

School-based prevention programs
  Approaches involving the social environment, including social influences
Community-based prevention programs
  May also enhance effects of school-based programs
State and federal prevention initiatives
  Antitobacco media campaigns
    May enhance school-based programs
  Restrictions on tobacco advertising
  Restrictions on tobacco availability to minors
  Restrictions on smoking in public places including schools
  Increased taxation
    Adolescents may be sensitive to price increases
Limited work in adolescent cessation
  School-based cessation approaches
  Adolescent cessation in managed care

TABLE 9–6   Adult Cessation Strategies

Strategy	Comments on Risk
Aversion (rapid smoking, oversmoking)	May pose significant risk, especially for smokers with existing CVD
Contingency contracting (rewards for abstinence)	
Social support (support from clinician, group support, support from family and friends)	
Relaxation techniques (progressive relaxation, deep breathing)	
Stimulus control and cue extinction (restricting where and when smoking takes place)	
Coping skills (problem solving, cognitive and behavioral strategies)	
Reduced smoking and nicotine fading (gradual reduction in numbers of cigarettes, switching to lower tar and nicotine brands)	
Multicomponent treatment programs (combinations of behavioral techniques)	
Hypnosis	
Acupuncture	
Nonprofit and proprietary programs	
Self-help (written materials, videos, tapes, hotlines/helplines)	
Computer-tailored messages	
Pharmacological intervention	
Nicotine patch	Skin rashes and irritation, usually mild
Nicotine polacrilex (nicotine gum)	Mouth soreness, hiccups, dyspepsia, jaw ache, generally mild and transient, often alleviated by correcting patients' chewing technique
Nicotine nasal spray	Nose and eye irritation is common, but usually disappears within 1 week
Nicotine inhaler	Few side effects, may cause mouth or throat irritation
Zyban (bupropion hydrochloride)	Slight risk of seizure, should not be used by patients with eating disorders, seizure disorders, or those taking certain other medications

The vast majority of the published work with adults has been limited not only to individual smokers but also to smokers who have sought assistance in quitting. Unfortunately, individual smokers who are ready to quit and who seek help represent a very small proportion of the overall smoking population.[66] Furthermore, even in these smokers, absolute long-term outcomes with formal smoking-cessation programs have tended to be disappointing. Intensive multisession group clinics generally produce no more than 30 percent of participants showing abstinence at 1 year.[57] Unaided quit attempts fare substantially less well: of the approximately 17 million smokers in the United States who attempt to quit on their own each year, fewer than 10 percent are successful.

Traditionally, interventions have focused on a single assisted quit attempt. A more effective approach may be to view smoking as a chronic disease and to support multiple quit attempts if necessary.[67] More recently, larger-scale public health efforts have been undertaken to address smoking cessation at the community level and to target adults who may not present for treatment or who may not be immediately interested in quitting.[68,69] For many years, smoking and other uses of tobacco were seen as essentially learned behaviors. More recently, however, cigarettes and other tobacco products have been recognized as physically addictive.[70]

Interventions Targeted at Individuals

There has been far more progress in developing effective smoking-cessation interventions with adults than with adolescents. An exhaustive review of the published smoking-cessation literature between 1975 and 1994 was undertaken by a panel appointed by the Agency for Health Care Policy and Research (AHCPR).[57] An overall conclusion of the panel was that effective smoking-cessation treatments are available for adults. More specific conclusions were that brief cessation treatments improve outcome and that a dose-response relationship exists between the intensity and duration of a program and effectiveness, with more intensive treatments generally producing better long-term abstinence. In addition, the panel recognized three specific treatment elements as effective: nicotine replacement therapy (nicotine patches or gum), social support (clinician-provided encouragement and assistance), and skills training/problem solving (techniques for achieving and maintaining abstinence).

Behavioral Treatments

Despite the addictive properties of nicotine, behavioral aspects of smoking are still seen as critical. The most effective intervention programs have included behavioral treatment components. The AHCPR guidelines report findings for a number of specific behavioral components, including aversive smoking, intratreatment social support, problem solving/skills training, quit day, extratreatment social support, motivation, weight/diet/nutrition, exercise/fitness, contingency contract, relaxation/breathing, and cigarette fading.[57] Most of these specific treatment compo-

nents have not been proven effective in isolation but may contribute to an overall multicomponent intervention.

Aversion Although the guideline found aversive smoking to be effective (and indeed to achieve the highest absolute abstinence levels), aversive techniques have largely gone out of favor. These techniques have included rapid smoking[71,72] and oversmoking or satiation.[73,74] Rapid smoking requires smokers to take very frequent puffs, typically every 6 s, for as long as they can tolerate the procedure. Oversmoking requires subjects to dramatically increase (perhaps double) their usual cigarette consumption for an arbitrary period, typically 1 week. Concerns have been expressed about the safety of rapid smoking and oversmoking.[75] Acceptability of these techniques to smokers has been an additional issue. Other options have included reduced aversion techniques,[76,77] including focused smoking (smoking at a regulated but slower rate) and smoke holding (retaining smoke in the mouth and throat while breathing through the nose).

Contingency contracting Several studies have required participants to submit monetary deposits that are refunded contingent upon maintained abstinence.[78,79] Contracts may also call for self-administered rewards for progressively longer periods of abstinence. Typically, contingency contracting has been included as part of multicomponent behavioral programs.

Social support Supportive intervention during direct contact with a clinician or in a group (intratreatment social support) increases smoking-cessation rates.[57] However, although social support from friends and family is strongly related to successful outcomes in smoking cessation treatments, efforts to systematically enhance natural social support as part of treatment intervention generally have proven unsuccessful.[80]

Relaxation techniques Progressive relaxation and deep breathing strategies have been employed for smoking cessation, although rarely in isolation. A major rationale for the use of these procedures is that smoking relapses are very likely to occur during negative emotional states.[81,82] Relaxation training allows an alternative response for coping with negative emotions or stressful situations and with the stress of quitting smoking and nicotine withdrawal effects. However, there is little evidence to support the efficacy of relaxation training as a stand-alone technique.[83]

Stimulus control and cue extinction Stimulus control and cue extinction procedures also have tended to produce weak results. These procedures have been used in an effort to reduce the huge number of environmental cues that have been associated with smoking.[84] In theory, if some of the cues governing smoking can be weakened or extinguished, quitting should be facilitated. One strategy has been to gradually reduce smoking consumption by progressively restricting the types of situations in which smoking is permitted. Another type of stimulus-control strategy permits smoking only at set times (e.g., every hour on the half hour) regardless of the individual's desire to smoke.[85]

Coping skills Favorable results have been found for specific training in coping skills. Coping skills include problem solving and methods for managing stress and preventing relapse. Shiffman found that a combination of cognitive (e.g., mentally reviewing benefits of quitting) and behavioral (e.g., physical activity, leaving a tempting situation) coping responses provided maximum protection against smoking in a potential crisis situation.[82]

Reduced smoking and nicotine fading Nicotine fading is a nonaversive preparation technique based on the logical premise that withdrawal discomfort might be ameliorated if nicotine consumption were progressively reduced prior to abstinence. This premise may appear to be in conflict with the results of gradual reduction or cigarette "tapering" procedures. Strategies that have emphasized cutting down the numbers of cigarettes smoked have been almost uniformly unsuccessful.[86] Smokers typically appear to reach a "stuck point," often at 10 to 12 cigarettes per day.[86] For the typical smoker of approximately a pack per day, compensatory changes in puffing can compensate for reduced numbers of cigarettes at this

level. Nicotine fading is an alternative in which smokers switch in a series of progressive steps over several weeks to cigarettes rated lower in tar and nicotine[87] or use commercially available nicotine-reduction filters.[88] These procedures have not proven successful in improving smoking-cessation outcomes.

Multicomponent treatment programs The most successful behavioral programs have incorporated multiple treatment components. Emphasis has been placed both upon initial preparation for quitting and longer-term maintenance. Reported long-term abstinence rates for these multicomponent treatment programs have approached 50 percent.[77,89] More recent outcomes have tended to be less successful, however.[90]

Hypnosis and Acupuncture

There are numerous approaches to smoking cessation that are not primarily behavioral or pharmacologic. Two commonly advertised methods include hypnosis and acupuncture. Unfortunately, there are few good studies of these methods and overall results tend to be disappointing. Telling, perhaps, was the fact that only three acceptable studies that examined hypnosis were found in preparation of the AHCPR guidelines, despite the widespread use of this technique.[57] Because the studies were of poor quality and their results were inconsistent, the evidence was insufficient to assess the effectiveness of hypnosis. Studies that have compared acupuncture at theoretically correct sites versus "incorrect" or sham sites have generally found no differences in outcome.

Nonprofit and Proprietary Programs

The oldest of the nonprofit programs are the Five-Day-Plans sponsored by the Seventh-Day Adventist Church.[91] An estimated 14 million smokers in more than 150 countries have attended Five-Day-Plans. This program considers both physical and psychological aspects of cigarette dependence but uses few cognitive-behavioral strategies. Treatment consists of five 90-min to 2-h sessions on consecutive days.

The Five-Day Plan has been revised and renamed The Breathe-Free Plan to Stop Smoking, which includes eight sessions over a 3-week period.

Both the American Cancer Society and the American Lung Association offer formal group programs. Lando et al. compared these two programs.[92] Smokers ($n = 1041$) in three Iowa communities were randomly assigned to American Cancer Society clinics, American Lung Association clinics, or to an intensive multicomponent behavioral program derived from laboratory research. Although results initially favored the laboratory program over both nonprofit clinics, differences between the laboratory program and the American Lung Association program were no longer significant after 1 year of follow-up. Sustained abstinence rates at 1 year were 22.2, 19.0, and 12.1 percent for the laboratory, American Lung Association, and American Cancer Society clinics respectively. The American Lung Association program (Freedom from Smoking) was more intensive than the American Cancer Society program (FreshStart) with the former program consisting of seven 90-min to 2-h group sessions in addition to an initial orientation over a 7-week period and the latter consisting of four 1-h group sessions over either 2 or 4 weeks. The content of the American Cancer Society FreshStart program has recently been revised.

A number of commercial programs are available, usually concentrated in larger metropolitan areas. Most programs tend not to be highly profitable and therefore do not remain active. In evaluating commercial methods, it again appears that the most successful are those that include multicomponent cognitive-behavioral techniques. A number of commercial products (e.g., lozenges, filters) have been introduced as aids to smoking cessation. Currently, none of these products other than nicotine replacement and Zyban are recognized as effective.

Self-Help

The AHCPR panel concluded that self-help interventions may increase abstinence rates relative to no intervention, but that the effect is modest. Simply handing smokers written self-help materials has not been demonstrated to be effective. There is evidence based on a limited number of studies that smoker-initiated calls to telephone hot lines/help lines for cessation counseling or assistance does improve abstinence rates.[57] Although results have been mixed, several studies have found good results for proactive telephone support in which calls are initiated by the help line rather than by the smoker.[93–95]

Computer-Tailored Messages

Computer-tailored messages or "expert systems" have the potential for individualizing cessation content to the individual smoker. Some encouraging preliminary results have been reported with these types of programs.[96–98]

Pharmacologic Intervention

Currently there are a number of pharmacologic aids that are recognized as effective by the Food and Drug Administration (FDA). Most of these aids involve some form of nicotine replacement: nicotine patch, nicotine gum, nicotine nasal spray, and nicotine inhaler. Each of these products has specific advantages and disadvantages. A good description of these is contained in the *Quit Smoking Action Plan* produced by the American Lung Association (Appendix 9–1)[99] and also available on line at http://www.lungusa.org. The information below on pharmacologic adjuncts is adapted from that guide. Guides for clinicians include a *Clinician's Guide* (Appendix 9–2), based on the *Clinical Practice Guideline on Smoking Cessation* prepared by a panel of experts convened by the AHCPR. These guides are also available on line at http://www.ahcpr.gov/guide/.

The patch is easy to use and needs to be applied only once each day. However, it does not allow very flexible dosing (e.g., once the patch is placed on the skin, the delivered dose is not controlled by the patient) and delivery of nicotine is relatively slow. The gum allows more flexible dosing but is somewhat harder to use correctly. Most gum users underdose with this medication. Nicotine nasal spray also has the advantage of flexible dosing, and it provides faster delivery of nicotine. However, many users are bothered by initial eye and nose irritation and frequent use is necessary to obtain adequate nicotine levels. The most recently approved product is the nicotine inhaler, which allows flexible dosing and at least partially mimics the hand-to-mouth behavior of smoking. The inhaler also has few side effects. A major limitation, however, may be the need to do far more puffing than on a cigarette. For optimal nicotine dosage, many hundreds of puffs may be needed as opposed to perhaps 200 for a regular pack-per-day smoker.

The only FDA-approved nonnicotine medication is bupropion hydrochloride (trade name Zyban). This product is available in tablet form. Its appears to act on brain chemistry to bring about some of the same effects that nicotine has when people smoke, although its action is not fully understood. The product is easy to use and can be combined with nicotine replacement. Preliminary evidence suggests that the combination of nicotine patch and Zyban may be more effective than either alone.[100] The main ingredient in Zyban has been available for many years as a treatment for depression under the trade name Wellbutrin. However, Zyban works well in smokers with no symptoms of depression. The major risk of this product is a very slight possibility of seizures.

The AHCPR guidelines reviewed extensive literature for both patch and gum. There were, however, few studies on other forms of nicotine replacement medication. Recent published reports have found good results for both nicotine nasal spray[101] and nicotine inhaler.[102]

Community and Public Health Approaches

Fewer than 1 percent of all smokers have attended formal group or individual treatment programs. Even if half of these smokers achieved permanent abstinence, the overall impact on smoking prevalence would be extremely modest. There is a need for a comprehensive public health approach to smoking that includes community and systems changes in addition to treatment programs of varying types and intensities.[66,103] These approaches are summarized in Table 9–7.

TABLE 9–7   Community and Public Health Approaches

Interventions in health systems
   Clinician advice (brief advice significantly increases quitting)
   Pharmacologic treatment
Work-site interventions (convenient access to large population of smokers, opportunities to capitalize on social support)
Community programs
   Overall mixed results
   "Quit and Win" contests widely disseminated
Policy changes

Health care approaches   Primary care and other clinicians have unique access to the smoking population. At least 70 percent of smokers see a physician each year.[57] Smokers cite physician advice to quit as an important motivator.[104,105] Unfortunately, however, only about half of current smokers report ever having been asked about their smoking status or urged to quit by physicians, and substantially fewer have received advice on how to quit smoking successfully. Brief physician advice alone has been associated with a 30 percent increase in the probability of quitting.[57] Although absolute abstinence rates were modest, universal application of physician or other clinician advice could have major public health impact. Combining brief advice with offers of pharmacologic treatment could further increase the likelihood of success.

A major issue in health system implementation is lack of reimbursement for smoking-cessation services. Curry and colleagues found that use of smoking-cessation services varies with the extent of coverage.[106] Full coverage of both behavioral intervention and nicotine replacement therapy led to highest rates of use of smoking-cessation services and to the greatest impact on the overall prevalence of smoking.

Work-site interventions   Work sites provide convenient access to a large population of smokers as well as the opportunity to capitalize on social support in this setting. Some very positive results have been reported for work-site interventions, although not all studies have been successful. Jeffery and colleagues[107] found modest but significant reductions in overall work-site smoking prevalence with an intervention that provided structured group programs and incentives (e.g., refundable payroll deductions) for quitting. The Working Well Trial, conducted in 111 work sites, was the largest work-site cancer-control trial in the United States.[108] Interventions addressed dietary patterns and smoking. Although reductions in tobacco use were in the predicted direction, differences in tobacco use between intervention and control work sites were not significant.

Community programs Several major community smoking interventions were offered as part of multicomponent heart disease prevention studies.[50,109,110] The Stanford Five-City Project reported significant smoking reductions in the intervention cohort relative to the control, but changes were not found in cross-sectional samples. The Pawtucket Heart Health Program failed to obtain differences in smoking prevalence between an intervention and a comparison city. The Minnesota Heart Health Program found mixed but primarily negative results for smoking intervention. The only evidence of a significant intervention effect was for women in cross-sectional survey data.[111]

Although the overall impact of these communitywide trials on smoking prevalence was disappointing, a useful innovation resulting from these programs was the "Quit and Win" smoking cessation contest. These contests have been successful at the community level in engaging relatively large proportions of the smoking population. Contests also have engaged large numbers of nonsmokers in support of smokers' quit efforts and have increased community awareness around issues of quitting. Community contests have enrolled as many as 7 percent of all eligible smokers and have involved many more in reported quit attempts during the contest period.[112] The Quit and Win contest model has been applied in communities in a number of countries around the world and also in national smoking cessation contests in the United Kingdom and in Finland.

A direct successor to these community trials was the COMMIT project, which focused only on smoking.[113,114] In contrast to the earlier studies, COMMIT randomly assigned communities to intervention or control conditions and included sufficient numbers of communities to allow use of the community as the unit of analysis. One community within each of 11 matched community pairs (10 in the United States, 1 in Canada) was randomly assigned to intervention. The initial target of COMMIT was heavy smokers, defined as those who smoked 25 or more cigarettes per day. Intervention channels focused upon public education through the media and communitywide events, health care providers, work sites and other organizations, and cessation resources.[113] No differences were found between intervention and comparison communities in quit rates among heavy smokers. There was a significant intervention effect on quitting in light-to-moderate smokers;[113] however, evaluation of overall smoking prevalence failed to indicate significant differences between intervention and comparison communities.[114] Results did indicate significant but overall rather modest differences between smokers in intervention and comparison communities in receipt of intervention activities.

More promising results have been reported for the American Stop Smoking Intervention Study (ASSIST). ASSIST is the largest tobacco-control project ever undertaken in the United States.[115] In this initiative, 17 U.S. states funded through ASSIST were compared with 32 others (California, which already had extensive tobacco control activities, was omitted). The primary goal of ASSIST was to reduce smoking prevalence and cigarette consumption among adults in ASSIST states. ASSIST was designed as a collaborative effort between the National Cancer Institute and the American Cancer Society (ACS). The primary contractors for ASSIST were state health departments. State health departments and ACS divisions formed coalitions with health organizations, health and social service agencies, and community groups to develop and implement comprehensive smoking-control plans.

ASSIST targeted those considered at higher risk for smoking—including youth, ethnic minorities, blue-collar workers, the unemployed, women, heavy smokers, and users of smokeless tobacco. Interventions were delivered to target populations through five channels: community environment, work sites, schools, health care settings, and community groups such as churches and chambers of commerce. Emphasis was primarily upon policy and media interventions with less emphasis on programmatic services. Per capita consumption was almost identical in intervention and comparison states before 1993, when full funding for ASSIST interventions began. By 1996, smokers in the intervention states were consuming approximately 7 percent fewer cigarettes per capita.[116]

Policy changes   Perhaps one of the largest impacts to society may be improvements in health that can result from policy changes, such as the passage of antitobacco legislation. An excellent example of this stems from a study of respiratory health before and after recent prohibition began in bars and taverns in California.[117] In a small study of 53 bartenders in San Francisco, 59 percent of those with respiratory symptoms at baseline no longer had symptoms at follow-up; of those with sensory irritations, 78 percent had resolution of symptoms (both $p < .001$). Further, a significant improvement (increase of 4.2 percent) in mean forced vital capacity (FVC) was reported after prohibition. Finally, after cessation of workplace environmental tobacco exposure (as compared with continued exposure), significant improvements both in FVC (6.8 percent increase) and mean forced expiratory volume in 1 s (FEV_1) (4.5 percent increase) were reported.

Summary

The evidence linking tobacco use to the incidence and mortality from cardiovascular diseases is substantial. Approximately a half-million deaths annually are attributed to cigarette smoking, and economic costs total some $100 billion in medical expenses and indirect costs. Environmental tobacco "secondhand" smoke is also an important culprit, responsible for some 35,000 to 40,000 deaths from heart disease annually. Important interventions among youth include school- and community-based prevention programs, state and federal initiatives, and cessation assistance. For adults, various behavioral treatments, self-help approaches, and pharmacologic therapies are available. Community and public health approaches, including health care and work-site programs, are invaluable. Physicians and other health care providers need to take greater initiative in reviewing and following up on tobacco use and in informing patients about appropriate community and health care resources for those needing help.

Although reductions in adult smoking will have the most immediate benefit in terms of reduced hospitalizations from myocardial infarction and stroke as well as saving associated medical costs of more than $3 billion over 7 years for a program reducing smoking prevalence by 1 percent per year,[118] the key to making future progress is primary prevention of smoking in children and teenagers. The fact that tobacco use is dangerous, lethal, and disabling when used as directed has resulted in the call by many experts for the FDA to take steps to regulate its sale and use.[119]

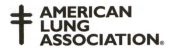

Quit Smoking Action Plan
Introduction

The American Lung Association developed this booklet under the guidance of a team of experts on cigarette smoking. It offers specific recommendations for selecting a personalized *Quit Smoking Action Plan* to free yourself of cigarettes and stay that way.

How To Use This Booklet

To help you better understand your options, the material in this booklet is presented in the following 3 Steps of a *Quit Smoking Action Plan*, along with charts to guide you through each step.

STEP 1 - **Preparing to Quit**

STEP 2 - **Using Medications**

STEP 3 - **Staying Smoke-Free**

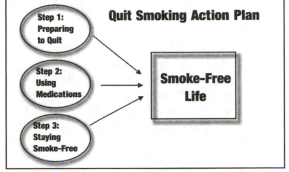

A Deadly Combination: Addiction and Behavior

Nicotine is a powerful drug that raises mood, reduces anxiety, and, in those accustomed to it, increases alertness. Over time, it causes changes in smokers' brains that make them need nicotine. Then, when they try to quit, smokers have unpleasant symptoms such as irritability, craving for cigarettes or difficulty concentrating.

An additional obstacle to quitting is the many daily behavior patterns that smokers may not even realize they have, such as morning or before-bed cigarette routines, or smoking with friends, co-workers or spouses. These links can be numerous and strong, but your *Quit Smoking Action Plan* should help you deal with them.

People who are fairly dependent on cigarettes need to incorporate multiple sources of help in their quitting plan to maximize their odds of success. Those who are less dependent on cigarettes may be successful by using only a few sources of help. However, the more help you have, the better your chances of quitting and staying smoke-free.

Be a Smart Quitter!

There are many programs to help you quit smoking. The cost of these programs may vary from almost nothing to hundreds of dollars. A higher cost does not guarantee success. Many health plans and worksites provide free quit-smoking programs and some health plans cover the cost of medications to help you quit. Check with your insurance carrier or employer for more information.

© 1998 American Lung Association

Before investing your time or money in a program, ask questions such as:

- ▶ Is there a cost to you?
- ▶ Is the program convenient for you?
- ▶ Is the staff well trained and professional?
- ▶ Does the program meet your needs?
- ▶ What is the success rate of this program?

A program representative should be able to answer your questions. If they can't, keep looking. There are no tricks or magic bullets to make you stop smoking. If a program seems too easy, guarantees you will quit, or claims a success rate that sounds unrealistic, look elsewhere.

Examining Your Options

The charts on the next few pages review your options for each of the 3 steps of your *Quit Smoking Action Plan*. Although there are many sources of help available, it's best to choose what feels right to you. The more comfortable you are with the methods you use, the better the chances that you will stick with them.

STEP #1: **Preparing to Quit**

What You Need to Do

1. Identify your personal reasons for quitting.
2. Set a quit date, usually within 10 days to several weeks. If you smoke mostly at work, try quitting on a weekend. If you smoke mostly when relaxing or socializing, quit on a weekday.

(From the American Lung Association,[99] with permission.)

3. Identify your barriers to quitting (such as your spouse smokes or you've relapsed before due to depression or weight gain). You'll find sources of help in this booklet to overcome these barriers.

4. Make SPECIFIC plans AHEAD OF TIME for dealing with temptations. Identify two or three coping strategies that work for you (such as taking a walk or calling a friend).

5. Get cooperation from family and friends. They can't quit for you but they can help by not smoking around you, providing a sympathetic ear and encouragement when you need it and leaving you alone when you need some space.

(see Step #1 chart, "Preparing to Quit," page 3)

STEP #2: Using Medications

What You Need To Know

When you smoke a cigarette, a high concentration of nicotine enters your body rapidly and travels to your brain. Nicotine medications provide you with a safer alternative source of nicotine that enters the body less rapidly and in a lower concentration than cigarettes. There is much unfounded concern about the safety of nicotine medications even though they have been extensively tested and used by millions of people. Unlike cigarettes, which contain thousands of harmful chemicals, nicotine medications contain small doses of nicotine alone to combat cravings and urges to smoke.

To optimize your chances of success, generally medications should be a component of your *Quit Smoking Action Plan*. However, not everyone who decides to quit smoking will want or need to use them. Depending on the medication you use, you may need a prescription. As with any medication, consult the package directions or your pharmacist before using. If you are pregnant, consult your physician; if you are taking other medications, consult the doctor who prescribed them or your pharmacist.

Your goal in using nicotine medication is to stop smoking completely. If you plan to take nicotine medications, begin using them on your quit date. If you continue to have strong urges to smoke or are struggling to stop smoking completely, ask your healthcare provider about additional help.

If you take the non-nicotine medication, it should be started about 7-10 days before your target quit date.

(See STEP #2 chart, "Using Medications" page 4)

Other Tips for Using Medications:

- Ask your physician or pharmacist for advice if you are uncertain about which medication to use.

- Learn to use the medication you choose (examples: apply patches properly, use nicotine gum, nasal spray or inhaler as recommended on package labeling).

- Many experts believe nicotine medications are often taken for too short a time to be of full benefit to users. For this reason, your healthcare provider may advise you to use your medication for a longer period of time or in combination with another medication. However, if you take these medications on your own, do not deviate from package directions.

STEP #3: **Staying Smoke-Free**

What You Need To Remember

After quitting and getting through the first couple of weeks, staying off cigarettes is critical—and not always easy. Research indicates that continued support and encouragement from health providers, family, friends and other sources are extremely helpful.

Your friends and family won't automatically know how to encourage you. Talk to them ahead of time about what they can do. Also, think about who you want to give you encouragement—someone who will stay positive even if you have some problems along the way.

(See STEP #3 chart, "Staying Smoke-Free," page 5)

The average person makes two to four attempts at quitting before they are able to stay smoke-free. If you return to smoking, it doesn't mean you can't quit. It just means you need to try again by figuring out what caused you to slip and improving your plan for next time.

You may want to use medications this time if you have tried to quit without them in the past. Or you may want to try a different group, individual counselor or other source of help if you've been unsuccessful at quitting on your own.

Some smokers wrongly believe they can reduce their health risks and continue to smoke by substituting other forms of tobacco. Low tar/nicotine cigarettes are not safer than cigarettes, nor do they reduce your risk of smoking-related disease. Smokeless tobacco, pipes and cigars also are not safe.

Step #1: Preparing to Quit

Description & Examples	Pros & Cons	Comments
Group Programs American Lung Association's Freedom From Smoking® group program offers seven sessions to help you set and follow your *Quit Smoking Action Plan*. Also offered by many hospitals, medical facilities and by voluntary agencies.	*Pros* • Supportive, encouraging environment • Opportunity for building skills needed to quit smoking *Cons:* • Meeting schedule may not be flexible enough for some • A group may not be available when you need it	*Comments/limitations:* Best for those who work well with others. The groups focus on helping you change your smoking behaviors. May also be helpful for those whose family or friends are unlikely to provide support. Usually meets for four to seven sessions with each session lasting one to two hours.
Individual Counseling From Healthcare Provider Many healthcare providers offer individual quit-smoking programs that help you develop a *Quit Smoking Action Plan*. They should also provide encouragement for staying smoke-free and plans for coping with relapse.	*Pros:* • Flexible • Personalized to your needs • Opportunity for building skills needed to quit smoking *Cons:* • No opportunity for peer support, sharing • Usually requires an appointment	*Comments/limitations:* This may be best if you have a good relationship with your healthcare provider. Best for people who prefer to work independently rather than in group settings. The more counseling sessions you attend, the better your chances of staying smoke-free.
Books, Manuals, Audiotapes, Video-tapes, and Internet Resources ALA's *7 Steps to a Smoke-Free Life* is one of many excellent sources available. These should be educational, informative and discuss the key parts of a *Quit Smoking Action Plan*. May be a starting point for additional help.	*Pros:* • Convenient • Private • May be especially appropriate for those who like to work on their own or enjoy "do-it-yourself" projects *Cons:* • Success depends on continued use • Many are superficial and do not provide needed key elements	*Comments/limitations:* Although you may prefer to quit on your own, quitting without preparing an action plan is unlikely to be successful. The American Lung Association provides a variety of materials and programs, including special programs for pregnant women, African-American smokers and other populations.
Telephone Counseling Many health providers and worksites offer telephone counseling to provide assistance in developing and following through with your *Quit Smoking Action Plan*. (Additionally, telephone counseling to provide encouragement for staying smoke-free is described later in this guide.) Many states have smokers' help lines. For more information, call: **American Lung Association 1-(800) LUNG-USA**	*Pros:* • Convenient • Flexible • Personal and private • Useful in rural areas or anywhere access to counseling services is limited *Cons:* • Phone counselor may change from contact to contact • Lack of fixed schedule may be discouraging to some	*Comments/limitations:* Telephone counseling services are also sometimes used to help you stay smoke-free. Ask your healthcare provider or check your phone book for availability of these services in your area.

Step #2: Using Medications

Description & Examples	Pros & Cons	Comments

Nicotine Patch
 	
    NicoDerm® CQ
    Nicotrol®
    Nicotine Transdermal Patch
    (prescription required)
    Habitrol® (prescription required)
    ProStep® (prescription required)
 	
Patches deliver nicotine through the skin in different strengths, over different lengths of time.
	Pros:
	• Easy to use
	• Only needs to be applied once a day
	• Some available without a prescription
	• Few side effects
	Cons:
	• Less flexible dosing
	• Slow onset of delivery
	• Mild skin rashes and irritation
		Comments/limitations: Patches vary in strengths and the length of time over which nicotine is delivered. Depending on the brand you use, may be left on for anywhere from 16 to 24 hours. Some smokers who use these products can stop them abruptly, while others prefer to reduce their dosage slowly.

Nicotine Polacrilex (nicotine gum) Nicorette® The term "gum" is misleading. Although it actually is a gum-like substance impregnated with small amounts of nicotine, nicotine gum is not chewed like regular gum. Instead, you chew it briefly and then "park" it between your cheek and gum. The nicotine is absorbed through the lining of the mouth.	**Pros:** • Convenient • Flexible dosing • Faster delivery of nicotine than the patches **Cons:** • May be inappropriate for people with dental problems and those with temporomandibular joint (TMJ) syndrome • Cannot eat or drink while the medication is in your mouth • Frequent use during the day required to obtain adequate nicotine levels	**Comments/limitations:** Many people use this medication incorrectly. Most of the time the gum is in your mouth, it should be "parked" between your cheek and gum. Read package directions carefully for a full explanation. To achieve greatest benefit, you generally should chew nine or more pieces per day.
Nicotine Nasal Spray Nicotrol® NS (prescription required) Delivers nicotine through the lining of the nose when you squirt it directly into each nostril.	**Pros:** • Flexible dosing • Can be used in response to stress or urges to smoke • Fastest delivery of nicotine of currently available products • Reduces cravings within minutes **Cons:** • Nose and eye irritation is common, but usually disappears within one week. • Frequent use during the day required to obtain adequate nicotine levels	**Comments/limitations:** Unlike nasal sprays used to relieve allergy symptoms, the nicotine spray is not meant to be sniffed. Rather, it is sprayed once into each nostril once or twice an hour. Take a deep breath, hold it, spray once into each nostril and exhale through the mouth. Ask your pharmacist for help in using the product correctly.
Nicotine Inhaler Nicotrol® Inhaler (prescription required) A plastic cylinder containing a cartridge that delivers nicotine when you puff on it. Although similar in appearance to a cigarette, the inhaler delivers nicotine into the mouth, not the lung, and enters the body much more slowly than the nicotine in cigarettes.	**Pros:** • Flexible dosing • Mimics the hand-to-mouth behavior of smoking • Few side effects • Faster delivery of nicotine than the patches **Cons:** • Frequent use during the day required to obtain adequate nicotine levels • May cause mouth or throat irritation	**Comments/limitations:** Puffing must be done frequently, far more often than your cigarette. Each cartridge lasts for 80 long puffs; each cartridge is designed for 20 minutes of use. A minimum of six cartridges per day is needed for three to six weeks, then the patient starts tapering off. You do not need to inhale deeply to achieve an effect. Small doses of nicotine provide a sensation in the back of the throat similar to cigarette smoke.

Step #2: Using Medications, continued

Non-nicotine medication	Pros:	Comments/limitations:
Zyban™ (bupropion hydrochloride) Sustained-Release Tablets (prescription required) Currently the only non-nicotine medication shown to be effective for quitting smoking. Treatment must be started at least one week before your target quit date.	• Easy to use • Pill form • Few side effects • Can be used in combination with nicotine patches *Cons:* • Should not be used by patients with eating disorders, seizure disorders or those taking certain other medications • Lack of flexibility of use	This is the first medication to help quit smoking that is available in tablet form. Its primary role is to act on brain chemistry to bring about some of the same effects that nicotine has when people smoke. A small risk of seizure is associated with use of this medication. The main ingredient in Zyban has been available for many years as a treatment for depression under the trade name Wellbutrin. However, it works well in people with no depression as an aid to quit smoking.

Step #3: Staying Smoke-Free

Source of Help	Pros & Cons
Preventing Relapse The group program, individual counseling from a healthcare provider, telephone counseling or self-help materials you choose should include information on how to prevent a relapse and what to do if a relapse occurs.	Refer to **Step #1**: Preparing to Quit
Encouragement from Family and Friends	Pros: • Convenient/available • Understand you well and can anticipate your needs • Reinforce your desire to quit when you feel tempted to smoke again Cons: • May become overly critical if your quit attempt fails • If they try to quit for you instead of for themselves, they may relapse and undermine your efforts
Worksite & Community Many worksites and communities offer quit-smoking programs. These often include group programs such as those offered by the American Lung Association or support programs such as Nicotine Anonymous. Smoke-free worksite and community promotional campaigns may also include "buddy systems" and other activities to help people stay smoke-free.	Pros: • Helpful to have encouragement in the places—your job or community—where you spend most of your time • Helpful—and healthful—to work in smoke-free workplace Cons: • Programs may not be available or may be hard to find in your area • Work site may not be smoke-free or may not encourage nonsmoking
Telephone Encouragement or "Health Lines" In addition to telephone counseling for developing a *Quit Smoking Action Plan*, many employers, HMOs, communities, and makers of nicotine and non-nicotine medications offer ongoing telephone counseling to encourage staying smoke-free.	Pros: • Convenient • Private • Provide support when family and friends do not or cannot Cons: • May not be available in your health plan, company, or community

Conclusion

The information you have just read is meant to provide the knowledge you need to prepare and use your *Quit Smoking Action Plan*. Some of the main messages to keep in mind are:

• You can quit! Millions—about half of all smokers in the U.S.—already have.
• The more dependent you are on cigarettes, the harder it is to quit.
• Don't be afraid to ask for help.
• The more sources of help you use, the better your chance of success.

By reading this booklet and understanding the roles of behavior, medications and support, you have taken a major step toward becoming smoke-free. You may want to show this information to your healthcare provider and make notes of any questions you have now.

In addition, a listing of national organizations has been included to provide you with more sources of help and guidance. Good luck and good health!

When You Can't Breathe, Nothing Else Matters®

Brought to you by an unrestricted educational grant from McNeil Consumer Products Company.
All rights reserved. No part of this book may be used or reproduced in any manner whatsoever
without written permission from the American Lung Association.
Printed in the United States of America, September 1998.

✝ **AMERICAN LUNG ASSOCIATION®**

For information write:
American Lung Association
1740 Broadway
New York, NY 10019-4374
Fax: (212) 265-5642
Phone: (212) 315-8700

National Web Site: http://www.lungusa.org

RESOURCES

American Lung Association
Call 1-800-LUNG-USA to contact your local
American Lung Association office.
Internet: http://www.lungusa.org
America Online: Keyword: ALA

The American Academy of Family Physicians
Department of Public Health & Scientific Affairs & Health Education
Kansas City, MO
(800) 274-2237, ext. 5500

Action on Smoking and Health
2013 H Street
Washington, D.C. 20077-2410
(202) 659-4310

American Academy of Otolaryngology Head and Neck Surgery
One Prince Street
Alexandria, VA 22314
(703) 836-4444

American Cancer Society
1599 Clifton Road, NE
Atlanta, GA 30329
(404) 320-3333

American Heart Association
7272 Greenville Avenue
Dallas, TX 75231
(800) AHA-USA1 (242-8721)

Centers for Disease Control and Prevention
National Center for Chronic Disease Prevention and Health Promotion
Office on Smoking and Health
Mailstop K-50
4770 Buford Highway, NE
Atlanta, GA 30341-3724
(800) CDC-1311

National Cancer Institute
Bethesda, MD 20894
(800) 4-CANCER (422-6237)

National Heart, Lung, and Blood Institute
Building 31, Room 4A21
Bethesda, MD 20892
(301) 496-4236

National Institute on Drug Abuse
Drug Abuse Information and Treatment Referral Line
11426 Rockville Pike, Suite 410
Rockville, MD 20852
(800) 662-4357
(800) 662-9832 (Spanish)
(800) 228-0427 (hearing impaired)

Nicotine Anonymous
P.O. Box 591777
San Francisco, CA 94159-1777
(415) 750-0328

THE AMERICAN LUNG ASSOCIATION QUIT SMOKING ACTION PLAN WAS DEVELOPED UNDER THE GUIDANCE OF AN EXPERT PANEL, INCLUDING:

Edwin B. Fisher, PhD, Panel Chair
Professor of Psychology, Medicine and Pediatrics
Division of Health Behavior Research
Washington University
St. Louis, MO

Donald J. Brideau, Jr., MD
Medical Director, Integrated Physician Services
Inova Health System
Assistant Clinical Professor, George Washington Medical School
Fairfax, VA

Jack L. Cox, MD
Director of Graduate Medical Education/
Regional Medical Director
Intermountain Healthcare, Inc.
Provo, UT

Norman H. Edelman, MD
Scientific Consultant, American Lung Association
Professor of Medicine, Dean of the School of Medicine
Health Science Center, State University of New York at Stony Brook

Richard D. Hurt, MD
Director, Nicotine Dependence Center
Mayo Clinic
Rochester, MN

Daniel A. Hussar, PhD
Remington Professor of Pharmacy
Philadelphia College of Pharmacy
University of the Sciences in Philadelphia
Philadelphia, PA

Harry Lando, PhD
Professor
University of Minnesota
Minneapolis, MN

Scott J. Leischow, PhD
Director, Arizona Program for Nicotine and Tobacco Research
The University of Arizona
Tucson, AZ

Edward Lichtenstein, PhD
Research Scientist
Oregon Research Institute
Eugene, OR

David P. L. Sachs, MD
Director, Palo Alto Center for Pulmonary Disease Prevention
Clinical Associate Professor, Department of Medicine
Stanford University Medical School
Palo Alto, CA

The information found on these pages is not intended to provide specific medical advice, or replace the continuing care, guidance and supervision provided by your doctor and other members of your healthcare team. All readers are encouraged to seek proper medical advice and maintain regular communications with their doctor.

HELPING SMOKERS QUIT

ASK ADVI

Every person who smokes should be offered smoking cessation treatment at every office visit.

Clinicians should ask about and record the tobacco-use status of every patient.

Cessation treatment even as brief as 3 minutes a visit is effective.

The more intense the treatment, the more effective it is in producing long-term abstinence from tobacco.

Nicotine replacement therapy (nicotine patches or gum), social support, and skills training are effective components of smoking cessation treatment.

Health care systems should be modified to routinely identify and intervene with all tobacco users at every visit.

A GUIDE FOR PRIMARY CARE CLINICIANS

Ask about smoking

Implement an officewide system that ensures that tobacco-use status is obtained and recorded for every patient at every office visit.

 Include tobacco use in vital signs data collected

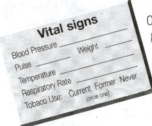

Vital signs
Blood Pressure _____
Pulse _____   Weight _____
Temperature _____
Respiratory Rate _____
Tobacco Use: Current   Former   Never
(circle one)

Or,
place tobacco-use status stickers on all patient charts, or indicate smoking status using computer reminder systems.

Advise tobacco users to quit

In a clear, strong, and personalized manner, urge every smoker to quit.

Be clear. ("I think it is important for you to quit smoking now, and I will help you.")

Speak strongly. ("As your clinician, I need you to know that quitting smoking is the most important thing you can do to protect your current and future health.")

Personalize your advice. ("You've already had one heart attack.") Mention the impact of smoking on children or others in the household. ("You know your children need you.")

Source: The Agency for Health Care Policy and Research

SE ASSIST

SMOKING KILLS MORE THAN 400,000 PERSONS A YEAR IN THE UNITED STATES. EVERY OFFICE VISIT IS AN OPPORTUNITY TO PROMOTE SMOKING CESSATION.

Assist the patient with a quit plan

Advise the smoker to:

- Set a quit date, ideally within 2 weeks.
- Inform friends, family, and coworkers of plans to quit, and ask for support.
- Remove cigarettes from home, car, and workplace and avoid smoking in these places.
- Review previous quit attempts—what helped, what led to relapse.
- Anticipate challenges, particularly during the critical first few weeks, including nicotine withdrawal.

Give advice on successful quitting:

- Total abstinence is essential—not even a single puff.
- Drinking alcohol is strongly associated with relapse.
- Having other smokers in the household hinders successful quitting.

Encourage use of nicotine replacement therapy:*

- Both the nicotine patch and nicotine gum are effective pharmacotherapies for smoking cessation.
- The nicotine patch may be easier to use than the gum in most clinical settings.

Make culturally and educationally appropriate materials on cessation techniques readily available in your office.

* For more information on prescribing, precautions, and side effects, see the *Clinical Practice Guideline.*

This *Clinician's Guide* is based on the *Clinical Practice Guideline on Smoking Cessation.* It was prepared by a panel of experts convened by the Agency for Health Care Policy and Research, and reflects a thorough review of evidence from clinical studies spanning 1978 to 1994.

For more copies of this guide, the complete *Clinical Practice Guideline*, a *Quick Reference Guide for Smoking Cessation Specialists*, a *Consumer Version* (available in English and Spanish), or a list of other AHCPR guidelines, call 800-358-9295 or write:

AHCPR Publications Clearinghouse
P.O. Box 8547
Silver Spring, MD 20907

These and other guidelines are available through the Internet (http://www.ahcpr.gov/guide/). Copies of this and other brochures are free through InstantFAX, which operates all day every day. Using a fax machine equipped with a touchtone telephone, dial 301-594-2800, push 1, and then press the start button for instructions and a list of publications.

U.S. Department of Health and Human Services
Public Health Service
Agency for Health Care Policy and Research
2101 East Jefferson Street, Suite 501
Rockville, MD 20852

Clinical Practice Guideline No. 18
AHCPR Publication No. 96-0693
April 1996

For sale by the U.S. Government Printing Office
Superintendent of Documents, Mail Stop: SSOP, Washington, DC 20402-9328

A GUIDE FOR PRIMARY CARE CLINICIANS

Intensive Programs

Offer intensive smoking cessation programs.

If your patient prefers intensive treatment or you think such a program is appropriate, refer him or her to an intensive smoking cessation program administered by a specialist. Always follow up with the patient about quitting.

- ◆ Intensive programs are strongly correlated with cessation success.
- ◆ Information obtained in the assessment (e.g., comorbidity, stress level) is useful in counseling.
- ◆ Many different types of clinicians (e.g., nurses, dentists, psychologists) are effective in increasing quit rates.
- ◆ Intensive programs should offer 4–7 sessions, each at least 20–30 minutes in length, lasting at least 2 weeks.
- ◆ Counseling should offer problem solving and skills training as well as social support.
- ◆ Counseling should reinforce motivation to quit and relapse prevention. Individual and group counseling are both effective.
- ◆ Every smoker should be offered nicotine replacement therapy (patch or gum), except when medically contraindicated.

Key Treatment Strategies

Three treatment strategies are particularly effective:

- ◆ Nicotine replacement therapy—should be encouraged for most patients. Although the patch and gum are both effective, the patch is associated with fewer compliance problems and requires less effort to train patients in its use.

  Patch: Plan on 8 weeks of therapy. Starting on the quit day, place a new patch, each morning, on a relatively hairless place between the neck and the waist. Consult package insert for dosing suggestions and precautions.

  Gum: Use for up to 3 months. Patients often do not use enough gum to get maximum benefit. Use one piece every 1–2 hours. Chew and "park" gum (between cheek and gum) intermittently for about 30 minutes to allow nicotine absorption. Use 4-mg (vs. 2-mg) dose for highly dependent smokers.

  Nasal Spray: Recently approved by FDA. Consult package insert for dosing and precautions.

- ◆ Clinician-provided social support—communicate caring and concern by being open to the patient's fears and difficulties.
- ◆ Skills-training/problem-solving techniques—review previous quit successes and failures, anticipate relapse risk situations, and stress total abstinence starting on the quit day.

If a smoker doesn't want to quit, clinicians should ask questions at each visit that help the patient identify (1) reasons to quit and (2) barriers to quitting. Pledge to assist the patient when he or she is ready to quit.

Follow Up

Schedule followup contact, either in person or by telephone.

Timing

- First followup contact within 2 weeks of the quit date, preferably during the first week.
- Second contact within the first month.
- Further followup contacts as needed.

Actions during followup visits:

- Congratulate success.
- If a lapse occurred, ask for recommitment to total abstinence.
- Remind the patient that a lapse can be used as a learning experience and review the circumstances that caused it. Suggest alternative behaviors.
- Identify problems encountered and anticipate challenges in the immediate future.

All treatment strategies apply to **adolescents** who smoke. Clinicians should be empathetic and nonjudgmental, and should personalize the encounter to the adolescent's individual situation. Nicotine replacement therapy may be considered in adolescents addicted to nicotine.

Prevent Relapse

To prevent relapse, offer ex-smokers reinforcement.

- Congratulate, encourage, and stress importance of remaining abstinent.
- Review the benefits, including potential health benefits, to be derived from cessation.
- Review the patient's success in quitting.
- Inquire about problems encountered in maintaining abstinence and offer possible solutions.
- Anticipate problems or threats to maintaining abstinence.

Discuss specific problems, such as:

- Weight gain
- Negative mood/depression
- Prolonged nicotine withdrawal
- Lack of support for cessation

Fear of **weight gain** is an impediment to smoking cessation. Inform smokers that many people gain weight when they stop smoking. Tell them that weight gain is a minor risk compared with the risks of continued smoking. Tell patients to tackle one problem at the time—first be confident that they have quit smoking for good, then work on reducing weight gain. Nicotine gum may delay weight gain.

References

1. U.S. Department of Health and Human Services: *Targeting Tobacco Use: The Nation's Leading Cause of Death: At-A-Glance.* Bethesda, MD, Centers for Disease Control and Prevention, 1998.

2. U.S. Public Health Service: *The Health Consequences of Smoking: Cardiovascular Disease: A Report of the Surgeon General.* DHHS Publication No. (PHS) 84–50204. Rockville, MD, U.S. Department of Health and Human Services, 1983.

3. U.S. Department of Health and Human Services: *The Health Consequences of Involuntary Smoking: A Report of the Surgeon General.* Rockville, MD, Office on Smoking and Health, 1986.

4. Lam TH, He Y: Passive smoking and coronary heart disease: a brief review. *Clin Exp Pharmacol Physiol* 1997; 24:993–996.

5. Steenland K, Thun M, Lally C, et al: Environmental tobacco smoke and coronary heart disease in the American Cancer Society CPS-II cohort. *Circulation* 1996; 94:622–628.

6. U.S. Department of Health and Human Services: *Changes in Cigarette-Related Disease Risks and Their Implication for Prevention and Control.* Monograph 8. NIH Publication No. 97–4213. Rockville, MD, U.S. Department of Health and Human Services, Public Health Services, National Institutes of Health, National Cancer Institute, 1997.

7. Keys A, Menotti A, Aravanis C, et al: The Seven Countries Study: 2,289 deaths in 15 years. *Prev Med* 1984; 13:141–154.

8. Kawachi I, Colditz GA, Stampfer MJ, et al: Smoking cessation and time course of decreased risks of coronary heart disease in middle-aged women. *Arch Intern Med* 1994; 154:169–175.

9. Centers for Disease Control: *The Health Benefits of Smoking Cessation: A Report of the Surgeon General.* DHHS Publication No. (CDC) 90–8416. Washington, DC, Public Health Service, Office on Smoking and Health, 1990.

10. Neaton JD, Wentworth D, for the Multiple Risk Factor Intervention Trial Research Group: Serum cholesterol, blood pressure, cigarette smoking, and death from coronary heart disease: overall findings and differences by age for 316,099 white men. *Arch Intern Med* 1992; 152:56–64.

11. The Multiple Risk Factor Intervention Trial Research Group: Mortality after 16 years for participants randomized to the Multiple Risk Factor Intervention Trial. *Circulation* 1996; 94:946–951.

12. Escobedo LG, Caspersen CJ: Risk factors for sudden coronary death in the United States. *Epidemiology* 1997; 8:175–180.

13. Rosenberg L, Miller DR, Kaufman DW, et al: Myocardial infarction in women under 50 years of age. *JAMA* 1983; 250:2801–2806.

14. Kannel WB, McGee DL, Castelli WP: Latest perspectives on cigarette smoking and cardiovascular disease: the Framingham study. *J Cardiac Rehabil* 1984; 4:267–277.

15. Miettinen TA, Gulling H: Mortality and cholesterol metabolism in familial hypercholesterolemia: long-term follow-up of 96 patients. *Arteriosclerosis* 1988; 8:163–167.

16. Pooling Project Research Group: Relationship of blood pressure, serum cholesterol, smoking habit, relative weight, and ECG abnormalities to incidence of major coronary events: final report of the Pooling Project. *J Chronic Dis* 1978; 31:201–306.

17. Suarez L, Barrett-Connor E: Interaction between cigarette smoking and diabetes mellitus in the prediction of death attributed to cardiovascular disease. *Am J Epidemiol* 1984; 120:670–675.

18. Mishell DR: Use of oral contraceptives in women of older reproductive age. *Am J Obstet Gynecol* 1988; 158:1652–1657.

19. Williams RR, Hasstedt SJ, Wilson DE, et al: Evidence that men with familial hypercholesterolemia can avoid early coronary death: an analysis of 77 gene carriers in four Utah pedigrees. *JAMA* 1986; 255:219–224.

20. Hermanson B, Omenn GS, Kronmal RA, et al: Beneficial six-year outcome of smoking cessation in older men and women with coronary artery disease: results from the CASS registry. *N Engl J Med* 1988; 319:1365–1369.

21. Rosenberg L, Kaufman DW, Helmrich SP, et al: The risk of myocardial infarction after quitting smoking in men under 55 years of age. *N Engl J Med* 1985; 313:1511–1514.

22. McGill HC, McMahan CA, Malcom GT, et al, for the PDAY Research Group: Effects of serum lipoproteins and smoking on atherosclerosis in young men and women. *Arterioscler Thromb Vasc Biol* 1997; 17:95–106.

23. Zimmerman M, McGeachie J: The effect of nicotine on aortic endothelium: a quantitative ultrastructural study. *Atherosclerosis* 1987; 63:33–41.

24. Fried LP, Moore RD, Pearson TA: Long-term effects of cigarette smoking and moderate alcohol consumption on coronary artery diameter: mechanisms of coronary artery disease independent of atherosclerosis or thrombosis. *Am J Med* 1986; 80:37–44.

25. Meade TW, Imeson J, Stirling Y: Effects of changes in smoking and other characteristics on clotting factors and the risk of ischaemic heart disease. *Lancet* 1987; 2:986–988.

26. Maouad J, Fernandez F, Barrillon A, et al: Diffuse or segmental narrowing (spasm) of coronary arteries during smoking demonstrated on angiography. *Am J Cardiol* 1984; 53:354–355.

27. Gori GB: Environmental tobacco smoke and coronary heart syndromes: absence of an association. *Regul Toxicol Pharmacol* 1995; 21:281–295.

28. Kawachi I, Colditz GA, Speizer FE, et al: A prospective study of passive smoking and coronary heart disease. *Circulation* 1997; 95:2374–2379.

29. Steenland K, Sieber K, Etzel RA, et al: Exposure to environmental tobacco smoke and risk factors for heart disease among never smokers in the Third National Health and Nutrition Examination Survey. *Am J Epidemiol* 1998; 147:932–939.

30. Wells AH: Heart disease from passive smoking in the workplace. *J Am Coll Cardiol* 1998; 31:1–9.

31. Kritz H, Schmid P, Sinzinger H: Passive smoking and cardiovascular risk. *Arch Intern Med* 1995; 155:1942–1948.

32. Glantz SA, Parmley WW: Passive smoking and heart disease: mechanisms and risk. *JAMA* 1995; 273:1047–1053.

33. Weiss ST: Cardiovascular effects of environmental tobacco smoke. *Circulation* 1996; 94:599.

34. U.S. Department of Health and Human Services: *Preventing Tobacco Use among Young People: A Report of the Surgeon General.* Atlanta, GA, U.S. Department of Health and Human Services, Public Health Service, Centers for Disease Control and Prevention, National Center for Chronic Disease Prevention and Health Promotion, Office on Smoking and Health, 1994.

35. DiFranza JR, Richards JW, Paulman PM, et al: RJR Nabisco's cartoon camel promotes camel cigarettes to children. *JAMA* 1991; 266:3149–3153.

36. Johnston LD, O'Malley PM, Bachman JG: *National Survey Results on Drug Use from the Monitoring the Future Study, 1968–1974: Vol 1. Secondary School Students.* Rockville, MD, National Institutes on Drug Abuse.

37. Centers for Disease Control: Surveillance for selected tobacco-use behaviors—United States, 1900–1994. *MMWR* 1994; 43:1–43.

38. Centers for Disease Control and Prevention: *Chronic Diseases and Their Risk Factors.* Atlanta, GA, Centers for Disease Control and Prevention, 1998.

39. Wechsler H, Rigotti NA, Gledhill-Hoyt J, Lee H: Increased levels of cigarette use among college students—cause for national concern. *JAMA* 1998; 280:1673–1678.

40. Arnett DK, Sprafka JM, McGovern PG, et al: Trends in cigarette smoking: the Minnesota Heart Survey, 1980 through 1992. *Am J Public Health* 1998; 88:1230–1233.

41. Thompson EL: Smoking education programs 1960–1976. *Am J Public Health* 1978; 68:250–257.

42. Botvin GJ, Wills TA: Personal and social skills training: cognitive-behavioral approaches to substance abuse prevention. In: Bell CS, Battjes R (eds): *Prevention Research: Deterring Drug Abuse among Children and Adolescents.* Monograph No. 63. DHHS Publication No. (ADM). Bethesda, MD, U.S. Department of Health and Human Services, Public Health Service, Alcohol, Drug Abuse, and Mental Health Administration, National Institute on Drug Abuse, 1985:85–1334.

43. Tobler NS: Meta-analysis of 143 adolescent drug prevention programs: quantitative outcome results of program participants compared to a control or comparison group. *J Drug Issues* 1986; 16:537–567.

44. Tobler NS: Drug prevention programs can work: research findings. *J Addict Dis* 1992; 11:1–28.

45. Rundall TG, Bruvold WH: A meta-analysis of school-based smoking and alcohol use prevention programs. *Health Educ Q* 1988; 15:317–334.

46. Rooney B: A meta-analysis of smoking-prevention programs after adjustment for study design (dissertation). Minneapolis, MN; University of Minnesota, 1992.

47. Bruvold WH: A meta-analysis of adolescent smoking-prevention programs. *Am J Public Health* 1993; 83:872–880.

48. Glynn TJ: Essential elements of school-based smoking-prevention programs. *J Sch Health* 1989; 59:181–188.

49. Perry CL, Kelder SH, Murray DM, et al: Community-wide smoking prevention: long-term outcomes of the Minnesota Heart Health Program and the class of 1989 study. *Am J Public Health* 1992; 82:1210–1216.

50. Luepker RV, Murray DM, Jacobs DR, et al: Community education for cardiovascular disease prevention: risk factor changes in the Minnesota Heart Health Program. *Am J Public Health* 1994; 84:1383–1393.

51. Flynn BS, Worden JK, Secker-Walker RH, et al: Prevention of cigarette smoking through mass media intervention and school programs. *Am J Public Health* 1992; 82:827–834.

52. Forster JL, Murray DM, Wolfson M, et al: The effects of community policies to reduce youth access to tobacco. *Am J Public Health* 1998; 88:1193–1198.

53. Rigotti NA, DiFranza JR, YuChiao C, et al: The effect of enforcing tobacco-sales laws on adolescents' access to tobacco and smoking behavior. *N Engl J Med* 1997; 337:1044–1051.

54. Centers for Disease Control: Incidence of initiation of cigarette smoking—United States, 1965–1996. *MMWR* 1998; 47:837–840.

55. Sussman S, Dent CW, Burton D, et al: *Developing School-Based Tobacco Use Prevention and Cessation Programs.* Thousand Oaks, CA, Sage Publications, 1995.

56. Hollis JF, Vogt TM, Stevens V, et al: The tobacco reduction and cancer control (TRACC) program: team approaches to counseling in medical and dental settings. *Tobacco and the Clinician: Interventions for Medical and Dental Practice.* Smoking and Tobacco Control Monograph No. 5. NIH Publication No. 94–3693. Rockville, MD, U.S. Department of Health and Human Services, 1994.

57. Fiore MC, Bailey WC, Cohen SJ, et al: *Smoking Cessation. Clinical Practice Guideline No. 18.* AHCPR Publi-

cation No. 96-0692. Rockville, MD, U.S. Department of Health and Human Services, Public Health Service, Agency for Health Care Policy and Research, 1996.

58. Smith TA, House RF Jr, Crogham IT, et al: Nicotine patch therapy in adolescent smokers. *Pediatrics* 1996; 98:659–667.

59. Colby S, Monti P, Barnett N, et al: Motivational interviewing with teen smokers in a hospital setting: 3-month treatment outcome results. *Ann Behav Med* 1997; 19:S049.

60. Miller WR, Rollnick S: *Motivational Interviewing: Preparing People to Change Addictive Behavior.* New York, Guilford Press, 1991.

61. Sussman S, Lichtman K, Ritt A, et al: Effects of thirty-four adolescent tobacco use and prevention trials on regular users of tobacco products. *Substance Use and Misuse.* (Still in press.)

62. Barker D: Reasons for tobacco use and symptoms of nicotine withdrawal among adolescent and young adult tobacco users—United States. *MMWR* 1993; 43:745–750.

63. Klesges R, Haddock K, Lando H, et al: Efficacy of forced smoking cessation and an adjunctive behavioral treatment on long-term smoking rates. *J Consult Clin Psychol.* (Still in press.)

64. U.S. Department of Health and Human Services: *Tobacco Use Among U.S. Racial/Ethnic Minority Groups—African Americans, American Indians and Alaska Natives, Asian Americans and Pacific Islanders, and Hispanics: A Report of the Surgeon General.* Atlanta, GA, U.S. Department of Health and Human Services, Centers for Disease Control and Prevention, National Center for Chronic Disease Prevention and Health Promotion, Office on Smoking and Health, 1998.

65. Lam TH, He Y, Li LS, et al: Mortality attributable to cigarette smoking in China. *JAMA* 1997; 278:1505–1508.

66. Lichtenstein E, Glasgow RE: Smoking cessation: what have we learned over the past decade? *J Consult Clin Psychol* 1992; 60:518–527.

67. Lando H, Rolnick S, Klevan D, et al: Telephone support as an adjunct to transdermal nicotine. *Am J Public Health* 1997; 87:1670–1674.

68. Lichtenstein E, Glasgow RE: A pragmatic framework for smoking cessation: implications for clinical and public health programs. *Psychol Addict Behav* 1997; 11:142–151.

69. DiClemente C, Prochaska J, Fairhurst S, et al: The process of smoking cessation: an analysis of precontemplation, contemplation, and preparation stages of change. *J Consult Clin Psychol* 1991; 59:295–304.

70. U.S. Department of Health and Human Services: *The Health Consequences of Smoking: Nicotine Addiction: A Report of the Surgeon General.* Rockville, MD, U.S. Department of Health and Human Services, Public Health Service, Centers for Disease Control, Center for Health Promotion and Education, Office on Smoking and Health, 1994.

71. Lichenstein E, Harris DE, Birchler GR, et al: Comparison of rapid smoking, warm, smoky air, and attention placebo in the modification of smoking behavior. *J Consult Clin Psychol* 1973; 40:92–98.

72. Poole AD, Sanson-Fisher RW, German GA: The rapid-smoking technique: therapeutic effectiveness. *Behav Res Ther* 1981; 389–397.

73. Resnick JH: Effects of stimulus satiation on the over-learned maladaptive response of cigarette smoking. *J Consult Clin Psychol* 1968; 32:501–505.

74. Lando HA: A comparison of excessive and rapid smoking in the modification of chronic smoking behavior. *J Consult Clin Psychol* 1975; 43:350–355.

75. Hauser R: Rapid smoking as a technique of behavior modification: caution in selection of subjects. *J Consult Clin Psychol* 1974; 42:625.

76. Powell DR, McCann BS: The effects of a multiple treatment program and maintenance procedures on smoking cessation. *Prev Med* 1981; 10:94–104.

77. Tiffany ST, Martin EM, Baker TB: Treatments for cigarette smoking: an evaluation of the contributions of aversion and counseling procedures. *Behav Res Ther* 1986; 24:437–452.

78. Elliott R, Tighe T: Breaking the cigarette habit: effects of a technique involving threatened loss of money. *Psychol Rec* 1968; 18:503–513.

79. Lando HA: Aversive conditioning and contingency management in the treatment of smoking. *J Consult Clin Psychol* 1976;44:312.

80. Lichenstein E, Glasgow RE, Abrams DB: Social support in smoking cessation: in search of effective interventions. *Behav Res Ther* 1986; 17:607–619.

81. Brandon TH, Tiffany ST, Baker TB: The process of smoking relapse, in Tims FM, Leukefeld CG (eds): *Relapse and Recovery in Drug Abuse.* NIDA Research Monograph 72. DHHS Publication No. (ADM) 86-1473, Rockville, MD, U.S. Department of Health and Human Services, Public Health Service, Alcohol, Drug Abuse, and Mental Health Administration, National Institute on Drug Abuse, 1986.

82. Shiffman S: Relapse following smoking cessation: a situational analysis. *J Consult Clin Psychol* 1982; 50:71–86.

83. Hatsukami D, Lando H: Smoking cessation. In: Ott PJ, Tartar RE, Ammerman RT (eds): *Sourcebook on Substance Use and Abuse. Etiology, Epidemiology, Assessment, and Treatment.* Needham Heights, MA, Allyn & Bacon, 1999:399–415.

84. Abrams DB: Roles of psychosocial stress, smoking cues and coping in smoking-relapse prevention. *Health Psychol* 1986; 5(suppl):91–92.

85. Shapiro D, Tursky B, Schwartz GE, et al: Smoking on cue: a behavioral approach to smoking reduction. *J Health Soc Behav* 1971; 12:108–113.

86. Flaxman J: Quitting smoking now or later: gradual, abrupt, immediate, and delayed quitting. *Behav Res Ther* 1978; 9:260–270.

87. Foxx RM, Brown RA: A nicotine fading and self-monitoring program to produce cigarette abstinence or controlled smoking. *J Appl Behav Anal* 1979; 12:111–125.

88. McGovern PG, Lando HA: Reduced nicotine exposure and abstinence outcome in two nicotine fading methods. *Addict Behav* 1991; 16:11–20.

89. Hall SM, Rugg D, Tunstall C, et al: Preventing relapse to cigarette smoking by behavioral skill training. *J Consult Clin Psychol* 1984; 52:372–382.

90. Lando H, Sipfle CL, McGovern PG: A statewide public service smoking cessation clinic. *Am J Health Promotion* 1995; 10:9–11.

91. McFarland MI: When five became twenty-five: a silver anniversary of the five-day plan to stop smoking. *Adventist Heritage* 1986; 11:57–64.

92. Lando H, McGovern P, Barrios F, et al: Comparative evaluation of American Cancer Society and American Lung Association smoking cessation clinics. *Am J Public Health* 1990; 80:554–559.

93. Lando H, Johnson K, McGovern P, et al: Smoking patterns and interest in quitting in Urban American Indians. *Public Health Rep* 1992; 107:340–344.

94. Orleans CT, Schoenbach VJ, Wagner EH, et al: Self-help quit smoking intervention: effects of self-help materials, social support intervention, and telephone counseling. *J Consult Clin Psychol* 1991; 59:439–448.

95. Zhu S-H, Stretch V, Balabanis M, et al: Telephone counseling for smoking cessation: effects of single-session and multiple-session interventions. *J Consult Clin Psychol* 1996; 64:202–221.

96. Velicer WF, Prochaska JO, Bellis JM, et al: An expert system intervention for smoking cessation. *Addict Behav* 1993; 18:269–290.

97. Strecher VJ, Kreuter M, Den Boer DJ, et al: The effects of computer-tailored smoking cessation messages in family practice settings. *J Fam Pract* 1994; 39:262–270.

98. Pallonen UE, Velicer WF, Prochaska JO, et al: Computer-based smoking cessation interventions in adolescents: description, feasibility, and six-month follow-up findings. *Subst Use Misuse* 1998; 33:1–31.

99. American Lung Association: *Quit Smoking Action Plan.* New York: American Lung Association, 1998.

100. Hurt RD, Sachs DPL, Glover ED, et al: Comparison of sustained-release bupropion and placebo for smoking cessation. *N Engl J Med* 1997; 337:1195–1202.

101. Stapleton JA, Sutherland G, Russell MAH: How much relapse after one year erode effectiveness of smoking cessation treatments? Long term follow up of randomised trial of nicotine nasal spray. *BMJ* 1998; 316:830–831.

102. Hjalmarson A, Nisson F, Sjostrom L, et al: Nicotine inhaler smoking cessation. *Arch Intern Med* 1997; 157:1721–1728.

103. Abrams DB, Orleans CT, Niaura RS, et al: Integrating individual and public health perspectives for treatment of tobacco dependence under managed health care: a combined stepped-care and matching model. *Ann Behav Med* 1996; 18:290–304.

104. National Cancer Institute: Tobacco and the clinician: interventions for medical and dental practice. NIH Publication No. 94–3693. *Monogr Natl Cancer Inst* 1994; 5:1–22.

105. Ockene JK: Smoking intervention: the expanding role of the physician. *Am J Public Health* 1994; 77:782–783.

106. Curry SJ, Grothaus LC, McAfee T, et al: Use and cost effectiveness of smoking-cessation services under four insurance plans in a health maintenance organization. *N Engl J Med* 1998; 339:673–679.

107. Jeffery RW, Forster JL, French SA, et al: The Healthy Worker Project: a work-site intervention for weight control and smoking cessation. *Am J Public Health* 1993; 83:395–401.

108. Sorenson G, Thompson B, Glanz K, et al, for the Working Well Trial: Work site–based cancer prevention: primary results from the Working Well Trial. *Am J Public Health* 1996; 86:939–947.

109. Carleton RA, Lasater TM, Assaf AR, et al, and the Pawtucket Heart Health Program Writing Group: The Pawtucket Heart Health Program: community changes in cardiovascular risk factors and projected disease risk. *Am J Public Health* 1995; 85:777–785.

110. Farquhar JW, Fortmann SP, Flora JA, et al: Effects of community-wide education on cardiovascular disease risk factors. *JAMA* 1990; 264:359–365.

111. Lando H, Pechacek TF, Pirie PL, et al: Changes in adult cigarette smoking in the Minnesota Heart Health Program. *Am J Public Health* 1995; 85:201–208.

112. Pechacek TF, Lando HA, Nothwehr F, et al: Quit and Win: a community-wide approach to smoking cessation. *Tobacco Control* 1994; 3:236–241.

113. The COMMIT Research Group: Community Intervention Trial for Smoking Cessation (COMMIT): I. Cohort results from a four-year community intervention. *Am J Public Health* 1995; 85:183–192.

114. The COMMIT Research Group: Community Intervention Trial for Smoking Cessation (COMMIT): II. Changes in adult cigarette smoking prevalence. *Am J Public Health* 1995; 85:193–200.

115. Manley M, Lynn W, Epps RP, et al: The American Stop Smoking Intervention Study for cancer prevention: an overview. *Tobacco Control* 1997; 6:S5-S11.

116. Manley MW, Pierce JP, Gilpin EA, et al: Impact of the American Stop Smoking Intervention Study on cigarette consumption. *Tobacco Control* 1997; 6:S12–S16.

117. Eisner MD, Smith AK, Blanc PD: Bartenders' respiratory health after establishment of smoke-free bars and taverns. *JAMA* 1998; 280:1909–1914.

118. Lightfoot JM, Glantz SA: Short-term economic and health benefits of smoking cessation. Myocardial infarction and stroke. *Circulation* 1997; 96:1089–1096.

119. Kannel WB: Curbing the tobacco menace. *Circulation* 1997; 96:1070.

120. Centers for Disease Control and Prevention: Perspectives in disease prevention and health promotion: smoking. *MMWR* 1997; 46:444–451.

121. Hirayama T: Lung cancer in Japan: effects of nutrition and passive smoking. In: Mizell M, Correa P (eds): *Lung Cancer: Causes and Prevention*. New York, Verlag Chemie International, 1984: 175–195.

122. Garland C, Barrett-Connor E, Suarez L, et al: Effects of passive smoking on ischemic heart disease mortality of non-smokers. *Am J Epidemiol* 1985; 121:645–650.

123. Svendsen KH, Kuller LH, Martin MJ, Ockene JK: Effects of passive smoking in the Multiple Risk Intervention Trial. *Am J Epidemiol* 1987; 126:783–795.

124. Helsing KJ, Sandler DP, Comstock GW, Chee E: Heart disease mortality in nonsmokers living with smokers. *Am J Epidemiol* 1988; 127:915–922.

125. Hole DJ, Gillis CR, Chopra C, Hawthorne VM: Passive smoking and cardiorespiratory health in a general population in the west of Scotland. *BMJ* 1989; 299:423–427.

126. Layard MW: Ischemic heart disease and spousal smoking in the National Mortality Followback Survey. *Regul Toxicol Pharmacol* 1995; 21:180–183.

127. Tunstall-Pedoe H, Brown CA, Woodward M, Travendale R: Passive smoking by self report and serum cotinine and the prevalence of respiratory and coronary heart disease in the Scottish Heart Health Study. *J Epidemiol Community Health* 1995; 49:139–143.

128. Everett SA, Husten CG, Warren CW, et al: Trends in tobacco use among high school students in the United States, 1991–1995. *J Sch Health* 1998; 69:137–140.

CHAPTER 10

Obesity, Weight Control, and Cardiovascular Disease

Karen C. McCowen
George L. Blackburn

Obesity is a factor of significant etiologic importance in the development of cardiovascular disease (CVD).[1] Statistics available for the prevalence of obesity in Western (especially U.S.) societies indicate that it is a health hazard of staggering proportion, despite an ever-increasing pursuit of thinness among certain sections of the population.[2] Since 1985, when its first consensus conference on the topic was convened, the National Institutes of Health (NIH) has recognized that obesity prevention and treatment should be medical priorities. In response to the mounting evidence relating adiposity to coronary heart disease (CHD), the American Heart Association recently reclassified obesity as a major, modifiable risk factor for CHD.[3]

Obesity is a risk factor for the development of hypertension, diabetes mellitus, and hyperlipidemia, classic contributors to coronary and vascular disease.[4] In an Australian study, cross-sectional analysis of a large population of blood donors demonstrated that being overweight was associated with high cholesterol, triglycerides (TG), and systolic blood pressure in men and with high cholesterol and systolic blood pressure in women.[5] There was marked clustering of elevated values of these variables in the heavier subjects, while the leanest were remarkably free of high values. In contrast, a Scottish study of untreated hypertensives found a relation between adiposity and blood pressure only in male nonsmokers.[6] Other obesity-associated factors that may have deleterious effects on coronary atherosclerosis include obstructive sleep apnea and hem-

orrheological abnormalities such as low levels of plasminogen activator inhibitor-1 (PAI-1) and higher blood viscosity (Table 10–1). Obesity also engenders insulin resistance, with consequent hyperinsulinemia; elevated insulin levels may be linked to atherosclerosis, although this is controversial. Of increasing importance is the role of intraabdominal fat, estimated by waist circumference, which may relate to the insulin-resistance syndrome and inflammation. In addition, weight gain during young adult life may be one of the most important determinants of cardiovascular risk.[7]

Obesity: Epidemiology, Assessment, and Relation to Risk

Definition and Prevalence of Obesity

Obesity, meaning an excess of total body fat, is most typically defined by body mass index (BMI). This is calculated by dividing an individual's weight (in kilograms) by the square of the height (in square meters) for both men and women. Table 10–2 documents the range of normal, overweight, and underweight according to standard criteria for BMI.

The National Health and Nutrition Examination Survey (NHANES) has been documenting heights and weights of representative samples of the population for several decades.[8] NHANES has usually defined overweight as a BMI equal to or greater than 27.8 for men and equal to or greater than 27.3 for women, representing sex-specific 85th percentile

TABLE 10–1 Risk Factors for Atherosclerosis and Vascular Disease Associated with Obesity

Hypertension
Dyslipidemia
Diabetes mellitus (type 2)
Hyperinsulinemia
Obstructive sleep apnea
Low levels of plasminogen activator inhibitor
Hyperviscosity

TABLE 10–2 Standard Criteria for Body Mass Index (BMI)

	BMI, kg/m^2
Underweight	18.5
Healthy weight	18.5–24.9
Overweight	25.0–29.9
Obese	30–39.9
Morbid obesity	≥40

values for the survey of 1976–1980. However, desirable weight is probably lower than this. The U.S. Department of Health and Human Services and the American Heart Association define overweight as a BMI above 25 and obesity as a BMI above 30.[3,9] But it is recognized that the measurement of excess weight is not an exact science. The BMI definition does not take into account body fat distribution; those with a central or abdominal body fat pattern are generally at higher cardiovascular risk.[3]

Figure 10–1 depicts the increasing prevalence of both overweight and obesity from the early 1960s through 1994, when the most recent NHANES was completed. As can be seen, the most recent information indicates that almost 60 percent of men and 50 percent of women are obese or overweight for the population as a whole, although certain ethnic minorities (notably African Americans and Mexican-Americans) have an even higher prevalence of this problem. From the same survey, 20 percent of males and 25 percent of females were found to have a BMI above 30, thus falling into the "obese" category.

Most epidemiologic studies have shown that being overweight or obese is associated with higher mortality.[10–12] The Nurses' Health Study showed that in women who were "never smokers" without a recent history of weight loss, a BMI of 27 to 29 was associated with a relative risk (RR) of death of 1.6 [95 percent confidence intervals (CI) = 1.1 to 2.5], a BMI of 29 to 32 with a RR of 2.1 (95 percent CI = 1.4 to 3.2), and a BMI equal to or greater than 32 with a RR of 2.2 (95 percent CI = 1.4 to 3.4) as compared with the leanest cohort, with a BMI below

19.[12] Similarly in never-smoking male alumni of Harvard University, a BMI equal to or greater than 26 was associated with a RR of 1.67 (95 percent CI = 1.29 to 2.17), compared with those with a BMI below 22.5.[13] In these studies, risk of death was greater with higher BMI. Mortality was lowest in the leanest participants, without evidence for a J- or U-shaped curve when smokers and those with intercurrent illnesses were excluded. With advancing age, the relationship between obesity and mortality is less apparent, as weight loss related to illness becomes increasingly important.[14] It is less clear that obesity in ethnic minorities in the U.S. is associated with the same increase in overall mortality, as good longitudinal data are sparse.

Obesity and Hypertension

There are many cross-sectional and longitudinal studies that delineate the association between obesity and the presence of hypertension. The etiology of the link between excess body weight and elevation in blood pressure has not been completely explained.[15] Across the spectrum of epidemiologic studies, the existence of this relationship is consistent. In the Nurses' Health Study, excess weight and even modest weight gain substantially increased the risk for hypertension.[16] For each 1 kg/m^2 increment in current BMI, the relative risk of hypertension was 12 percent. Women with a BMI above 31 had a relative risk of 6.3 (95 percent CI = 5.8 to 6.9) compared with the leanest women. Weight gain after age 18 of 1 kg elevated the risk of hypertension by 5 percent. The INTERSALT[17]

FIGURE 10–1 Increasing prevalence of overweight (BMI > 25 kg/m²) in U.S. adults (*A*) and of obesity (*B*) (BMI > 30 kg/m²). (Adapted from Kuczmarski et al.,[8] with permission.)

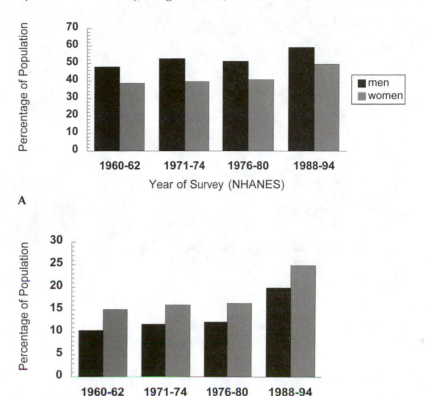

and NHANES cross-sectional studies showed a direct correlation between BMI and blood pressure. The National Heart Foundation of Australia surveyed over 5500 persons and showed almost identical findings.[18] In addition, they noted that overweight hypertensives were less likely to achieve normal blood pressure control on treatment. The Intersalt study has shown that an additional 10 kg of body mass is associated with higher systolic (3 mmHg) and diastolic (2.2 mmHg) blood pressures.[17]

One pathophysiologic explanation for the association between hypertension and obesity may be hyperinsulinemia. Skeletal muscle resistance to the action of insulin is present in obesity. In order to maintain normal glucose homeostasis, a compensa-

tory elevation in plasma insulin concentrations is seen. Fasting and postprandial hyperinsulinemia is well described in the obese. Insulin may elevate blood pressure by affecting renal sodium retention and, through activation of the sympathetic nervous system, raising peripheral resistance. Accordingly, many cross-sectional studies demonstrate that insulin concentrations correlate with blood pressure.

Obesity and Diabetes

Obesity is also a major risk factor for the development of type 2 diabetes. Underlying (possibly inherited) insulin resistance is compounded by the fact that obesity worsens insulin sensitivity. Ultimately,

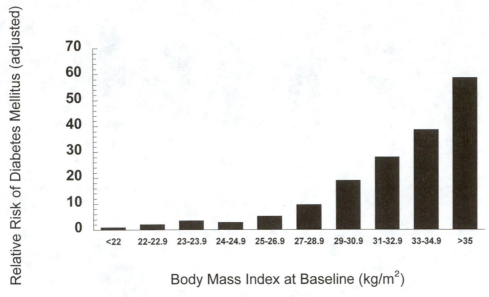

FIGURE 10–2 The risk of developing diabetes mellitus over 8 years is increased for each increment in BMI. Note that the risk was significantly elevated for all BMI ranges ≥22. (Data from the Nurses' Health Study,[22] with permission.)

pancreatic production of insulin becomes exhausted, with the occurrence of hyperglycemia and frank diabetes mellitus. Obesity may account for 50 percent or more of the variance in insulin sensitivity in the general population; abdominal fat bears a particularly strong relation to insulin resistance.[7]

The association of higher BMI with increased rates of type 2 diabetes has been shown in diverse populations, both those with high[19,20] and low[21] rates of diabetes. Studies of the Pima Indian tribe, in which diabetes is rampant, show the importance of this association. The incidence of diabetes was strongly related to preceding obesity, with approximately 0.8 cases per 1000 person-years for BMI below 20, in comparison with 72 cases for BMI above 40. Interestingly, diabetes was extremely rare in this tribe in the 1940s, when the diet consisted of complex carbohydrates with very low amounts of fat. Exposure of the Pima Indians to a more sedentary lifestyle and a change in their diet to a more typical "American"

high-calorie, high-fat type has led to obesity, and a prevalence of diabetes that exceeds 50 percent in adults.

In the Nurses' Health Study, even among women of average BMI, 23 to 23.9, the relative risk of developing diabetes was 3.6 (2.3 to 5.1) times that of women with a BMI below 22.[22] The risk continued to increase above this level in proportion to the BMI (Fig. 10–2). Weight at age 18 bore no relation to future rate of diabetes; instead, weight gain after this age was a major determinant of risk. For an increase of 20 to 35 kg, the relative risk was 11.3, and for an increase of more than 35 kg, the relative risk rose to 17.3. Thus, even for women of average weight, the relation between BMI and risk of diabetes is continuous. Similarly, in the Health Professionals Study of more than 50,000 male health professionals, BMI was strongly linked to risk of diabetes.[23] From multivariate analysis controlling for smoking, age, and family history, a BMI above 35 yielded a relative risk of 42 (95 percent CI = 22.0 to 80.6) for the development of diabetes.

Obesity and Dyslipidemia

Obesity strongly affects lipoprotein metabolism and is related to higher low-density-lipoprotein cholesterol (LDL) and triglycerides (TGs) and lower levels of high-density-lipoprotein cholesterol (HDL). Weight loss reduces TGs, increases HDL, and lowers LDL, but with HDL increases being more pronounced in women and LDL changes of greater magnitude in men.[7] Body weight is possibly the most important determinant of rates of cholesterol synthesis in obese persons. Rates of cholesterol production correlate with excess body mass;[24] one study determined that each kilogram increase in body fat was associated with increased synthesis of cholesterol, 20 mg/dL.[25] There is also some evidence that the activity of the rate-limiting enzyme for cholesterol synthesis, HMG-CoA reductase, is reduced after energy restriction. The "low HDL, high TG" phenotype is the most frequently described dyslipidemia among the obese in both longitudinal and cross-sectional studies.[26,27] In the Framingham Offspring Study, increased levels of BMI are associated with lower HDL and higher LDL, as seen in Fig. 10–3. A 10-kg/m^2 increment in BMI is associated with a 3.2-mg/dL (in women) to 10 mg/dL (in young men) lower HDL cholesterol level.[28] Cross-sectional data indicate that this magnitude of weight difference may cause a 10-mg/dL rise in LDL cholesterol and is associated with a more atherogenic (small and dense) LDL particle.[29]

Obesity in Childhood

In children as in adults, obesity is associated with a clustering of metabolic risk factors that increase the chance of CVD in later life. In a recent Taiwanese study of over 1300 school-age children, about 70 percent of obese boys had one cardiovascular risk factor; the prevalence of two or more risk factors was consistently higher among obese than among non-obese children.[30] NHANES has documented increasing prevalence of overweight between the ages of 4

and 17 years (Fig. 10–4), although children younger than this are not so affected.[31,32]

Obesity and Vascular Disease

Although obesity is associated with cardiovascular risk factors, a pertinent question is whether obesity is a risk factor for CHD and stroke *themselves*.[33]

The Nurse's Health Study has observed rates of incident CHD in a large (>115,000) group of female nurses since the 1970s, using frequent questionnaires. Over 14 years of follow-up, almost 1300 cases of CHD were ascertained.[34,35] After controlling for age, smoking, menopausal status, estrogen therapy and family history, it was determined that risk of CHD rose with increasing BMI above 23 (Fig. 10–5A). This was striking because it indicated elevated risk even within the "normal" range for BMI. For women with a BMI above 29, the relative risk compared with those whose BMI was below 21 was 3.6. Similarly, a history of weight gain, even in women of normal weight, was strongly associated with the development of CHD (Fig. 10–5B). For stroke, which has been studied less intensively than heart attack, events caused by ischemia (i.e., not by hemorrhage) are associated with overweight in a variety of studies.[36–38]

NHANES reported a relative risk of 1.5 for CVD in later life for a woman with a BMI above 29 versus the referent population (BMI < 21).[39] Similar findings have been reported for men[40] and many other populations, with the notable exception of the Pima Indian tribe, in which rates of CHD are strangely low, despite obesity and the plethora of other risk factors endemic in this group.[41]

In addition, obesity has been associated with myocardial hypertrophy independent of hypertension and with higher rates of heart failure in the Framingham cohort.[1] Moderate impairment of diastolic function was found in over 50 percent of a group with morbid obesity studied by echocardiography.[42] A different study found an incidence of approximately 50 percent for increased thickness of the septum and left ventricular wall, cardiac chamber enlargement, and impaired contractility.[43]

FIGURE 10–3 Effect of change in weight over 10 years on HDL (*A*) and LDL (*B*) cholesterol for men and women. (Data from the Framingham Offspring Study,[28] with permission.)

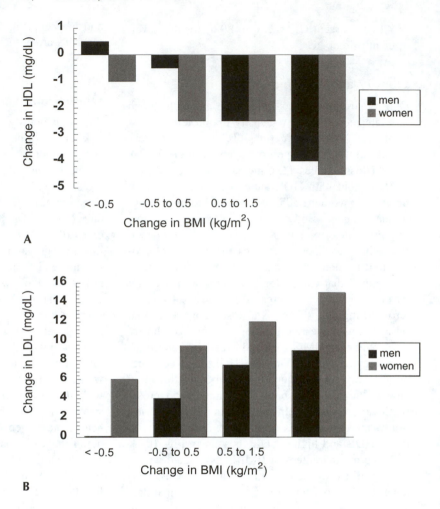

Visceral Adiposity: A Better Predictor of Risk?

An increasingly recognized part of the spectrum of obesity is the concept of central or visceral obesity. Knowledge of BMI gives an incomplete picture of the magnitude of risk, since BMI cannot discriminate between persons with adiposity that is predominantly subcutaneous in site and those with excessive fat depots located in the abdomen. In addition, short stature in itself has been associated with higher morbidity and mortality. Thus, among obese persons, BMI reflects the negative effects of being both fat and/or short. However, central adiposity is associated with greater levels of insulin resistance and hyperinsulinemia, higher blood pressure, and exaggerated dyslipidemia.[44,45]

Among the largest studies to date examining the relation of central obesity to CHD is the Nurses' Health Study, where a waist-hip ratio (WHR) of 0.88

FIGURE 10–4   Increasing prevalence of overweight in U.S. children and adolescents. Overweight was defined here as >85 centile for a population surveyed in the 1960s for the National Health Education Survey.[31]

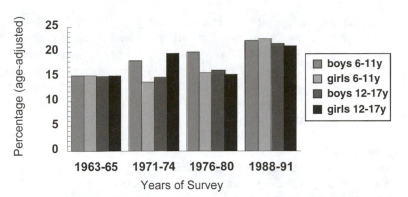

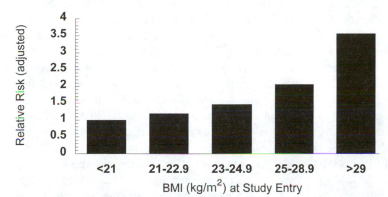

FIGURE 10–5   Effect of obesity on rates of coronary disease. Baseline BMI is correlated with risk over the subsequent 14 years of the development of coronary disease (*A*), and history of weight gain after the age of 18 years is also associated with increased risk (*B*). Note that the risk is significantly increased for BMI ≥23 and weight gain ≥5 kg. (Data adapted from a report of the Nurses' Health Study.[34])

A

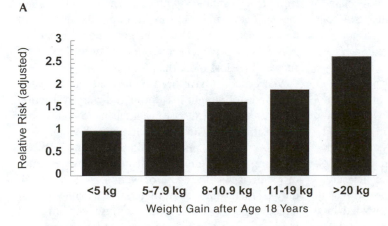

B

or higher was associated with a relative risk of 3.25 (95 percent CI = 1.78 to 5.95) for CHD compared with a WHR of less than 0.72. A waist circumference of 38 in. or more was associated with a relative risk of 3.06 (95 percent CI = 1.54 to 6.10).[46]

In another study, trunkal obesity and the size of fat cells in the abdomen displayed highly significant correlations with insulin and glucose levels following a glucose challenge, whereas thigh and subcutaneous fat did not.[47] The same workers studied a group of obese, premenopausal women and showed negative correlations between deep abdominal fat mass and HDL, or HDL/LDL ratio.[48] The presence of increased abdominal fat is an important predictor of cardiac risk in the absence of obesity.[49] Abdominal obesity as determined by waist circumference but not BMI predicted risk of stroke in the Physician's Health Study.[50] The pathophysiologic basis for this difference is likely that visceral adipocytes have higher rates of lipolysis; thus portal vein free fatty acid (FFA) concentration is increased. When the liver sees a large pool of FFA, both gluconeogenesis and very low density lipoprotein (VLDL) secretion are increased. Insulin clearance is also diminished, which leads to systemic hyperinsulinemia. Hyperlipidemia in the peripheral circulation is associated with decreased rates of glucose uptake. This combination of insulin resistance and increased gluconeogenesis can lead to impairment in glucose tolerance and, ultimately, to the development of diabetes. Syndrome X is the name given to a constellation of these metabolic risk factors associated with central adiposity.

The Measurement of Visceral Adiposity

Clinical markers of visceral adiposity include increased waist circumference or WHR above population means. Many of the early studies in this field used WHR to define abdominal obesity. However, waist circumference is a more accurate reflection of abdominal fat and, of course, is easier to measure. Studies have compared waist circumference with abdominal fat as measured directly by computed tomography or magnetic resonance imaging and found the former to be a reasonable substitute for the latter. It is probably unnecessary to invest in more sophis-

ticated measures of obesity such as total body electrical conductivity, bioelectrical impedance, or dual-energy x-ray absorptiometry, since they are costly and time-consuming. A major advantage of simple weight and circumference measures is the potential for patients to perform these themselves and track their own progress. In addition, the studies that have helped us gauge the extent of weight loss required all involved measurement of BMI or waist circumference.[51]

Weight Control and Risk Reduction

For an individual patient interested in disease prevention, initial measures of height, weight, and waist circumference should be performed. Criteria for normal BMI are defined in Table 10–2. Waist circumference above 35 in. in women or 40 in. in men has been shown to be associated with increased risk for CHD. The presence of high BMI or waist circumference, in the presence of willingness to lose weight, should prompt consideration of a hypocaloric diet. While the patient follows such a diet, both body weight and waist circumference should be monitored. The only randomized controlled study of weight loss with cardiac morbidity and mortality as endpoints was performed in Indian coronary patients following myocardial infarction who were randomized to either (1) a diet that was low in saturated fat and rich in fruits and vegetables with frequent weight-loss advice or (2) to a "usual care" group. This resulted in approximately a 50 percent reduction in cardiac events and 45 percent lower mortality in those who successfully lost more than 5 kg over the year.[52]

Many studies have been performed that focus on the effects of weight loss through dietary restriction (with or without exercise) as a means to control hypertension and dyslipidemia. In general, weight loss in obese persons results in improvement in blood pressure, dyslipidemia, and diabetes. However, rates of recidivism with regain of weight are substantial; only a small minority of dieters are capable of sustained success. Those who exercise concurrently, however, appear to maintain weight loss better.

Consequently, many obese people have had recurrent cycles of loss followed by regain of weight.

Recent articles have demonstrated that a history of weight cycling in itself may be a risk factor for cardiac events, although this is controversial.[53,54] In a prospective longitudinal study of over 33,000 women in Iowa who were sent questionnaires over a 30-year period, increasing cardiovascular risk factors were seen across the quartiles of increasing weight cycling.[55] To some extent, however, this was confounded by unhealthy behaviors in those who cycled frequently, although statistical significance remained when these behaviors were factored out. Therefore, methods of weight control that have prolonged results would be of immense value for the overweight population for permanent reduction of coronary risk factors.

Weight Control and Dyslipidemia

Weight reduction through caloric restriction has been associated with significant reductions in LDL cholesterol in many studies. A meta-analysis of more than 70 randomized controlled trials found a correlation between fall in LDL and the amount of weight lost.[56] The effects of diet and weight loss on changes in HDL cholesterol have been more variable. It is clear that the institution of a diet low in saturated fat causes a fall in HDL as well as LDL.[57,58] However, when such a diet is prolonged, weight loss occurs and is maintained, and HDL returns to baseline and may subsequently rise.[59,60] The ultimate effect in most studies is a sizable improvement (decrease) in the LDL/HDL ratio.

There are many studies of dietary intervention for hyperlipidemia in the published literature. However, many of these were carried out over just weeks to months without long-term follow up. Although such studies have demonstrated sizable reductions in lipids (TG reductions between 2 and 36 percent, LDL reductions between 3 and 32 percent, and HDL changes from -7 to $+18$ percent compared with control groups), such short-term data are of little practical use to the clinician facing an overweight or obese patient with a lifelong health problem. What is notable is that, in those studies in which results have been analyzed by gender, the rise in HDL by dietary restriction alone is consistently less for

women than for men. In one typical example, moderately overweight sedentary persons were assigned randomly to one of three interventions: control; a hypocaloric diet comprising 55 percent carbohydrate, 30 percent total fat—with saturated fat 10 percent or less—and cholesterol below 300 mg/dL; or the same diet in combination with exercise. This study lasted for 1 year and resulted in significant weight loss and reduction in body fat in both intervention groups.[61] However, the combined program effected greater loss of weight and fat. For men, exercise plus diet increased HDL significantly more than diet alone. In contrast, HDL decreased in the women who dieted, although exercise prevented that fall in the combination group.

Reduction in HDL has unfortunately been a consistent finding, especially in women who start a diet that is low in saturated fat.[59] Often this is of sufficient magnitude that the overall effect on lipid status is to worsen (increase) the LDL/HDL ratio. What remains unclear is whether this is bad for cardiovascular health. In women, HDL has been shown in some analyses to be a stronger risk factor for coronary disease than LDL.[62–64] However, if it is lowered in conjunction with an LDL-lowering diet, the overall effect may be beneficial. While it is true that, within a population, level of HDL is clearly inversely correlated with the chance of developing CHD, ecologic studies[65] demonstrate that populations with naturally low-fat diets have lower levels of both LDL and HDL, and correspondingly lower rates of heart attack and cardiac death.

The efficacy of aerobic exercise alone to alter lipid profiles has been controversial. One meta-analysis indicated that exercise training alone *without* weight loss yielded no overall change in HDL.[66] Weight loss was compared with exercise training in a study of 170 obese, middle-aged men over a 9-month period randomized to diet with weight loss, exercise without weight loss, or a control group.[67] The diet group lost 10 percent of their body weight; the exercisers lost body fat without alteration in BMI. A reduction was seen in the dieters' LDL (7 percent), fasting insulin (18 percent), and TGs (18 percent), whereas HDL rose 13 percent. Exercise alone had a lesser benefit on these parameters: LDL and fasting insulin, no change; TGs, 7 percent decrease; and HDL, 5 percent increase—although only the LDL was different from that of controls. In the subsequent multivariate analysis, the major independent predictor of improvement in HDL was the amount of body fat lost. Interestingly, older men saw fewer beneficial changes than younger. In a different study of middle-aged men matched for age, endurance training was carried out over 9 months with improvements in $\dot{V}_{O_2max}$.[68] When stratified for body weight, HDL rose by the end of the program in lean and moderately obese participants (BMI < 30) but did not change in those with a BMI of 31 to 37. Thus, especially in the obese population, weight loss may be mandatory in addition to exercise to improve the lipid profile.

There have been fewer published trials of the effect of weight loss on lipid profiles in obese children; however, in general the results are close to those observed in adults.[69,70] In one study, 32 children received dietary and exercise counseling over a period of one year and were observed over the second year.[71] An average of 15 kg was lost initially and maintained for 2 years. Fasting hyperinsulinemia was reduced, and favorable effects were seen on HDL cholesterol and the total/HDL cholesterol ratio. Other studies of weight reduction in adolescents indicate that those

with abdominal obesity exhibit more beneficial changes in the atherogenic risk-factor profile than do those with gluteal-femoral obesity.[72]

Weight Control and Hypertension

For hypertension, even moderate weight loss in overweight and obese persons can effect reductions in both systolic and diastolic blood pressure. There are several large population studies in which normotensive but overweight individuals have had lowering of blood pressure and reduction in the incidence of hypertension with a hypocaloric diet.[73–77] These trials are described more fully in Table 10–3. With successful dieting and weight reduction, left ventricular mass has been shown to regress.[78] One possible confounder is that hypocaloric diets are often low in sodium. However, it is clear that when comparisons have been made between overweight subjects randomized to low-salt versus low-calorie diets, salt reduction is relatively ineffective without weight loss.[79] Several studies have compared weight reduction with pharmacotherapy for hypertension. In general, blood pressures were lower with drug treatment; however, it is clear that the addition of lifestyle modification reduced the need for medication and had an overall effect to reduce vascular risk.[80]

TABLE 10–3 Effect of Weight Loss on Blood Pressure and Incidence of Hypertension as Compared with "Usual Diet" Group in Recent Clinical Trials

Reference Number	Trial Number	Number of Patients	Duration, months	Weight Loss versus Usual Care, kg	BP Difference (mmHg) from "Usual Diet"	Percent Remaining Normotensive versus Placebo
77	TOHP*	2250	48	1.9	1.1 / 1	62% versus 56%
76	HCP†	189	48	1.8	0.6 / 1.5	39% versus 5%
75	HPT‡	841	36	3.4	2.4 / 1.8	61.3% versus 71.8%¶
73	TAIM§	878	6	4.76	2.8 / 2.5	

*Trials of Hypertension Prevention.
†Hypertension Control Program.
‡Hypertension Prevention Trial.
§Trial of Antihypertensive Interventions and Management Study.
¶ p = not significant.

Also notable about these trials, so many of which were relatively long-term, was the fact that regain of lost weight was the rule—not unexpectedly—with return of blood pressure toward baseline values. Recently, a clinical trial evaluating the effects of dietary patterns on blood pressure (Dietary Approaches to Stop Hypertension, or DASH) was published and showed that the addition of low-fat dairy and generous helpings of fruits and vegetables to the diet was associated with lowering of both systolic and diastolic blood pressures (by 5.5 and 3.0 mmHg, respectively, in the entire sample, and by 11.4 and 5.5 mmHg, respectively, in those with preexisting hypertension, relative to the control diet low in fruits, vegetables, and diary products, all $p < .001$).[81] By maximizing palatability, this occurred without undue perturbation of cultural dietary norms. Participants in the treatment group received the same salt allowance as the control group. Striking improvements in blood pressure were seen with the diet intervention. Such a diet is probably one that could be maintained for long periods of time with reasonable compliance. For obese patients with hypertension as their main cardiac risk factor, in whom weight loss through a hypocaloric regime with exercise has failed repeatedly, consideration should be given to the institution of a diet such as DASH rather than further half-hearted attempts to lose weight (see also Chap. 6).

Weight Control, Diabetes Mellitus, and Impaired Glucose Tolerance

The patient with type 2 diabetes has everything to gain by weight reduction. Such persons are almost uniformly overweight. Dietary therapy is one of the cornerstones of blood sugar management. Weight loss not only lessens hyperglycemia but, in some patients with diabetes, and with sufficient weight loss, can make possible the discontinuation of insulin or oral therapy.[82] Diabetes-related mortality was shown to be reduced in a cohort of women who intentionally lost weight over a 12-year period.[83] This area is discussed in more detail in Chap. 8.

In normoglycemic overweight persons, several randomized trials of lifestyle modification versus standard dietary advice showed measurable improvements in glucose and insulin levels with weight loss.[67,84,85] When impairment in glucose tolerance is already present, diet or diet plus exercise can reduce the incidence of diabetes in overweight persons.[86]

Fat Restriction

Since recommendations to consume no more than 30 percent of total calories from fat have been launched over the past three decades, dietary consumption from fat has been reduced from 40 to 42 percent of total calories to about 34 percent. But recent data suggest that we are consuming more calories overall despite a decrease in the percentage of calories from fat. The message of calorie restriction, coupled with a reduction in dietary fat and emphasis on increased fruit and vegetable consumption, needs to be more effectively disseminated.[3] The greater availability of low-fat and fat-free foods allows for greater choices and substitution away from traditional, higher-fat alternatives. While general recommendations are provided by the American Heart Association steps 1 and 2 diets,[87] fat and calorie restriction must be individualized according to the patient's needs and risk-factor profile. Details of individualized nutritional approaches to cardiovascular disease prevention are provided in Chap. 13.

Hypocaloric diet

Hypocaloric dieting, whether or not a low-fat diet is employed, invariably produces both weight loss and a decrease in abdominal adiposity. In general, such diets allow 1000 to 1200 kcal per day. A more stringent approach is the very low-calorie diet that permits only 400 to 500 kcal per day. Initial weight loss is more rapid, although the amount of weight lost over a year, is similar with either plan.[88] The very low calorie diet is probably more likely to be associated with dropout and failure of adherence. The issue of how low a diet should be in fat content is unclear. It is usually easier to consume fewer calories on an ad libitum regime when fat is minimized; this can become self-defeating if palatability decreases. In addition, contrary to common belief, reduction of fat content of the diet *without* attention to calories will not result in weight loss.[89] It has not been examined whether consumption of a low-fat diet independent of caloric restriction can influence visceral adiposity. Adoption of an exercise program without a hypocaloric diet has produced weight loss in some but not all trials. To summarize a number of studies comparing modalities of weight loss, the combination of low-calorie diet and aerobic exercise can be more successful than either strategy alone.

Physical Activity

The importance of incorporating regular physical activity concurrently with a dietary program is well documented. One recent study showed that, although diet combined with various types of exercise or no exercise provided weight losses ranging from 13.5 to 17.4 kg over 48 weeks, participants regained 35 to 55 percent of their weight in the year after treatment. However, those who reported exercising regularly in the 4 months preceding the follow-up assessment regained significantly less weight than the nonexercisers.[90] In addition, a meta-analysis of studies published in the past 25 years has recently shown that, on average, a 15-week diet or diet-plus-exercise program produces a weight loss of about 11 kg, with about a 6.6 kg loss maintained after 1 year in the diet-only group but an 8.6 kg maintenance in the diet-plus-exercise group.[91]

Efforts should be made to encourage individuals to take small steps toward increasing physical activity, such as walking up steps instead of taking elevators as well as parking farther away from one's destination. A brisk walk of 30 minutes daily or on most days should be recommended when possible. Also, state and local authorities should be encouraged to provide more opportunities for safe, community-based physical activity programs, including walking and biking paths and other community facilities.[3] Chapter 12 provides additional details regarding physical activity recommendations.

Social Support

Effective maintenance of weight loss requires ongoing contact with the physician or counselor, help in problem solving, and enhancing interactions. While personal contact is best, mail or phone contacts can suffice in most cases. Participants should be encouraged to bring in a spouse or friends. Maintaining a good quality of life is also important, which involves physical functioning, psychological functioning, and social functioning as well as overall life satisfaction and perceptions of health status. Focus groups can provide insight into patients' perceptions of why obesity is a problem and psychological issues such as lack of control and depression.[7]

Pharmacotherapy and Bariatric Surgery

Since long-term weight loss through dieting is so uniformly unsuccessful, two main alternatives have been popularized. One involves gastrointestinal surgery (bariatric surgery), which aims to reduce the amount of food it is possible to ingest and/or induce mild malabsorption.[92] The alternative involves medication used to reduce appetite.[93] Unfortunately, with the latter approach, lost weight is regained when medications are discontinued; thus there are no good long-term data. The implication is that such drugs would most likely need to be taken for a protracted period. Recent experience with the popular combination fenfluramine/phenteramine and its possible association with cardiac valvular disease has led to caution in the medical treatment of obesity.[94] The most exciting new drug to the market, sibutramine, is a serotonin and norepinephrine reuptake blocker and has been approved by the Food and Drug Administration (FDA) for weight control in those with marked adult weight gain or a BMI equal to or greater than 27. There is a dose-related effect on weight loss.[95] It increases satiety and thermogenesis of brown adipose tissue in animal models and has not been associated with neurotoxicity or pulmonary hypertension. Orlistat, a newly approved inhibitor of intestinal lipases, works by inhibiting fat absorption. Several trials involving 1 to 2 years on treatment demonstrate its efficacy.[96] Although research is under way in the search for drugs "without toxicity" that can be used as anorexigens, it is difficult to embrace this approach without evidence that pharmacotherapy has long-lasting beneficial effects.

Bariatric surgery is a major undertaking; however, it can produce a significant loss of weight with reports of more than 50 percent of the excess lost over the first 2 years.[97] Because of the serious nature of the intervention, most series include only persons with BMI above 35. The most common surgical procedure in use is the banded gastroplasty; distal small bowel bypass surgery has largely been abandoned because of unpleasant diarrhea, higher rates of surgical complications, and the development of micronutrient deficiencies.

In a randomized trial, in which 168 morbidly obese persons had gastric restriction surgery, weight maintenance was found to be more successful with gastroplasty than that after dieting.[98] By reaching 75 percent reduction of their excess weight (over a mean time of 10 months), those who had undergone surgery experienced dramatic changes in their metabolic profiles: an increase in HDL by 24 percent and a decrease in fasting insulin by 62 percent.[98,99] Gastric restriction is also effective therapy for hypertension associated with obesity, with preoperative hypertension resolving in 66 percent at least 1 year later and the amount of weight lost predicting the degree of reduction in blood pressure.[100] Cardiac ventricular compliance and function were significantly improved in a group of 12 obese persons studied before and after surgery with an average weight loss of 55 kg.[101] Similarly, a gastric stapling procedure produced improvements in cardiac chamber size and left ventricular function in a study of 34 patients.[41] While there have been no long-term randomized trials of reduction of morbidity and mortality with this approach, observational studies have demonstrated that the incidence of diabetes, hypertension, and dyslipidemia can be reduced significantly.[102–104] In a patient population of almost 500, the prevalence of diabetes and impaired glucose tolerance fell precipitously from 34 percent to 5 percent postoperatively.[105]

Conclusions

In summary, obesity is a rampant problem with serious health consequences, being linked to increases in hypertension, dyslipidemia, and diabetes. Rates of CHD and stroke as well as overall mortality are significantly increased in obese persons. Even those who are mildly overweight have higher rates of these diseases.[8] Weight loss by whatever means is clearly associated with less comorbidity; however, there are few good long-term studies in the medical literature.

The challenge remains of how to reduce the increasing prevalence of obesity and its sequelae in both children and adults.[7] Unfortunately, since rates of recidivism are so high after initial periods of success, particularly if initial weight loss occurs rapidly, emphasis must be placed on lifestyle alterations that are personally and culturally acceptable, if there is to be any chance of permanency. Diets need to be palatable and varied, with such approaches as "low-fat" and "low-salt" deemphasized in favor of "low-calorie" with plenty of fruits, vegetables, and dairy products. Perhaps the greatest challenge for weight-loss practitioners is to target obese children and adolescents, who will grow up to become the obese hypertensive, diabetic, hypercholesterolemic patients in the offices of tomorrow's physicians. Finally, both a population approach and an individual approach are needed. The population-based effort should focus on the community, including schools and the media, while the individual strategy best consists of a multidisciplinary approach consisting of physicians, exercise specialists, dietitians, nurses, and other health care personnel. Such an approach is crucial to obtaining long-term success. Further, management of associated risk factors—including dyslipidemia, hypertension, and insulin resistance—will help to prevent the cardiovascular complications of diabetes.[7]

References

1. Hubert HB, Feinleib M, McNamara PM, Castelli WP: Obesity as an independent risk factor for cardiovascular disease: a 26-year follow-up of participants in the Framingham Heart Study. *Circulation* 1983; 67:968–977.
2. National Obesity Education Initiative: *Clinical Guidelines on the Identification, Evaluation and Treatment of Overweight and Obesity in Adults: The Evidence Report.* 1998. NIH Pub. No. 98–4083, National Heart, Lung and Blood Institute, Bethesda, MD.
3. Eckel RH, Krauss RM for the AHA Nutrition Committee: American Heart Association call to action: obesity as

a major risk factor for coronary heart disease. *Circulation* 1998; 97:2099–2100.

4. Sjostrom LV: Mortality of severely obese subjects. *Am J Clin Nutr* 1992; 55:516S–523S.

5. Brennan PJ, Simpson JM, Blacket RB, McGilchrist CA: The effects of body weight on serum cholesterol, serum triglycerides, serum urate and systolic blood pressure. *Aust NZ J Med* 1980; 10:15–20.

6. Ballantyne D, Devine BL, Fife R: Interrelation of age, obesity, cigarette smoking, and blood pressure in hypertensive patients. *BMJ* 1978; 1:880–881.

7. Krauss RM, Winston M, Fletcher BJ, Grundy SM: Obesity: impact on cardiovascular disease. AHA conference proceedings. *Circulation* 1998; 98: 1472–1476.

8. Kuczmarski RJ, Carroll MD, Flegal KM, Troiano RP: Varying body mass index cutoff points to describe overweight prevalence among U.S. adults: NHANES III (1988 to 1994). *Obesity Res* 1997; 5:542–548.

9. U.S.Department of Agriculture and U.S. Department of Health and Human Services: *Nutrition and Your Health: Dietary Guidelines for Americans.* Home and Garden Bulletin No. 232. Washington, DC, U.S. Government Printing Office, 1995.

10. Manson JE, Stampfer MJ, Hennekens CH, Willett WC: Body weight and longevity: a reassessment. *JAMA* 1987; 257:353–358.

11. Bender R, Trautner C, Spraul M, Berger M: Assessment of excess mortality in obesity. *Am J Epidemiol* 1998; 147:42–48.

12. Manson JE, Willett WC, Stampfer MJ: Body weight and mortality among women. *N Engl J Med* 1995; 333:677–685.

13. Lee IM, Manson JE, Hennekens CH, Paffenbarger RS: Body weight and mortality: a 27-year follow-up of middle-aged men. *JAMA* 1993; 270:2823–2828.

14. Stevens J, Cai J, Pamuk ER, et al: The effect of age on the association between body-mass index and mortality. *N Engl J Med* 1998; 338:1–7.

15. Hsueh WA, Buchanan TA: Obesity and hypertension. *Endocrinol Metab Clin North Am* 1998; 23:405–427.

16. Huang Z, Willett WC, Manson JE, et al: Body weight, weight change, and risk for hypertension in women. *Ann Intern Med* 1998; 128:81–88.

17. Dyer AR, Elliott P: The Intersalt study: relations of body mass index to blood pressure: Intersalt Co-operative Research Group. *J Hum Hypertens* 1989; 3:299–308.

18. MacMahon SW, Blacket RB, Macdonald GJ, Hall W: Obesity, alcohol consumption and blood pressure in Australian men and women: the National Heart Foundation of Australia Risk Factor Prevalence Study. *J Hypertens* 1984; 2:85–91.

19. Knowler WC, Pettitt DJ, Savage PJ, Bennett PH: Diabetes incidence in Pima indians: contributions of obesity and parental diabetes. *Am J Epidemiol* 1981; 113:144–156.

20. Lee ET, Howard BV, Savage PJ, et al: Diabetes and impaired glucose tolerance in three American Indian populations aged 45–74 years: the Strong Heart Study. *Diabetes Care* 1995; 18:599–610.

21. Larsson B, Bjorntorp P, Tibblin G: The health consequences of moderate obesity. *Int J Obesity* 1981; 5:97–116.

22. Colditz GA, Willett WC, Stampfer MJ, et al: Weight as a risk factor for clinical diabetes in women. *Am J Epidemiol* 1990; 132:501–513.

23. Chan JM, Rimm EB, Colditz GA, et al: Obesity, fat distribution, and weight gain as risk factors for clinical diabetes in men. *Diabetes Care* 1994; 17:961–969.

24. Nestel PJ, Whyte HM, Goodman DS: Distribution and turnover of cholesterol in humans. *J Clin Invest* 1969; 48:982–991.

25. Schreibman PH, Dell RB: Cholesterol localization, synthesis and turnover. *J Clin Invest* 1975; 55:986–993.

26. Despres JP, Moorjani S, Tremblay A, et al: Relation of high plasma triglyceride levels associated with obesity and regional adipose tissue distribution to plasma lipoprotein-lipid composition in premenopausal women. *Clin Invest Med* 1989; 12:374–380.

27. Denke MA, Sempos CT, Grundy SM: Excess body weight: an under-recognized contributor to dyslipidemia in white American women. *Arch Intern Med* 1994; 154:401–410.

28. Anderson KM, Wilson PW, Garrison RJ, Castelli WP: Longitudinal and secular trends in lipoprotein cholesterol measurements in a general population sample: the Framingham Offspring Study. *Atherosclerosis* 1987; 68:59–66.

29. Reaven GM, Chen YD, Jeppesen J, et al: Insulin resistance and hyperinsulinemia in individuals with small, dense low density lipoprotein particles. *J Clin Invest* 1993; 92:141–146.

30. Chu NF, Rimm EB, Wang DJ, et al: Clustering of cardiovascular disease risk factors among obese schoolchildren: the Taipei Children Heart Study. *Am J Clin Nutr* 1998; 67:1141–1146.

31. Troiano RP, Flegal KM, Kuczmarski RJ, et al: Overweight prevalence and trends for children and adolescents: the National Health and Nutrition Examination Surveys, 1963 to 1991. *Arch Pediatr Adolesc Med* 1995; 149:1085–1091.

32. Ogden CL, Troiano RP, Briefel RR, et al: Prevalence of overweight among preschool children in the United States, 1971 through 1994. *Pediatrics* 1997; 99:e1.

33. Solomon CG, Manson JE: Obesity and mortality: a review of the epidemiologic data. *Am J Clin Nutr* 1997; 66:1044S–1050S.

34. Willett WC, Manson JE, Stampfer MJ, et al: Weight, weight change, and coronary heart disease in women: risk within the "normal" weight range. *JAMA* 1995; 273:461–465.

35. Manson JE, Colditz GA, Stampfer MJ, et al: A prospective study of obesity and risk of coronary heart disease in women. *N Engl J Med* 1990; 322:882–889.

36. Prineas RJ, Folsom AR, Kaye SA: Central adiposity and increased risk of coronary artery disease mortality in older women. *Ann Epidemiol* 1998; 3:35–41.

37. Terry RP, Page WF, Haskell WL: Waist hip ratio, body mass index and premature mortality in U.S. army veterans during a 23-year follow-up study. *Int J Obesity* 1992; 16:417–422.

38. Rexrode KM, Hennekens CH, Willett WC, et al: A prospective study of body mass index, weight change, and risk of stroke in women. *JAMA* 1997; 277:1539–1545.

39. Harris TB, Ballard-Barbasch R, Madans J, et al: Overweight, weight loss, and risk of coronary heart disease in older women: the NHANES I Epidemiologic Follow-up Study. *Am J Epidemiol* 1993; 137:1318–1327.

40. Harris TB, Launer LJ, Madans J, Feldman JJ: Cohort study of effect of being overweight and change in weight on risk of coronary heart disease in old age. *BMJ* 1997; 314:1791–1794.

41. Nelson RG, Sievers ML, Knowler WC, et al: Low incidence of fatal coronary heart disease in Pima Indians despite high prevalence of non-insulin-dependent diabetes. *Circulation* 1990; 81:987–995.

42. Zarich SW, Kowalchuk GJ, McGuire MP, et al: Left ventricular filling abnormalities in asymptomatic morbid obesity. *Am J Cardiol* 1991; 68:377–381.

43. Alpert MA, Terry BE, Kelly DL: Effect of weight loss on cardiac chamber size, wall thickness and left ventricular function in morbid obesity. *Am J Cardiol* 1985; 55:783–786.

44. Reeder BA, Senthilselvan A, Despres JP, et al: The association of cardiovascular disease risk factors with abdominal obesity in Canada: Canadian Heart Health Surveys Research Group. *Can Med Assoc J* 1997; 157(suppl 1):S39–45.

45. Vanhala MJ, Pitkajarvi TK, Kumpusalo EA, Takala JK: Obesity type and clustering of insulin resistance–associated cardiovascular risk factors in middle-aged men and women. *Int J Obes Relat Metab Disord* 1998; 22:369–374.

46. Rexrode KM, Carey CJ, Hennekens CH, et al: Abdominal obesity and coronary heart disease in women. *JAMA* 1998; 280:1843–1848.

47. Despres JP, Nadeau A, Tremblay A, et al: Role of deep abdominal fat in the association between regional adipose tissue distribution and glucose tolerance in obese women. *Diabetes* 1989; 38:304–309.

48. Despres JP, Moorjani S, Ferland M, et al: Adipose tissue distribution and plasma lipoprotein levels in obese women: importance of intra-abdominal fat. *Arteriosclerosis* 1989; 9:203–210.

49. Freedman DS, Williamson DF, Croft JB, et al: Relation of body fat distribution to ischemic heart disease: the National Health and Nutrition Examination Survey I (NHANES I) Epidemiologic Follow-up Study. *Am J Epidemiol* 1995; 142:53–63.

50. Walker SP, Rimm EB, Ascherio A, et al: Body size and fat distribution as predictors of stroke among U.S. men. *Am J Epidemiol* 1996; 144:1143–1150.

51. Van der Kooy K, Seidell JC: Techniques for the measurement of visceral fat: a practical guide. *Int J Obesity* 1993; 17:187–196.

52. Singh RB, Rastogi SS, Verma R, et al: Randomised controlled trial of cardioprotective diet in patients with recent acute myocardial infarction: results of one year follow up. *BMJ* 1992; 304:1015–1019.

53. Prentice AM, Jeff SA, Goldberg GR, et al: Effects of weight cycling on body composition. *Am J Clin Nutr* 1992; 56:209S–216S.

54. Phinney SD: Weight Cycling and cardiovascular risk in obese men and women. *Am J Clin Nutr* 1992; 56:781–782.

55. Folsom AR, French SA, Zheng W, et al: Weight variability and mortality: the Iowa Women's Health Study. *Int J Obesity Relat Metab Disord* 1996; 20:704–709.

56. Dattilo AM, Kris-Etherton PM: Effects of weight reduction on blood lipids and lipoproteins: a meta-analysis. *Am J Clin Nutr* 1992; 56:320–328.

57. Cole TG, Bowen PE, Schmeisser D, et al: Differential reduction of plasma cholesterol by the American Heart Association Phase 3 Diet in moderately hypercholesterolemic, premenopausal women with different body mass indexes. *Am J Clin Nutr* 1992; 55:385–394.

58. Nicklas BJ, Katzel LI, Bunyard LB, et al: Effects of an American Heart Association diet and weight loss on lipoprotein lipids in obese, postmenopausal women. *Am J Clin Nutr* 1997; 66:853–859.

59. Leenen R, van der Kooy K, Meyboom S, et al: Relative effects of weight loss and dietary fat modification on serum lipid levels in the dietary treatment of obesity. *J Lipid Res* 1993; 34:2183–2191.

60. Schaefer EJ, Lichtenstein AH, Lamon-Fava S, et al: Body weight and low-density lipoprotein cholesterol changes after consumption of a low-fat ad libitum diet. *JAMA* 1995; 274:1450–1455.

61. Wood PD, Stefanick ML, Williams PT, Haskell WL: The effects on plasma lipoproteins of a prudent weight-reducing diet, with or without exercise, in overweight men and women. *N Engl J Med* 1991; 325:461–466.

62. Schenk-Gustafsson K: Risk factors for cardiovascular disease in women: assessment and management. *Eur Heart J* 1996; 17(suppl D):2–8.

63. Rifkind BM: High density lipoprotein cholesterol and coronary artery disease: survey of the evidence. *Am J Cardiol* 1990; 66:3a–6a.

64. Miller M, Kwiterovich PO Jr: Isolated low HDL cholesterol as an important risk factor for coronary heart disease. *Eur Heart J* 1990; 11(suppl H): 9–14.

65. Connor WE, Cerqueira MT, Connor RW, et al: The plasma lipids, lipoproteins and diet of the Tarahumara Indians of Mexico. *Am J Clin Nutr* 1978; 31:1131–1142.

66. Tran ZV, Weltman A, Glass GV, Mood DP: The effects of exercise on blood lipids and lipoproteins: a meta-analysis of studies. *Med Sci Sports Exerc* 1983; 15:393–402.

67. Katzel LI, Bleecker ER, Colman EG, et al: Effects of weight loss vs aerobic exercise training on risk factors for coronary disease in healthy, obese, middle-aged and older men: a randomized controlled trial. *JAMA* 1995; 274:1915–1921.

68. Nicklas BJ, Katzel LI, Busby-Whitehead J, Goldberg AP: Increases in high-density lipoprotein cholesterol with endurance exercise training are blunted in obese compared with lean men. *Metabolism* 1997; 46:556–561.

69. Widhalm K, Maxa E, Zyman H: Effect of diet and exercise upon the cholesterol and triglyceride content of plasma lipoproteins in overweight children. *Eur J Pediatr* 1978; 127:121–126.

70. Epstein LH, Kuller LH, Wing RR, et al: The effect of weight control on lipid changes in obese children. *Am J Dis Child* 1989; 143:454–457.

71. Nuutinen O, Knip M: Weight loss, body composition and risk factors for cardiovascular disease in obese children: long-term effects of two treatment strategies. *J Am Coll Nutr* 1992; 11:707–714.

72. Wabitsch M, Hauner H, Heinze E, et al: Body-fat distribution and changes in the atherogenic risk-factor profile in obese adolescent girls during weight reduction. *Am J Clin Nutr* 1994; 60:54–60.

73. Wassertheil-Smoller S, Oberman A, Blaufox MD, et al: The Trial of Antihypertensive Interventions and Management (TAIM) Study: final results with regard to blood pressure, cardiovascular risk, and quality of life. *Am J Hypertens* 1992; 5:37–44.

74. The Treatment of Mild Hypertension Research Group: The treatment of mild hypertension study: a randomized, placebo-controlled trial of a nutritional-hygienic regimen along with various drug monotherapies. *Arch Intern Med* 1991; 151:1413–1423.

75. Hypertension Prevention Trial Research Group: The Hypertension Prevention Trial: three-year effects of dietary changes on blood pressure. *Arch Intern Med* 1990; 150:153–162.

76. Stamler R, Stamler J, Grimm R, et al: Nutritional therapy for high blood pressure. Final report of a four-year randomized controlled trial—The Hypertension Control Program. *JAMA* 1987; 257:1484–1491.

77. The Trials of Hypertension Prevention Collaborative Research Group: Effects of weight loss and sodium reduction intervention on blood pressure and hypertension incidence in overweight people with high-normal blood pressure: The Trials of Hypertension Prevention, phase II. *Arch Intern Med* 1997; 157:657–667.

78. Himeno E, Nishino K, Nakashima Y, et al: Weight reduction regresses left ventricular mass regardless of blood pressure level in obese subjects. *Am Heart J* 1996; 131:313–319.

79. Eliahou HE, Erdberg A, Blau A: Energy restriction or salt restriction in the treatment of overweight hypertension: which one? A point of view. *Clin Exp Hypertens* 1990; 12:795–802.

80. Fagerberg B, Berglund A, Andersson OK, Berglund G: Weight reduction versus antihypertensive drug therapy in obese men with high blood pressure: effects upon plasma insulin levels and association with changes in blood pressure and serum lipids. *J Hypertens* 1992; 10:1053–1061.

81. Appel LJ, Moore TJ, Obarzanek E, et al: A clinical trial of the effects of dietary patterns on blood pressure: DASH Collaborative Research Group. *N Engl J Med* 1997; 336:1117–1124.

82. Paisey RB, Harvey P, Rice S, et al: An intensive weight loss programme in established type 2 diabetes and controls: effects on weight and atherosclerosis risk factors at 1 year. *Diabetes Med* 1998; 15:73–79.

83. Williamson DF, Pamuk E, Thun M, et al: Prospective study of intentional weight loss and mortality in never-smoking overweight U.S. white women aged 40–64 years. *Am J Epidemiol* 1995; 141:1128–1141.

84. Nilsson PM, Lindholm LH, Schersten BF: Life style changes improve insulin resistance in hyperinsulinaemic subjects: a one-year intervention study of hypertensives and normotensives in Dalby. *J Hypertens* 1992; 10:1071–1078.

85. Hjermann I, Leren P, Norman N, et al: Serum insulin response to oral glucose load during a dietary intervention trial in healthy coronary high risk men: the Oslo study. *Scand J Clin Lab Invest* 1980; 40:89–94.

86. Pan XR, Li GW, Hu YH, et al: Effects of diet and exercise in preventing NIDDM in people with impaired glucose tolerance: the Da Qing IGT and Diabetes Study. *Diabetes Care* 1997; 20:537–544.

87. American Heart Association: *Dietary Treatment of Hypercholesterolemia: A Manual for Patients.* Dallas, American Heart Association, 1988.

88. Wadden TA, Foster GD, Letizia KA: One-year behavioral treatment of obesity: comparison of moderate and severe caloric restriction and the effects of weight maintenance therapy. *J Consult Clin Psychol* 1994; 62:165–171.

89. Ernst ND, Obarzanek E, Clark MB, et al: Cardiovascular health risks related to overweight. *J Am Diet Assoc* 1997; 97:S47–S51.

90. Wadden TA, Vogt RA, Foster GD, Anderson DA: Exercise and the maintenance of weight loss: 1-year follow-up of a controlled clinical trial. *J Consult Clin Psychol* 1998; 66:429–433.

91. Miller WC, Koceja DM, Hamilton EJ: A meta-analysis of the past 25 years of weight loss research using diet,

exercise, or diet plus exercise intervention. *Int J Obesity Rel Metab Disord* 1997; 21:941–947.

92. Pories WJ, MacDonald KG: The surgical treatment of morbid obesity. *Curr Opin Gen Surg* 1993; 195–205.

93. Bray GA: Use and abuse of appetite-suppressant drugs in the treatment of obesity. *Ann Intern Med* 1993; 119:707–713.

94. Connolly HM, Crary JL, McGoon MD, et al: Valvular heart disease associated with fenfluramine-phentermine. *N Engl J Med* 1997; 337:581–588.

95. Bray GA, Ryan DH, Gordon D, et al: A double-blind randomized placebo controlled trial of sibutramine. *Obesity Res* 1996; 4:263–270.

96. Davidson MH, Hauptman J, DiGirolamo M, et al: Weight control and risk factor reduction in obese subjects treated for 2 years with orlistat: a randomized controlled trial. *JAMA* 1999; 281:235–242.

97. Macgregor AM, Rand CS: Gastric surgery in morbid obesity: outcome in patients aged 55 years and older. *Arch Surg* 1993; 128:1153–1157.

98. Andersen T, Backer OG, Stokholm KH, Quaade F: Randomized trial of diet and gastroplasty compared with diet alone in morbid obesity. *N Engl J Med* 1984; 310:352–356.

99. Wolf AM, Beisiegel U, Kortner B, Kuhlmann HW: Does gastric restriction surgery reduce the risks of metabolic diseases? *Obes Surg* 1998; 8:9–13.

100. Foley EF, Benotti PN, Borlase BC, et al: Impact of gastric restrictive surgery on hypertension in the morbidly obese. *Am J Surg* 1992; 163:294–297.

101. Alaud-din A, Meterissian S, Lisbona R, et al: Assessment of cardiac function in patients who were morbidly obese. *Surgery* 1990; 108:809–818.

102. Long SD, O'Brien K, MacDonald KG Jr, et al: Weight loss in severely obese subjects prevents the progression of impaired glucose tolerance to type II diabetes: a longitudinal interventional study. *Diabetes Care* 1994; 17:372–375.

103. Benotti PN, Bistrain B, Benotti JR, et al: Heart disease and hypertension in severe obesity: the benefits of weight reduction. *Am J Clin Nutr* 1992; 55:586S–590S.

104. Lardinois F, Jacquet P, Belachew M: Gastroplasty as a surgical treatment of obesity: experience of over 400 operations. *Acta Chir Belg* 1994; 94:75–79.

105. Pories WJ, MacDonald KG Jr, Morgan EJ, et al: Surgical treatment of obesity and its effect on diabetes: 10-y follow-up. *Am J Clin Nutr* 1992; 55:582S–585S.

CHAPTER 11

Thrombosis, Inflammation, and Infection

Nathan D. Wong
Paul M. Ridker

Although modifiable risk factors such as dyslipidemia, hypertension, and diabetes are associated with increased risk for coronary heart disease (CHD), a substantial number of individuals experiencing coronary events often do not have well-recognized standard risk factors. Identification of high-risk individuals through traditional risk-factor assessment often fails to identify many individuals at high risk for future coronary thrombosis.[1]

Epidemiologic studies done over the past two decades have suggested possibly important roles for thrombosis, local or systemic inflammation, and chronic infection in the initiation and progression of CHD.[1,2] The relation of increased fibrinogen levels, platelet aggregation, and other markers of thrombosis to coronary event risk have been well-documented. In the past decade, clinical trials documenting the role of antithrombotic and antiplatelet agents have been important for setting standards of care in secondary prevention. More recently, there has been increasing evidence for a role of local and systemic inflammation in the initiation and progression of atherosclerosis and its complications. The possibility that infectious serology may play a role in this inflammatory process has also been an evolving area of investigation.[3]

This chapter reviews the evidence relating thrombotic factors to CHD risk as well as the role of antithrombotic and antiplatelet agents (especially aspirin) in the primary and secondary prevention of CHD. The state of knowledge regarding inflammatory and infectious factors, including possible prevention therapies, is also discussed.

Thrombosis

Thrombus formation is a critical factor in the precipitation of unstable angina, acute myocardial infarction, and thrombotic coronary occlusion during or following coronary angioplasty.[4] Although coronary atherosclerosis is present in most instances of coronary thrombosis,[5] a thrombus often develops at sites of coronary artery stenosis of only mild to moderate severity.[6,7] The concept of evolving coronary thrombosis in unstable angina and in occlusive thrombosis producing myocardial infarction has been established from early studies.[8-11] Subsequently, evidence has implicated platelet aggregation, activation of the coagulation system, and eventually coronary thrombosis in the development of unstable angina, acute myocardial infarction, and sudden coronary death.[4] Occlusive coronary thrombosis is an early event in more than 80 percent of transmural myocardial infarctions.[12] Roughly, 95 percent of sudden death victims can be shown to have coronary thrombosis, plaque injury, or both.[13]

The chronic inflammatory nature of atherosclerosis eventually leads to breakdown of connective tissue and plaque fissuring and rupture, activating platelets and stimulating formation of thrombin. The platelets undergo a "release reaction" culminating in the synthesis of thromboxane A_2, an extremely potent vasoconstrictor and platelet aggregant. Platelet aggregation becomes irreversible, accompanied or followed by thrombin generation, incorporation of fibrin and red blood cells, and formation of a red thrombus.[4] Markers of platelet activation such as thromboxane A_2 are often elevated in the course of unstable coronary artery disease.[14]

Fibrinogen

Fibrinogen appears to contribute to atherosclerosis by several mechanisms: (1) by promoting atherosclerosis, (2) as an essential component of platelet aggregation, (3) in relation to fibrin deposited and the size of the clot, both of which are directly related to the plasma fibrinogen level, and (4) as a result of increasing plasma viscosity.[15] Recent evidence also suggests that the association of fibrinogen to CHD may relate to its role in inflammation.[16]

Observational data indicate that patients with angina pectoris frequently have higher levels of fibrinogen and that plasma levels of fibrinogen increase with severity of CHD.[17] The Leigh Clinical Research Unit[18] showed, in 297 men followed for 7 years, that plasma fibrinogen was the strongest independent indicator of future coronary occlusion. The Northwick Park Heart Study[19] demonstrated higher baseline levels of fibrinogen in those who subsequently experienced a nonfatal or fatal cardiovascular event. Studies done in Goteborg,[20] Framingham,[21] and Caerphilly,[22] taken together, show about a 1.6-fold increased incidence of cardiovascular disease for each standard deviation increase in fibrinogen levels independent of other risk factors. Among 965 patients with unstable angina or non-Q-wave myocardial infarction, comparing the highest ($\geq$4.0 g/L) versus lowest (<3.38 g/L) tertile of fibrinogen, death was significantly more common (6.9 versus 1.6 percent), as was combined death and/or myocardial infarction (19.1 versus 9.3 percent) within 5 months.[23] Others have also shown increased fibrinogen levels measured after angioplasty to be significantly associated with restenosis, where those with a fibrinogen measurement of greater versus less than 3.5 g/L had twofold or greater restenosis rates, depending on how restenosis was defined.[24]

Among the largest studies to report a prospective relation of fibrinogen to CHD is the Atherosclerosis Risk in Communities (ARIC) study, involving 14,477 adults aged 45 to 64 years followed for 5.2 years. Elevated levels of fibrinogen were associated with significant relative risks for CHD of 1.76 in men and 1.54 in women, which were attenuated (to 1.48 and 1.21, respectively) after adjustment for other risk factors.[25] The Scottish Heart Health Study, involving 5095 men and 4860 women,[26] showed fibrinogen to be an independent risk factor for new coronary events both in men and women, with and without prior CHD—with hazard ratios ranging from 1.93 to 4.86—comparing the highest to the lowest quintile of fibrinogen level. Hazard ratios ranged from 2.2 to 3.4 for coronary death and all-cause mortality in men and women. The Prospective Cardiovascular Munster (PROCAM) study in 2116 healthy men showed the incidence of coronary events to be 2.4-fold greater in the upper versus lower tertile of fibrinogen levels, which remained significant after adjusting for other risk factors.[27] Also, cross-sectional analysis of 3571 elderly Japanese-American men showed a significant association between fibrinogen levels and CHD after adjustment for major risk factors, with the highest prevalence (34 percent) of CHD seen in past and current smokers in the highest quintile of fibrinogen.[28] A recent study among nearly 700 hypercholesterolemic men free of clinical CHD demonstrated increased fibrinogen levels (upper versus lowest fibrinogen tertile) to be significantly associated with an increased likelihood of atherosclerotic lesions in the carotid, femoral, aorta, and coronary arteries (odds ratios of 2.2 to 3.6).[29]

A recent metanalysis of 18 studies involving 4018 CHD cases showed a combined relative risk (RR) for CHD of 1.8 [95 percent confidence intervals (CI) 1.6 to 2.0] comparing the top versus bottom tertile of fibrinogen levels (mean 0.35 versus 0.25 g/dL) (Fig. 11–1).[30]

Fibrinogen levels increase with age and body mass index, and are also associated with higher cholesterol levels. Smoking can reversibly elevate fibrinogen levels; individuals who exercise, eat vegetarian di-

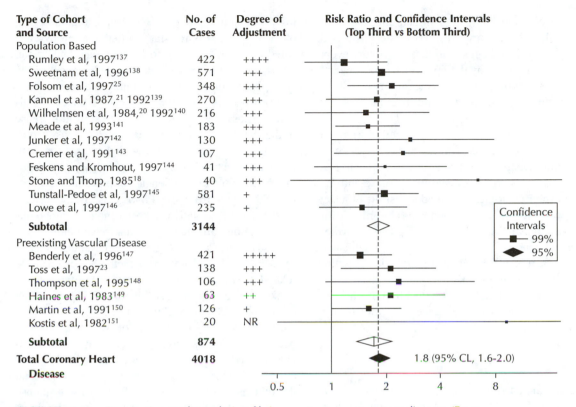

Type of Cohort and Source	No. of Cases	Degree of Adjustment	Risk Ratio and Confidence Intervals (Top Third vs Bottom Third)
Population Based			
Rumley et al, 1997[137]	422	++++	
Sweetnam et al, 1996[138]	571	+++	
Folsom et al, 1997[25]	348	+++	
Kannel et al, 1987,[21] 1992[139]	270	+++	
Wilhelmsen et al, 1984,[20] 1992[140]	216	+++	
Meade et al, 1993[141]	183	+++	
Junker et al, 1997[142]	130	+++	
Cremer et al, 1991[143]	107	+++	
Feskens and Kromhout, 1997[144]	41	+++	
Stone and Thorp, 1985[18]	40	+++	
Tunstall-Pedoe et al, 1997[145]	581	+	
Lowe et al, 1997[146]	235	+	
Subtotal	**3144**		
Preexisting Vascular Disease			
Benderly et al, 1996[147]	421	+++++	
Toss et al, 1997[23]	138	+++	
Thompson et al, 1995[148]	106	+++	
Haines et al, 1983[149]	63	++	
Martin et al, 1991[150]	126	+	
Kostis et al, 1982[151]	20	NR	
Subtotal	**874**		
Total Coronary Heart Disease	**4018**		1.8 (95% CL, 1.6-2.0)

Confidence Intervals
— ■ — 99%
— ◆ — 95%

0.5   1   2   4   8

FIGURE 11–1 Prospective studies relating fibrinogen to coronary artery disease. (From Danesh et al.,[30] with permission.)

ets, and consume alcohol have been noted to have lower levels.[31] The Caerphilly and Speedwell studies[22] show that those with the highest levels of blood viscosity or fibrinogen face more than four times the risk of CHD as compared to those with lower levels.

Plasma fibrinogen is also a marker of increased risk for stroke, but risk may be attenuated when adjusted for standard risk factors. One study involving fibrinogen levels measured after the acute-phase following a stroke showed a twofold increased risk in those with levels above 3.6 g/L after adjustment for other risk factors.[20]

In smokers, cigarette smoking cessation is associated with lower fibrinogen levels. There is also evidence that exercise may lower levels of fibrinogen[32] as well as plasma viscosity.[33] Regarding pharmaco-

logic therapy, one recent study among patients with familial combined hyperlipidemia and CHD showed combined simvastatin-ciprofibrate therapy to significantly lower plasma fibrinogen levels by 24 percent,[34] suggesting that HMG-CoA reductase-fibrate combinations may be helpful. HMG-CoA reductase inhibitors may serve to reduce coronary event risk, partly by inhibiting platelet aggregation and maintaining a favorable balance between prothrombotic and fibrinolytic mechanisms. Some studies involving these medications show reductions in platelet aggregation, reduced plasma viscosity, and lowered fibrinogen levels; however, these findings are not consistent.[35] The Postmenopausal Estrogen/Progestin Interventions (PEPI) study did show estrogen replacement therapy in postmenopausal women to reduce levels of fibrinogen.[36] In addition, the Benzafibrate Infarction Prevention (BIP) study showed fibrinogen levels to be decreased, but coronary event risk not to be reduced by therapy with benzafibrate.[37] Despite these promising data, measurement of fibrinogen remains complicated and its clinical utility limited.[38]

The consistent relation of increased fibrinogen levels to the occurrence of initial and recurrent cardiovascular events has argued for its inclusion as a major risk factor for cardiovascular disease and the need for intervention trials aimed to test the efficacy of lowering fibrinogen in individuals at high risk for cardiovascular disease.[39] But while plasma fibrinogen contributes to risk over and above established risk factors, it is difficult, because of the lack of clinical trials on drugs to selectively lower plasma fibrinogen levels, to determine whether high fibrinogen levels are a cause or consequence of cardiovascular disease (CVD).[15]

Factors VII and VIII

There are mixed reports relating a possible role of coagulation factor VIIc in cardiovascular disease. The PROCAM study in 2116 healthy male subjects showed no association between factor VIIc and coronary events, although a trend toward higher factor VIIc levels was noted when fatal events were taken into account.[28] A study of 401 consecutive patients undergoing coronary angiography did not show an association between factor VIIc and previous myocardial infarction. Activated factor VIIa, however, was lower in those with a previous myocardial infarction and in those who had undergone a prior coronary angioplasty.[40] Among elderly subjects in the Cardiovascular Health Study, fibrinogen and to a lesser extent, factor VIII, but not factor VII, were associated with evidence of subclinical cardiovascular disease from a variety of examination and ultrasound measures.[41]

Factor V Leiden

Another factor related to hypercoagulability is factor V Leiden, a single point mutation in the gene coding for coagulation factor V, which results in a form of factor V_a that is resistant to degradation by activated protein C, leading to a hypercoagulable state. This is present in approximately 4 to 6 percent of the U.S. population. A review of published case-control and prospective cohort studies shows factor V Leiden to be associated with a three- to sixfold increase in the risk for primary and recurrent venous thromboembolism, with risks being higher in those with other risk factors such as advanced age, hyperhomocysteinemia, or deficiencies of protein C and protein S.[42] Data from the Physicians' Health Study shows a greater relative risk of venous thromboembolism among affected versus unaffected individuals with advancing age.[43] Regarding arterial thrombosis, the same study did not show factor V Leiden to be related to future risk of myocardial infarction or stroke.[44] Further, the Cardiovascular Health Study did not show factor V Leiden to be associated with the future risk (over 3.4 years of follow-up) of myocardial infarction, angina, stroke, or transient ischemic attack.[45] The lack of a demonstrated association of factor V Leiden mutation with arterial thrombosis and the unknown effect of more intense or prolonged anticoagulant therapy raises the question of the utility of screening for this disorder.[42]

Endogenous Fibrinolytic Capacity: tPA and PAI-1

Systemic fibrinolytic balance between thrombosis and hemorrhage is mediated by two proteins, endogenous tissue-type plasminogen activator (tPA) and a fast-acting inhibitor, plasminogen activator inhibitor type 1 (PAI-1).[1] PAI-1 has also been shown to be expressed most frequently in fibrous and calcified plaques and to be increased with the severity of coronary atherosclerotic lesions.[46]

Some studies have linked high levels of tPA and PAI-1 with increased cardiovascular risk.[1] In healthy persons, the only controlled prospective study relating baseline levels of tPA and PAI-1 showed no association between baseline fibrinolytic state and the risk of venous thrombosis.[47] Among patients with coronary artery bypass surgery, those with subsequent graft occlusion within 10 days had significantly higher PAI-1 levels than those without occlusion and also had reduced fibrinolytic response and tPA activity.[48] Among diabetic patients with CHD, a disproportionate elevation of PAI-1 is observed as compared with nondiabetic patients with CHD—thus providing further evidence of an association of increased PAI-1 with insulin resistance and diabetes.[49]

Other observations show a relation of PAI-1 deficiency with bleeding, while high levels are associated with frank arterial thrombosis.[50] Increased plasma PAI-1 is present among young survivors of myocardial infarction, and other studies show elevated PAI-1 or tPA levels in those with angina, severe CHD, and recurrent ischemia—which represent situations where endothelial dysfunction may be present.[1]

The Physician's Health Study showed plasma levels of endogenous tPA to be significantly higher among those who experienced a first myocardial infarction (RR = 2.81, 95 percent CI 1.47 to 5.37) or stroke (RR = 3.51, 95 percent CI 1.72 to 7.17) among those in the fifth versus first quintile).[51,52] A nested case-control study within the Rotterdam study showed increased levels of tissue plasminogen activator antigen to be associated with an increased risk of myocardial infarction (odds ratios of 1.7; 95 percent CI 0.9 to 3.3; 12.3, 95 percent CI 1.2 to 4.4; and 2.0, 95 percent CI 1.0 to 3.8 for the second, third, and fourth quartiles compared with the first), but these risks were attenuated after adjustment for other risk factors.[53] With regard to possible interventions to treat impaired fibrinolysis, some studies involving angiotensin-converting enzyme inhibitors do show significant reductions in PAI-1 or TPA antigen levels; however, these findings are by no means consistent.[35,54,55]

The possible role of activation of the endogenous fibrinolytic system as a marker of future CVD risk is partly supported by studies of D-dimer, a breakdown product of fibrinogen, which has been noted to be elevated in those with the highest risk of myocardial infarction.[56,57] In the Physicians' Health Study,[57] those with D-dimer concentrations above the 95th percentile ($\geq$107 ng/mL) were at more than twice the risk of myocardial infarction than those with levels at or below the 50th percentile (<38 ng/mL). Recently, Lowe et al.[58] showed, in the prospective Caerphilly Study cohort, that those with levels of D-dimer in the top quintile had an adjusted relative odds of ischemic heart disease events of 3.5 (95 percent CI 1.8 to 6.9).

Platelet Size, Function, and Aggregation

Platelet hyperreactivity as measured by spontaneous platelet aggregation (SPA) has been noted to be a marker for survival and secondary coronary events post–myocardial infarction. Those who were SPA-positive were found to have a fivefold greater risk of death in one limited study of 120 patients.[59] This was consistent with previous observations of a shortened bleeding time being the best clinical marker of platelet reactivity. Cross-sectional data from the Caerphilly Collaborative Heart Disease Study[60] showed a strong relation between platelet function and past history of myocardial infarction. Platelet reactivity may be reduced by diets high in the ratio of polyunsaturated to saturated fat[61] and increased n-3 fatty acids,[62] and by smoking cessation.[1]

Platelet size (volume) has also been shown to be a sensitive marker of future thrombotic risk. Platelet volume measured 6 months post–myocardial infarction in 1716 men was greater in those who suffered a recurrent infarction or death.[63] A Norwegian study of 487 men showed those with the highest platelet counts to have a significant 2.5-fold increased risk for cardiovascular mortality.[64] A more recent case-control study, however, indicated platelet volume not to differ between patients with versus those without previous myocardial infarction.[65]

Aspirin and Other Antiplatelet Therapy

Aspirin

In platelets, aspirin prevents the formation of thromboxane A_2, thereby preventing platelet aggregation. Aspirin has also been reported to improve endothelial function, which can then improve vasodilation, reduce thrombosis, and help to inhibit progression of atherosclerosis.[66] Evidence exists from epidemiologic studies for a protective effect for coronary events; there is also clinical trial evidence in both primary and secondary prevention (Table 11–1).

The largest trial of primary prevention is the Physicians' Health Study,[67] where more than 22,000 male physicians aged 40 to 84 were assigned to 325 mg aspirin or placebo every other day for 5 years. A highly significant 44 percent reduction (2.55 versus 4.4/1000 per year) ($p < .0001$) in risk for myocardial infarction was observed, in conjunction with a nonsignificant increased incidence of stroke (2.18 versus 1.79/1000 per year). Overall, bleeding was more common in aspirin users, as was bleeding requiring transfusion. The British Doctors' Study of 5000 male physicians aged 50 to 78 years on 500 mg aspirin per day or placebo for 6 years showed little effect on either myocardial infarction or stroke.[68] Al-

though the Physicians' Health Study and the British Doctors' Study provide evidence of the efficacy of aspirin in men, results from trials done specifically in women are not yet available.

The largest prospective cohort study reported involving aspirin use is the Nurses' Health Study[69] of 87,678 U.S. registered nurses aged 34 to 65, free of diagnosed coronary heart disease, stroke, and cancer at baseline. Among women who took one to six aspirins per week, there was a significant 32 percent lower risk of first myocardial infarction among those aged 50 or older. No benefits or harm was seen for stroke risk among them or among women taking more than six aspirins per week. In older women, however, the Cardiovascular Health Study[70] showed frequent or infrequent aspirin use in women to be associated with an 80 percent increased risk of ischemic stroke (RR = 1.8, 95 percent CI 1.2 to 2.8) and a fourfold increased risk of hemorrhagic stroke

TABLE 11–1   Major Clinical Trials of Aspirin Use and Cardiovascular Disease

Reference	Population	Result
Primary prevention		
U.S. Physicians' Health Study[67]	22,071 male physicians aged 40–84 years	44% ↓ in risk of MI 13% ↑ in risk of stroke (N.S.)
British Doctors' Study[68]	5139 male physicians aged 50–78 years	3% ↓ in risk of MI (N.S.) 13% ↑ in risk of stroke (N.S.)
Hypertension Optimal Treatment (HOT)[74]	18,790 hypertensive patients (53% male)	15% ↓ CVD events 36% ↓ MI 2% ↓ risk of stroke (N.S) 7% ↓ risk of mortality (N.S.)
Women's Health Study[71]	40,000 female health professionals	Ongoing
Secondary prevention		
Antiplatelet Trialists' Collaboration[85]	54,000 patients with CVD (10 trials post-MI)	31% ↓ risk of nonfatal MI 42% ↓ risk of nonfatal stroke 13% ↓ risk of total vascular mortality
International Study of Infarct Survival[84]	17,187 patients with evolving MI	49% ↓ risk of reinfarction 26% ↓ risk of nonfatal stroke 23% ↓ risk of total vascular mortality

Key: CVD, cardiovascular disease; MI, myocardial infarction; N.S., nonsignificant.

(95 percent CI = 1.6 to 10.0) after adjustment for other risk factors. These findings did not hold in men, however.

The currently ongoing Women's Health Study involving low-dose aspirin use (100 mg every other day) among 40,000 female nurses aged 45 and over will provide data on the efficacy of aspirin use in women.[71] Considering a higher baseline risk of stroke versus myocardial infarction (MI) in women and overall risk/benefit considerations, recommendations regarding low-dose aspirin use for primary prevention in women must await results of this trial.[72,73]

In the Hypertension Optimal Treatment (HOT) study,[74] among the nearly 9400 hypertensive patients (47% women) randomized to 75 mg/day of aspirin as compared with a nearly equivalent number assigned to placebo, all major cardiovascular events were reduced by 15 percent ($p = .03$) and MI by 36 percent ($p = .002$), but there was no effect on stroke. Unfortunately, nonfatal bleeds remained nearly twice as common in the aspirin group (RR = 1.8, $p < .001$).

A recently reported metanalysis of 16 trials with 55,462 subjects involving a mean dosage of 273 mg/day of aspirin and mean duration of treatment for 37 months showed aspirin use to be associated with an absolute risk reduction in MI of 137 events/10,000 persons (95 percent CI 107 to 167) and, for ischemic stroke, a risk reduction of 39 events/10,000 persons (95 percent CI 17 to 61) (both $p < .001$). A significant increase in risk of hemorrhagic stroke of 12 events/10,000 persons (95 percent CI 5 to 20) ($p < .001$), however, was reported.[75]

For secondary prevention, there have been six large, randomized, double-blind clinical trials of aspirin alone following MI.[76–81] Five of these trials used dosages of 300 to 1500 mg of aspirin daily and showed favorable trends for a reduction of total mortality. The Aspirin Myocardial Infarction Study (AMIS)[80] showed a trend against aspirin for mortality but a nonsignificant reduction in risk for recurrent MI. In patients with unstable angina, the VA Cooperative Trial[82] in 1266 men showed aspirin to be associated with a 51 percent reduction in death and acute MI (10.1 to 5 percent). The Montreal Heart Institute Study showed a 72 percent lower risk.[83]

Aspirin has also been shown to be necessary in the acute phase following MI, when thrombolytic therapy is used. The best evidence for this derives from the Second International Study of Infarct Survival (ISIS-2),[84] where a 40 percent reduction in the risk of 5-week vascular mortality was noted in those on the combination of aspirin and streptokinase as compared with only a 23 percent risk reduction in those given streptokinase and a 21 percent reduction in those receiving aspirin alone.

The Antiplatelet Trialists' Collaboration reported an updated metanalysis of 145 randomized trials conducted in 70,000 high-risk patients with occlusive vascular disease and 30,000 low-risk patients from the general population, most commonly using aspirin as the antiplatelet agent.[85] Among the high-risk patients receiving antiplatelet therapy, significant reductions were seen in overall mortality (18 percent), nonfatal MI (35 percent), and nonfatal stroke (31 percent). Among 20,000 patients with a history of MI, there was a 29 percent lower risk of new vascular events in those receiving aspirin (10.6 percent) versus the control regimen (14.4 percent) (Table 11–1).

Other Antiplatelet Therapy

Ticlopidine is a platelet antiaggregatory agent that inhibits the formation of arterial thrombi, prolongs bleeding time, and normalizes shortened platelet survival. The Canadian American Ticlopidine Study (CATS)[86] showed a 30.2 percent reduction in the risk of stroke, MI, or vascular death among 1053 patients assigned to ticlopidine or placebo 1 to 17 weeks after thromboembolic stroke. The Ticlopidine Aspirin Stroke Study (TASS)[87] showed a slight advantage of ticlopidine over aspirin in reducing death from any cause or nonfatal stroke (20 versus 23 percent of patients) over 6 years.

Clopidogrel, a new thienopyridine derivative similar to ticlopidine, also inhibits platelet aggregation. As shown in the trial of Clopidogrel versus Aspirin in Patients at Risk of Ischaemic Events (CAPRIE)[88] among over 19,000 patients with either ischemic stroke, MI, or peripheral vascular disease followed for nearly 2 years, there was a significant 8.7 percent reduction in risk (95 percent CI 0.3 to 16.5) favoring clopidogrel over aspirin. The overall safety profile was at least as good in the clopidogrel group versus those on aspirin.

Recommendations for Aspirin/Antiplatelet Therapy

Antiplatelet therapy is effective in reducing vascular events, including nonfatal MI, stroke, or vascular death in patients with preexisting coronary artery disease or stroke. Aspirin is effective in dosages of 75 to 325 mg. When thrombolytic therapy is used, concomitant aspirin therapy provides substantial additional risk reduction.[84] In such high-risk patients, aspirin reduces vascular events by about one-fourth, nonfatal MI by one-third, nonfatal stroke by one-third, and vascular death by one-sixth. For secondary prevention of stroke, there is evidence that ticlopidine may be more effective than aspirin, but its greater cost and more frequent and serious adverse effects warrant its careful consideration only for select groups of stroke patients.[4] For aspirin-intolerant patients, clopidogrel may be an option and has been shown to be efficacious in patients with MI, stroke, and peripheral vascular disease.[88] With benefits clear and aspirin use clearly recommended post–myocardial infarction, based on these data, utilization rates appear to be 95 percent or higher overall but slightly less in men, the elderly, and among those with health maintenance organization insurance.[89] This contrasts with surveys done about 5 years earlier showing aspirin use to be substantially lower.[90,91] The argument has been made that some 5000 to 10,000 additional lives annually could be saved if aspirin were administered to all patients after acute MI.[92]

The efficacy of lower dosages of aspirin is under investigation in order to determine the optimal dose of aspirin to provide cardiovascular benefits while minimizing side effects such as gastrointestinal bleeding. The ability of 100 mg alternate-day aspirin to inhibit platelet function has been documented, with decreases in mean thromboxane and prostacyclin levels to 7.5 and 15.6 percent of baseline, respectively (both $p < .001$).[93] In the HOT study, while showing the continued efficacy of low-dose (75 mg/day) aspirin therapy in reducing cardiovas-

cular events and MI with no increase in stroke, nonfatal bleeds remained twice as common.[74] The clinical efficacy of this dosage in the primary prevention of cardiovascular events is being evaluated in the ongoing Women's Health Study.[71] Data from the Physicians' Health Study suggest that alternate-day aspirin could yield lower benefits. While those with excellent adherence (at least 95 percent of prescribed tablets) showed a significant 51 percent reduction in the risk of MI, poor adherers (less than 50 percent of prescribed tablets) showed a nonsignificant 17 percent reduction in risk.[94] Others have argued that dosages in secondary prevention as low as 30 mg/day may be sufficient for the prevention of MI through inhibition of thromboxane synthesis, arguing for more extensive clinical trials on low-dose formulations.[95]

Recommendations for aspirin use in primary prevention are based on the careful weighing of risks versus benefits, considering criteria such as age and general risk of the patient for cardiovascular events. In those free of CHD and younger than 50 years, aspirin is not recommended, considering evidence of no benefit in those younger than 50 years of age and an increased risk of bleeding, transfusion, and trend toward more hemorrhagic stroke.[72] Aspirin use may be considered, however, in those older than 50 years of age who have at least an additional risk factor for CHD and who are free of contraindications for its use, based on evidence of increasing benefits with advancing age and presence of hypertension, diabetes, cigarette smoking, and lack of exercise.[67,69] More recently, groups such as the American Diabetes Association have recommended aspirin use in diabetics with at least one other coronary risk factor or preexisting CHD.[96]

Inflammation and C-Reactive Protein

Local and systemic inflammation may play a role in the initiation and progression of atherosclerosis. C-reactive protein (CRP) is an acute-phase reactant marker for underlying systemic inflammation, with levels increasing 100-fold or more in response to severe bacterial infection, physical trauma, or other inflammatory conditions. A level of 10 mg/L or higher generally signifies clinically important levels.[97]

Studies over the past two decades[98-100] show CRP to be significantly higher in patients with MI or CHD and, more recently, demonstrate the predictive value of CRP for subsequent coronary events in patients with preexisting CHD.[100-102] A recent review presented seven studies with relative risks ranging from approximately 2 to 5 (Fig. 11–2).[103]

In the Physicians' Health Study,[104] CRP was measured in 543 initially healthy men who developed MI or stroke and in an equivalent number of controls not reporting events. Baseline CRP was significantly higher in those experiencing versus not experiencing subsequent MI (1.51 versus 1.13 mg/L) or ischemic stroke (1.38 versus 1.13 mg/L). In comparing those in the highest versus lowest quartile for CRP, the relative risk for MI was 2.9 and for stroke

1.9. Most interestingly, aspirin use was associated with a significantly reduced risk of MI (by 56 percent) in those in the highest quartile of CRP but with only a modest, nonsignificant reduction in risk (of 14 percent) among those in the lowest quartile of CRP. It was concluded that CRP may provide a method for identifying those where anti-inflammatory agents such as aspirin may prove most effective. In a second report from the Physicians' Health Study, CRP provided significantly better prediction of first MI when added to models including total and HDL cholesterol alone, further suggesting its utility in the prediction of CHD.[105]

A recent report from the Women's Health Study[106] showed substantially higher baseline CRP levels in women developing CVD events than in those remaining disease free, with a 7.4-fold increased risk of MI or stroke (4.8-fold for any CVD event) among

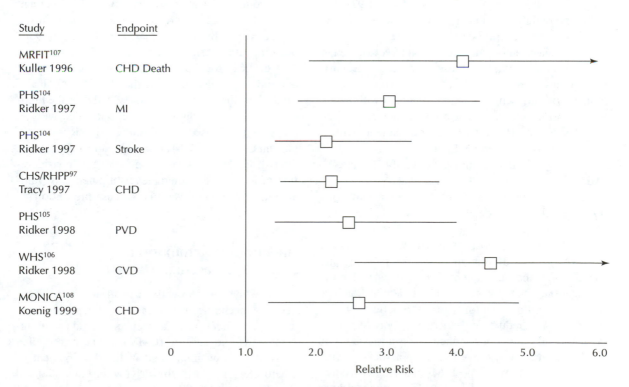

FIGURE 11–2 Prospective studies of C-reactive protein and CVD. Relative rates for highest versus lowest quartile of C-reactive protein levels are presented. (From Ridker and Haughie,[103] with permission.)

those with the highest levels of CRP. It was also determined that risk-prediction models including CRP provided significantly better prediction than models excluding CRP.

From population-based studies, evidence of an association of CRP to an increased risk of CHD mortality derives from the Multiple Risk Factor Intervention Trial (MRFIT), where a nested case-control study of 98 cases of MI, 148 CHD deaths, and 491 controls showed that over 17 years of follow-up, deaths from CHD among smokers were 4.3-fold greater (95 percent CI 1.74 to 10.8) among those in the fourth versus the first quartile of CRP.[107] Most recently, in a population-based random sample of 936 men who participated in the MONICA Augsburg Cohort Study, the relative risk (RR) associated with a 1 standard deviation increase in log-CRP level was 1.67 (95 percent CI 1.29 to 2.17), which was essentially unaffected after adjusting for age and smoking (RR = 1.50, 95 percent CI = 1.14 to 1.97). No other potential confounders were identified or entered the prediction models[108]

CRP measurement may also be an effective means for risk stratification of those with acute coronary syndromes. A recent study of 110 patients admitted with suspected ischemic heart disease but without elevated serum creatine-kinase levels showed an elevated level of CRP in 59 percent of patients with a final diagnosis of acute MI but in only 5 percent of patients with a final diagnosis of unstable angina.[109] Additionally, CRP levels are associated with a poor prognosis in patients with unstable angina or non-Q-wave MI; risks of death within 5 months were 2.2, 3.6, and 7.5 percent by tertiles of CRP level (<2, 2 to 10 and >10 mg/L, respectively) ($p < .01$).[110]

The role of different therapies for reducing inflammation and subsequent CHD risk is under investigation. One promising report demonstrated a possible nonlipid, anti-inflammatory effect of the HMG-CoA reductase therapy pravastatin.[111] Whereas inflammation, defined as elevations both in CRP and serum amyloid A levels, was associated with risk of recurrent events post–MI in those not receiving pravastatin (RR = 2.1, $p < .05$), individuals receiving pravastatin had this risk attenuated to where it was no longer significant (RR = 1.3, $p = .5$).

Recently, it has been recommended that a marker of inflammation, namely CRP, be considered in the list of measures used in cardiovascular risk assessment in middle-aged men. Levels of CRP are relatively stable over time and are affected by little other than inflammation; prediction is independent of other known risk factors and is additive to subclinical measures of atherosclerosis; and sensitive, inexpensive assays are becoming widely available.[97]

The role of circulating adhesion molecules as cellular mediators of inflammation is of increasing interest. In a nested case-control study of the Atherosclerosis Risk in Communities (ARIC) longitudinal cohort study, increased levels of endothelial-leukocyte adhesion molecule-1 (E-selectin) and intercellular adhesion molecule-1 (ICAM-1) were seen in patients with incident CHD or carotid artery atherosclerosis as compared with control subjects. Odds ratios for CHD of 5.53 (95 percent CI = 2.51 to 12.21) and carotid artery atherosclerosis of 2.03 (95 percent CI = 1.14 to 3.25) were observed for those in the highest versus the lowest quartile of ICAM-1. Odds of carotid atherosclerosis were 2.03 (95 percent CI = 1.14 to 3.62) for those in the highest versus lowest quartile of E-selectin.[112] In the Physicians' Health Study, baseline levels of soluble CAM-1 in the highest quartile (>260 ng/mL) were associated with an 80 percent increased risk of future MI (RR = 1.8, 95 percent CI = 1.1 to 2.8) after multivariate adjustment for risk factors.[113] These results suggest consideration of antiadhesion therapies as a potentially valuable means of cardiovascular disease prevention.[113]

Infection, Inflammation, and Cardiovascular Disease

Local or systemic infections resulting from gram-negative bacteria such as *Chlamydia pneumoniae* and *Helicobacter pylori* as well as of viral origin, including cytomegalovirus (CMV), and herpes simplex virus, have been implicated in the development of atherosclerosis, partly by driving inflammation.[114] Systemic antibody titers show previous exposure to infectious pathogens with persistently positive serology and represent markers for chronic, persistent infection. Over a dozen retrospective serologic studies have reported a positive relation of infectious pathogens with CHD, including angiographic restenosis; however, these studies are subject to substantial bias and confounding. In contrast, prospective studies in which the exposure is ascertained before the onset of cardiovascular events have not provided strong evidence of an association. A summary of these prospective studies appears in Table 11-2.

Saikku et al.[115] first reported a relation of *C. pneumoniae* to CHD and acute MI in 1988. They found 68 percent of patients with acute MI had elevated IgG and/or IgA titers against *C. pneumoniae* as compared with only 17 percent of control subjects. An overall association of 70 to 100 percent between *C. pneumoniae* and atherosclerosis is seen from immunocystochemistry and staining techniques. *C. pneumoniae* is uncommon in childhood but increases in prevalence to 70 percent in men and 50 percent in women.[116] It has been detected in fatty streaks and in atheromatous lesions from autopsy[117]

as well as in plaques from the coronary and carotid arteries in several studies, including those in young adults with atherosclerosis.[118, 119] One study of 60 autopsies showed 36 of 42 severe atherosclerotic cases to be seropositive, as compared with only 1 of 18 with mild disease.[120] The Helsinki Heart Study showed an odds for developing CHD of 2.6 (not significant) in those with elevated *C. pneumoniae* antibody titers versus controls.[121]

Additional evidence of the link between *C. pneumoniae* and inflammation derives from a recent report documenting increased titers of the former to be associated with elevated concentrations of fibrinogen, C-reactive protein, and troponin T.[122] The association between persistent *C. pneumoniae* infection and increased fibrinogen remained independent of other risk factors.

A recently reported prospective follow-up of the Physicians' Health Study, however, casts doubt as to the prospective relation of *C. pneumoniae* with CHD risk.[123] Chlamydial IgG seropositivity (as an indicator of *C. pneumoniae* with CHD exposure) was

TABLE 11–2 Summary of Major Prospective Studies of Infectious Pathogens and Coronary Artery Disease

Reference	N (w/endpoint) / N (controls)		RR (95% CI)
Chlamydia pneumoniae			
Saikku 1992[121]	103, CHD	103	2.3 (0.9–6.2)*
Ridker 1998[123]	343	343	1.1 (0.8–1.5)*
Helicobacter pylori			
Whincup 1996[124]	135, MI	136	1.31 (0.70–2.43)*
Strandberg 1997[125]	127, CVD death	497	1.07 (0.73–1.5)
Aromaa 1996[127]	441, MI	842	1.29 (0.94–2.00)
Wald 1997[126]	648, CHD death	1296	1.06 (0.86–1.31)*
Folsom 1998[128]	217, CHD	498	0.85 (0.43–1.69)*
Strachan 1998[129]	1796 (total),		
	IHD incidence		1.05 (0.80–1.39)†
	All-cause death		1.46 (1.12–1.92)†
	Fatal IHD		1.54 (1.03–2.30)†
Cytomegalovirus			
Ridker 1998[135]	643, MI / stroke	643	0.94 (0.7–1.2)*
Herpes simplex virus			
Ridker 1998[135]	643, MI / stroke	643	0.72 (0.6–0.9)*

Key: CHD, coronary heart disease; MI, myocardial infarction; CVD, cardiovascular disease; IHD, ischemic heart disease.

*Adjusted for other coronary risk factors.

†Did not retain statistical significance when adjusted for other risk factors.

virtually identical among those subsequently experiencing first MI and age- and smoking-matched controls. In addition, there was no relation of *C. pneumoniae* with CRP.

H. pylori seropositivity also shows mixed results in relation to CHD (Table 11-2). Whincup et al.[124] showed an association of *H. pylori* with MI (OR = 1.8), but this diminished to 1.3 (not significant) after adjustment for risk factors. Three other prospective studies have also not documented a relation of *H. pylori* seropositivity with CHD death[125,126] or MI.[127] Most recently, within the large, longitudinal ARIC study, there was no association of *H. pylori* seropositivity with incident CHD occurring over a 3.3-year follow-up period among middle-aged men and women.[128] The smaller but longer-term Caerphilly Prospective Heart Disease Study showed, among 1796 men followed for a mean of 13.7 years, no association of incident ischemic heart disease with *H. pylori* (OR = 1.05, 95 percent CI = 0.80 to 1.39) but a stronger relation with all-cause mortality (OR = 1.46, 95 percent CI = 1.12 to 1.92) and fatal ischemic heart disease (OR = 1.54, 95 percent CI = 1.03 to 2.30).[129] However, those seropositive for both *C. pneumoniae* and *H. pylori* had an OR = 2.6 for coronary artery disease (CAD) and 2.0 for MI and also tended to have higher CRP levels.[114] Also, in a case-control study, *H. pylori* infection was significantly higher among CHD patients than among matched controls (62 versus 40 percent, p < .01; OR 2.8, 95 percent CI = 1.3 to 7.4) and was mediated through cytotoxin-associated gene-A (Cag A), an indicator of more virulent *Helicobacter* strains.[130]

Herpes simplex and cytomegalovirus (CMV) are associated with mixed results regarding the risk for CHD (Table 11–2). CMV genomes are seen more frequently in those with severe versus mild or no atherosclerosis.[131] CMV seropositivity has been shown to be a significant risk factor (OR = 3.6) for pretransplant atherosclerosis in a cardiac transplant population.[132] Also, from a transplant study,[133] CMV positive versus negative patients showed lower 5-year survival (32 versus 68 percent), higher rate of graft loss due to atherosclerosis (69 versus 37 percent), and higher death due to 50 percent or greater

obstruction (8 versus 1 percent). The longitudinal ARIC study provides the strongest evidence, with a graded relation between odds of intimal-medial thickness and serum CMV antibody titer, even after adjustment for risk factors.[134] A large, nested case-control study among nearly 1300 participants of the Physicians' Health Study, however, actually showed an unexpected inverse relation between CMV seropositivity and risk for MI or stroke over 12 years (RR = 0.72, 95 percent CI 0.6 to 0.9), which the authors attributed to chance; nevertheless, this study does not support a relation of CMV seropositivity to increased vascular event risk.[135]

Caution must be applied, however, in interpreting findings of many studies that suggest a link between infection and CHD risk. For several of these studies, it is difficult to exclude the possibility that the observed associations may be the result of selection bias or confounding on the basis of age, smoking, socioeconomic status, or other factors. Individuals with greater infectious burdens may be at greater risk, partly because they are older, have poorer health habits, or have less access to care.[2] Additional data from emerging prospective studies and clinical trials involving various treatments are accumulating to further establish the role of infection in CHD risk. One should not assume that antibiotic therapy for CHD is yet appropriate or acceptable. Only large, properly designed trials will provide the evidence as to whether and which treatment is appropriate.[136]

Summary

As we begin the new millennium, we are faced with the challenge of identifying individuals who may be prone to initial or recurrent cardiovascular events but who do not have typical risk factors normally used in cardiovascular risk assessment. While data are promising regarding the role of thrombosis in increasing coronary event risk, only for aspirin and other selected antithrombotic agents is the evidence available to recommend their use in selected populations. Although fibrinogen levels generally confer increased risk for coronary events, studies show they do not add to the prediction of coronary events beyond that of more established risk factors. Also, there are no interventions yet available or recommended specifically to lower fibrinogen levels to reduce risk. Markers of local or systemic inflammation—such as C-reactive protein, an acute phase reactant, for which elevated levels correlate with increased risks for cardiovascular events—suggest a promising means for risk stratification. There are, however, no established guidelines regarding its routine measurement or use in risk stratification. Finally, the role that bacterial or viral infection may play in atherosclerosis is uncertain. Most data are observational, possibly subject to selection and other biases, and there are few prospective studies. Nevertheless, the possibility remains that further research will help define a role for measurement of thrombotic, inflammatory, and infectious factors in cardiovascular risk assessment as well as establish effective treatment strategies for individuals that would benefit from intervention.

References

1. Ridker PM: The pathogenesis of atherosclerosis and acute thrombosis: relevance to strategies of cardiovascular disease prevention. In: Manson JE, Ridker PM, Gaziano JM, Hennekens CH (eds): *Prevention of Myocardial Infarction*. New York, Oxford University Press, 1996, pp 32–54.
2. Ridker PM: Inflammation, infection, and cardiovascular risk. How good is the clinical evidence? (editorial). *Circulation* 1998; 97:1671–1674.
3. Libby P, Egan D, Skarlatos S: Roles of infectious agents in atherosclerosis and restenosis: an assessment of the evidence and need for future research. *Circulation* 1997; 96:4095–4103.
4. Cairns JA, Lewis D, Meade TW, et al: Antithrombotic agents in coronary artery disease. Fourth ACCP Consensus Conference on Antithrombotic Therapy. *Chest* 1995; 108 (suppl):380S–400S.
5. Sanz G, Castanev A, Bertrui A, et al: Determinants of prognosis in survivors of myocardial infarction: a prospective clinical angiographic study. *N Engl J Med* 1982; 306:1065–1071.
6. Ambrose J, Tannenbaum M, Alexopoulos D, et al: Angiographic progression of coronary artery disease and the development of myocardial infarction. *J Am Coll Cardiol* 1988; 12:56–62.
7. Little WC, Constantinescu M, Applegate RJ, et al: Can coronary angiography predict the site of a subsequent myocardial infarction in patients with mild-to-moderate

8. Parkinson J, Bedford DE: Cardiac infarction and thrombosis. *Lancet* 1928; 14:195–239.
9. Levine SA, Brown CL: Coronary thrombosis: its various clinical features. *Medicine* 1929; 8:245–418.
10. Sampson JJ, Eliaser M: The diagnosis of impending acute coronary artery occlusion. *Am Heart J* 1937; 13:676–686.
11. Feil H: Preliminary pain in coronary thrombosis. *Am J Med Sci* 1937; 193:42–48.
12. DeWood MA, Spores J, Notske R, et al: Prevalence of total coronary occlusion during the early hours of transmural myocardial infarction. *N Engl J Med* 1980; 303:897–902.
13. Davies MJ, Thomas AC: Plaque fissuring: the cause of acute myocardial infarction, sudden ischaemic death, and crescendo angina. *Br Heart J* 1988; 60:459–464.
14. Fitzgerald DJ, Roy L, Catella F, et al: Platelet activation in unstable coronary disease. *N Engl J Med* 1986; 315:983–989.
15. Heinrich J, Assmann G: Fibrinogen and cardiovascular risk. *J Cardiovasc Risk* 1995; 2:197–205.
16. Andreotti F, Burzotta F, Maseri A: Fibrinogen as a marker of inflammation: a clinical view. *Blood Coagul Fibrinolysis* 1999; 10 (suppl 1): S3–S4.
17. Rainer C, Kawanishi DT, Chandraranta AN, et al: Changes in blood rheology in patients with stable angina pectoris as a result of coronary artery disease. *Circulation* 1987; 76:15–20.
18. Stone MC, Thorpe JM: Plasma fibrinogen: a major coronary risk factor. *JR Coll Gen Pract* 1985; 35:565–569.
19. Meade TW, Mellows S, Brozovic M, et al: Haemostatic function and ischemic heart disease: principle results of the Northwick Park Heart Study. *Lancet* 1986; 2:533–537.
20. Wilhelmsen L, Svardsudd K, Korsan-Bengtsen K, et al: Fibrinogen as a risk factor for stroke and myocardial infarction. *N Engl J Med* 1984; 311:501–505.
21. Kannel WB, Wolf PA, Castelli WP, D'Agostino RB: Fibrinogen and risk of cardiovascular disease: the Framingham study. *JAMA* 1987; 258:1183–1186.
22. Yarnell JWG, Baker IA, Sweetnam PM, et al: Fibrinogen, viscosity, and white blood cell count are major risk factors for ischemic heart disease: the Caerphilly and Speedwell Collaborative Heart Disease Studies. *Circulation* 1991; 83:836–844.
23. Toss H, Lindahl B, Siegbahn A, Wallentin L: Prognostic influence of increased fibrinogen and C-reactive protein levels in unstable coronary artery disease: FRISC Study Group. Fragmin during Instability in Coronary Artery Disease. *Circulation* 1997; 96:4202–4210.
24. Montalescot G, Ankri A, Vicaut E, et al: Fibrinogen after coronary angioplasty as a risk factor for restenosis. *Circulation* 1995; 92:31–38.

coronary artery disease? *Circulation* 1988; 78:1157–1166.

25. Folsom AR, Wu KK, Rosamond WD, et al: Prospective study of hemostatic factors and incidence of coronary heart disease: the Atherosclerosis risk in Communities (ARIC) study. *Circulation* 1997; 96:1102–1108.

26. Woodward M, Loew GD, Rumley A, Tunstall-Pedoe H: Fibrinogen as a risk factor for coronary heart disease and mortality in middle-aged men and women: the Scottish Heart Health Study. *Eur Heart J* 1998; 19:55–62.

27. Henrich J, Balleisen L, Schulte H, et al: Fibrinogen and factor VII in the prediction of coronary risk: results from the PROCAM study in healthy men (published errarum appears in *Arterioscler Thromb* 1994; 14:392). *Arterioscler Thromb* 1994; 14:54–59.

28. Sharp DS, Abbott RD, Burchfiel CM, et al: Plasma fibrinogen and coronary heart disease in elderly Japanese-American men. *Arterioscle Thromb Vasc Biol* 1996; 16: 262–268.

29. Levenson J, Giral P, Megnien JL, et al: Fibrinogen and its relations to subclinical extracoronary and coronary atherosclerosis in hypercholesterolemic men. *Arterioscler Thromb Vasc Biol* 1997; 17:45–50.

30. Danesh J, Collins R, Appleby P, Peto R: Association of fibrinogen, C-reactive protein, albumin, or leukocyte count with coronary heart disease: a meta-analysis of prospective studies. *JAMA* 1998; 279:1477–1482.

31. Ernst E: Plasma fibrinogen: an independent cardiovascular risk factor. *J Intern Med* 1990; 27:365–372.

32. Stratton JR, Chandler WL, Schwartz RS, et al: Effects of physical conditioning on fibrinolytic variables and fibrinogen in young and old healthy adults. *Circulation* 1991; 83:1692–1697.

33. Koenig W, Sund M, Doring A, Ernst E: Leisure-time physical activity but not work-related physical activity is associated with decreased plasma viscosity. *Circulation* 1997; 95:335–341.

34. Kontopoulos AG, Athyros VG, Papageorgiou AA, et al: Effects of simvastatin and ciprofibrate alone and in combination on lipid profile, plasma fibrinogen and low density lipoprotein particle structure and distribution in patients with familial combined hyperlipidemia and coronary artery disease. *Coron Artery Dis* 1996; 7:843–850.

35. Rosenson RS, Tagney CC: Antiatherothrombotic properties of stations: implications for cardiovascular event reduction. *JAMA* 1998; 279:1643–1650.

36. The Writing Group of the PEPI Trial: Effects of estrogen or estrogen/progestin regimens on heart disease risk factors in postmenopausal women. *JAMA* 1995; 273:199–208.

37. Behar S, for the Benzafibrate Infarction Prevention Study Group: Lowering fibrinogen levels: clinical update. *Blood Coagul Fibrinolysis* 1999; 10:41–43.

38. Ridker PM: Evaluating novel cardiovascular risk factors: can we predict better heart attacks? *Ann Intern Med* 1999; 130:933–937.

39. Kannel WB: Influence of fibrinogen on cardiovascular disease. *Drugs* 1997; 54(suppl 3):32–40.

40. Danielsen R, Onundarson PT, Thors H, et al: Activated and total coagulation factor VII, and fibrinogen in coronary artery disease. *Scand Cardiovasc* 1998; 32:87–95.

41. Tracy RP, Bovill EG, Yanez D et al: Fibrinogen and factor VIII, but not factor VII, are associated with measures of subclinical cardiovascular disease in the elderly. Results from The Cardiovascular Health Study *Arterioscler Thromb Vasc Biol* 1995; 15:1269–1279.

42. Price DT, Ridker PM: Factor V Leiden mutation and the risks for thromboembolic disease: a clinical perspective. *Ann Intern Med* 1997; 127:895–903.

43. Ridker PM, Glynn RJ, Miletich JP, et al: Age-specific incidence rates of venous thromboembolism among heterozygous carriers of factor V Leiden mutation. *Ann Intern Med* 1997; 126:528–531.

44. Ridker PM, Hennekens CH, Lindpaintner K, et al: Mutation in the gene coding for coagulation factor V and the risk of myocardial infarction, stroke, and venous thrombosis in apparently healthy men. *N Engl J Med* 1995; 332:912–917.

45. Cushman M, Rosendaal FR, Psaty BM, et al: Factor V Leiden is not a risk factor for arterial vascular disease in the elderly: results from the Cardiovascular Health Study. *Thromb Haemostas* 1998; 79:912–915.

46. Padro T, Steins M, Li CX, et al: Comparative analysis of plasminogen activator inhibitor-1 expression in different types of atherosclerotic lesions in coronary arteries from human heart explants. *Cardiovasc Res* 1997; 36:28–36.

47. Ridker PM, Vaughan DE, Stampfer MJ, et al: Baseline fibrinolytic state and the risk of venous thrombosis: a prospective study of endogenous tissue-type plasminogen activator and plasminogen activator inhibitor. *Circulation* 1992: 85:1822–1827.

48. Rifon J, Paramo JA, Panizo C, et al: The increase of plasminogen activator inhibitor activity is associated with graft occlusion in patients undergoing aorto-coronary bypass surgery. *Br J Haematol* 1997; 99:262–267.

49. Sobel BE, Woodcock-Mitchell J, Schneider DJ: Increased plasminogen activator inhibitor type 1 in coronary artery atherectomy specimens from type 2 diabetic compared with nondiabetic patients: a potential factor predisposing to thrombosis and its persistence. *Circulation* 1998; 97:2213–2221.

50. Erickson LA, Rici GJ, Lund JE, et al: Development of venous occlusions in mice transgenic for the plasminogen activator inhibitor-1 gene. *Nature* 1990; 346:74–76.

51. Ridker PM, Vaughan DE, Stampfer MJ, et al: Endogenous tissue-type plasminogen activator and risk of myocardial infarction. *Lancet* 1993; 341:1165–1168.

52. Ridker PM, Hennekens CH, Stampfer MJ, et al: A prospective study of endogenous tissue plasminogen activator and the risk of stroke. *Lancet* 1994; 343:940–943.

53. van der Bom JG, de Knijff P, Haverkate F, et al: Tissue plasminogen activator and risk of myocardial infarction: the Rotterdam Study. *Circulation* 1997; 95:2623–2627.

54. Ridker PM, Gaboury CL, Conlin PR, et al: Stimulation of plasminogen activator inhibitor in vivo by infusion of angiotensin II: evidence of a potential interaction between the rein angiotensin system and fibrinolytic function. *Circulation* 1993; 87:1969–1973.

55. Vaughan DE, Rouleau JL, Ridker PM, et al: Effects of ramipril on plasma fibrinolytic balance in patients with acute anterior myocardial infarction: HEART Study Investigators. Circulation 1997; 96:442–447.

56. Fowkes FGR, Lowe GDO, Housley E, et al: Cross-lined fibrin degradation products, progression of peripheral arterial disease, and risk of coronary heart disease. *Lancet* 1993; 342:84–86.

57. Ridker PM, Hennekens CH, Cerskus A, Stampfer MJ: Plasma concentration of cross linked fibrin degradation product (D-dimer) and the risk of future myocardial infarction. *Circulation* 1994; 90:2236–2240.

58. Lowe GD, Yarnell JW, Sweetnam PM, et al: Fibrin D-dimer, tissue plasminogen activator, plasminogen activator inhibitor, and the risk of major ischaemic heart disease in the Caerphilly Study. *Thromb Haemostas* 1998; 79:129–133.

59. Trip MD, Manger Cats V, van Capelle FJL, Vreeken J. Platelet hyperreactivity and prognosis in survivors of myocardial infarction. *N Engl J Med* 1990; 322:1549–1554.

60. Elwood PC, Renaud S, Sharp DS, et al: Ischemic heart disease and platelet aggregation: the Caerphilly Collaborative Heart Disease Study. *Circulation* 1991; 83:38–44.

61. Beswick AD, Fehily AM, Sharp DS, et al: Long-term diet modification and platelet activity. *J Intern Med* 1991; 229:511–515.

62. Nelson GL, Schmidt PC, Corlash L: The effect of a salmon diet on blood clotting, platelet aggregation, and fatty acids in normal adult men. *Lipids* 1001; 26:87–96.

63. Martin JF, Bath PMW, Burr ML: Influence of platelet size on outcome after myocardial infarction. *Lancet* 1991; 338:1409–1411.

64. Traulow E, Erikssen J, Sandvik L, et al: Blood platelet count and function are related to total and cardiovascular death in apparently healthy men. *Circulation* 1991; 84:613–617.

65. Halbmayer WM, Haushofer A, Radek J, et al: Platelet size, fibrinogen and lipoprotein (a) in coronary heart disease. *Coron Artery Dis* 1995; 6:397–402.

66. Husain S, Andrews NP, Mulcahy D, et al: Aspirin improves endothelial dysfunction in atherosclerosis. *Circulation* 1998; 97:716–720.

67. The Steering Committee of the Physicians' Health Study Research Group: Final report on the aspirin component of the ongoing Physicians' Health Study. *N Engl J Med* 1989; 321:129–135.

68. Peto R, Gray R, Collins R, et al: Randomized trial of prophylactic daily aspirin in British male doctors. BMJ 1988; 296:313–316.

69. Manson JE, Stampfer J, Colditz GA, et al: A prospective study of aspirin use and primary prevention of cardiovascular disease in women. *JAMA* 1991; 266:521–527.

70. Kronmal RA, Hart RG, Manolio TA, et al: Aspirin use and incident stroke in the Cardiovascular Health Study: CHS Collaborative Research Group. *Stroke* 1998; 29:887–894.

71. Buring JE, Hennekens CH, for the Women's Health Study Research Group: The Women's Health Study: summary of the study design. *J Myocardial Ischemia* 1992; 4:27–29.

72. Hennekens CH, Dyken ML, Fuster V: AHA scientific statement on aspirin as a therapeutic agent in cardiovascular disease: a statement for healthcare professionals from the American Heart Association. *Circulation* 1997; 96:2751–2753.

73. Meade TW: Aspirin, myocardial infarction, and gastrointestinal bleeding. *Lancet* 1999; 353:676.

74. Hansson L, Zanchetti A, Carruthers SG, et al for the HOT Study Group. Effects of intensive blood-pressure lowering and low-dose aspirin in patients with hypertension: principal results of the Hypertension Optimal Treatment (HOT) randomised trial. *Lancet* 1998; 351:1755–1762.

75. He J, Whelton PK, Vu B, Klag MJ: Aspirin and risk of hemorrhagic stroke. *JAMA* 1998; 280:1930–1935.

76. Elwood PC, Cochrane AL, Burr ML, et al: A randomized controlled trial of acetylsalicylic acid in the secondary prevention of mortality from myocardial infarction. *BMJ* 1974; 1:436–440.

77. The Coronary Drug Project Research Group: Aspirin in coronary heart disease. *J Chronic Dis* 1976; 29:625–642.

78. Breddin K, Loew D, Lechner K, et al: Secondary prevention of myocardial infarction: a comparison of acetylsalicylic acid, placebo, and phenprocoumon. *Hemostasis* 1980; 9:325–344.

79. Elwood PC, Sweetnam PM: Aspirin and secondary mortality after myocardial infarction. *Lancet* 1979; 2:1313–1315.

80. Aspirin Myocardial Infarction Study Research Group: A randomized, controlled trail of aspirin in persons recovered from myocardial infarction. *JAMA* 1980; 243:661–669.

81. The Persantine-Aspirin Reinfarction Study Research Group: Persantine and aspirin in coronary heart disease. *Circulation* 1980; 62:449–461.

82. Lewis HD, Davis JW, Archibald DG, et al: Protective effects of aspirin against acute myocardial infarction and death in men with unstable angina: result of a Veterans Administration Cooperative Study. *N Engl J Med* 1983; 309:396–403.

83. Cairns JA, Gent M, Singer J, et al: Aspirin, sulfinpyrazone, or both, in unstable angina: results of a Canadian multicenter clinical trial. *N Engl J Med* 1985; 313:1369–1375.

84. ISIS-2 (Secondary International Study of Infarct Survival) Collaborative Group: Randomized trial of intravenous streptokinase, oral aspirin, both, or neither among 17,187 cases of suspected acute myocardial infarction: ISIS-2. Lancet 1988; 2:349–360.

85. Antiplatelet Trialists' Collaboration: Collaborative overview of randomised trials of antiplatelet therapy: 1. Prevention of death, myocardial infarction, and stroke by prolonged antiplatelet therapy in various categories of patients. *BMJ* 1994; 308:81–106.

86. Gent M, Blakely JA, Easton JD, et al: The Canadian American Ticlopidine Study (CATS) in thromboembolic stroke. *Lancet* 1989; 1:1215–1220.

87. Hass WK, Easton JD, Adams HP, et al: A randomized trial comparing ticlopidine hydrochloride with aspirin for the presentation of stroke in high-risk patients. *N Engl J Med* 1989; 321:501–507.

88. CAPRIE Steering Committee: A randomised, blinded, trial of clopidogrel versus aspirin in patients at risk of ischaemic events (CAPRIE). *Lancet* 1996; 348:1323–1339.

89. Hill JW, Roglieri JL, Warburton SW: Aspirin treatment after myocardial infarction: are health maintenance organization members, women, and the elderly undertreated? *Am J Managed Care* 1996; 4:51–58.

90. Rogers WJ, Bowlby LJ, Chandra NC, et al: Treatment of myocardial infarction in the United States (1990 to 1993): observations from the National Registry of Myocardial Infarction. *Circulation* 1994; 90:2103–2114.

91. Krumholz HM, Radford MJ, Ellerbeck EF, et al: Aspirin in the treatment of acute myocardial infarction in elderly Medicare beneficiaries: patterns of use and outcomes. *Circulation* 1995; 92:2841–2847.

92. Hennekens CH, Jonas MA, Buring JE: The benefits of aspirin in acute myocardial infarction: still a well-kept secret in the United States. Arch Intern Med 1994; 154:37–39.

93. Ridker PM, Hennekens CH, Tofler GH, et al: Antiplatelet effects of 100 mg alternate day oral aspirin: a randomized, double-blind, placebo-controlled trial of regular and enteric coated formulations in men and women. *J Cardiovasc Risk* 1996; 3:209–212.

94. Glynn RJ, Buring JE, Manson JE, et al: Adherence to aspirin in the prevention of myocardial infarction: the Physician's Health Study. *Arch Intern Med* 1994; 154:2649–2657.

95. Forster W, Parratt JR: The case of low-dose aspirin for the prevention of myocardial infarction: but how low is low? *Cardiovasc Drugs Ther* 1997; 10:727–734.

96. American Diabetes Association: Aspirin therapy in diabetes: position statement. *Diabetes Care* 1997; 20:1772–1773.

97. Tracy RP: Inflammation in cardiovascular disease: cart, horse, or both? (editorial) *Circulation* 1998; 97:2000–2002.

98. de Beer FC, Hind CR, Fox KM, et al: Measurement of C-reactive protein concentration in myocardial ischemia and infarction. *Br Heart J* 1982: 47:239–243.

99. Pietila K, Marmoinen A, Hermens W, et al: Serum C-reactive protein concentration in myocardial infarct patients with a closed versus an open infarct-related coronary artery after thrombolytic therapy. *Eur Heart J* 1993; 14:915–919.

100. Gaspardone A, Crea F, Versaci F, et al: Predictive value of C-reactive protein after successful coronary-artery stenting in patients with stable angina. *Am J Cardiol* 1998; 82:515–518.

101. Morrow DA, Rifai N, Antman EM, et al: C-reactive protein is a potent predictor of mortality independently of and in combination with troponin T in acute coronary syndromes: a TIMI11a substudy. Thrombolysis in Myocardial Infarction. *J Am Coll Cardiol* 1998; 31:1460–1465.

102. Thompson SG, Kienast J, Pyke SDM, et al: Hemostatic factors and the risk of myocardial infarction or sudden death in patients with angina pectoris. *N Engl J Med* 1995; 332:635–642.

103. Ridker PM, Haughie P: Prospective studies of C-reactive protein as a risk factor for cardiovascular disease. *J Invest Med* 1998; 46:391–395.

104. Ridker PM, Cushman M, Stampfer MJ, Tracy RP: Inflammation, aspirin, and the risk of cardiovascular disease in apparently healthy men. *N Engl J Med* 1997; 336:973–979.

105. Ridker PM, Glynn RJ, Hennekens CH: C-reactive protein adds to the predictive value of total and HDL-cholesterol in determining risk of first myocardial infarction. *Circulation* 1998; 97:2007–2011.

106. Ridker PM, Buring JE, Shih J, et al: Prospective study of C-reactive protein and the risk of future cardiovascular events among apparently healthy women. *Circulation* 1998; 98:731–733.

107. Kuller LH, Tracy RP, Shaten J, Meilahn EN: Relation of C-reactive protein and coronary heart disease in the MRFIT nested case-control study. Multiple Risk Factor Intervention Trial. *Am J Epidemiol* 1996; 144:537–547.

108. Koenig W, Sund M, Frohlich M, et al: C-reactive protein, a sensitive marker of inflammation, predicts future risk of coronary heart disease in initially healthy middle-aged men. Results form the MONICA (Monitoring Trends and Determinants in Cardiovascular Disease) Augsburg Cohort Study, 1984–1992. *Circulation* 1999; 99:237–242.

109. Mach F, Lovis C, Gaspoz JM, et al: C-reactive protein as a marker for acute coronary syndromes. *Eur Heart J* 1997; 18:1897–1902.

110. Toss H, Lindahl B, Siegbahn A, Wallentin L: Prognostic influence of increased fibrinogen and C-reactive protein levels in unstable coronary artery disease. FRISC Study Group. Fragmin during Instability in Coronary Artery Disease. *Circulation* 1997; 96:4204–4210.

111. Ridker PM, Rifai N, Pfeffer MA, et al: Inflammation, pravastatin, and the risk of coronary events after myocardial infarction in patients with average cholesterol levels. Cholesterol and Recurrent Events (CARE) investigators. *Circulation* 1998; 98:839–844.

112. Hwang S-J, Ballantyne CM, Sharrett AR, et al: Circulating adhesion molecules VCAM-1, ICAM-1, and E-selectin in carotid atherosclerosis and incident coronary heart disease cases: the Atherosclerosis Risk in Communities (ARIC) study. *Circulation* 1997; 96:4219–4225.

113. Ridker PM, Hennekens CH, Roitman-Johnson B, et al: Plasma concentration of soluble intercellular adhesion molecule 1 and risks of future myocardial infarction in apparently healthy men. *Lancet* 1998; 351:88–92.

114. Anderson JL, Carlquist JF, Muhlestein JB, et al: Evaluation of C-reactive protein, an inflammatory marker, and infectious serology as risk factors for coronary artery disease and myocardial infarction. *J Am Coll Cardiol* 1998; 32:35–41.

115. Saikku P, Mattila K, Nieminen S, et al: Serological evidence of an association of a novel chlamydia, TWAR, with chronic coronary heart disease and acute myocardial infarction. *Lancet* 1988; 1:983–985.

116. Grayston JT, Campbel LA, Kuo CC, et al: A new respiratory pathogen: *Chlamydia pneumoniae* infection and atherosclerosis. *J Invest Med* 1997; 45:168–174.

117. Shor A, Kuo CC, Patton DL: Detection of *Chlamydia pneumoniae* in coronary arterial fatty streaks and atheromatous plaques. *S Afr Med J* 1992; 82:158–161.

118. Kuo CC, Grayston JT, Campbell LA, et al: *Chlamydia pneumoniae* (TWAR) in coronary arteries of young adults (15–34 years old). *Proc Natl Acad Sci USA* 1995; 92:6911–6914.

119. Campbell LA, O'Brien ER, Cappuccio AL, et al: Detection of *Chlamydia pneumoniae* TWAR in human coronary atherectomy tissues. *J Infect Dis* 1995; 172:585–588.

120. Mehta JL, Saldeen TG, Rand K: Interactive role of infection, inflammation, and traditional risk factors in atherosclerosis and coronary artery disease. *J Am Coll Cardiol* 1998; 31:1217–1225.

121. Saikku P, Leinonen M, Tenkanen L, et al: Chronic *Chlamydia pneumoniae* infection as a risk factor for coronary heart disease in the Helsinki Heart Study. *Ann Intern Med* 1992; 116:273–278.

122. Toss H, Gnarpe J, Gnarpe H, Siegbahn A, et al: Increased fibrinogen levels are associated with persistent *Chlamydia pneumoniae* infection in unstable coronary artery disease. *Eur Heart J* 1998; 19:570–577.

123. Ridker PM, Kundsin RB, Stampfer MJ, et al: A prospective study of *Chlamydia pneumoniae* IgG seropositive and risks of future myocardial infarction (abstr). Presented at the 71st Scientific Sessions, American Heart Association, Dallas, November 1998.

124. Whincup PH, Mendall MA, Perry IJ, et al: Prospective relations between *Helicobacter pylori* infection, coronary heart disease, and stroke in middle-aged men. *Heart* 1996; 75:568–572.

125. Strandberg TE, Tilvis RS, Vuoristo M, et al: Prospective study of *Helicobacter pylori* seropositivity and cardiovascular diseases in a general elderly population. *BMJ* 1997; 314:1317–1318.

126. Wald NJ, Law MR, Morris JK, Bagnall AM: *Helicobacter pylori* infection and mortality from ischaemic heart disease: negative result from a large, prospective study. *BMJ* 1997; 315:1199–1201.

127. Aromaa A, Knekt P, Reunanen A, et al: *Helicobacter* infection and the risk of myocardial infarction (abstr). *Gut* 1996; 39(suppl 2):A91.

128. Folsom AR, Nieto J, Sorlie P, et al: *Helicobacter pylori* seropositivity and coronary heart disease incidence. *Circulation* 1998; 98:845–850.

129. Strachan DP, Mendall MA, Carrington D, et al: Relation of *Helicobacter pylori* infection to 13-year mortality and incident ischemic heart disease in the Caerphilly Prospective Heart Disease Study. *Circulation* 1998; 98:1286.

130. Pasceri V, Cammarota G, Patti G, et al: Association of virulent *Helicobacter pylori* strains with ischemic heart disease. *Circulation* 1998; 97:1675–1679.

131. Hendricks MGR, Salimens MMM, Vauboven CPA, Bruggerman CA: High prevalence of latently present cytomegalovirus in arterial walls of patients suffering from grade III atherosclerosis. *Am J Pathol* 1990; 136:23–28.

132. Dummer S, Lee A, Breinig MK, et al: Investigation of cytomegalovirus infection as a risk factor for coronary atherosclerosis in the explanted hearts of patients undergoing heart transplantation. *J Med Virol* 1994; 44:305–309.

133. Grattan MT, Moreno-Cabral CE, Starnes VA, et al: Cytomegalovirus infection is associated with cardiac allograft rejection and atherosclerosis. *JAMA* 1989; 261:3561–3566.

134. Neito FJ, Adam E, Sorlie P, et al: Cohort study of cytomegalovirus infection as a risk factor for carotid intimal-medial thickening, a measure of subclinical atherosclerosis. *Circulation* 1996; 94:922–927.

135. Ridker PM, Hennekens CH, Stampfer MJ, Wang F: Prospective study of herpes simplex virus, cytomegalovirus, and the risk of future myocardial infarction and stroke. *Circulation* 1998; 98:2796–2799.

136. Grayston JT: Antibiotic treatment of *Chlamydia pneumoniae* for secondary prevention of cardiovascular events (editorial). *Circulation* 1998; 97:1669–1670.

137. Rumley A, Lowe GDO, Norrie J, et al: Blood rheology and outcome in the west of Scotland coronary prevention study. *Br J Haematol* 1997; 97(suppl 1):78.

138. Sweetnam PM, Thomas HF, Yarnell JWG, et al: Fibrinogen, viscosity and the 10-year incidence of ischaemic heart disease. *Eur Heart J* 1996; 17:1814–1820.

139. Kannel WB: Fibrinogen: a major cardiovascular risk factor. In: Ernst E, Koenig W, Lowe GDO, Meade TW, eds. *Fibrinogen: A "New" Cardiovascular Risk Factor.* Vienna, Austria: Blackwell-MZV; 1992:101–109.

140. Eriksson H, Wilhelmsen L, Welin L, et al: 21-year follow-up of CVD and total mortality among men born in 1913. In: Ernst E, Koenig W, Lowe GDO, Meade TW (eds.): *Fibrinogen: A "New" Cardiovascular Risk Factor.* Vienna, Austria: Blackwell-MZV; 1992:115–119.

141. Meade T, Ruddock V, Stirling Y, et al: Fibrinolytic activity, clotting factors, and long-term incidence of ischaemic heart disease in the Northwick Park Heart Study. *Lancet* 1993; 342:1076–1079.

142. Junker R, Heinrich J, Schulte H, et al: Coagulation factor VII and the risk of coronary heart disease in healthy men. *Arterioscler Thromb Vasc Biol* 1997; 17:1539–1544.

143. Cremer P, Nagel D, Bottcher B, Seidel D: Fibrinogen: ein koronärer Risikfaktor. *Diagn Labor* 1991; 42:28–35.

144. Feskens EJM, Kromhout D: Fibrinogen and factor VII activity as risk factors for cardiovascular disease in an elderly cohort. *Can J Cardiol* 1997; 13(suppl B):282B.

145. Tunstall-Pedoe H, Woodward M, Tavendale R, et al: Comparison of the prediction by 27 different risk factors of coronary heart disease and death in men and women of the Scottish Heart Health Study. *BMJ* 1997; 315:722–729.

146. Lowe GDO, Lee AJ, Rumley A, et al: Blood viscosity and risk of cardiovascular events: the Edinburgh Artery Study. *Br J Haematol* 1997; 96:168–173.

147. Benderly M, Graff E, Reicher-Reiss H, et al: Fibrinogen is a predictor of mortality in coronary heart disease patients. *Arterioscler Thromb Vasc Biol* 1996; 16:351–356.

148. Thompson SG, Kienast J, Pyke SDM, et al: Hemostatic factors and the risk of myocardial infarction or sudden death in patients with angina pectoris. *N Engl J Med* 1995; 332:634–641.

149. Haines AP, Howarth D, North WRS, et al: Haemostatic variables and outcome of myocardial infarction. *Thromb Haemostas* 1983; 50:800–803.

150. Martin JF, Bath PMW, Burr ML: Influence of platelet size on outcome after myocardial infarction. *Lancet* 1991; 338:1409–1411.

151. Kostis JB, Baughman DJ, Kuo PT: Association of recurrent myocardial infarction with hemostatic factors: a prospective study. *Chest* 1982; 81:571–575.

CHAPTER 12

Physical Activity

Nathan D. Wong
Stanley L. Bassin

All parts of the body which have a function, if used in moderation and exercised in labors in which each is accustomed, become thereby healthy, well developed, and age more slowly, but if unused and left idle, they become liable to disease and defective in growth and age quickly.

—Hippocrates

Physical activity has played a prominent role in the development of Western civilization, but only recently has the absence of regular physical exercise been shown to affect our life span. Physical activity is a natural aspect of human life that has evolved over the last 2 million years. Early human life involved a nomadic lifestyle, searching for food across wide distances. Once our ancestors settled in and began to raise animals and other food, followed by the industrial revolution, with further specialization of work, less physical labor was required. Eventually, powered public and private transportation became available, further reducing the required amount of physical activity. In the latter part of this century, advances in modern technology have enabled our society to function in such a way that hard physical work is hardly needed for our work or daily living.

Over the last few decades, studies have shown a sedentary lifestyle to be associated with an increased risk of coronary heart disease (CHD),[1] cardiovascular disease (CVD),[2–5] and all-cause mortality.[5–6] Physical activity as part of daily living is associated with a decreased risk for CVD, stroke, diabetes, obesity, and all-cause mortality.[7] Even those who are moderately active have lower mortality rates than those who are least active. Unfortunately, the U.S. population is becoming increasingly sedentary, with recent estimates indicating that only 15 percent of

Americans older than 18 years of age get regular vigorous activity (three times a week for at least 20 min), and 60 percent reporting no regular leisure-time activity (with 25 percent not active at all).[8] There is great potential for reducing CVD risk in those initially sedentary who become moderately active,[6] but those who remain sedentary have the highest risk for CVD and all-cause mortality.[1]

This chapter reviews the evidence relating leisure-time and occupational physical activity to morbidity and mortality from CVD and its risk factors. Practical recommendations for initiating and maintaining a physical activity routine for primary and secondary prevention of CVD are also discussed.

Prevalence and Trends in Physical Activity

Only 22 percent of adults report regular sustained physical activity of any intensity lasting 30 min or more five times per week (although more recent standards of 30 min daily at least 3 times per week have been used as a minimum standard). The percentage of adults with a sedentary lifestyle (from the Behavioral Risk Factor Surveillance Study, 1991–1992) ranged from 51 to 68 percent, depending on ethnicity and gender (Fig. 12–1).[9] In 1996, the

Percent (%)

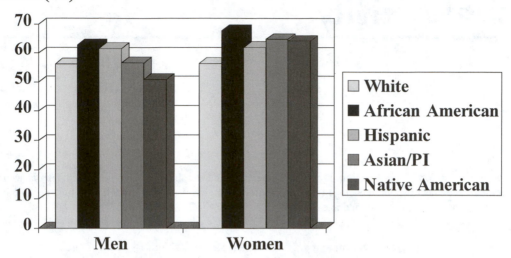

FIGURE 12–1 Estimated percentage of adults with sedentary lifestyle by race and sex, United States: 1991–1992. (From the American Heart Association,[9] with permission.)

percentage of adults reporting no leisure-time physical activity (no exercise, recreation, or physical activities other than regular job duties during the past month) varied from 17.5 percent in Utah to 51.1 percent in Georgia,[10] although a recent survey in California estimates this figure to be as high as 55 percent.[11] Physical inactivity is more prevalent among women than men, among blacks and Hispanics than whites, among older than younger adults, and among the less affluent than the more affluent.[8]

Among American youth ages 12 to 21 years, nearly half are not vigorously active on a regular basis, and daily enrollment in physical activity classes has declined among high school students from 42 percent in 1991 to 27 percent in 1997. From the 1997 Youth Risk Behavior Survey,[12] while nearly two-thirds (63.8 percent) of U.S. high school students reported participating in three or more bouts of vigorous physical activity (e.g., sufficient to cause heavy breathing or sweating, such as basketball or jogging) during the past 7 days, there appears to be a substantial decline with age. While 66.1 percent of females in grade 9 report such activity, this declines to 43.6 percent by grade 12; in males, the figures de-

cline from 78.7 to 68.4 percent over the same ages. There is also significant variation in the reported prevalence of physical activity among youth by gender and ethnicity (Fig. 12–2).

Significant reductions in the frequency of reported physical activity have been shown over recent years, especially in white males, with nearly a doubling in the prevalence of those reporting no leisure-time physical activity from 1988 to 1991 (12.9 percent) to 1992 (25.3 percent).[9] Data from the Behavioral Risk Factor Surveillance System survey in 26 states conducted between 1986 and 1990 reports a slight increase (2.1 percent) overall in those regularly active (with intense activity). Women and older adults made the most beneficial changes, while nonwhites and the least educated had unfavorable changes.[13] Others report, in young adults, a decrease in energy expenditure over 7 years of approximately 30 percent. Although some of the reduction was related to age, a secular trend was responsible for 38 percent of this decrease in black men, 43 percent in black women, 52 percent in white men, and 81 percent in white women.[14] There may be many reasons for this, including possibly a reduction in the perceived soci-

---

Percent (%)

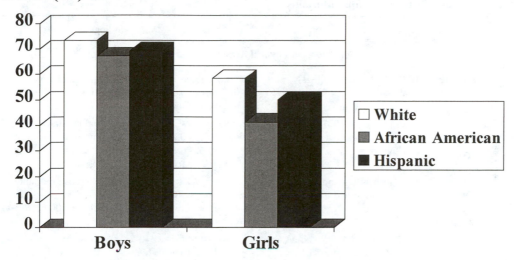

FIGURE 12–2   Percentage of high school students who participated in vigorous physical activity, by sex and race ethnicity—United States, 1997. (From the Centers for Disease Control and Prevention.[12])

etal value of regular physical activity. These low activity levels suggest young adults to be an important target group for physical activity promotion programs in an effort to reverse individual and population-wide declines occurring prior to middle age.

Evidence Relating Physical Activity to Cardiovascular Disease and All-Cause Mortality

Multiple prospective studies published over the past 35 years have shown a strong, consistent, and graded relation between self-reported occupational[15–20] and leisure-time physical activity and CVD events, CVD mortality, and all-cause mortality.[2–7,21–43]

Occupational Physical Activity

Initial observations among London busmen suggested a relation between increased levels of occupational physical activity and risk of myocardial infarction.[15] These investigators found that the most highly active conductors on London's double-decker buses were at lower risk of coronary heart disease (CHD) and tended to suffer less severe heart attacks than those who worked sitting at the wheel. Other studies of occupationally physically active cohorts, such as farmers,[16] railroad trackmen and clerks,[17,18] cargo handlers and warehousemen,[19] and letter carriers and mail clerks[20] have also generally shown lower CHD risk with higher levels of physical activity but have not addressed potential confounders such as other CHD risk factors. Large metanalyses have summarized these earlier studies and confirm an inverse relation between physical activity and CHD risk.[21,22]

Leisure-Time Physical Activity

Recent studies documenting an inverse relation of leisure-time physical activity with CHD incidence and mortality as well as all-cause mortality are summarized in Table 12–1.

Paffenbarger and colleagues' landmark investigations showed habitual physical activity to be inversely related to the risk of coronary heart disease (CHD) in approximately 17,000 male college alumni

TABLE 12–1   Selected Recent Studies of Association between Self-Reported Physical Activity or Measured Fitness and Cardiovascular Disease and Total Mortality

Author	Population	Findings
Self-Reported Physical Activity		
Paffenbarger et al., 1986[24]	16,936 U.S. male college alumni aged 35–74 followed for 12–16 years	28% lower risk of all-cause mortality among those expending 2000 kcal/week or more versus less ($p < .0001$)
Kujala et al.,[34] 1998	7925 men and 7,977 women in Finland followed for 17 years	RR (95% CI) for all-cause mortality 0.57 (0.45–0.74) in conditioning exercisers and 0.71 (0.62–0.81) in occasional exercisers, versus sedentary
Haapanen et al.,[35] 1996	1072 men in Finland aged 35–63 followed for 11 years	RR = 2.74 (1.46–5.14) for all-cause mortality and 3.58 (1.45–8.85) for cardiovascular mortality for those expending <800 kcal/week versus >2100 kcal week
Haapanen et al.,[36] 1997	1340 men and 1500 women aged 35–63 followed for 10 years	RR = 1.98 (1.22–3.23) for those in lowest versus highest tertile of physical activity
Leon et al.,[37] 1997	12,138 middle-aged U.S. men followed for 16 years	29% reduction in CHD mortality and 22% reduction in all-cause mortality for those least versus moderately active
Rosengren et al.,[38] 1997	7142 men in Sweden aged 47 to 55 followed for 20 years	RR = 0.72 (0.56–0.92) for CHD death and RR = 0.70 (0.61–0.80) for total mortality in most versus least active
Eaton et al.,[39] 1995	8463 Israeli government employees followed for 21 years	RR = 0.79 (0.66–0.95) for CHD mortality and 0.91 (0.83–0.99) for all-cause mortality in those with greatest versus least leisure-time physical activity; no relation to work-related physical activity
Wannamethee et al.,[40] 1998	4311 British men (mean age 63) followed for 4 years	RR = 0.61 (0.48–0.86) for light, 0.50 (0.31–0.79) for moderate, and 0.65 (0.45–0.94) for moderately vigorous/vigorous exercisers versus sedentary

aged 35 to 74 years.[23] Their more recent report[24] showed those expending 2000 kcal or more per week (compared to those expending less) to have a 28 percent reduced risk of death from all causes ($p < .0001$) over a follow-up period of 12 to 16 years. There was a steady decline in death rates as physical activity increased from less than 500 kcal/week to 3500 kcal/week. Also, total energy expenditure from vigorous activities [requiring 6 or more resting metabolic equivalents (METs), such as brisk walking, running, or swimming], but not from nonvigorous activities, was associated with reduced mortality.[5]

Morris et al.[25] showed, among 3590 middle-aged male civil servants followed for 10 years, nearly a threefold higher incidence of both fatal myocardial infarction ($p < .001$) and sudden death ($p < .01$) among sedentary men as compared to men who participated in vigorous exercise sports. This study was also noteworthy in showing that exercise must be current; rates of CHD were as high in those who never played vigorous sports as in those who had previously (20 to 40 years prior) participated, but did not currently.[3]

A number of other recent reports provide further evidence regarding the inverse relation between self-

Author	Population	Findings
Kaplan et al.,[41] 1996	6131 U.S. adults followed for 28 years	RR = 0.84 (0.77–0.92) for all-cause mortality and 0.81 (0.71–0.93) for CVD mortality comparing those in 75th versus 25th percentile of activity, risk factor–adjusted
Rodriguez et al.,[42] 1994	8006 Japanese-American men aged 45–68 followed for 23 years	RR = 0.83 (0.70–0.99) for CHD incidence and 0.74 (0.56–0.97) for CHD mortality, attenuated after adjustment for risk factors
Folsom et al.,[43] 1997	7459 U.S. men and women aged 45–64 followed for 4–7 years	RR = 0.73 for women and RR = 0.82 for men for CHD incidence/standard deviation increment in physical activity, risk factor–adjusted; no relation to occupational physical activity
	Measured Physical Fitness	
Blair et al.,[4] 1989	10,224 men and 3120 women in U.S. followed for 8 years by the Cooper Clinic	RR (95% CI) for all-cause mortality in those in lowest versus highest fitness quintile 1.58 (1.32–1.89) in men and 1.94 (1.30–2.88) in women, risk factor–adjusted
Ecklund et al.,[28] 1988	4276 men aged 30–69 in the Lipid Research Clinics Mortality Follow-up Study followed for 10 years	RR (95% CI) for CVD mortality 2.7 (1.4–5.1) and CHD death 3.2 (1.5–6.7) per increment of 35 beats per minute at submaximal treadmill testing
Slattery et al.,[29] 1988	3043 white middle-aged men aged 22–79 followed for up to 20 years	RR = 1.43 (age-adjusted) and 1.20 (age- and risk factor–adjusted) for CHD death per 30 beats per minute heart rate at submaximal treadmill testing

reported physical activity and CHD morbidity and mortality and total mortality. The Finnish Twin Cohort[34] showed, among 7925 men and 7977 women who were initially healthy, a significantly reduced rate of death in those who were classified as conditioning exercisers [relative risk (RR) = 0.57, 95 percent confidence interval [(CI) 0.45 to 0.74] or occasional exercisers (RR = 0.71, 95% CI = 0.62 to 0.81). Findings remained at least as pronounced after adjusting for genetic factors and familial aggregation of health habits during childhood. In middle-aged Finnish men, those with an estimated leisure time physical activity energy expenditure of less than 800 kcal/week, as compared to 2100 kcal/week, were found to be at approximately a threefold greater risk for both cardiovascular and all-cause mortality after adjustment for age, smoking, and certain social characteristics.[35] These investigators also showed in

middle-aged men and women a significant inverse relation of physical activity to 10-year incidence of coronary heart disease.[36]

Several studies also show the inverse relation of physical activity with CHD to be independent of major, potentially confounding risk factors. A 20-year follow-up of 7142 men in Goteborg, Sweden, aged 47 to 55 years at baseline without symptomatic CHD,[38] showed, after adjustment for a wide range of risk factors, the most active men (as compared to the least active men) to have a significant 28 percent reduction in the risk of CHD death and 30 percent reduction in total mortality. The Israeli Ischemic Heart Disease Study[39] of nearly 8500 government employees showed self-reported leisure-time physical activity (but not work-related physical activity) also to be related to a significant 21 percent reduction in CHD mortality and a 9 percent reduction in all-cause mortality. These findings persisted after adjustment for potential confounding risk factors. Finally, the Alameda County Study,[41] involving follow-up of 6131 adults for 28 years, showed those at the 75th percentile (compared to those at the 25th percentile) of physical activity, after adjusting for other risk factors, to be at a 19 percent lower risk of CVD mortality and a 16 percent lower risk of all-cause mortality.

The possibility that the greatest cardiovascular benefits from physical activity may occur at moderate levels of exercise has also been noted. Sixteen-year follow-up of 12,138 middle-aged men at high risk of CHD participating in the Multiple Risk Factor Intervention Trial (MRFIT)[37] showed men in the least-active decile (0 to 9 min/day) of leisure-time physical activity to have a significant, excess age-adjusted mortality of 29 and 22 percent for CHD and all causes, respectively, as compared to those in deciles 2 to 4 (10 to 36 min/day). Higher deciles of activity, however, were not associated with further reductions in mortality. Also, in a British cohort of more than 4000 older men (mean age 63 years), compared to those sedentary, a 50 percent lower risk of incident CHD was found in moderate exercisers whereas only a 35 percent risk reduction was observed in more vigorous exercisers.[40] These findings suggest that cardiovascular benefits may be maximized at moderate levels of physical activity without further benefit at higher activity levels.

Other data suggest that the association of increased levels of physical activity to CHD incidence and mortality may be due to risk-factor differences between exercisers and nonexercisers. In 8006 Japanese-American men initially aged 45 to 68 years and followed for 23 years,[42] those in the highest tertile of physical activity had a significant 17 percent lower risk of incident CHD and 26 percent lower CHD mortality; however, these findings were attenuated after adjustment for cardiovascular risk factors. Also, among both men and women aged 45 to 64 years enrolled in the Atherosclerosis Risk in Communities (ARIC) study,[43] significant CHD risk reductions of 18 to 27 percent (depending on gender and physical activity measure used) were noted but were attenuated after adjustment for other risk factors. The impact of physical activity on CHD may be mediated at least in part by its effects on improving risk factors such as hypertension, diabetes, cholesterol, and body-mass index. These potential cardiovascular risk factor benefits of physical activity are discussed below.

Fitness Level and Cardiovascular Risk

Physical fitness measured by an exercise treadmill test has also been shown to be inversely related to all-cause mortality among more than 10,000 men and 3000 women followed for an average of slightly more than 8 years.[4] Age-adjusted all-cause mortality rates (per 10,000 person-years) declined significantly across fitness quintiles (least fit to most fit) from 64.0 to 18.6 in men and from 39.5 to 8.5 in women. Comparing those in the lowest to those in the highest quintile, relative risks (and 95 percent confidence intervals) were 1.58 (1.32 to 1.89) for men and 1.94 (1.30 to 2.88) for women after adjusting for other coronary risk factors. In addition, 8.5-year follow-up of 4276 men initially aged 30 to 69 who participated in the Lipid Research Clinics Mortality Follow-up Study provides further support to this. In these individuals, a lower level of physical fitness was associated with a higher risk of death (per increment of 35 beats per minute in heart rate during submaximal treadmill testing) from CVD (RR = 2.7, $p < .01$) or CHD (RR = 3.2, $p < .01$).[28] Finally, in 3043 U.S. railroad workers followed for up to 20 years, an increment of 30 beats per minute heart rate upon submaximal treadmill testing was associated with an age-adjusted relative risk for CHD of 1.43 (1.20 after adjusting for other risk factors).[29]

Cardiovascular Benefits of Physical Activity and Fitness

A wide range of studies conducted in youth, women, men, older persons, and different ethnic groups document increased levels of physical activity to be related to decreased or improved cardiovascular risk factors. Many of the benefits of exercise training from endurance and resistance activities diminish within 2 weeks if physical activity is significantly reduced and disappear entirely within 2 to 8 months.[8]

Children and Young Adults

In children and young adults aged 9 to 24, the Young Finns Study ($n = 2358$) showed level of physical activity to be positively associated with overall high-density lipoprotein-cholesterol (HDL-C) and HDL_2-C levels and negatively associated with triglycerides, apolipoprotein B, and insulin levels in males. In females, only a negative association with triglyceride levels was noted.[44] An inverse association of physical activity with obesity, but not blood pressure, was also observed. Among over 1500 Singapore youth aged 6 to 18, self-reported physical activity was significantly correlated (inversely) with total cholesterol and triglycerides in boys and with body fat and body-mass index in girls.[45] Amount of television watched as a marker of physical inactivity (among other unhealthful behaviors) has been shown to be significantly associated with body weight both in boys and girls and additionally with body-mass index and systolic blood pressure in boys[46] in a study of over 1000 youth in Belgium. In another study, amount of television watched was the strongest indicator of the likelihood of having total cholesterol levels of 200 mg/dL or higher after adjusting for other risk factors, including a family history of premature heart disease or hyperlipidemia.[47] Increasing usage of computers and the Internet could also be associated with reduced physical activity and should be the subject of future investigation.

Adults

Numerous studies document the relation of increased physical activity or fitness levels with an improved cardiovascular risk factor profile in adults. The Cooper Clinic showed increases in treadmill time to be associated with beneficial changes in several cardiovascular risk factors.[48] Others have shown aerobic exercise to be associated with decreases of 8 to 10 mmHg in systolic and diastolic blood pressure.[49-51]

The Pawtucket Heart Study found, in 381 men and 556 women, that both estimated maximal oxygen consumption and self-reported physical activity were significantly associated with blood pressure, body-mass index, and HDL-C, although the correlations were, in fact, stronger for oxygen consumption ($r = 0.24$ to 0.65) than for self-reported physical activity ($r = 0.09$ to 0.14).[52]

Among 1206 adults aged 35 to 64 living in rural Shanghai, China, significant inverse trends with physical activity were found in men for hypertension, total cholesterol, body-mass index, and heart rate and in women for hypertension, systolic and diastolic blood pressure, body-mass index, and heart rate. However, these findings (except for heart rate) were attenuated after adjustment for body mass index. HDL-C and current smoking, however, were not related to physical activity.[53]

Among 3331 adult Japanese men, frequency of physical activity was independently and inversely related to HDL-C levels, and those in the sedentary group had a greater number of coronary risk factors present than those who exercised 1, 2, and 3 or more days per week (mean number of risk factors: 1.38, 1.19, 1.19, and 0.99, respectively).[54] Finally, a pooled analysis among three European cohorts consisting of a total of 402 men aged 69 to 90 years demonstrated a significant inverse relation of total physical activity with HDL-C.[55]

Women

Recent studies of women document important protective associations of level of physical activity and cardiovascular risk factors. Increased levels of HDL-C seen as a result of exercise are related to changes in body weight, and those who exercise at higher levels also have greater increases in HDL-C.[56-58] In the Postmenopausal Estrogen/Progestins Intervention Trial among 851 women aged 45 to 64, leisure-time self-reported physical activity was positively associated with levels of HDL-C ($p = .001$) and inversely associated with insulin and fibrinogen levels (both $p < .05$). Moderate and heavy leisure activities were associated with the highest HDL-C levels.[59] A large cohort of 4576 Dutch women aged 49 to 70 showed blood pressure (systolic/diastolic) to be inversely associated with time spent in sports after adjustment for age, education, and smoking (128.9/77.8 mmHg in the highest sports tertile and 132.1/79.0 mmHg in the lowest sports tertile). Body-mass index, waist/hip ratio, and waist circumference also showed an inverse relation with certain physical activities.[60] Finally, intraabdominal adipose tissue, determined by computed tomography, appears to be negatively related to level of physical activity.[61]

Other Benefits of Physical Activity

Improved exercise performance with training is the result of (1) increased ability to use oxygen in deriving energy for work and (2) increased maximum ventilatory oxygen uptake related to increasing both maximum cardiac output and the ability of muscles to extract and use oxygen from blood. There are also beneficial changes in hemodynamic, hormonal, metabolic, neurologic, and respiratory function that occur with increased exercise capacity.[1]

Physical activity may favorably affect body fat distribution, while physical inactivity results in fewer kilocalories expended, leading to obesity.[8] In overweight persons, regular physical activity enhances the effects on blood lipoprotein levels of a diet low in saturated fat and cholesterol.[62] Exercise training has beneficial effects on adipose tissue distribution[63] and on insulin sensitivity.[64] There may also be a beneficial effect in the prevention of other diseases, including certain cancers and osteoporosis.[65]

Resistance training, while having only modest effects on most cardiovascular risk factors as compared to aerobic training, does aid carbohydrate metabolism through the development or maintenance of muscle and the effects on basal metabolism.[66–67]

Finally, longitudinal studies have shown that exercise training appears to result in improvement in psychological functioning, including reducing depression,[68–70] improving self-confidence and self-esteem,[71] and attenuating cardiovascular and neurohumoral responses to mental stress.[72] Physical activity also improves health-related quality of life by enhancing psychological well-being and improving physical functioning in those impaired by poor health.[8]

Assessment of Physical Activity and Fitness

Self-Report Techniques

Diaries, logs, recall surveys, retrospective quantitative histories, and global self-reports are frequently used to give an overall estimate of physical activity, often taking into account intensity, duration, frequency, and type of activity:[8]

1. *Diaries* detail nearly all physical activity performed in a given (usually short) period and usually involve a summary index derived by summing the total duration of time spent in an activity multiplied by the estimated rate of energy expenditure or intensity, or listing the accumulated time across all activities.
2. *Logs* provide a record of participating in specific types of activities. Both diaries and logs are frequently time-intensive to complete.
3. *Recall surveys* are generally useful for assessing physical activity in large populations because they are easy to administer, not costly, and generally acceptable to study participants. They are used for time frames ranging from 1 week to a lifetime and may assess either precise or more general estimates of usual participation.
4. A *retrospective quantitative history* is the most comprehensive type of physical activity recall survey, requiring detailed information on frequency and duration of participation for a given list of activities performed for up to the past year.
5. *Global self-reports* involve asking respondents to rate their level of physical activity in relation to the adult population in general or to a specific age/gender group. One drawback is that there is often actually greater variation inherent in persons giving similar ratings.[8]

Appendixes 12–1 and 12–2 provide examples of self-reported physical activity surveys that are practical to administer to a general adult population.

Direct Monitoring

Physical activity can also be measured more directly by behavioral observation, the use of mechanical or electronic devices, or physiologic measurements. Although not subject to the limitations of memory and biases, as in self-reporting, these methods are usually quite expensive and burdensome on participants and staff and have been traditionally used mainly for small-scale studies.

Mechanical or electronic measurement involves devices such as those used to monitor heart rates and can provide a continuous recording of a physiologic process, representing both the duration and intensity of activity. Estimated daily energy expenditure, such as oxygen update, for a given physical activity can be obtained; however, there are limitations. The heart rate–energy expenditure curve is different for each individual and variable for low-intensity physical activities. Furthermore, wearing of such monitors for

extended periods of time can be inconvenient. Other methods involve the use of motion sensors, such as pedometers, or *physiologic measures of energy expenditure* such as calorimetry, where measurement of expired air is obtained.[8]

Measurement of Physical Activity Intensity

The intensity of physical activity can be characterized using qualitative terms such as *light* or *low, moderate* or *mild, hard* or *vigorous,* or *very hard* or *strenuous.*[8] For example, one validated instrument, as used in the Coronary Artery Risk Development in Young Adults (CARDIA) study,[73] allows for the calculation of estimated energy expenditure (EEE) for each of several activity groups based on known intensities in metabolic units or METs (ratio of metabolic rate during activity to resting metabolic rate) (Table 12–2 and Appendix 12–2). From the

TABLE 12–2   One-Year Physical Activity Recall: Activity Groups and Metabolic Equivalent (MET) Values

Activity Groups and Sample Activities*	METs
Vigorous home-related activities [e.g., snow shoveling, moving or lifting heavy objects (>9 kg), chopping wood]	6.0
Vigorous work-related activities [e.g., lifting and carrying heavy loads (>9 kg), digging ditches, heavy carpentry, heavy construction, heavy ranching, [such as working irrigation ditches]	8.0
Jogging, running, vigorous hiking, cross-country skiing	8.0
Vigorous racket sports	8.0
Vigorous bicycling (>16 km/h), rowing machine, jumping rope	8.0
Swimming, other vigorous water activities (e.g., water-skiing)	6.0
Vigorous exercise class, jazz exercise, vigorous dancing	6.0
Other strenuous sport (e.g., downhill skiing, roller skating, soccer, basketball)	7.0
Vigorous conditioning exercises (e.g., vigorous calisthenics, universal workout, weight lifting)	6.0
Less strenuous home maintenance, gardening	5.0
Indoor household chores (e.g., painting, cleaning, child care)	4.5
Less strenuous work-related activities (e.g., waitressing, nursing, lifting, carrying >9 kg)	4.5
Less strenuous home exercise, calisthenics	4.0
Less strenuous sports (e.g., hunting, badminton)	4.0
Bowling, golf	3.5
Other brisk walking (not covered in previous questions), hiking	4.0

*"Vigorous" activities were defined as those with a MET level of 6 or more.
Source: Adapted from Sidney et al.,[73] with permission.

frequency and duration spent on each activity, EEE per year can be calculated by summing across all activity groups, plus the energy spent in sleep (assigned a MET value of 1.0), plus the EEE from light activities (assigned a MET value of 1.5—e.g., sitting). The EEE per year is then estimated by subtracting all the time not spent in moderate (MET grouping 3.5 to 5.0) or vigorous (MET grouping ≥6.0) activity.

Assessment of Physical Fitness

Physical fitness assessment is more highly developed and relies on measurements of endurance (or cardiorespiratory fitness), muscular fitness, and body composition, often with excellent accuracy and reliability. Maximal oxygen uptake or aerobic power ($\dot{V}_{O_2 max}$) is the most established criterion of cardiorespiratory fitness and is measured in healthy persons during large-muscle dynamic activity such as walking, running, or cycling. It is most accurately determined by measuring expired air composition and respiratory volume during maximal exertion but requires expensive equipment, trained technicians, and cooperation from the participant. It can also be estimated from peak exercise workload during a maximal exercise test without measuring respiratory gases; this requires a calibrated exercise device, adherence to a protocol, and cooperation from the participant.[8]

Health behaviors such as physical activity are difficult to measure accurately and their validity is often in question. It is often uncertain how well self-reported physical activity represents an individual's habitual activity, considering factors such as incomplete recall, exaggeration of the amount of activity, and unrepresentative time intervals frequently sampled. Little work has been published validating self-reports with various measures of physical fitness. Misclassification using invalid measures would tend to bias studies toward finding no association; the consistent finding of the association of physical activity with lower risk of several diseases suggests that such measures do have at least some validity and that more precise measures would show even stronger associations.[8]

Recommendations for Physical Activity in Adults

Recommendations in Healthy Persons for Primary Prevention of Coronary Heart Disease

In 1996, the National Institutes of Health convened a consensus development conference[74] that resulted in the following recommendations:

1. All Americans should engage in regular physical activity at a level appropriate to their capacity, needs, and interests.
2. Children and adults alike should set a goal of accumulating at least 30 min of moderate-intensity physical activity on most and preferably all days of the week.
3. For those with known cardiovascular disease, cardiac rehabilitation programs that combine physical activity with reduction in other risk factors should be more widely used.

These recommendations were based on the premise that most Americans have little or no physical activity in their daily lives (largely because of changes in the work environment). The evidence to date suggests physical inactivity to be a major risk factor for CVD. Also, even moderate levels of physical activity can confer strong benefits, and those already meeting goals can derive additional benefit by becoming more physically active or including more vigorous activity.[75] Public health recommendations have evolved from emphasizing vigorous aerobic activity for cardiorespiratory fitness to moderate levels of activity for a wide variety of health benefits; cardiorespiratory endurance activities should be supplemented with strength-development exercises at least twice per week to improve musculoskeletal health and maintain the ability to perform normal activities.[8]

In the health care setting or at the work site, only trained and experienced personnel should discuss physical activity and provide exercise prescriptions for patients and their families. Untrained but well-intentioned personnel frequently offer improper information and are not prepared to supervise or monitor patient activity. Physicians and their staff have the responsibility to promote regular physical activity as well as the reduction of other risk factors. Although many delegate the task of providing these services to other members of the health care team, physicians must set up and support the agenda and determine what is medically appropriate. Exercise specialists, including appropriately trained nurses, can also work with the physician in physical activity assessment, prescription, and monitoring. Medical training programs should now begin to prepare physicians to recommend physical activity and to assess it as part of every medical history.[1] Consideration should be given to intensity, duration, and frequency as well as mode and progression of all types of physical activity programs.[76] Sedentary men over the age of 40 or women over the age of 50 are advised to consult a physician before beginning a vigorous physical activity program.[8]

The President's Council on Physical Fitness and Sports[77] provides, as an initial classification, five different levels of physical activity (Table 12–3). These include activities that are universally recommended and depend on the individual's current level of activity. For those pursuing a modest level of activity, recommendations are provided for additional activ-

TABLE 12–3 Model for Physical Activity Recommendations

Activities recommended for everyone

Activities for sedentary individuals

Activities for moderately active individuals interested in health
  Cardiovascular
  Bone
  Low back
  Psychological

Activities for moderately active individuals interested in physical fitness
  Aerobic fitness
  Relative leanness
  Muscular strength and endurance
  Flexibility

Activities for vigorously active individuals interested in performance
  Sport(s)
  Physical task(s)

Source: From the Department of Health and Human Services.[76]

ity based largely on the individual's specific health, fitness, and/or performance goals.

Activities for everyone promote general health and well-being and can be done as part of the individual's daily living routine. Examples include walking rather than riding whenever possible, climbing stairs instead of taking an elevator, parking further away from one's destination (e.g., workplace or store), and other alternatives to the daily routine that will improve incidental physical activity.

For sedentary individuals who are currently engaging in no physical activity or those who cannot walk for 30 min continuously without discomfort or pain (those unable to walk can substitute other activities, such as moving in a wheelchair or swimming), 30 min of moderate-intensity activity is recommended, in addition to the universally recommended activities mentioned above. This may involve walking, yard work, cycling, or low-impact exercise broken into two to four 10-min segments during the workday and/or in the morning or evening.

A moderately active individual, in contrast, should be able to accumulate 30 min of activity daily (e.g., 30 min of walking continuously without pain or discomfort) in addition to those activities recommended for sedentary individuals. Such an individual would typically not be able to jog 3 mi (or walk 6 mi at a brisk pace, cycle 12 mi, or swim $\frac{3}{4}$ mi) continuously without discomfort or undue fatigue. These individuals should be encouraged to include 30 min of moderate-intensity activity in their daily routine (Table 12–4).

Moderately active individuals with fitness goals should continue to accumulate the recommended 30 min of daily activity as described above. In addition, specific types of activity should be considered, depending on the goal desired (Table 12–5). For example, if aerobic fitness is desired, at least 20 min of high-intensity activity should be preceded and followed by 5 to 10 min of moderate-intensity activity, 3 to 4 days per week. The heart rate during these vigorous activities should be 70 to 85 percent of the age-predicted maximum, calculated as follows: target heart rate = (0.70 to 0.85) × (220 beats per minute − age in years). For example a 40-year-old individual would have an estimated maximum heart rate of 180 beats per minute, with a target heart rate of 126 to 153 beats per minute. Other goals, such as achieving muscular strength and endurance, require resistance activities to maintain muscle mass.

TABLE 12–4   Physical Activity for Health Goals*

Health Goal	Recommended Activity
Cardiovascular	Accumulate at least 30 min of daily moderate-intensity activities
	Include longer duration and/or higher intensity
Bone	Weight-bearing activities
	Resistance exercises
Low Back	Static stretching in midtrunk and thigh regions
	Abdominal curl ups
Psychological	Enjoyable activities and fun atmosphere

*These activities should be considered *after* an individual is already doing those activities recommended in Table 12–3. These activities should be done *in addition* to Table 12–3 activities.
Source: From the Department of Health and Human Services.[76]

TABLE 12–5   Physical Fitness Goals and Recommended Activities*

Physical Fitness Goals	Recommended Activities
Aerobic fitness	20–30 min of vigorous-intensity activity, 3–5 days per week
Relative leanness, too little fat	Eat more calories, especially carbohydrates
	Include resistance exercise
Too much fat	Reduce calories, especially fat
	Increase duration of aerobic activities
	Include resistance exercise
Muscular strength/ muscle endurance	Include resistance exercise: one to two sets, 10–15 repeats, each group 2–3 days per week
Flexibility	Daily static stretching, 10–30 s two to three times, each joint

*These activities should be considered only *after* an individual is doing the activities in Table 12–4. These activities should be done *in addition* to Table 12–4 activities.
Source: From the Department of Health and Human Services.[76]

A vigorously active individual can run 3 mi (or walk fast 6 mi, cycle 12 mi, or swim $\frac{3}{4}$ mi) continuously within his or her target heart rate, three to four times per week without discomfort or pain (Table 12–6). For those with performance goals, a variety of sport and performance activities should be considered depending on level of interest—such as soccer, basketball, racquetball, or high-intensity exercise to music—in addition to accumulating 30 min of daily moderate-intensity activity, including vigorous activity at target heart rate during the days when no sport/performance activities are planned.

The long-term success of any physical activity program is determined by compliance. While one is on business or vacation, there must be a plan for incorporating physical activities, as for other aspects of the trip (meals, social functions, etc.). Although many lodging facilities do provide exercise or fitness facilities, this is not always the case. Exercise facilities may not always be convenient or available; as a substitute, one can bring portable exercise equipment, such as walking or jogging shoes.[76]

Important influences on physical activity patterns both in adults and in younger people include confidence in one's ability to engage in certain activities (self-efficacy), enjoyment of the activity, support from others, positive beliefs concerning the benefits

TABLE 12–6   Recommended Activity for Performance Goals*

Performance Goals	Recommended Activities
Sport or physical task(s)	Develop and/or maintain fitness levels
	Interval training
	Motor tasks related to performance
	Specific skills related to performance
	Strategy and mental readiness

*These activities should be considered only *after* an individual is doing activities recommended in Table 12–5. These activities should be done *in addition* to activities in Table 12–5.
Source: From the Department of Health and Human Services.[76]

of physical activity, and the lack of any perceived barriers to being physically active.[8]

Physical Activity in Secondary Prevention

In persons with CVD or diabetes or at high risk for these diseases, a consultation with a physician is recommended before beginning a new physical activity program.[8] For promotion of physical activity in those who have recently suffered a cardiac event, walking is the recommended mode of early activity unless the individual is recommended to attend supervised exercise classes, where other activities can be provided. Limited walking can begin with gradual increases in duration until 5 to 10 min of continuous movement is achieved. In the first 2 weeks after myocardial infarction or coronary artery bypass surgery, the emphasis should be on offsetting the effects of bed rest or prior periods of physical inactivity. Initial activities should be supervised, with symptoms, rating of perceived exertion, heart rate, and blood pressure monitored. When safety and tolerance have been documented, activity can be performed unsupervised. Such activity is usually safe; however, patients should be instructed regarding precautions—such as awareness of chest discomfort, faintness, and dyspnea—and should appropriately consult their physicians.[76]

After the patient's condition has stabilized, usually 2 to 6 weeks after the coronary event, a symptom-limited exercise test is performed; this is essential prior to the beginning of a physical activity program. In most cases, a conditioning program can be initiated, with careful prescription of activity based on the results of the exercise test and consultation. Conditioning will generally involve the use of large-muscle-group activities, initially performed for 10 min, with the goal of building up to 20 to 30 min at a time. Supervised group sessions are generally recommended to enhance the educational process, ensure tolerability, confirm progress, and provide medical supervision in high-risk situations. Low-risk persons who are highly motivated and understand the principles of exercise training may undertake unsupervised home programs.[76]

In the absence of ischemia or significant arrhythmias (low-risk patients), exercise intensity should approximate 50 to 80 percent of the maximal oxygen capacity based on the exercise test or 20 beats per minute above resting heart rate until such a test is performed. The exercise training heart rate should be 50 to 75 percent of the heart rate reserve, as follows:

$$[(\text{Maximal heart rate} - \text{resting heart rate}) \times 50 \text{ to } 75\%] + \text{resting heart rate}$$

Activities can be prescribed on the basis of the work intensity at which this training heart rate is achieved after 5 to 10 min at the same workload (steady state). Widely available heart rate counters can be used as aids.[76]

The intensity of exercise can also be judged by the individual using a perceived exertion rating scale consisting of 15 categories ranging from 6 to 20, with a verbal description at every odd number beginning with 7 (very, very light) progressing to 19 (very, very hard). As a general guideline, less than 12 is perceived as light intensity (40 to 60 percent of maximal heart rate), 12 to 13 as moderate intensity (60 to 75 percent of maximal heart rate), and 14 to 16 as high intensity (75 to 90 percent of maximal heart rate). Several training sessions using this perceived exertion scale will be needed to validate an activity's difficulty. Normally, individuals may begin at moderate intensity levels—although some may need to begin at light intensity levels. After safe levels have been established, increments in duration of 5 min can be made each week. With increased strength and decreases in exercise heart rate with conditioning, intensity levels can be eventually increased and some resistance exercises added.[76]

In moderate- to high-risk individuals, such as those with ischemia or arrhythmias, an exercise test and medical supervision are essential. The conditioning work intensity is derived from the heart rate associated with the abnormality, with the recommended peak training heart rate usually 10 beats per minute below the heart rate where the abnormality occurs. If exercise continues to a high level of effort, a heart rate of 50 to 60 percent of the maximum can be used if it falls at least 10 beats below where the abnormality occurs. Ideally, these individuals should be enrolled in a cardiac rehabilitation program that can risk-stratify them appropriately, and exercise testing should be repeated at least annually.[76]

Recommendations for Physical Activity in Youth

Physical activity should begin early in the school years and continue throughout an individual's lifetime. The early years are most important for developing positive attitudes toward physical activity. Schools must designate physical education programs with trained teachers for children at an early age. Recreational sports—including running, dancing, swimming, and certain resistance exercises using free weights or specific equipment—can be used with supervision. There must also be a supportive environment both at school and in the home conducive to physical activity.[77]

Interventions that target physical education in elementary schools can increase the amount of time that students spend engaging in physical activity.[8] Children at higher levels of cardiovascular risk may see significant benefits in the reduction or control of risk factors from physical activity of appropriate quantity and intensity. For some children, participation in physical activity is a way of life, but for an increasing number, this is not true. The increasing trend of obesity demonstrates that a greater effort needs to be made to promote participation in physical activity.

The President's Council on Physical Fitness and Sports has also recently published guidelines for physical activity in children[77,78] (Table 12–7). These guidelines are intended to aid teachers, coaches, parents, and others who work with children, helping children to make decisions that are in their best interest. Guidelines 1 and 2 specify more activity for children than for adults because children are inherently active, need activity for normal growth and development, and need time in activity to develop lifetime physical activity skills. Because children are by nature active intermittently and not necessarily captivated by longer, sustained exercise, as are adults, Guideline 3, specifying intermittent exercise, is provided. The rationale of Guideline 4, which discourages extended periods of inactivity for children, is based on the observation that children become less active over time, and childhood inactivity tracks to adulthood inactivity. Therefore, avoiding long periods of inactivity and engaging in frequent periods of activity during the day would hopefully prevent inactivity in adults. Finally, Guideline 5 encourages a wide variety of physical activities that build upon all parts of health-related physical fitness, including cardiovascular fitness, strength, muscular endurance, flexibility, and healthy body composition.

Summary guidelines (Table 12–8)[79] specific for adolescents are also published. Although these guidelines are more similar to adult guidelines than the guidelines for children, much of the activity for teens will be associated with school and community activities. A wide variety of activities should be en-

---

TABLE 12–7 Physical Activity for Children: Guidelines Summary

Guideline 1. Elementary school–aged children should accumulate at *least 30 to 60 min* of age-appropriate physical activity from a variety of physical activities on all or most days of the week.

Guideline 2. An accumulation of more than 60 min and up to several hours per day of age- and developmentally appropriate activity is encouraged for elementary school–aged children.

Guideline 3. Some of the child's physical activity each day should be in periods lasting 10 to 15 min or more and include moderate to vigorous physical activity. This activity will typically be intermittent in nature, involving alternating moderate to vigorous activity with *brief periods* of rest and recovery.

Guideline 4. *Extended periods of inactivity are inappropriate* for children.

Guideline 5. A variety of physical activities is recommended for elementary school children.

Source: Adapted from the National Association of Sport and Physical Education,[78] with permission.

couraged to provide a foundation that can serve for a lifetime.

A comprehensive set of guidelines for the promotion of physical activity among young people and adolescents has also been published (Table 12–9),[80]

TABLE 12–8 Physical Activity for Adolescents: Guidelines Summary

Guideline 1. All adolescents should be physically active daily or nearly every day as part of play, games, sports, work, transportation, recreation, physical education, or planned exercise in family, school, and community activities.

Guideline 2. Adolescents should engage in three or more sessions per week of activities that last 20 min or more at a time and require moderate to vigorous levels of exertion.

Source: Adapted from Sallis et al.,[79] with permission.

suggesting that initiatives that can be implemented in schools and communities, giving attention to the roles of parents, community organizations, and health care professionals. These guidelines are based on the premise that youth are most likely to develop physically active lifestyles if they are provided with experiences they enjoy and can be successful at, and which are developmentally appropriate and matched to the individual or group's interests.

Conclusions

There is an increasing trend toward a sedentary lifestyle among most age, gender, and ethnic groups in the United States. A significant proportion of the population does not engage in recommended levels of physical activity. Physical inactivity has been determined to be a major independent risk factor for

TABLE 12–9 Guidelines for Promoting Physical Activity Among Youth

1. **Policy:** Schools and communities should establish policies that promote enjoyable, lifelong physical activity among young people.

2. **Environment:** Schools and communities should provide physical and social environments that encourage and enable safe and enjoyable physical activity.

3. **Physical Education:** Schools should implement physical education programs that emphasize enjoyable participation in physical activity and that help students develop the knowledge, attitudes, motor skills, behavioral skills, and confidence needed to adopt and maintain physically active lifestyles.

4. **Health Education:** Schools should implement health education programs that help students develop the knowledge, attitudes, behavioral skills, and confidence needed to adopt and maintain physically active lifestyles.

5. **Extracurricular Activities:** Schools should provide extracurricular physical activity programs that meet the needs and interests of all students.

6. **Parental Involvement:** Parents and guardians should be in physical activity instruction programs and in extracurricular and in community physical activity programs, and they should be encouraged to support their children's participation in enjoyable physical activity.

7. **Personnel Training:** Schools and communities should provide training for education, coaching, recreation, and health-care personnel that imparts the knowledge and skills needed to effectively promote enjoyable, lifelong physical activity among young people.

8. **Health Services:** Health care professionals should assess physical activity patterns among young people, counsel them about physical activity, refer them to appropriate programs, and advocate for physical activity instruction and programs for young people.

9. **Community Programs:** Communities should provide a range of developmentally appropriate community sports and recreation programs that are attractive to all young people.

10. **Evaluation:** Schools and communities should regularly evaluate physical activity instruction, programs, and facilities.

Source: Adapted from Centers for Disease Control and Prevention.[80]

CVD and all-cause mortality. Increased levels of physical activity leads to improvements in blood pressure, diabetes, lipoprotein levels, and obesity. It is well established that some activity is better than inactivity, and excessive amounts of physical activity may not lead to incremental benefit in the risk reduction of CVD risk beyond a certain point.

Physical activity should begin sooner rather than later within one's life span for increased health and longevity. Parents, schools, and community organizations need to provide a supportive environment that encourages and integrates physical activity into the daily lifestyle. Children must be introduced to the principles of regular physical activity and be provided with opportunities and skills that they can enjoy for many years. Parents need to be educated regarding the health benefits of regular physical activity and its contribution to quality of life and given the skills to incorporate activity into their daily lives involving the entire family.[1] As our society continues to perform less work-related physical activity, the population will require new ways to obtain adequate and regular physical activity to promote a healthy life.

APPENDIX 12–1   THE AEROBICS CENTER LONGITUDINAL STUDY PHYSICAL ACTIVITY QUESTIONNAIRE

Activity component(s) assessed:
  Leisure and household
Time frame of recall:
  Past 3 mo
Original mode of administration:
  Self-administered by mail
Primary source of information:
  Dr. Steven N. Blair
  Cooper Institute for Aerobics Research
  12330 Preston Road
  Dallas, TX 75230
Primary reference:
  Kohl, H. W., S. N. Blair, R. S. Paffenbarger, Jr., C. A. Macera, and J. J. Kronenfeld. A mail survey of physical activity habits as related to measured physical fitness. *Am J. Epidemiol.* 127:1228–1239, 1988.

Reliability and Validity Studies

TABLE 1   Validation studies of the Aerobics Institute Longitudinal Study Questionnaire

References	Method	Sample	Summary Results	
Kohn et al. (1)	Relationships between treadmill time and various physical activity parameters from the survey (Pearson correlations)	374 male patients of the Cooper Clinic with an average age of 47.1 years	Racket sports	0.01
			Bicycling	0.06
			Swimming	−0.11
			Other strenuous sports	0.19*
			Frequency of sweating	0.51*
			Runners, joggers, and walkers	
			Miles/workout	0.35*
			Workouts/wk	0.29*
			Average time/mile	−0.39*
Oliveria et al. (3)	Relationships between weekly energy expenditure from physical activity and maximal exercise treadmill time (correlation coefficients†)	7570 predominantly white, married, college-educated men between the ages of 20 and 80 yr	Baseline physical activity	0.41
			Follow-up physical activity in 1982	0.32

*$p < 0.05$.

†No p value reported.

Source: Reprinted with permission from Dr. Steven N. Blair, Cooper Institute for Aerobics Research, Dallas, TX.

In this section we would like to ask you about your current physical activity and exercise habits that you perform regularly, at least once a week. Please answer as accurately as possible. Circle your answer or supply a specific number when asked.

Exercise/Physical Activity

1. For the last three months, which of the following moderate or vigorous activities have you performed regularly? *(Please circle YES for all that apply and NO if you do not perform the activity; provide an estimate of the amount of activity for all marked YES. Be as complete as possible.)*

Walking

    NO   YES ⟶   How many sessions per week?   _____

                        How many miles (or fractions) per session?   _____

                        Average duration per session?   _____ (minutes)

What is your usual pace of walking? *(Please circle one)*

CASUAL or STROLLING (<2 mph)	AVERAGE or NORMAL (2 to 3 mph)	FAIRLY BRISK (3 to 4 mph)	BRISK or STRIDING (4 mph or faster)

Stair Climbing

    NO   YES ⟶   How many flights of stairs do you   _____

                        climb UP each day? (1 flight = 10 steps)

Jogging or Running

    NO   YES ⟶   How many sessions per week?   _____

                        How many miles (or fractions) per session?   _____

                        Average duration per session?   _____ (minutes)

Treadmill

    NO   YES ⟶   How many sessions per week?   _____

                        Average duration per session?   _____

                        Speed? _____ (mph) Grade? _____ (%)

Bicycling

    NO   YES ⟶   How many sessions per week?   _____

                        How many miles per session?   _____

                        Average duration per session?   _____ (minutes)

Swimming Laps

    NO   YES ⟶   How many sessions per week?   _____

                        How many miles per session?

                         (880 yds = 0.5 miles)   _____

                        Average duration per session?   _____ (minutes)

Aerobic Dance/Calisthenics/Floor Exercise
  NO   YES ⟶   How many sessions per week?   _____
                Average duration per session?   _____ (minutes)

**Moderate Sports (e.g. Leisure volleyball, golf
(not riding), social dancing, doubles tennis)**
  NO   YES ⟶   How many sessions per week?   _____
                Average duration per session?   _____ (minutes)

**Vigorous Racquet Sports (e.g. Racquetball,
singles tennis)**
  NO   YES ⟶   How many sessions per week?   _____
  NO   YES ⟶   Average duration per session?   _____ (minutes)

**Other Vigorous Sports or Exercise Involving
Running (e.g. Basketball, soccer)**
  NO   YES ⟶   Please specify: _____
                How many sessions per week?   _____
                Average duration per session?   _____ (minutes)

Other Activities
  NO   YES ⟶   Please specify: _____
                How many sessions per week?   _____
                Average duration per session?   _____ (minutes)

Weight Training (Machines, free weights)
  NO   YES ⟶   How many sessions per week?   _____
                Average duration per session?   _____ (minutes)

**Household Activities (Sweeping, vacuuming,
washing clothes, scrubbing floors)**
  NO   YES ⟶   How many hours per week?   _____

Lawn Work and Gardening
  NO   YES ⟶   How many hours per week?   _____

2. How many times a week do you engage in vigorous physical activity long enough to work up a sweat? _____ *(times per week)*

Instructions:

Instructions for the recipient are listed on the first page of the questionnaire.

Calculations:

Scoring has been done by assigning MET values to reported activities as shown below (1). The scores can also be converted to kilocalories (3).

$$(\text{sessions/wk}) \times (\text{min/session}) \times (\text{h/min}) \times (\text{METs}) = \text{MET-h/wk}$$

Example:

Hypothetical raw data from the ACLS questionnaire:
  Bicycling: 3 sessions/wk, 10 miles/session, 30 min/session
Swimming: 2 session/wk, 1 mile/session, 60 min/session
  Bicycling is assigned a MET value of 4.0, and swimming is assigned a MET value 10.0 (1).
  Bicycling: (3 sessions/wk) × (30 min/session) × (1 h/60 min × 4.0 METs) = 6.0 MET-h/wk
Swimming: (2 sessions/wk) × (60 min/session) × (1 h/60 min × 10.0 METs) = 20.0 MET-h/wk
  Total = 26.0 MET-h/wk

Other Studies Using the Questionnaire

In addition to the references cited above, at least one additional study has used the ACLS Questionnaire (2).

References

1. Kohl, H.W., S. N. Blair, R. S. Paffenbarger, Jr., C. A. Macera, and J. J. Kronenfeld. A mail survey of physical activity habits as related to measured physical fitness. *Am. J. Epidemiol.* 127:1228–1239, 1988.
2. Macera, C. A., K. L. Jackson, D. R. Davis, J. J. Kronenfeld, and S. N. Blair. Patterns of non-response to a mail survey. *J. Clin. Epidemiol.* 43:1427–1430, 1990.
3. Oliveria, S. A., H. W. Kohl, III, D. Trichopoulos, and S. N. Blair. The association between cardiorespiratory fitness and prostate cancer. *Med. Sci. Sports Exerc.* 28:97–104, 1996.

APPENDIX 12–2   CARDIA PHYSICAL ACTIVITY HISTORY

Activity component(s) assessed:
   Leisure, job, and home/household
Time frame of recall:
   Past 12 mo
Original mode of administration:
   Interviewer-administered in person or by telephone
Primary source of information:
   Dr. David R. Jacobs, Jr.
   Division of Epidemiology,
   University of Minnesota
   1300 South 2nd Street, Suite 300,
   Minneapolis, MN 55454
Primary reference:
   Jacobs, D. R. Jr., L. P. Hahn, W. L. Haskell, P. Pirie, and S. Sidney. Reliability and validity of a short physical activity history: CARDIA and the Minnesota Heart Health Program. *J. Cardiopulm. Rehab.* 9:448–459, 1989.

Reliability and Validity Studies

TABLE 6   Reliability studies of the CARDIA Physical Activity History

Reference	Methods	Sample	Summary Results	
Jacobs et al. (1)	Relationships between moderate intensity, heavy intensity, and total activity units at baseline and 2-wk retest (Pearson correlations[†])	129 men and women between the ages of 18 and 74 yr; 46% male, 80% employed, 19% homemaker, 37% high school graduate or less education	Moderate Heavy Total	0.77 0.79 0.84
Jacobs et al. (2)	Relationships between moderate intensity, heavy intensity, and total activity units at first test and 1-mo retest (correlation coefficients)	28 men and 50 women, predominantly Caucasian between the ages of 20 and 59 yr	Moderate Heavy Total	0.66* 0.91* 0.88*

*$p < 0.05$.
[†]No p value reported.

CARDIA PHYSICAL ACTIVITY HISTORY

Now I'll be asking you about some specific activities and the amount of time you spend doing each. Only include the time spent actually doing the activity. For example, sitting by the pool does not count as time swimming; sitting in a chair lift does not count as time skiing.

First I'll ask you about vigorous activities. Vigorous activities increase your heart rate or make you sweat when doing them or make you breathe hard or raise your body temperature. If you do an activity but not vigorously, please include it later when I ask you about other non-strenuous sports.

1. The first vigorous activity is running or jogging. Did you run or jog in the past 12 months for at least one hour total time in any month? For instance, you might have done three 20-minute sessions in the month. (VIGOROUS BACKPACKING, HIKING, MOUNTAIN CLIMBING)

___ Yes → 2. How many months did you do this activity?   _____

___ No ↓ 3. (How many of these months/In this month)
           did you do this activity for at least 1 hour a week?   _____

        4. (How many of these months/In this month)
           did you do this activity for at least 2 hours a week?   _____

5. Did you do vigorous racquet sports in the past 12 months for at least one hour total time in any month? (TENNIS, BADMINTON, PADDLE BALL, RACQUETBALL, HANDBALL, SQUASH)

___ Yes → 6. How many months did you do this activity?   _____

___ No ↓ 7. (How many of these months/In this month)
           did you do this activity for at least 1 hour a week?   _____

        8. (How many of these months/In this month)
           did you do this activity for at least 3 hours a week?   _____

9. Did you bicycle faster than 10 miles an hour or exercise hard on an exercise bicycle (in the past 12 months for at least one hour total time in any month)? (ROWING MACHINE)

___ Yes ➔   10. How many months did you do this activity?   _____

___ No ⬇   11. (How many of these months/In this month)
            did you do this activity for at least **1** hour a week?   _____

         12. (How many of these months/In this month)
            did you do this activity for at least **2** hours a week?   _____

13. Did you swim in the past 12 months for at least one hour total time in any month? (SNORKELING, SCUBA DIVING)

___ Yes ➔   14. How many months did you do this activity?   _____

___ No ⬇   15. (How many of these months/In this month)
            did you do this activity for at least **1** hour a week?   _____

         16. (How many of these months/In this month)
            did you do this activity for at least **2** hours a week?   _____

17. Did you do a vigorous exercise class or vigorous dancing (in the past 12 months for at least one hour total time in any month)? (JAZZERCISE, JANE FONDA-TYPE WORKOUT, AEROBIC DANCING, BALLET)

___ Yes ➔   18. How many months did you do this activity?   _____

___ No ⬇   19. (How many of these months/In this month)
            did you do this activity for at least **1** hour a week?   _____

         20. (How many of these months/In this month)
            did you do this activity for at least **3** hours a week?   _____

21. Did you do a vigorous job activity such as lifting, carrying, or digging in the past 12 months for at least one hour total time in any month? (LOADING TRUCKS, STACKING LUMBER)

___ Yes ➜ 22. How many months did you do this activity? _____

___ No ↓ 23. (How many of these months/In this month) did you do this activity for at least **2** hour a week? _____

24. (How many of these months/In this month) did you do this activity for at least **5** hours a week? _____

25. Did you do home or leisure activity such as snow shoveling, moving heavy objects, or weight lifting (in the past 12 months for at least one hour total time in any month)? (SHOVELING SAND OR GRAVEL, NAUTILUS WORKOUT, MOVING FURNITURE)

___ Yes ➜ 26. How many months did you do this activity? _____

___ No ↓ 27. (How many of these months/In this month) did you do this activity for at least **1** hour a week? _____

28. (How many of these months/In this month) did you do this activity for at least **3** hours a week? _____

29. Did you do other strenuous sports such as basketball, football, skating, or skiing in the past 12 months for at least one hour total time in any month? (MARTIAL ARTS, SOCCER, RUGBY, LAND OR WATER SKIING, ICE OR ROLLER SKATING)

___ Yes ➜ 30. How many months did you do this activity? _____

___ No ↓ 31. (How many of these months/In this month) did you do this activity for at least **1** hour a week? _____

32. (How many of these months/In this month) did you do this activity for at least **3** hours a week? _____

Now, I'd like to ask you about more leisurely activities.

33. Did you do nonstrenuous sports such as softball, shooting baskets, volleyball, ping pong, leisurely jogging, swimming or biking which we haven't included before (in the past 12 months for at least one hour total time in any month)? (HORSEBACK RIDING, FISHING FROM BANK OR BOAT, ARCHERY, NONVIGOROUS ROWING OR SAILING, NONVIGOROUS BIKING)

___ Yes ➜   34. How many months did you do this activity?   _____

___ No ⬇   35. (How many of these months/In this month) did you do this activity for at least **1** hour **a** week?   _____

         36. (How many of these months/In this month) did you do this activity for at least **3** hours a week?   _____

37. Did you take walks or hikes or walk to work in the past 12 months for at least one hour total time in any month? (STREAM FISHING, HUNTING)

___ Yes ➜   38. How many months did you do this activity?   _____

___ No ⬇   39. (How many of these months/In this month) did you do this activity for at least **2** hour a week?   _____

         40. (How many of these months/In this month) did you do this activity for at least **4** hours a week?   _____

41. Did you bowl or play golf (in the past 12 months for at least one hour total time in any month)?

___ Yes ➜   42. How many months did you do this activity?   _____

___ No ⬇   43. (How many of these months/In this month) did you do this activity for at least **1** hour a week?   _____
             ___ Always use motorized cart
         44. (How many of these months/In this month) did you do this activity for at least **3** hours a week?   _____
             ___ Always use motorized cart

45. Did you do home exercises or calisthenics in the past 12 months for at least one hour total time in any month? (NONVIGOROUS EXERCISE OR ROWING MACHINE)

___ Yes ➔ 46. How many months did you do this activity? _____

___ No ⬇ 47. (How many of these months/In this month) did you do this activity for at least **1** hour a week? _____

48. (How many of these months/In this month) did you do this activity for at least **3** hours a week? _____

49. Did you do home maintenance and gardening, including carpentry, painting, raking or mowing (in the past 12 months for at least one hour total time in any month)? (HANGING WALLPAPER, WEEDING, GARDENING)

___ Yes ➔ 50. How many months did you do this activity? _____

___ No ⬇ 51. (How many of these months/In this month) did you do this activity for at least **2** hour a week? _____

52. (How many of these months/In this month) did you do this activity for at least **5** hours a week? _____

53. List sports or other activities not elsewhere classified

SPORT:_____

54. Have you already counted this in any other category?

___ Yes (if yes, do not record here) ___ No

55. How many months? _____ 56. Average hrs. in those months? _____

57. List sports or other activities not elsewhere classified

SPORT:_____

58. Have you already counted this in any other category?

_ Yes (if yes, do not record here) ___ No

59. How many months? _____ 60. Average hrs. in those months? _____

TABLE 7   Validation studies of the CARDIA Physical Activity History

Reference	Method	Sample		Summary Results			
Jacobs et al. (1)	Relationships between total activity units and four skinfolds (SKIN), caloric intake (CAL), treadmill test (TRM), and HDL cholesterol (HDL-C) (Pearson correlations[†])	5069 men and women between the ages of 18 and 30 yr. 52% Black, 54% female; 40% ≤ 12 yr of education	Men Women	SKIN −0.12 −0.15	CAL 0.21 0.07	TRM 0.25 0.36	HDL-C 0.11 0.13
Jacobs et al. (2)	Relationships between moderate and heavy intensity activity units and maximum oxygen consumption (V_{O_2max}). % body fat (BF), Caltrac (CAL; MET-min/d), and total 4-wk activity history (FWH; MET-min/d) Spearman correlations)	28 men and 50 women predominantly Caucasian between the ages of 20 and 59 yr	Moderate Heavy	V_{O_2max} 0.08 0.63*	BF −0.09 −0.35*	CAL 0.11 0.31*	FWH 0.08 0.54*

*$p < 0.05$.

[†]No p value reported.

Source: Reprinted with permission from Dr. David R. Jacobs, Jr., Division of Epidemiology, Univ. of Minnesota, Minneapolis, MN.

Instructions

Instructions are listed on the questionnaire. Individuals are asked to specify any activities from a list of 13 activity categories that they participated in for at least 1 h (total time) during any of the last 12 mo (1). For specific activities, the individual reports the number of months of participation and the number of months of frequent participation. Frequent participation is defined as follows.

2 h or more for activity categories A (jogging or running), C (cycling), and D (swimming)

3 h or more for activity categories B (vigorous racket sports), E (vigorous exercise class or vigorous dancing), F (home or leisure activity such as snow shoveling, moving, lifting), H (strenuous sports such as basketball, football, skating, and skiing), I (nonstrenuous sports, bowling, golf), and L (home exercises, calisthenics)

4 h or more for category J (walks or hikes)

5 h or more for activity categories G (vigorous job activity) and M (home maintenance)

Calculations

Exercise units = sum (for moderate, heavy, or all activities) of:

$$(intensity) \times [(months\ of\ infrequent\ activity) + (3 \times months\ of\ frequent\ activity)]$$

Exercise units can be computed for moderate, heavy, or all activities separately: 100 exercise units is approximately equivalent to engaging in a heavy intensity activity (such as jogging) for 4 mo of the year. The intensity levels are listed in Table 8.

TABLE 8 Intensity levels for activities in the CARDIA Physical Activity History

	Intensity (METS/min)*	Cutpoint for Frequent Participation (h/wk)
Heavy intensity activities		
A. Jog or run	8	2
B. Vigorous racket sports	8	3
C. Bicycle faster than 10 mi/h	6	2
D. Swimming	6	2
E. Vigorous exercise class or vigorous dancing	6	3
F. Nonjob activity such as shoveling, weight lifting, and moving heavy objects	6	3
G. Vigorous job activity such as lifting, carrying, or digging	5	5
H. Other strenuous sports such as basketball, football, skating, or skiing	8	3
Moderate intensity activities		
J. Take walks or hikes or walk to work	4	4
K. Bowling or golf	3	3
L. Home exercises, calisthenics	4	3
M. Home maintenance and gardening, including carpentry, painting, raking, or mowing	4	5

*Approximately equal to kilocalories for a 70-kg man.

Reprinted by permission of the publisher from Jacobs, D. R. Jr., L. P. Hahn, W. L. Haskell, P. Pirie, and S. Sidney. Reliability and validity of a short physical activity history: CARDIA and the Minnesota Heart Health Program. J. Cardiopul. Rehabil. 9:448–459, 1989. Copyright 1989 by Lippincott-Raven Publishers.

Example

Activities of a hypothetical individual:

Weight-lifting:	< 3 h/wk for 2 mo and ≥ 3 h/wk for 1 mo
Golf:	< 3 h/wk for 3 mo
Walking:	< 4 h/wk for 6 mo and ≥ 4 h/wk for 6 mo
Moderate score:	$4 \times [6 + (3 \times 6)]$ for walks $+ 3 \times (3 + 0)$ for golf $= 105$
Heavy score:	$6 \times [2 + (3 \times 1)]$ for weight lifting $= 30$
Total score:	$105 + 30 = 135$ exercise units

References

1. Jacobs, D. R. Jr., L. P. Hahn, W. L. Haskell, P. Pirie, and S. Sidney. Reliability and validity of a short physical activity history: CARDIA and the Minnesota Heart Health Program. *J Cardiopul Rehabil* 9:448–459, 1989.

2. Jacobs, D. R. Jr., B. E. Ainsworth, T. J. Hartman, and A. S. Leon. A simultaneous evaluation of 10 commonly used physical activity questionnaires. *Med Sci Sports Exerc* 25:81–91, 1993.

3. Sidney, S., D. R. Jacobs, Jr., W. L. Haskell, et al. Comparison of two methods of assessing physical activity in the Coronary Artery Risk Development in Young Adults (CARDIA) Study. *Am J Epidemiol* 133:1231–1245, 1991.

4. Slattery, M. L. and D. R. Jacobs, Jr. Assessment of ability to recall physical activity of several years ago. *Ann Epidemiol* 5:292–296, 1995.

References

1. Fletcher GF, Balady G, Blair SN, et al: Statement on exercise: benefits and recommendations for physical activity programs for all Americans—a statement for health professionals by the Committee on Cardiac Rehabilitation of the Council on Clinical Cardiology, American Heart Association. *Circulation* 1996; 94:857–862.

2. Powell KE, Thompson PD, Caspersen CJ, Kendrick JS: Physical activity and the incidence of coronary heart disease. *Annu Rev Public Health* 1987; 8:253–287.

3. Morris JN, Clayton DJ, Everitt MG, et al: Exercise in leisure time: coronary attack and death rates. *Br Heart J* 1990; 63:325–334.

4. Blair SN, Kohl HW III, Paffenbarger RS Jr, et al: Physical fitness and all-cause mortality: a prospective study of healthy men and women. *JAMA* 1989; 262:2395–2401.

5. Lee IM, Hsieh CC, Paffenbarger RS Jr: Exercise intensity and longevity in men: the Harvard Alumni Health Study. *JAMA* 1995; 273:1179–1184.

6. Blair SN, Kohl HW III, Barlow CE, et al: Changes in physical fitness and all-case mortality: a prospective study of healthy and unhealthy men. *JAMA* 1995; 273:1093–1098.

7. Pate RR, Pratt M, Blair SN, et al: Physical activity and public health: a recommendation from the Centers for Disease Control and Prevention and the American College of Sports Medicine. *JAMA* 1995; 273:402–407.

8. *Physical Activity and Health: A Report of the Surgeon General.* Washington, DC, U.S. Department of Health and Human Services, Centers for Disease Control and Prevention, National Center for Chronic Disease Prevention and Health Promotion, The President's Council on Physical Fitness and Sports, 1996.

9. American Heart Association: *Physical Inactivity Biostatistical Fact Sheets, 1999.* Dallas, AHA, 1999.

10. Centers for Disease Control: *Chronic Diseases and Their Risk Factors: The Nation's Leading Causes of Death.* Washington, DC, U.S. Department of Health and Human Services, 1998.

11. Gazzaniga JM, Kao C, Cowling DW, et al: *Cardiovascular Disease Risk Factors among California Adults, 1984–1996.* Sacramento, CA, CORE Program, University of California San Francisco and California Department of Health Services, 1998.

12. Centers for Disease Control and Prevention: Youth risk behavior surveillance—United States, 1997. *MMWR* 1998; 47:1–89.

13. Caspersen CJ, Merritt RK: Physical activity trends among 26 states, 1986–1990. *Med Sci Sports Exerc* 1995; 27:713–720.

14. Anderssen N, Jacobs DR Jr, Sidney S, et al: Change and secular trends in physical activity patterns in young adults: a seven-year longitudinal follow-up in the Coronary Artery Risk Development in Young Adults Study (CARDIA). *Am J Epidemiol* 1996; 143:351–362.

15. Morris JN, Kagan A, Pattison DC, Gardner MJ: Incidence and prediction of ischaemic heart disease in London busmen. *Lancet* 1966; 2:552–559.

16. Pomrehn PR, Wallace RB, Burmeister LF: Ischemic heart disease mortality in Iowa farmers: the influence of lifestyle. *JAMA* 1982; 248:1073–1076.

17. Taylor HL, Blackburn H, Keys A, et al: Coronary heart disease in seven countries: IV. Five-year follow-up of employees of selected U.S. railroad companies. *Circulation* 1970; 41(suppl 1): 20–39.

18. Menotti A, Puddu V: Ten-year mortality from coronary heart disease among 172,000 men classified by occupational physical activity. *Scand J Work Environ Health* 1979; 5:100–108.

19. Paffenbarger RS Jr, Hale WE: Work activity and coronary heart mortality. *N Engl J Med* 1975; 292:545–550.

20. Kahn HA: The relationship of reported coronary heart disease mortality to physical activity of work. *Am J Public Health* 1963; 53:1058–1067.

21. Berlin JA, Colditz GA: A meta-analysis of physical activity in the prevention of coronary heart disease. *Am J Epidemiol* 1990; 132:612–628.

22. Karvonen MJ: Physical activity in work and leisure time in relation to cardiovascular diseases. *Ann Clin Res* 1983; 14(suppl 34):118–123.

23. Paffenbarger RS Jr, Wing AL, Hyde RT: Physical activity as an index of heart attack risk in college alumni. *Am J Epidemiol* 1978; 108:161–175.

24. Paffenbarger RS, Hyde RT, Wing AL, Hsieh C-C: Physical activity, all-cause mortality, and longevity of college alumni. *N Engl J Med* 1986; 314:605–613.

25. Morris JN, Everitt MG, Pollard R, Chave SPW: Vigorous exercise in leisure-time: protection against coronary heart disease. *Lancet* 1980; 2:1207–1210.

26. Leon AS, Connett J, Jacobs DR, Rauramaa R: Leisure-time physical activity levels and risk of coronary heart disease and death: the Multiple Risk Factor Intervention Trial. *JAMA* 1987; 258:2388–2395.

27. Pekkanen J, Marti B, Nissinen A, et al: Reduction of premature mortality by high physical activity: a 20-year follow-up of middle-aged Finnish men. *Lancet* 1987; 1:1473–1477.

28. Ekelund LG, Haskell WL, Johnson JL, et al: Physical fitness as a predictor of cardiovascular mortality in asymptomatic North American men: the Lipid Research Clinics Mortality Follow-up Study. *N Engl J Med* 1988; 319:1379–1384.

29. Slattery ML, Jacobs DR, Nichaman MZ: Leisure time physical activity and coronary heart disease death: the US Railroad Study. *Circulation* 1989; 79:304–311.

30. Shaper AG, Wannamethee G: Physical activity and ischemic heart disease in middle-aged British men. *Br Heart J* 1991; 66:384–394.

31. Paffenbarger RS Jr, Hyde RT, Wing AL, et al: The association of changes in physical activity level and other

lifestyle characteristics with mortality among men. *N Engl J Med* 1993; 328:538–545.

32. Lakka TA, Venalainen JM, Rauramaa R, et al: Relation of leisure-time physical activity level and cardiorespiratory fitness to the risk of acute myocardial infarction in men. *N Engl J Med* 1994; 339:1549–1554.

33. Blair SN, Kampert JB, Kohl HW, et al: Influences of cardiorespiratory fitness and other precursors on cardiovascular disease and all-cause mortality in men and women. *JAMA* 1996; 276:205–210.

34. Kujala UM, Kaprio J, Sarna S, Koskenvuo M: Relationship of leisure-time physical activity and mortality. *JAMA* 1998; 279:440–444.

35. Haapanen N, Miilunpalo S, Vuori I, et al: Characteristics of leisure time physical activity associated with decreased risk of premature all-cause and cardiovascular disease mortality in middle-aged men. *Am J Epidemiol* 1996; 143:870–880.

36. Haapanen N, Miilunpalo S, Vuori I, et al: Association of leisure time physical activity with the risk of coronary heart disease, hypertension, and diabetes in middle-aged men and women. *Int J Epidemiol* 1997; 26:739–747.

37. Leon AS, Myers MJ, Connett J: Leisure time physical activity and the 16-year risks of mortality from coronary heart disease and all-causes in the Multiple Risk Factor Intervention Trial (MRFIT). *Int J Sports Med* 1997; 18(suppl 3):S208–S215.

38. Rosengren A, Wilhelmsen L: Physical activity protects against coronary death and deaths from all causes in middle-aged men: evidence from 20-year follow-up of the primary prevention study in Goteborg. *Ann Epidemiol* 1997; 7:69–75.

39. Eaton CB, Medalie JH, Flocke SA, et al: Self-reported physical activity predicts long-term coronary heart disease and all-cause mortalities: twenty-one-year follow-up of the Israeli Ischemic Heart Disease Study. *Arch Fam Med* 1995; 4:323–329.

40. Wannamethee SG, Shaper AG, Walker M: Changes in physical activity, mortality, and incidence of coronary heart disease in older men. *Lancet* 1998; 351:1630–1638.

41. Kaplan GA, Strawbridge WJ, Cohen RD, Hungerford LR: Natural history of leisure-time physical activity and its correlates: associations with mortality from all-causes and cardiovascular disease over 28 years. *Am J Epidemiol* 1996; 144:793–797.

42. Rodriguez BL, Curb JD, Burchfiel CM, et al: Physical activity and 23-year incidence of coronary heart disease morbidity and mortality among middle-aged men: the Honolulu Heart Program. *Circulation* 1994; 89:2540–2544.

43. Folsom AR, Arnett DK, Hutchinson RG, et al: Physical activity and incidence of coronary heart disease in middle-aged women and men. *Med Sci Sports Exerc* 1997; 29:901–909.

44. Raitakari OT, Taimela S, Porkka KV, et al: Associations

between physical activity and risk factors for coronary heart disease: the Cardiovascular Risk in Young Finns Study. *Med Sci Sports Exerc* 1997; 29:1055–1061.

45. Schmiedt GJ, Walkuski JJ, Stensel DJ: The Singapore Youth Coronary Risk and Physical Activity Study. *Med Sci Sports Exerc* 1998; 30:105–113.

46. Guillaume M, Lapidus L, Bjorntorp P, Lambert A: Physical activity, obesity, and cardiovascular risk factors in children: the Belgian Luxembourg Child Study II. *Obesity Res* 1997; 5:549–556.

47. Wong ND, Hei TK, Qaqundah PY, et al: Television viewing as a marker for pediatric hypercholesterolemia. *Pediatrics* 1992; 90:75–79.

48. Blair SN, Cooper KH, Gibbons LW, et al: Changes in coronary heart disease risk factors associated with increased treadmill time in 753 men. *Am J Epidemiol* 1983; 118:352–359.

49. Hagberg JM, Montain SJ, Martin WH III, Ehsani AA: Effect of exercise training in 60–69 year old persons with essential hypertension. *Am J Cardiol* 1989; 64:348–353.

50. Jennings GL, Deakin G, Dewar E, et al: Exercise, cardiovascular disease and blood pressure. *Clin Exp Hypertens [A]* 1989; 11:1035–1052.

51. Braith RW, Pollock ML, Lowenthal DT, et al: Moderate- and high-intensity exercise lowers blood pressure in normotensive subjects 60–79 years of age. *Am J Cardiol* 1994; 73:1124–1128.

52. Eaton CB, Lapane KL, Garber CE, et al: Physical activity, physical fitness, and coronary heart disease risk factors. *Med Sci Sports Exerc* 1995; 27:340–346.

53. Hong Y, Bots ML, Pan X, et al: Physical activity and cardiovascular risk factors in rural Shanghai, China. *Int J Epidemiol* 1994; 23:1154–1158.

54. Hsieh SD, Yoshinaga H, Muto T, Sakurai Y: Regular physical activity and coronary risk factors in Japanese men. *Circulation* 1998; 97:661–665.

55. Bijnen FC, Feskens EJ, Caspersen CJ, et al: Physical activity and cardiovascular risk factors among elderly men in Finland, Italy, and the Netherlands. *Am J Epidemiol* 1996; 143:553–561.

56. Tran ZV, Weltman A: Differential effects of exercise on serum lipid and lipoprotein levels seen with changes in body weight: a meta-analysis. *JAMA* 1985; 254:919–924.

57. King AC, Haskell WL, Young DR, et al: Long-term effects of varying intensities and formats of physical activity on participation rates, fitness, and lipoproteins in men and women aged 50 to 65 years. *Circulation* 1995; 91:2596–2604.

58. Williams PT: High-density lipoprotein cholesterol and other risk factors for coronary heart disease in female runners. *N Engl J Med* 1996; 334:1298–1303.

59. Greendale GA, Bodin-Dunn L, Ingles S, et al: Leisure, home, and occupational physical activity and cardiovascular risk factors in postmenopausal women: the Postmenopausal Estrogens/Progestins Intervention (PEPI)

study. *Arch Intern Med* 1996; 156:418–424.

60. Pols MA, Peeters PH, Twisk JW, et al: Physical activity and cardiovascular disease risk profile in women. *Am J Epidemiol* 1997; 146:322–328.

61. Hunter GR, Kekes-Szabo T, Treuth MS, et al: Intra-abdominal adipose tissue, physical activity and cardiovascular risk in pre-and postmenopausal women. *Int J Obesity Rel Metab Disord* 1996; 20:860–865.

62. Wood PD, Stefanick ML, Williams PT, Haskell WL: The effects on plasma lipoproteins of a prudent weight-reducing diet, with or without exercise, in overweight men and women. *N Engl J Med* 1991; 325:461–465.

63. Schwartz RS, Shuman WP, Larson V, et al: The effect of intensive endurance exercise training on body fat in young and older men. *Metabolism* 1991; 40:545–551.

64. King DS, Dalsky GP, Clutter WE, et al: Effects of exercise and lack of exercise on insulin sensitivity and responsiveness. *J Appl Physiol* 1988; 64:1942–1946.

65. Lee IM: Physical activity, fitness, and cancer. In: Bouchard C, Shephard RJ, Stephens T (eds): *Physical Activity, Fitness, and Health: International Proceedings and Consensus Statement.* Champaign, IL, Human Kinetics Publishers, 1994, pp 814–831.

66. Kohrt WM, Holloszy JO: Loss of skeletal muscle mass with aging: effect on glucose tolerance. *J Gerontol A Biol Sci Med Sci* 1995; 50:68–72.

67. Evans WJ: Effects of exercise on body composition and functional capacity of the elderly. *J Gerontol A Biol Sci Med Sci* 1995; 50:147–150.

68. Blumenthal JA, Emery CF, Madden DJ, et al: Cardiovascular and behavioral effects of aerobic exercise training in healthy older men and women. *J Gerontol* 1989; 44:M147-M157.

69. Kavanaugh T, Shephard RJ, Tuck JA, Quershi S: Depression following myocardial infarction: the effects of distance running. *Ann NY Acad Sci* 1977; 301:1029–1038.

70. Martinsen EW, Medhus A, Sandvik L: Effects of aerobic exercise on depression: a controlled study. *Br Med J (Clin Res Ed)* 1985; 291:109.

71. Folkins CH, Sime WE: Physical fitness training and mental health. *Am J Psychol* 1981; 36:373–389.

72. Blumenthal JA, Fredrikson M, Kuhn CM, et al: Aerobic exercise reduces levels of cardiovascular and sympatho-adrenal responses to mental stress in subjects without prior evidence of myocardial ischemia. *Am J Cardiol* 1990; 65:93–98.

73. Sidney S, Jacobs DR, Haskell WL, et al: Comparison of two methods of assessing physical activity in the Coronary Artery Risk Development in Young Adults (CARDIA) study. *Am J Epidemiol* 1991; 133:1231–1245.

74. NIH Consensus Development Panel on Physical Activity and Cardiovascular Health: Physical activity and cardiovascular health. *JAMA* 1996; 276:241–246.

75. Fletcher GF: American Heart Association Medical/Scientific Statement—How to implement physical activity in primary and secondary prevention. *Circulation* 1997, 96:355–357.

76. Department of Health and Human Services: *Personalizing Physical Activity Prescriptions.* The President's Council on Physical Fitness and Sports Research Digest, 1997, Series 2(9):1–8. Washington, DC, DHHS, 1997.

77. Department of Health and Human Services: *Physical Activity for Young People.* The President's Council on Physical Fitness and Sports Research Digest, 1998; Series 3(3): 1–7. Washington, DC, DDHS, 1998.

78. National Association for Sport and Physical Education: *Physical Activity for Children: A Statement of Guidelines.* Reston, VA, NASPE Publications, 1998.

79. Sallis JF, Patrick K, Long BL: An overview of the international consensus conference on physical activity guidelines for adolescents. *Pediatr Exerc Sci* 1994; 6:299–301.

80. Centers for Disease Control and Prevention: Guidelines for school and community programs to promote lifelong physical activity among young people. *MMWR* 1997; 46(RR-6):1–36.

CHAPTER 13

Nutrition

Geeta Sikand
Penny Kris-Etherton
Gail C. Frank

It is well established that diet affects important factors related to coronary heart disease (CHD). For decades the focus has been on lowering low-density-lipoprotein cholesterol (LDL-C) by reducing saturated fat and cholesterol as well as achieving and maintaining a healthy body weight. Lowering of LDL-C has been shown to significantly decrease the incidence of CHD in primary and secondary prevention trials.[1,2] Current dietary recommendations target total fat, saturated fat, dietary cholesterol, dietary fiber, and weight control. Ample amounts of fruits, vegetables, grain products, nuts, and fish further confer cardioprotective effects.[3]

In this chapter, we review the evidence and means by which dietary restriction of fat, consumption of fatty acids, fiber, and other nutrients may reduce risk for CHD. We also describe the approach to medical nutrition therapy for the health care provider. Table 13–1 summarizes the risk-reducing effects of a wide range of nutritional factors, reviewed below.

Beneficial Effects of Diet on Coronary Heart Disease

Effects on Cholesterol and Lipids

The importance of saturated fat in elevating blood cholesterol levels has been widely demonstrated. In the Seven Countries Study,[4] there was a significant positive correlation between saturated fat intake and blood cholesterol levels (Fig. 13–1). Moreover, numerous controlled clinical studies have shown that both saturated fat and cholesterol raise blood cholesterol levels.[5] A metanalysis of randomized controlled trials evaluating the effects of Step 1 and Step 2 dietary interventions on plasma lipids and lipoproteins has reported that lowering saturated fat and cholesterol reduces total and LDL-C levels, by approximately 10 to 15 percent.[6] The impact on cholesterol levels from dietary saturated fat and cholesterol has been quantified by the equations of Keys et al.[4] and Hegsted et al.[7] These equations show that for every 1 percent increase in energy intake from saturated fat, blood cholesterol levels increase approximately 2 mg/dL. The impact of dietary cholesterol is less. Weight reduction also decreases blood cholesterol levels.[8]

Effects of Thrombosis

Omega-3 fatty acids have antithrombogenic and antiarrhythmic effects,[9,10] and they lower triglyceride levels.[11] The classic observational studies of the Greenland Eskimos showed that a diet rich in cold-water fish was associated with prolonged bleeding times and a low rate of myocardial infarction (MI).[12,13] Subsequent epidemiologic studies also established that fish consumption was inversely related to incidence of MI in other countries, including Japan, the Netherlands and England.[14–16] Nordoy and Goodnight[17] have reviewed the published clinical studies evaluating the antithrombotic effects of fish oil or omega-3 fatty acids. Subjects given omega-3 fatty acids consistently show a mild

TABLE 13–1 Cardiovascular Effects of Selected Dietary Components

Lower saturated fat and cholesterol intake:		
Step 1 Diet (8–10% of calories from saturated fat, <300 mg cholesterol)	↓ Total cholesterol	↓ LDL-C
Step 2 Diet (<8% calories from saturated fat, <200 mg cholesterol)	↓ ↓ Total cholesterol	↓ ↓ LDL-C
Moderate to very low fat diet (<20% calories from fat)	↓ ↓ ↓ Total cholesterol	↓ ↓ ↓ LDL-C
Omega-3 fatty acids	↓ ↓ Triglycerides	↓ Platelet aggregation
Soluble fiber (including oat bran)	↓ Total cholesterol	↓ LDL-C
Vitamin E	↓ LDL oxidative susceptibility	
	*↓ ↓ Risk of myocardial infarction, CVD events, and progression of atherosclerosis	
Vitamin C	Recycles vitamin E	
Vitamin A	No effect on CHD events from clinical trials	
Folic acid	↓ Homocysteine levels	
Alcohol	↑ HDL-C levels	
	↓ Blood clotting/coagulation	
	↑ Hypertension/stroke from high intake	
	†↓ ↓ CHD risk	
Soy protein	↓ Triglycerides	↓ LDL-C
Phytosterols	↓ Total cholesterol	↓ LDL-C
Garlic	↓ Total cholesterol	

*From secondary prevention trials.
†From observational studies.

prolongation of bleeding time and decreased reactivity to platelet aggregation as well as reduced platelet adhesion to surfaces. Moreover, the Lyon Diet-Heart Study[18] reported that survival rates were markedly increased in patients with coronary disease who followed a Mediterranean diet (with fish) that was high in linolenic acid. Interestingly, there was no difference in plasma lipids between the experimental and control groups, suggesting that the diet effects were mediated by alterations in platelet function.

Two fatty acids found in fish oil, EPA and DHA, are thought to account for much of the beneficial effect on CHD. Benefits have been observed when as little as one fish meal is included in the diet per week. Based on this evidence, many nutritionists have recommended inclusion of one or two fish-containing meals per week in the diet to reduce risk of CHD.[19]

Fiber

The AHA Dietary Guidelines for Healthy American Adults recommend a total dietary fiber intake of 25 to 30 g/day from foods—not supplements—to promote an eating pattern that is high in complex carbohydrates and low in total fat, saturated fat, and cholesterol.[20] Presently, average fiber intake in the United States is approximately 15 g/day.[21]

Observational studies report a significant inverse association between total fiber intake and cardiovascular disease (CVD) mortality, all-cause mortality,[22–25] and risk of MI.[26] After controlling for energy[23,24] and other factors,[25] the association between

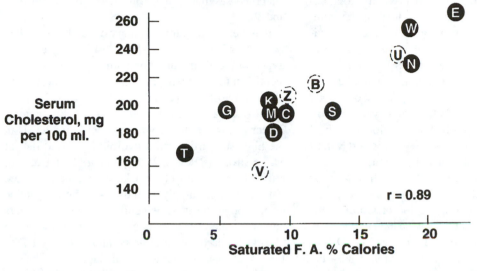

Average Percentage of Total Calories from Saturated Fatty Acids in the Diets Plotted Against the Median Serum Cholesterol Values of the Cohorts

Keys, 1970

B = Belgrade

E = East Finland

N = Zutphen

U = U. S. railroad

C = Crevalcore

G = Corfu

S = Slavonia

V = Velika Krsna

D = Dalmatia

M = Montegiorgio

T = Tanushimaru

W = West Finland

Z = Zrenjanin

FIGURE 13-1 Evidence from the Seven Countries Study showing the relationship between saturated fat intake and serum cholesterol levels. (Adapted from Keys,[4] with permission.)

fiber intake and CVD risk was lessened, illustrating the complexity of evaluating this association.[26]

Controlled clinical studies have reported a cholesterol-lowering effect of soluble fiber (provided by oats, beans, and/or psyllium) together with a low-fat diet of 10 to 15 percent of total caloric intake.[26] The effects of fiber alone (from two servings of oats) appear to account for an additional 2 to 3 percent of the response reported as a result of a low-fat diet.[27] Psyllium exerts a similar cholesterol-lowering effect.

Antioxidant Vitamins

Oxidative modification of low density lipoprotein (LDL) is thought to be the initiating event in the ath-

erosclerotic process. Vitamin E and beta-carotene are both transported in the LDL particle. Vitamin C serves to help recycle vitamin E. Enrichment of LDL with vitamin E, but not beta-carotene, reduces LDL oxidative susceptibility.[28]

Among 121,000 female nurses initially aged 30 to 55, after 8 years of follow-up, risk of MI was significantly lower among those in the highest versus lowest quintile of intake for vitamin E [relative risk (RR) = 0.66; 95 percent confidence interval (CI), 0.50 to 0.87],[29] which was attributed primarily to vitamin E supplementation rather than dietary intake. For beta-carotene, this study showed a trend toward lower MI risk associated with being in the highest versus lowest quintile of intake (RR = 0.78; 95 percent CI, 0.59 to 1.03; p for trend across quintiles =

.02). There was also a modest but nonsignificant risk reduction associated with vitamin C intake (RR = 0.80; 95 percent CI, 0.58 to 1.10). When a total antioxidant score was created by adding up the quintile levels of intake for beta-carotene, vitamin E, vitamin C, and riboflavin, the relative risk for CHD was 0.54 (95 percent CI, 0.40 to 0.73) among those in the highest versus lowest quintile of intake.[30] In the Health Professionals Follow-up Study of 39,000 men with no history of CVD, after 4 years of follow-up, there was a significant reduction in risk of coronary events among those in the highest versus lowest quintile of intake for both vitamin E (RR = 0.68; 95 percent CI, 0.51 to 0.90; p for trend = .01) and beta-carotene (RR = 0.75; 95 percent CI, 0.57 to 0.99, p for trend = .04), but not for vitamin C.[31] Only men with a high beta-carotene intake who were current or former smokers had a reduced CVD risk. Recently published primary prevention trials that have evaluated the effects of vitamin E and beta-carotene have not shown beneficial effects of antioxidant supplementation on CVD endpoints.[32,33]

Secondary prevention trials, however, have provided more encouraging results for vitamin E supplementation.[34,35] Risks of CVD events and MI have been shown to be reduced by 47 and 77 percent, respectively, with 400 or 800 IU of alpha-tocopherol.[34] Risk of nonfatal MI has been reportedly decreased by 38 percent among the group taking alpha-tocopherol.[35]

Recent recommendations from the American Heart Association (AHA)[36] support consumption of a balanced diet, emphasizing antioxidant-rich fruits and vegetables and whole grains. Although diet alone may not provide the levels of vitamin E intake that have been associated with risk reduction, the absence of efficacy and safety data from randomized trials precludes populationwide recommendations regarding vitamin E supplementation. If further studies in persons with CHD confirm the results of existing clinical trials, vitamin E supplementation in these individuals may be warranted.

Folic Acid, Vitamins B₆ and B₁₂

Homocysteine is a sulfur-containing amino acid that originates from intracellular metabolism of methio-

nine in liver, other organs, and red blood cells. It is rapidly oxidized in plasma to disulfide metabolites via processes that require folic acid and vitamins B_{12} and B_6.

In a metanalysis, the summary odds ratio for CHD was 1.7 (95 percent CI, 1.5 to 1.9) in subjects with hyperhomocysteinemia compared to control subjects.[37] In the Women's Health Study, a cohort study of 28,263 postmenopausal women with no history of cardiovascular disease or cancer at baseline, after a 3-year follow-up, those with homocysteine levels in the highest quartile had a twofold increased risk of MI or stroke (RR = 2.2; 95 percent CI, 1.1 to 4.6) after adjustment for other risk factors; the increased risks were due largely to those with homocysteine levels above the 95th percentile, however.[38] Others have reported a dose-response relationship between plasma levels of homocysteine and risk of CHD.[39] Levels of plasma homocysteine appear to be inversely associated with folate and B_6 intake.[40,41]

Although there is significant evidence for a relationship between plasma homocysteine and CVD, the AHA recommendations do not advocate populationwide screening of homocysteine levels until results of clinical trials become available.[42] Emphasis should be placed on meeting current recommended levels for folate, as well as vitamins B_6 and B_{12}, through intake of vegetables, fruits, legumes, meats, fish, and fortified grains and cereals. Screening for homocysteine, increased intake of vitamin-fortified foods, and possible supplemental vitamin intake (e.g., 0.4 mg of folic acid, 2 mg of vitamin B_6, and 6 μg of vitamin B_{12}) may be appropriate for high-risk groups (e.g., those with a personal or family history of premature CVD).[42]

Alcohol

Observational studies demonstrate a J-shaped curve relating alcohol consumption and total mortality,[43] with the point of lowest mortality occurring among those consuming one to two drinks per day.[44] Those seldom consuming alcohol have higher mortality rates, and total mortality increases in those consuming more than two drinks daily. Although there is a stepwise decline in the CHD death rate with increasing alcohol usage, mortality due to other diseases rises with the number of drinks consumed daily. Heavy alcohol consumption can have a number of adverse health effects, including hypertension and stroke.[45,46]

Consumption of one to two drinks per day is associated with about a 30 to 50 percent reduction in the risk of CHD,[47] and it has been suggested that about 50 percent of this protective effect is mediated through increased levels of high-density-lipoprotein cholesterol (HDL-C).[48] Several studies have shown that moderate consumption of alcohol raises HDL-C.[49] Other explanations for the benefit of alcohol use include beneficial effects on blood clotting, as by preventing coagulation or enhancing the breakup of clots when they form.[50] Also, recent data demonstrate that protection against CHD does not seem to differ according to the type of alcoholic beverage consumed (e.g., red wine, beer, etc.).[51]

Although moderate alcohol consumption (one or two drinks per day—one "drink equivalent" is equal to 12 oz of beer, 4 oz of wine, or a 1.5-oz shot of 80-proof spirit) is generally considered safe, those considering beginning or continuing alcohol use should consult a physician regarding the risks and benefits of its use. These considerations should be reviewed as part of regular medical care and revised if changes in health status may contraindicate its use. Alcohol use in adolescents and young adults should be carefully assessed and monitored, with appropriate advice given to prevent deleterious habits of consumption.[52]

Nuts

Several population studies have shown that frequent nut consumption is associated with a reduced incidence of coronary events.[53-55] In the Nurses' Health Study, consumption of five 1-oz servings of nuts per week was associated with a 40 percent reduction in coronary events. A dose-dependent association was observed, with consumption of two to four servings per week reducing relative risk by approximately 25 percent.[53] A study among Seventh Day Adventists showed a protective effect of nut consumption both in men and in women.[54]

Soy Protein

The collective effects of studies on soy protein in humans have been summarized in a metanalysis of 38 controlled clinical trials reported by Anderson et al.[56] In this analysis, the average intake of soy protein per day was 47 g, which resulted in a reduction in total cholesterol of 9.3 percent, 13 percent in LDL-C, and 11 percent in triglycerides. No significant effect was observed for soy protein on HDL-C levels. Consumption of soy protein (40 g/day) containing moderate or higher concentrations of isoflavones (1.39 or 2.25 mg/g protein) affected blood lipids similarly.[57] The active constituent that accounts for the lipid-lowering effect of soy protein is not clear. Nonetheless, isoflavonoids inhibit cell adhesion, alter growth factor activity, and inhibit cell proliferation, processes involved in lesion formation.[58] Genistein, a potent flavonoid, inhibits thrombin formation and platelet activation in vitro.[59]

Phytosterols (Plant Sterols)

Phytosterols occur naturally in plants. Although at least 44 plant sterols have been identified, the most abundant is β-sitosterol. Phytosterols have variable effects on total and LDL-C lowering, ranging from 0.2 to 26 percent for total cholesterol and 2 to 33 percent for LDL-C (average reduction 10 percent), even when a diet high in saturated fat and cholesterol is consumed. There has been interest in the development of phytosterol-supplemented foods such as sitostanol-supplemented margarine. A small amount—i.e., two servings per day—has been shown to lower LDL-C by approximately 10 percent or more.[60,61]

Garlic

Garlic, onions, and leeks are part of the allium family, associated with allium-containing sulfur compounds. There is evidence that these phytochemicals may influence plasma cholesterol and lower CHD risk. In a recent review, garlic was found to lower plasma lipids in 17 of 20 studies,[62] although studies with garlic oil or garlic powder have not shown an effect, possibly because the active compound(s) is not present.[63] A previous metanalysis of data from five garlic studies showed a mean reduction in cholesterol of 9 percent with a daily consumption of a half to one clove for 4 to 6 months.[64]

Rationale for Medical Nutrition Therapy

The National Cholesterol Education Program (NCEP) and the American Heart Association (AHA) consider dietary therapy, or medical nutrition therapy (MNT), as the primary approach for the prevention and treatment of hyperlipidemia.[3,65]

An important aim of MNT is to achieve the LDL-C reduction target, eliminating or reducing the need for antihyperlipidemic medications. According to the NCEP, a minimum of 6 months of dietary intervention, regular follow-up visits thereafter, and support from family and friends is necessary to achieve and maintain recommended dietary modifications. Some patients adhere poorly to MNT at first but will eventually modify their diet to achieve target LDL-C levels. Patients who have severe elevations of LDL-C often respond to dietary therapy but do not achieve their target LDL-C. For these patients, pharmacologic therapy is required in addition to MNT.[3]

There is marked heterogeneity in LDL-C response among individuals on cholesterol-lowering diets,[3] with the average LDL-C reduction expected from the Step 1 Diet being between 7 and 9 percent. The average population response to the Step 2 Diet is between 10 and 20 percent.[65] These estimates do not capture the magnitude of individual diet response. Schaefer et al.[66] reported a range of response in LDL-C from +3 to −55 percent in men and +13 to −39 percent in women on a Step 2 Diet. Baseline LDL-C concentrations and age accounted for 48 percent of the variability in LDL-C response to diet in men and age accounted for 13 percent in women.

In many cases, persons with elevated LDL-C levels do not receive referral to a registered dietitian for various reasons, including failure to consider the dyslipidemia a problem that should often be initially addressed by MNT. It has also been the impression that many patients with high blood cholesterol will be noncompliant, and therefore some physicians may not prescribe dietary intervention.[67] For example, in a recent study of 1934 hyperlipidemic patients with CHD in a managed care setting, approximately 88 percent had not been referred to a registered dietitian for MNT.[68]

Approaches to Medical Nutrition Therapy for Cardiovascular Disease Prevention

What Is Medical Nutrition Therapy?

Medical nutrition therapy (MNT) involves patient assessment and counseling by a qualified nutritional professional, integrating the scientific principles of food, nutrition, biochemistry, physiology, management, and behavioral and social sciences.[69] It is recommended for patients with at least one of the following cardiovascular risk factors[70]: dyslipidemia, hypertension, excess body weight, or diabetes.

MNT consists of four components: assessment, intervention, outcome measurement, and communication with the referring provider.[71]

Assessment An interview with the patient to obtain a nutrition history, assessment of nutrients that affect the condition or disease, baseline and follow-up change in dietary behaviors, lifestyle assessment including psychosocial and economic issues, exercise and smoking habits, clinical and biochemical data, past medical history including the physician's goals, any limitations, and medication information.

Intervention A nutritional care plan with treatment goals and a prescription with input from the patient. Self-management training with interactive and individualized education/counseling can assist the patient in developing skills and habits to change behaviors and improve health status, control of the disease, or condition and quality of life.

Outcomes Specific measurable behavioral, clinical, and functional (if appropriate) outcome-goal evaluation of a patient's knowledge of the plan and a time line for further follow-up. Outcomes expected by the next session also are defined.

Communication   Contact with the patient and referring provider as well as recording of summary notes in the medical record. The expected outcomes, type of intervention provided to meet goals, compliance potential, and goals achieved are also included.

The assessment tools range from the relatively simple, such as the MEDFICTS questionnaire (Appendix 13–1), to the more formal detailed dietary history forms accompanied by a 24-h food recall (Appendix 13–2), or a detailed food-frequency questionnaire or review of a 3- to 4-day food record.[3,71]

Effective Physician-Patient Communication regarding Medical Nutrition Therapy

Physician attitudes, interest, and involvement are key predictors of a patient's success with dietary intervention.[3] What health care providers say to their patients at the outset of an MNT referral is extremely important to the success of MNT. The physician's goal is to encourage patients to seek assistance from a registered dietitian because it will help them explore and choose the best options for diet and lifestyle change.

Maintaining Standards of Care for Medical Nutrition Therapy

High-quality MNT by registered dietitians can be implemented at a reasonable cost using algorithms and protocols for dyslipidemia (Appendix 13–3) and hypertension (Appendix 13–4) that have been published by the American Dietetic Association (ADA)[71] and the American Heart Association (AHA).[72] The NCEP treatment guidelines have emphasized that registered dietitian intervention should remain an important initial step in lipid reduction.[3,73] Several studies have reported that total and LDL-C are lowered from 5 to 15 percent with dietary intervention.[74–81]

Dietary Approaches for Cardiovascular Disease Prevention

Diets used for the prevention and treatment of cardiovascular disease include the following[71]:

(1) NCEP Step 1 Diet; (2) NCEP Step 2 Diet; (3) very low fat, high-carbohydrate diet; (4) diet high in monounsaturated fatty acids (high-MUFA diet); (5) diet high in soluble fiber; (6) vegetarian diets; (7) sodium-restricted diets; and (8) the cardiac diet.

The NCEP Step 1 and Step 2 Diets facilitate the gradual reduction of saturated fat and dietary cholesterol while the dieter is attaining or maintaining ideal weight. Depending on LDL-C levels, other modifications include changes in monounsaturated fatty acids (MUFA), polyunsaturated fatty acids (PUFA), and saturated fatty acids (SFA); addition of fiber; a recommendation to consume alcohol in moderation for those who do include alcohol in their diets; and sodium restriction.[3,71] Although national advisory groups have recommended a reduction in total fat with a compensatory increase in carbohydrates, these diets can raise triglycerides and lower HDL-C concentrations in some individuals.[82–84]

The Step I and II Diets

General Considerations   The primary goal of dietary therapy is to reduce saturated fat and cholesterol sufficiently to reduce LDL-C levels without compromising nutritional status and food palatability. The second goal of dietary therapy is to modulate weight, because obesity contributes to high cholesterol and triglycerides.[3,85,86] Levels of LDL-C for initiation of dietary therapy and goals of therapy based on the presence of CHD and risk factors are provided in Table 13–2.

Primary goals of dietary therapy are to guide hypercholesterolemic patients to (1) lower their intake of saturated fat (Step 1 = 8 to 10 percent of caloric intake, Step 2 ≤ 7 percent of caloric intake); (2) lower dietary cholesterol (Step 1 = ≤300 mg/day, Step 2 = ≤200 mg/day); and (3) restore caloric balance to achieve and maintain a healthy body weight (Table 13–3). Appendix 13–5 provides information on the maximum daily intake of total fat and saturated fat allowed to remain in compliance to a Step 1 or Step 2 Diet. Sample menus are also provided, based on 1600 calories a day consistent with a Step 1 Diet (Appendix 13–6) and Step 2 Diet (Appendix 13–7).

TABLE 13–2 Initiation and Goal LDL-Cholesterol Levels for Dietary Therapy

	LDL Cholesterol		
	Initiation Level	Goal of Therapy	Total Cholesterol Monitoring Goal
Without CHD and with fewer than two risk factors	≥160 mg/dL	≤160 mg/dL	<240 mg/dL
Without CHD and with two or more risk factors	≤130 mg/dL	<130 mg/dL	<200 mg/dL
With CHD	>100 mg/dL	≤100 mg/dL	≤160 mg/dL

TABLE 13–3 Dietary Therapy of High Blood Cholesterol

Nutrient	Step 1 Diet	Recommended Intake	Step 2 Diet
Total Fat		30% or less of total calories	
Saturated fatty acids	8–10% of total calories		Less than 7% of total calories
Polyunsaturated fatty acids		Up to 10% of total calories	
Monounsaturated fatty acids		Up to 15% of total calories	
Carbohydrates		55% or more of total calories*	
Protein		Approximately 15% of total calories	
Cholesterol	Less than 300 mg/day		Less than 200 mg/day
Total calories		To achieve and maintain desirable weight	

*Calories from alcohol not included.

The Step 1 Diet is recommended for all healthy individuals over the age of 2 and emphasizes fruits, vegetables, grains, cereals, legumes, lean meat, poultry, or fish, and low-fat dairy products (Table 13–4). It supports a moderate reduction in saturated fat and dietary cholesterol while emphasizing a nutritious and balanced diet. The primary goal is to target LDL-C levels with modest dietary changes so as to reduce the intake of saturated fat and dietary cholesterol. In addition, there is an emphasis on weight reduction, because obesity contributes importantly to high blood cholesterol.[3,86]

The Step 2 Diet is recommended for individuals with known CVD or those who do not respond adequately (e.g., do not reach LDL-C goals) after 8 to 12 weeks of a Step 1 Diet. A Step 2 Diet has been shown to decrease plasma LDL-C by 15 to 20 percent.

Considerations for Weight Reduction Both the Step 1 and Step 2 Diets include a weight-reduction component for overweight patients.[3] Obesity is a chronic and debilitating disease associated with increased morbidity and mortality from CVD and is a metabolic disorder often manifest by glucose intolerance, insulin resistance, dyslipidemia, and hypertension.[86,87]

The *Clinical Guidelines for the Identification, Evaluation, and Treatment of Obesity and Overweight in Adults*[86] recommend the use of body mass

TABLE 13–4   Examples of Foods to Choose or Decrease for Step 1 and Step 2 Diets*

Food Group	Choose	Decrease
Lean meat, poultry, Fish, ≤5–6 oz per day	Beef, pork, lamb—lean cuts trimmed before cooking	Beef, pork, lamb—regular ground beef, spare ribs, organ meats
	Poultry without skin	Poultry with skin, fried chicken
	Fish, shellfish	Fried fish, fried shellfish
	Processed meat—prepared lean meat, e.g., lean ham, lean frankfurters, lean meat with soy protein or carrageenan	Regular luncheon meat—e.g., bologna, salami, sausage, frankfurters
Eggs, ≤4 yolks per week, Step 1 ≤2 yolks per week, Step 2	Egg whites (two whites can be substituted for one whole egg in recipes), cholesterol-free egg substitute	Egg yolks (if more than four per week on Step 1 or if more than two per week on Step 2); includes eggs used in cooking and baking
Low-fat dairy, 2–3 servings/day	Milk—skim, 1/2% or 1% fat (fluid, powdered, evaporated) buttermilk	Whole milk (fluid, evaporated, condensed), 2% fat milk (lowfat), imitation milk
	Yogurt—nonfat or low-fat or yogurt beverages	Whole milk yogurt, whole milk whole milk yogurt beverages
	Cheese—low-fat natural or processed cheese	Regular cheeses (American, blue, Brie, cheddar, Colby, Edam, Monterey, whole-milk mozzarella, Parmesan, Swiss), cream cheese, Neufchatel cheese
	Low-fat or nonfat varieties, e.g., cottage cheese—low-fat, nonfat or dry curd (0–2% fat)	Cottage cheese (4% fat)
	Frozen dairy dessert—ice milk, frozen yogurt (low-fat or nonfat)	Ice cream
	Low-fat coffee creamer Low-fat or nonfat sour cream	Cream, half & half, whipping cream, nondairy creamer, whipped topping, sour cream
Fats and oils, ≤6–8 teaspoons per day	Unsaturated oils—safflower, sunflower, corn, soybean, cottonseed, canola, olive, peanut	Coconut oil, palm kernel oil, palm oil
	Margarine—made from unsaturated oils listed above, light or diet margarine, soft or liquid forms especially	Butter, lard, shortening, bacon fat, hard margarine
	Salad dressings—made with unsaturated oils listed above, low-fat or fat-free	Dressings made with egg yolk, cheese, sour cream, whole milk
	Seeds and nuts—peanut butter, other nut butters	Coconut
	Cocoa powder	Milk chocolate

(continued)

TABLE 13–4 (continued)

Food Group	Choose	Decrease
Breads/cereals, 6 or more servings daily	Breads—whole-grain bread, English muffins, bagels, buns, corn or flour tortillas	Breads in which eggs, fat, and/or butter are a major ingredient; croissants
	Cereals—oat, wheat, corn, Multigrain	Most granolas
	Pastas	
	Rice	
	Dry beans and peas	
	Crackers, low-fat—animal-type, graham, soda crackers, melba toasts, breadsticks	High-fat crackers
	Homemade baked goods using unsaturated oil, skim or 1% milk, and egg substitute—quick breads, biscuits, cornbread muffins, bran muffins, pancakes, waffles	Commercial baked pastries, muffins, biscuits
Soups	Reduced or low-fat and reduced-sodium varieties—e.g., chicken or beef noodle, minestrone, tomato vegetable, potato, reduced-fat soups made with skim milk	Soup containing whole milk, meat fat, poultry fat, or poultry skin
Vegetables, 3–5 servings/day	Fresh, frozen, or canned, without added fat or sauce	Vegetable fried or prepared with butter, cheese, or cream sauce
Fruits, 2–4 servings/day	Fruit—fresh, frozen, canned, or dried	
	Fruit juice—fresh, frozen, or canned	
Sweets and modified-fat desserts	Beverages—fruit flavored drinks, lemonade, fruit punch	
	Sweets—sugar, syrup, honey, jam, preserves, candy made without fat (candy corn, gumdrops, hard fruit-flavored gelatin	Candy made with milk chocolate, coconut oil, palm kernel oil, palm oil
	Frozen desserts—low-fat and nonfat yogurt, ice milk, sherbet sorbet, fruit ice, popsicles	Ice cream and frozen treats made with ice cream
	Cookies, cake, pie, pudding—Prepared with egg whites, egg substitute, skim milk or 1% milk and saturated oil or margarine; ginger snaps; fig and other fruit-bar cookies, fat-free cookies; angel food cake	Commercial baked pies, cakes, doughnuts, high-fat cookies, cream pies

*Careful selection of processed foods is necessary to stay within the sodium ≤2400-mg guideline.

index (BMI) to assess overweight and obesity. The BMI is calculated as follows: BMI = weight (kg)/ height squared (m²). BMI can be used to classify overweight and obesity (Table 13–5) and to estimate relative risk for disease compared to normal weight (Table 13–6). Patients should be weighed with shoes off and clad only in light clothing. For adult patients with a BMI of 25 to 34.9 kg/m², sex-specific waist circumferences cutoffs should be used in combination with BMI to identify those at increased disease risk. The waist circumferences for men and women at which there are increased relative risks for CHD are as follows: men above 102 cm (40 in.) and women above 88 cm (35 in.).

Treatment strategies used for weight reduction have, in general, not achieved the desired long-term effectiveness for most people.[88] Unsuccessful dieting can lead to negative health and psychological consequences.[89] A 32-year follow-up from the Framingham Heart Study showed that persons with higher fluctuations in body weight had a higher risk of CHD than individuals with stable weight histories.[90] A 16-year follow-up from the Nurses' Health Study showed that a weight gain of 10 kg or more since age 18 was associated with increased CHD mortality.[91] A 10 percent reduction in body weight may achieve

beneficial health consequences to counteract hypercholesterolemia, hypertension, and diabetes. In a 48-week study, 66 obese women given a low-fat diet lowered their serum cholesterol by 15.7 percent and triglycerides by 22.7 percent, with only an 11 percent reduction in body weight. Although the participants

TABLE 13–5   Classification of Overweight and Obesity by BMI[*]

	Obesity Class	BMI, kg/m²
Underweight		<18.5
Normal		18.5–24.9
Overweight		25.0–29.9
Obesity	I	30.0–34.9
	II	35.0–39.9
Extreme obesity	III	≥40

[*]Pregnant women who, on the basis of their prepregnant weight, would be classified as obese may encounter certain obstetrical risks. However, the inappropriateness of weight reduction during pregnancy is well recognized. Hence this guideline specifically excludes pregnant women.

Source: Adapted from *Preventing and Managing the Global Epidemic of Obesity*. Report of the World Health Organization Consultation of Obesity. Geneva, WHO, June 1997.

TABLE 13–6   Classification of Overweight and Obesity by Body-Mass Index (BMI), Waist Circumference, and Associated Disease Risk[*]

	BMI, kg/m²	Obesity Class	*Disease Risk[*] Relative to Normal Weight and Waist Circumference*	
			Men ≤102 cm (≤40 in.) Women ≤88 cm (<35 in.)	>102 cm (>40 in.) >88 cm (>35 in.)
Underweight	<18.5		—	—
Normal	18.5–24.9		—	—
Overweight	25.0–29.9		Increased	High
Obesity	30.0–34.9	I	High	Very High
	35.0–39.9	II	Very high	Very high
Extreme Obesity	≥40	III	Extremely high	Extremely high

[*]Disease risk for type 2 diabetes, hypertension, and cardiovascular disease.

[†]Increased waist circumference can also be a marker for increased risk even in persons of normal weight.

Source: Adapted from *Preventing and Managing the Global Epidemic of Obesity*. Report of the World Health Organization Consultation of Obesity. Geneva, WHO, June 1997.

started the program obese and finished obese, their lipid reduction was significant.[92] Also, a metanalysis showed an 11-lb weight loss to be associated with a decline of 10 mg/dL in total cholesterol.[93] Even less weight loss (5 to 10 lb) in overweight patients can double the LDL-C reduction achieved by reducing saturated fat and dietary cholesterol.[94–97] Weight loss in overweight individuals can also decrease triglycerides and increase HDL-C.[98–101]

Low-Fat and Very Low Fat, High-Carbohydrate Diets

Diets with less than 15 percent of energy from fat (33 g for a 2000-calorie diet, 50 g for a 3000-calorie diet) often contain fat calories distributed equally among saturated, monounsaturated, and polyunsaturated fats, with carbohydrates making up at least 70 percent and protein 15 percent of energy. Although this may lead to reduced HDL-C and elevated triglyceride levels,[71,102] such diets maximize reduction of SFAs and cholesterol.[102] Higher-fat diets have been associated with new atherosclerotic lesion formation[103]; diets low in cholesterol and with 20 percent or less of fat combined with exercise or stress management have been shown to slow progression and promote regression of atherosclerosis.[104,105] Ornish et al.[106] have reported that a very low fat diet (<10 percent of calories) combined with other lifestyle changes promoted the regression of lesions in 82 percent of subjects with coronary atherosclerosis assigned to the intervention group, along with a substantial reduction in angina. Despite this, there were no differences in the number of events between the two groups, possibly because of the small number of subjects studied and relatively short duration (1 year) of the study.

Patients most likely to benefit from very low fat, high-carbohydrate diets are those with diagnosed CVD and high-risk patients with genetic hyperlipidemia (familial hypercholesterolemia). Overweight patients are also likely to benefit; however, this diet may worsen the clinical profile of normal-weight and/or hypertriglyceridemic individuals.

These diets typically provide 65 percent of energy from carbohydrates and less than 20 percent from fat. Low-fat grains, legumes, nonfat dairy products, vegetables, and fruits are the primary food sources, along with 3 to 6 oz of lean meat, fish, or poultry.[71]

The major benefits of a very low fat, high-carbohydrate diet (<20 percent fat) are to obviate the need for antihyperlipidemic medications and possibly bypass surgery and to realize the benefits associated with a higher intake of fruits and vegetables.[71] A very low fat diet may facilitate weight loss. But the drawbacks are that (1) long-term maintenance can be challenging in a culture and environment where high-fat foods are plentiful, (2) there may be a reduction in HDL-C but an increase in serum triglycerides in individuals in the absence of weight reduction, and (3) glucose tolerance and lipids in patients with diabetes or hypertriglyceridemia may be impaired in the absence of weight loss.[107]

Very low fat diets should be reserved for motivated, high-risk persons with elevated LDL-C levels and/or preexisting CVD; support and careful supervision from a health care provider should be provided.[71,102] These diets, however, are not recommended for very young children, older persons, pregnant women, and persons with eating disorders because of the potential nutritional inadequacies.

A major low-fat dietary intervention study in conjunction with hormone replacement therapy (HRT) is being conducted (from 1994 to 2007) under the auspices of the Women's Health Initiative Clinical Trial.[108] The objective of this trial is to examine the effectiveness of dietary modification (and HRT) on risk of CHD and cancer in 48,000 women, 50 to 79 years of age. The dietary goals of this trial are to reduce total dietary fat to 20 percent of energy, increase fruits and vegetables to five servings per day, and increase whole-grain foods to six servings per day. Intervention women attend 18 group sessions and 1 individual session with a registered dietitian during the first 12 months and quarterly sessions thereafter for 9 to 12 years. Appendix 13–8 outlines objectives as well as nutrition and behavioral topics for the first six weekly sessions. This trial will provide a powerful assessment of the beneficial effects on CVD of a low-fat diet.

Diets High in Monounsaturated Fatty Acids

Monounsaturated fatty acids (MUFAs) have a neutral effect on blood cholesterol levels.[109] Interestingly, numerous clinical studies have shown that they have cholesterol-lowering effects similar to those of PUFAs when they replace SFAs in the diet. At high PUFA (but not MUFA) intakes, there may be a decrease in HDL-C.

High levels of oleic acid have been consumed as olive oil in the Mediterranean region, where the rates of CHD and total mortality are lowest.[110] In laboratory animals, a high linoleic acid but not oleic acid intake promotes chemical carcinogenesis.[111,112] In addition, a high PUFA intake can result in an increased susceptibility of LDL-C to oxidative modification, leading to an increased rate of atherogenesis.[113,114] MUFAs, on the other hand, do not facilitate LDL-C oxidation. Diets rich in MUFAs can be as effective as the AHA Step 1 Diet in modestly lowering LDL-C. The reduction of LDL-C is due to a decrease in dietary SFA.[115]

A high-MUFA diet can be of benefit in the management of dyslipidemia in patients with diabetes and insulin resistance.[116,117] Patients likely to benefit from a high-MUFA dietary regimen include those with: (1) hypertriglyceridemia and/or low HDL-C, (2) insulin-resistance syndrome (syndrome X), (3) type 2 diabetes with dyslipidemia, (4) familial combined hyperlipidemia (CHL), or (5) adherence difficulties on a Step 1 Diet.

Primary food sources of MUFAs include olive oil, olives, canola oil, nuts, and seeds as well as avocado, safflower, and sunflower oils, which are genetically selected to be high in oleic acid.[71] Some key characteristics of a high-MUFA diet are (1) a total fat intake of 35 percent or less of energy, although higher fat intakes may be justified on an individual basis (for example, on a 2000-calorie diet, the following would need to be consumed daily: 2 tbsp of olive oil, 1 medium avocado, 2 oz of peanuts, or 2 oz of almonds); (2) at least 15 percent of energy derived from MUFAs; (3) both SFAs and PUFAs are consumed at 10 percent of energy or less, and (4) energy intake is adjusted to maintain ideal body weight. Fat exchanges for SFAs, MUFAs, and PUFAs appear in Table 13–7.

Diets High in Soluble Fiber

A diet high in soluble fiber has a cholesterol-lowering effect and is also associated with more efficacious weight management, because high-fiber foods are generally lower in fat and cause a feeling of satiety by suppressing plasma insulin levels and increasing fullness.[118–120]

Glore and colleagues reviewed 77 studies on soluble fiber and determined that 69 (88 percent) demonstrated significant reductions in total cholesterol, 41 of 49 (84 percent) reported significant reductions in LDL-C, 43 of 57 (75 percent) reported no change in HDL-C, and 50 of 58 (86 percent) reported no change in triglyceride levels. The average reduction in total cholesterol from a Step 1 Diet with soluble fiber was 11 percent.[121]

Adequate soluble fiber equates to six or more servings of whole-grain products, six servings of fruits and/or vegetables, and one serving of beans daily.[71] Soluble fiber derived from pectin and guar gum has some cholesterol-lowering potential.[122] Beta-glycan is a gum found in oat products and psyllium and has been shown to reduce LDL-C levels.[123] Soluble fiber from two servings of oats increased the magnitude of cholesterol reduction an additional 2 to 4 percent.[124,125]

Patients are advised to increase their fiber intake gradually (5 to 10 g per week accompanied by adequate fluid). A total fiber intake of 20 to 30 g with 25 percent (6 to 10 g) to 33 percent derived from soluble fiber with a 1:3 ratio of soluble to insoluble fiber is recommended. Bulk laxatives containing psyllium seed husks have been shown in patients with hypercholesterolemia to reduce LDL-C by 8 percent with a dose of 1 tsp three times per day (10 g of soluble fiber).[123] The best sources of soluble fiber include oats, legumes, beans, and dried peas. Fruits, vegeta-

TABLE 13–7   SFA, MUFA, and PUFA Fat Exchanges

SFA exchange = 5 g total fat, 3 g SFA, 1 g MUFA, 1 g PUFA		
Bacon, cooked		1 slice (20 slices/lb)
Bacon, grease		1 tsp
Butter:	Stick	1 tsp
	Whipped	2 tsp
	Reduced-fat	1 tbsp
Chitterlings, boiled		1 tbsp
Coconut, sweetened, shredded		2 tbsp
Cream, half and half		2 tbsp
Cream cheese:	Regular	1 tbsp (1/2 oz)
	Reduced-fat	2 tbsp (1 oz)
Shortening or lard		1 tsp
Sour cream:	Regular	2 tbsp
	Reduced-fat	3 tbsp

MUFA exchange = 5 g total fat, 1 g SFA, 3 g MUFA, 1 g PUFA		
Avocado, medium		1/8 (1 oz)
Oil (canola, olive, peanut)		1 tsp
Olives	Ripe (black)	8 large
	Green (stuffed)	10 large
	Almonds, cashews	6 nuts
	Mixed (50% peanuts)	6 nuts
	Peanuts	10 nuts
	Pecans	4 halves
Peanut butter, smooth or crunchy		1 tbsp
Tahini paste		2 tsp

PUFA exchange = 5 g total fat, 1 g SFA, 1 g MUFA, 3 g PUFA		
Margarine:	Stick, tub or squeeze	1 tsp
	Lower-fat (30–50% veg. oil)	1 tbsp
Mayonnaise	Regular	1 tsp
	Reduced-fat	1 tbsp
Nuts	Walnuts, English	4 halves
Oil (corn, safflower, soybean)		1 tsp
Salad dressings:	Regular*	1 tbsp
	Reduced-fat*	2 tbsp
Miracle Whip Salad Dressing	Regular	2 tsp
	Reduced-fat	1 tbsp
Seeds	Pumpkin, sunflower	1 tbsp

Key: SFA, saturated fatty acid; MUFA, monounsaturated fatty acid; PUFA, polyunsaturated fatty acid.

*400 mg or more of sodium per exchange.

Source: Adapted from *Exchange Lists for Weight Management.* American Diabetes Association, and American Dietetic Association, 1995, Chicago, IL.

bles, and barley contain both soluble and insoluble fiber. Fiber supplements made from pectin, guar gum, locust bean gum, and psyllium husks provide another source; however, viscosity, taste characteristics, and gastrointestinal side effects may be deterrents to their long-term use.[119]

A diet high in soluble fiber (Appendix 13–9) can be incorporated into any of the lipid-lowering diets to enhance cholesterol reduction. The high-fiber foods generally suggested are low in fat and energy and high in nutrient density, such as antioxidants, phytochemicals, calcium, and iron. Some disadvantages are that those patients with digestive and gastrointestinal problems or chewing and swallowing difficulties may require additional guidance. As fiber is increased, side effects such as flatulence, abdominal bloating, and loose stools may occur until a tolerance is acquired with prolonged use. Dietary fibers may also bind with certain minerals, possibly reducing their bioavailability. A multivitamin and mineral supplement may be used to compensate for potential losses.[71]

Vegetarian Diets

Interest in vegetarian diets has increased because of their proposed cardiovascular health benefits. Vegetarian diets can be nutritionally adequate, tasty, and healthy,[126–128] but careful assessment and planning with a registered dietitian is necessary to prevent nutrient deficiencies. A vegetarian diet pattern is not inherently low in fat. Ideal candidates for this diet include individuals who are eager to discontinue meat consumption and who are willing to eat a variety of foods such as legumes and meat alternatives, including beans, lentils, and soy proteins combined with fruits, vegetables, and whole grains. Variation in vegetarian diets can occur due to individual differences and philosophies. Although there is no one "vegetarian diet," most can be classified as one of the following[128,129]:

Semivegetarian A diet consisting mainly of plant products and only occasional animal products such as red meat, poultry, seafood, and eggs.

Lacto-ovo-vegetarian A diet free of red meat, fish, and poultry but including milk and eggs. A lacto-ovo-vegetarian diet can be high in saturated fat and cholesterol from butter, cream, whole milk, eggs, cheese, sweets, desserts, and fried foods.

Lacto-vegetarian A diet free of red meat, fish, poultry, and eggs but containing milk products.

Vegan A diet that excludes any animal-derived products including red meat, fish, poultry, eggs, and milk.

Guidelines for implementation of a vegetarian diet consistent with the Step 1 and Step 2 Diets include the following[71,126,130]:

1. Fat intake should be 30 percent or less of energy intake. More than the two to four egg yolks per week may be included in a vegetarian meal plan of ovo-vegetarians as long as the target dietary cholesterol goals (<300 mg for a Step 1, <200 mg for a Step 2 diet) are met.
2. Adequate amounts of iron, zinc, calcium, vitamin B_{12}, and vitamin D from food should be provided.
3. Supplementation with a vitamin B_{12} source such as fortified soy milk, cereals, meat analogs, blackstrap molasses, and yeast.
4. For those living in areas of limited sunshine, fortified cereals, and milk can provide vitamin D.

All other nutrients can be obtained in a vegetarian diet. A vitamin and mineral supplement may be recommended on an individual basis. Protein needs can be met by consuming a variety of plant foods in amounts sufficient to meet energy requirements. Legumes, grains, vegetables, seeds, and nuts can be combined to provide complementary proteins, although—contrary to popular belief—these need not be eaten at the same meal. Some 50 percent or more of the grains consumed in a vegetarian diet should be from a whole-grain source.[131,132] In 1997, the Third International Congress on Vegetarian Nutrition proposed a vegetarian food guide pyramid (Fig. 13–2).[133]

Strict vegetarian diets can slow or halt the progression of atherosclerosis as well as play a role

FIGURE 13–2 Proposed vegetarian food guide pyramid. (From Krummel et al.,[70] with permission.)

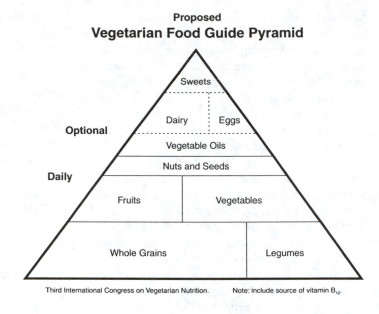

Proposed
Vegetarian Food Guide Pyramid

Sweets

Optional | Dairy | Eggs

Vegetable Oils

Nuts and Seeds

Daily | Fruits | Vegetables

Whole Grains | Legumes

Third International Congress on Vegetarian Nutrition.   Note: include source of vitamin B_{12}.

in regression of atheromatous plaque.[132,133] Less restrictive vegetarian approaches benefit lipid management, weight reduction, and blood pressure control as well as reducing the risk of osteoporosis, gallstones, kidney disease, and cancer.[134,135]

Sodium-Restricted Diets

Hypersensitive patients who are salt-sensitive and those with congestive heart failure are most likely to benefit from a sodium-restricted diet. Currently, there are no biological markers to identify those who are salt-sensitive. As a general guideline, people who are older, overweight, have low renin levels, or are of African-American ethnicity tend to be salt-sensitive.[136] It is important to maintain an adequate intake of calcium, magnesium, and potassium to prevent hypertension in humans and to identify food sources of these nutrients. Strategies to educate people to increase intake of these minerals, rather than to restrict sodium chloride, may be important to reduce the risk of salt-induced essential hypertension.[137] A diet including 2 to 3 g of sodium per day is used to treat mild congestive heart failure; 1 to

2 g per day is prescribed for moderate to severe congestive heart failure.[138] The level of sodium and fluid restriction is individualized on the basis of medications and symptoms.

The recommended amount of sodium in a restricted diet ranges from 2300 to 3000 mg per day. To achieve this target, salt use should be limited and replaced with herbs, spices, natural flavorings, and lower-sodium seasonings and condiments (Table 13–8).[71]

The DASH Diet

The Dietary Approaches to Stop Hypertension (DASH) Study has shown that a diet high in fruits and vegetables (nine servings per day) and low-fat dairy products elicits a hypotensive effect in both normotensive and hypertensive individuals comparable to that of drug therapy.[139] Importantly, the DASH diet exerts a more potent hypotensive effect than a sodium-restricted diet. Presently, the DASH diet is being widely endorsed by many health professionals for both the prevention and treatment of hypertension.

TABLE 13–8   High-Sodium Foods

Each item listed contains approximately 400 mg of sodium and should be used with care.

Miscellaneous items

1/4 tsp salt
1 tsp soy sauce
4 tsp Worcestershire sauce
2 1/3 tbsp catsup
2 tbsp mustard, chili sauce, or barbecue sauce
4 2/3 tbsp tartar sauce
4 2/3 tbsp mayonnaise
4 tbsp thousand island dressing
3 tbsp Russian salad dressing
2 tbsp French salad dressing
1 1/3 tbsp Italian salad dressing
4 medium, 3 extra large, or 2 giant green olives (16 g)
4 tbsp sweet pickle relish (60 g)

Meat or dairy item

1 small hot dog
1 slice luncheon meat
4 slices bacon
1 1/2 oz cooked pork sausage
1 1/2 oz ham or corned beef
1 1/2 oz regular canned tuna
3 oz regular canned salmon
1 1/2 oz regular canned crab
3/4 cup cottage cheese
2 oz cheese
1/4 of a 12-in. thin-crust pizza

Bread, cereal, dessert items

20 pretzels, small
2 twisted medium pretzels
1 Dutch or soft pretzel

Vegetable items

2 servings (1/2 cup each) regular canned vegetables
1/3 cup canned regular sauerkraut, drained
1/2 large dill pickle (30 g)
1 oz (approximately 20) potato chips

Soup items*

2/3 cup beef broth or vegetarian vegetable 1/2 cup bisque of tomato, clam chowder (Manhattan style), chicken gumbo, cream of asparagus, cream of celery, tomato rice, or tomato
1/3 cup cream of mushroom

*All soups listed are canned soups diluted with equal amounts of water.

Source: From the *ADA Manual of Clinical Dietetics,* 4th ed. Chicago, IL, 1997 with permission.

Cardiac Diet

A cardiac diet may be appropriate for anyone who has had an MI, cardiovascular surgery, or other condition related to CHD, as it can help slow the progression of atherosclerosis. For reversing atherosclerosis, more rigorous dietary and lifestyle changes may be necessary.[103,104,134]

Existing CHD places patients at greater risk for recurrent cardiac events. Aggressive lipid-lowering therapy may be required to reduce LDL-C to ≤100 mg/dL. Significant LDL-C lowering may decrease the rate of progression of atherosclerosis and may even lead to a regression of lesions.[3,65,103]

Dietary intervention for these individuals consists of the following:

1. The Step 2 Diet.
2. As advised for managing fluid retention and hypertension, 2400 mg of sodium or less.
3. Restriction of caffeine.
4. Fluid restriction for managing fluid retention or congestive heart failure.
5. Adjustments in energy levels may be needed for weight maintenance, loss, or gain. Weight reduction is desirable in overweight patients and weight maintenance is usually indicated during recovery from surgery.
6. A high potassium intake or potassium supplementation may be necessary for patients receiving potassium-depleting medications. Table 13–9 provides a listing of foods high in potassium. Salt substitutes can be a significant source of potassium and should be avoided by patients on medications that elevate serum potassium levels, such as potassium-sparing diuretics and angiotensin-converting enzyme inhibitors.
7. Small, frequent feedings are suggested for the immediate postsurgical period, as larger meals can increase myocardial oxygen demand, cause abdominal distention, and interfere with breathing by impairing normal diaphragmatic motion.
8. Nutrition education: As the typical hospital stay for cardiac procedures can be as short as 1 day for angioplasty or 5 days for coronary artery bypass surgery, the time for diet

education in the acute care setting is limited. Optimally, patients should be referred to a registered dietitian for outpatient education after discharge.

TABLE 13–9 Potassium Content of Some Common Foods

Each item listed contains more than 300 mg of potassium

Breads/cereal

Concentrated bran cereal (1/2 cup)
Raisin bran (1 cup)

Dairy

Milk, any fluid (1 cup)
Yogurt (8 oz)

Fruit/juice

Banana (1 medium)
Canteloupe (1 cup)
Figs, dried (3 medium)
Honeydew (1 cup)
Orange juice (1/2 cup)
Prune juice (1/2 cup)
Prunes, dried (5 large)
Raisins (1/3 cup)
Tomato juice (1/2 cup)

Meats/poultry/fish

Flounder (2 oz)

Miscellaneous

Potato chips (1 oz)
French fries (1 cup)

Vegetables

Avocado, raw (1/3 whole)
Bamboo shoots (1/2 cup)
Beans, red (1/3 cup)
Beans, lima, cooked (1/2 cup)
Celery, raw (1 cup)
Potato, baked (1 medium)
Potato, boiled in skin (1 medium)
Spinach, cooked (1/2 cup)
Sweet potato, baked in skin (1 small)
Tomatoes, canned (1/2 cup)
Tomato, raw (1 medium)
Tomato sauce, 1/2 cup

Source: From the Clinical Center Nutrition Department, National Institutes of Health, 1996.

Practical Considerations in Dietary Modification

Expected Responses to Diet Therapies

Although dietary intervention may improve CVD risk factors significantly, individual patient responses vary. Some patients will be able to manage their risk factors with diet alone, while others may need medications in addition to diet therapy. According to the NCEP II treatment guidelines, medications must not be used in place of MNT but in addition to it. This will help to keep the drug dose low and the drug costs down. Expected responses to dietary therapy from the Step 1 and 2 Diets are provided in Table 13–10.[3]

The NCEP Adult Treatment Panel II[3] states four reasons for the inadequate response to dietary therapy: (1) limited involvement by the health professional in making dietary therapy a priority; (2) poor adherence, requiring up to a year with proper instruction, and—in addition to counseling—resistance on the part of the health professional of the temptation to prescribe drugs until maximal adherence is achieved; (3) diet resistance, whereby some patients do not respond to dietary therapy—instances wherein the dietitian should do his or her best to ensure that the patient is complying; and (4) severe LDL-C elevations, where drug therapy needs to be added in addition to dietary therapy.

Long-Term Monitoring

Nutrition education should be continued and reinforced by a dietitian. Ideally, the patient can be counseled quarterly in the first year of long-term monitoring and twice yearly thereafter. This suggests that continuous attention should be given to dietary adherence to avoid a relapse. If the patient experiences a relapse, more stringent MNT may have to be reinstituted.[3]

Clinical Effectiveness and Cost Savings with Medical Nutrition Therapy

Treatment of dyslipidemia with MNT can be a very cost-effective antihyperlipidemic therapy because

TABLE 13–10   Expected Response to Diet Therapy

	Step 1	Step 2	Very Low Fat % change	High-MUFA
Total cholesterol	5–15	5–20	>20	5–15
LDL-C	5–20	10–25	>20	5–20
HDL-C	0 to −10[*]	0 to −15[*]	With or without weight loss	Slight or no change
Triglycerides	+5 to −10[*]	+10 to −10[*]	With or without weight loss	No or slight change

Key: LDL-C, low-density lipoprotein cholesterol; HDL-C, high-density lipoprotein cholesterol; MUFA, monounsaturated fat.

[*]Without weight loss or increased exercise. With weight loss, total cholesterol and LDL-C will decrease more; HDL-C will increase and triglycerides will decrease.

[†]Compared with average American diet (high-fat/high-saturated-fat diet).

[‡]Compared with low-fat diet.

medication and medication-related monitoring costs are averted.[74,75,105,106,140] In ambulatory patients with combined hyperlipidemia (hypercholesterolemia and hypertriglyceridemia),[140] a cost savings of $3.03 for each dollar spent on MNT was shown. With three individualized dietitian sessions of 1 h each [total time ($\pm$SD) = 169 $\pm$ 19 min] over 7 weeks, 50 percent of the patients no longer required lipid-lowering medications per NCEP treatment algorithm. This outcome led to an annual cost savings of $638 per patient. In a previous study[75] in subjects with primary hypercholesterolemia, after three dietitian visits (totaling 144 $\pm$ 21 min), 51 percent of patients (34 out of 67) were no longer receiving lipid-lowering drug therapy. The result was an annual cost savings of $60,561.68 (1995 U.S. dollars), or $904 per patient. A cost savings of $4.28 was realized for each dollar spent on MNT. The average reduction in LDL-C was 13 percent in three individualized dietitian sessions of approximately 1 h each in 7 weeks. Moreover, subjects who received four dietitian intervention visits (180 min) versus two visits (150 min) during 8 weeks experienced a superior LDL-C reduction outcome (12 versus 22 percent, p = .027). Also, in a study of weight management in dyslipidemic veterans, 43 percent of the non-dietitian-treated group experienced weight gain versus no weight gain in the dietitian-treated group.[141]

An annual cost savings of $1500 per patient has been reported because of antihyperlipidemic medications avoided as a consequence of dietitian intervention, with beneficial outcomes reported when hypercholesterolemic patients received 134 $\pm$ 77 min of counseling over three or four visits with a dietitian. Fewer than two sessions with a dietitian was not found to be beneficial. The cost savings attributed to MNT should be substantial if these figures are applied to the large number of patients with elevated lipids.[75]

From a population approach, data from the Framingham Heart Study and the National Health and Nutrition Examination Survey (NHANES) estimate that reducing saturated fat intake by 1 to 3 percent would prevent 32,000 CHD events and yield a combined savings in medical expenditures and lost earnings of $4.1 billion over 10 years (estimates in 1993 U.S. dollars).[142]

Achieving Behavioral Change

Successful behavioral change is essential to achieving the goals of MNT. A behavioral change program must be individualized and theory-based. In addition, counseling techniques must be employed that increase compliance and continue to motivate patients.

An assessment of a patient's unique needs and goals by a dietitian will facilitate development of an appropriate behavior change plan that elicits desired outcomes. Six behavioral change theories that are applied in practice by dietitians are shown in Table 13–11.

Behavior-modification techniques are used widely in clinical practice by dietitians to help patients make desired dietary changes. Specific behavioral strategies[69] that have been shown to be effective in eliciting diet-related changes are:

1. *Self-monitoring* This technique makes the patient aware of his or her dietary behavior by writing down the when, what, where, and how of their food and beverage intake. Patients examine their eating habits and are encouraged to make changes over time in a nonpunitive and a nonjudgmental setting.
2. *Stimulus control* This involves educating patients to limit high-risk situations that trigger undesirable food behavior.
3. *Positive reinforcement* This tool is about giving reinforcement to the patient-centered change in dietary behaviors.
4. *Contingency contracting* Formal or informal contracts are used to facilitate a mutually agreed upon dietary behavioral change.
5. *Goal setting* Realistic and very specific behavioral change objectives are mutually agreed upon by the patient and the dietitian.

Two positive counseling techniques that increase dietary adherence are[143]: (1) employing more strategies that influence client behavior and (2) involving the patient more during the session. Dietitians are trained to help patients identify barriers to dietary adherence[144] and strategies for overcoming them. Numerous barriers to dietary adherence have been identified (Table 13–12).

Dietitians utilize motivational strategies for enhancing dietary compliance (Table 13–13). In addition, strategies for maintaining dietary change are important and must be utilized. Common dietary change maintenance strategies used in practice are shown in Table 13–14. Dietary adherence can be improved when the counselor is warm and empathetic and shows interest and genuine concern.

Thus, dietary adherence can be improved with a behavioral change road map that is theory-driven and individualized to each patient's unique needs. A plan that defines behavior modification and counseling techniques is essential for long-term adherence.

In addition to developing an individualized blueprint for diet-related behavior change, dietitians intervene after helping patients identify what stage they are in their behavior change process. The six stages of behavior change defined by Prochaska and DiClementi require different interventions to be efficacious. Knowing where the patient is on the stage continuum can be identified by asking the patient to respond to a set of statements applicable to each stage, as follows[145–147]:

1. *Precontemplation* "Patient has no intention of taking action within the next 6 months." Patients may be unaware of the need or benefits, may be in denial or just uninterested in changing. They may feel a situation is hopeless because they have tried before and failed. They may feel safe in the precontemplation stage because they cannot fail if they do not try. Although staying in denial keeps them from going forward, precontemplators are not ready to change. A strategy for precontemplators is consciousness raising to help them move on to the contemplation stage.
2. *Contemplation* "Patient intends to take action within the next 6 months." Contemplators accept or recognize they have a problem and are beginning to think seriously about it. It may take a long time (sometimes years) for an individual to move out of the contemplation stage. Treating a contemplator with more consciousness raising and emotional arousal may be beneficial.
3. *Preparation* "Patient intends to take action within the next 30 days and has taken some behavioral steps towards this goal." Most people in this stage are planning to take action within a month. They are more future-oriented than past, more concerned about the pros of a new behavior than about the cons of an old one. Preparers develop a firm, detailed strategy for action.
4. *Action* "Patient has adopted this behavior for up to 6 months." This is the busiest stage of

TABLE 13–11 Behavior Change Theories in Medical Nutrition Therapy

Theory	Description	Dietitian/Patient Role
1. Person-centered theory	Involves counselors trying to change dietary behaviors by being good listeners and being concerned with their clients' thoughts and feelings.[154]	Dietitian assesses the patient's perceptions around food and eating that influence the ability to make dietary changes. Patient learns to solve his or her own problems by assessing current dietary behavior and establishing realistic goals for change with positive reinforcement.[69,154–156]
2. Rationale-emotive therapy	Assumes that irrationality in self-talk is the major trigger of an individual's emotional problems.[157]	Dietitian teaches clients to look to themselves for positive reinforcement for behaviors. Patient counters negative self-talk with a positive thought.
3. Behavioral Therapy		
a. Operant conditioning	Consequences determine whether a patient's behavior will be repeated; positive consequences or need satisfaction will lead to a greater frequency of the new behavior.	Dietitians teach and implement new behaviors.
b. Mimicking	Trying a behavior that others implement.	See 3a
c. Modeling	Planned imitation of an action.	See 3a
4. Gestalt theory	Emphasizes confrontation to show how denial and not taking responsibility for one's behavior can contribute to dietary problems.	Nutrition counselors teach patients how to take responsibility for making dietary changes and set reasonable goals.[154,155]
5. Family therapy	Assumes that the patient's behavior is influenced by the family and therefore all behaviors occur within the context of relationships.[157]	Patient learns to seek social support for attaining his or her nutritional goals.[47]
6. Self-management approach	Based on the assumption that behavioral approaches support short-term change but usually fail to maintain change in the long run.[158]	Patient learns that maintaining a new behavior is a life-long process.[159]

TABLE 13–12 Barriers to Dietary Adherence

Restrictive dietary pattern

Required changes in lifestyle and behavior

Symptom relief may not be noticeable or may be temporary

Interference of diet with family or personal habits

Cost, access to proper foods, and effort necessary for food preparation

Barriers identified by registered dietitians:

Complications with life-style and competing demands

Denial or perceiving disease as not serious

Poor understanding of diet/disease relationship

Lack of self-efficacy

Misinformation from unreliable sources.

TABLE 13–13 Motivational Strategies to Enhance Dietary Compliance

Tailor the diet to the client's lifestyle

Involve client in the decision making

Promote exercise

Identify areas the client is willing to change

Use praise and reinforcement

Use feedback

Provide pamphlets/books/lists

Set goals/contracts

Sequence instructional steps

Provide guidelines for restaurant dining

Discuss barriers to compliance

Use food records.

Source: From Glanz,[159] with permission.

TABLE 13–14 Strategies for Maintaining Dietary Change

Tailoring the diet to the patient's needs

Using social support inside and outside the health care setting

Providing the patient and caretaker with skill and training in addition to education

Ensuring an effective patient-counselor relationship

Evaluation, follow-up, and reinforcement.

Source: From Brown et al.,[160] with permission.

finding people who will applaud and motivate them through their change process.

5. *Maintenance* "Patient has adopted this behavior for more than 6 months." This is often the most difficult stage because relapse is a possibility. It can last 6 months to a lifetime. Lapses or setbacks are common and are facilitated by complacence, a high-risk environment, and self-blame for lapses. Strategies such as commitment, reward, environmental control, and social support are important in this stage.

6. *Termination* "Patient's behavior pattern is now habitual and requires little conscious thought." The problem is no longer an issue because the behavior has become integrated into the individual's lifestyle. The commitment to the successful behavior is so powerful that there is no stopping now. Some experts believe that termination never happens, only that maintenance becomes less vigilant over time.

By recognizing that changing behavior is a challenge—a dynamic process—and that patients have different needs at different points of the process, dietitians can help them reach their goals and improve their chances of preventing CVD.[147] Interventions targeted to stage of change have the potential for accelerating the rate of change for dietary behaviors.[148]

Nutrition for Prevention across Life Cycles and Multiple Cultures

Accurate CHD risk identification throughout one's life (childhood, adolescence, adulthood, and senior

change. This is where the new behavior is being practiced in a visible way. Patients make their environments more change-friendly, as by having cut-up fruit in the house instead of a fatty snack. Also they reinforce their positive behaviors, as by not giving in to the desire to eat a fatty food while watching a favorite movie. They actively seek social support by years), followed by personal acceptance that risk profiling and medical nutrition therapy are natural parts of health care, is a proactive strategy. Prevention can become a decade-by-decade approach beginning in childhood. Such approaches include:

1. Establishing healthy eating behaviors early extends heart health well into the seventh and eighth decades of life.
2. Monitoring anthropometric measures—including height, weight, and head circumference—during infancy is a part of the "well-baby" evaluations in most pediatric clinics. Anthropometric measurement and lipoprotein profiles of children, teens, and young adults should be a routine part of their care.
3. Referring outliers (e.g., patients who are overweight or obese or whose blood pressure and serum total cholesterol are above the 75th age-specific percentile) to a registered dietitian for MNT is a front-line approach for reducing CVD morbidity.
4. Promoting weight management during the reproductive years is crucial for women to reduce their chance of adding excess body weight with each pregnancy.
5. Increasing surveillance and monitoring of hypertension and diabetes mellitus can reduce comorbidity.
6. Eliminating disparity in access to MNT and general nutrition education among multiethnic, multicultural groups provides individuals with the knowledge and skills needed to practice healthy food choices from childbearing to child-rearing to senior living.
7. Using the *Dietary Guidelines for Americans*[83] as the basis of nutrition education and primary prevention provides a standard message at any age and for any type of food preparation at home, school, business, or health care facility.

The greatest challenge may relate to other lifestyle, cultural, and health care characteristics, including (1) trends in health care, such as reticence in referral for MNT or less frequent referral for exercise; (2) reduced attendance by the patient once involved in a program; (3) increased dropout rate and loss to follow-up; (4) variation in the patient's level of readiness to make the necessary dietary changes;

(5) increased use of alternative approaches to nutritional well-being; and (6) psychological stress of the diagnosis, such as increased anxiety, depression, guilt.

An additional challenge in today's multicultural environment is the break from the traditional medical model of health care, which has taken second place to self-care, self-help groups, and alternative treatments. These alternatives include folk healing, acupuncture, herbalism, and massage.[149] Folk healing predominates in non-Western societies as the preferred approach for 70 to 90 percent of health care,[150,151] and folk healers are found in major U.S. cities in all ethnic communities. Religion has an important role in protecting Latinos. Folk healers for Mexican, Puerto Rican, and Cuban communities believe that illness is either God's intention or the act of supernatural forces. Success of MNT in these cultures is very difficult to nonexistent, and today's registered dietitians may have to adapt their role to provide alternative dietary therapies in the prevention and treatment of disease. An intersection of culture, class, condition, and the environment may dominate the paradigm for successful MNT.[152]

A format that blends cultural food preferences, age, gender, socioeconomic level, CHD risk level, and the readiness of the patient can be driven by the following guidelines[154]:

1. Choose the least intervention when counseling.
2. Identify patient goals and let them dominate the intervention.
3. Define the patient's level of readiness.
4. Develop a working relationship with the patient, family, significant others.
5. Know the cultural rules of the patient about foods, religion, and use of alternative approaches.
6. Obtain a commitment for change, even if a small step.
7. Think and talk positively about the dietary behavior change as a solution.
8. Seek flexibility by giving patient backup plans.
9. Establish a time line for continuing the counseling and for monitoring success.
10. Think and talk about the future with healthier eating.

Conclusions

The relation of dietary saturated fat, cholesterol, and other nutritional factors to risk of CHD is well established. There is also significant evidence that nutritional modification resulting in decreasing the amount of dietary saturated fat and cholesterol and increasing antioxidant or fiber intake may reduce risk. Ongoing clinical trials, including the Women's Health Initiative, will examine the long-term preventive impact of a low-fat, high-fiber diet.[108]

Approaches to medical nutrition therapy (MNT) for nutrition intervention in the prevention of CHD and ensuring long-term compliance involve (1) identifying who could benefit, (2) understanding the nutritional guidelines and the effects of risk factors on CHD, (3) understanding the variety of dietary approaches in use and their risks and their benefits, (4) understanding the expected response to dietary intervention and the factors that contribute to an inadequate response in some people to MNT, and (5) understanding the theories of nutritional counseling and being able to assess a patient's stage of change to target the most appropriate nutritional intervention for the prevention of CHD. The role of the dietitian in educating not only patients, but other members of the healthcare team needs to be expanded if opportunities for CHD prevention are to be maximized.

Name _____

Date _____

MEDFICTS: Dietary Assessment Questionnaire

(**M**eats, **E**ggs, **D**airy, **F**ried foods, **I**n baked goods, **C**onvenience foods, **T**able fats, **S**nacks)

Directions: For each food category for both Group 1 and Group 2 listings: Please check a box in the "Weekly Consumption" column and in the "Serving Size" column. If patient rarely or never eats the food listed, please check only the "Weekly Consumption" box.

FOOD CATEGORY			WEEKLY CONSUMPTION			SERVING SIZE			SCORE
			Rarely/Never	3 or less serv/wk	4 or more serv/wk	Small	Average	Large	For office use
M Meats • Average amount per day: 6 oz (equal in size to 2 decks of playing cards) **Group 1** • Base your estimate on the food you consume the most of				3 pts	7 pts	x 1 pts	2 pts	3 pts =	
Beef Ribs, Steak, Chuck blade, Brisket, Ground Beef, Meatloaf, Corned Beef	**Processed meats** Regular hamburger, Fast food hamburger, Bacon, Lunchmeat, Sausage, Hot dogs, Knockworst	**Pork & Others** Pork shoulder, Pork chops, roast, Pork ribs, Ground pork, Regular ham, Lamb steaks, ribs, chops, Organ meats, Poultry with skin							
Group 2 **Lean Cuts of Beef** Sirloin tip, Flank steak, Round steak, Rump roast, Chuck arm roast	**Low-fat Processed Meats** Low-fat lunchmeat, Low-fat hot dogs, Canadian bacon	**Poultry, Fish, Meat** Poultry without skin, Fish, seafood, Lamb flank, leg-shank, sirloin, roast, Lean ham cured and fresh, Pork loin chops, tenderloin, Veal chops, cutlets, roast, Venison						6 pts = +	

				How many eggs do you eat each time?			
E Eggs • Weekly consumption is expressed as <u>times</u>/week							
Group 1 Whole eggs, Yolks		3 pts	7 pts	x ≤1 1 pts	2 2 pts	≥3 3 pts =	
Group 2 Egg whites, Egg substitutes (1/2 cup = 2 eggs)				≤1	2	≥3	

FOOD CATEGORY	Rarely/Never	3 or less serv/wk	4 or more serv/wk	Small	Average	Large	SCORE
D Dairy							
Milk • Average serving: 1 cup							
Group 1 Whole milk, 2% milk, 2% buttermilk, Yogurt (whole milk)		3 pts	7 pts	x 1 pts	2 pts	3 pts =	
Group 2 Skim milk, 1% milk, Skim milk-buttermilk Yogurt (nonfat & low-fat)							
Cheese • Average serving: 1 oz.							
Group 1 Cream cheese, Cheddar, Monterey Jack, Colby, Swiss, American processed, Blue cheese Regular cottage cheese and Ricotta (1/2 cup)		3 pts	7 pts	x 1 pts	2 pts	3 pts =	
Group 2 Low-fat & fat-free cheeses, Skim milk mozzarella String cheese Low-fat & fat-free cottage cheese, and Skim milk ricotta (1/2 C)							
Frozen Desserts • Average serving: 1/2 cup							
Group 1 Ice cream, Milk shakes		3 pts	7 pts	x 1 pts	2 pts	3 pts =	
Group 2 Ice milk, Frozen yogurt							

+ Score 6 points if this box is checked.

Comments: _____

Total

Source: From the National Cholesterol Education Program.[3]

MEDFICTS

FOOD CATEGORY	WEEKLY CONSUMPTION			SERVING SIZE			SCORE
	Rarely/ Never	3 or less serv/wk	4 or more serv/wk	Small	Average	Large	For office use
F Fried Foods • Average serving: see below **Group 1** French fries, Fried vegetables: (1/2 cup) *Fried chicken, fish, and meat: (3 oz.) *Check meat category also	☐	3 pts	7 pts	x 1 pts	2 pts	3 pts =	
Group 2 Vegetables, - not deep fried Meat, Poultry, or fish - prepared by baking, broiling, grilling, poaching, roasting, stewing	☐	☐	☐	☐	☐	☐	
I In Baked Goods Average serving: 1 serving **Group 1** Doughnuts, Biscuits, Butter rolls, Muffins, Croissants, Sweet rolls, Danish, Cakes, Pies, Coffee cakes, Cookies	☐	3 pts	7 pts	x 1 pts	2 pts	3 pts =	
Group 2 Fruit bars, Low-fat cookies/cakes/pastries, Angel food cake, Homemade baked goods with vegetable oils	☐	☐	☐	☐	☐	☐	
C Convenience Foods • Average Serving: see below **Group 1** Canned, Packaged, or Frozen dinners; e.g., Pizza (1 slice), Macaroni & cheese (about 1 cup), Pot pie (1), Cream soups (1 cup)	☐	3 pts	7 pts	x 1 pts	2 pts	3 pts =	
Group 2 Diet/Reduced calorie or reduced fat dinners (1 dinner)	☐	☐	☐	☐	☐	☐	
T Table Fats • Average serving: see below **Group 1** Butter, Stick magarine: 1 pat Regular salad dressing or mayonnaise, Sour cream: 1 - 2 Tbsp	☐	3 pts	7 pts	x 1 pts	2 pts	3 pts =	
Group 2 Diet and tub magarine, Low-fat & fat-free salad dressings Low-fat & fat-free mayonnaise	☐	☐	☐	☐	☐	☐	
S Snacks • Average serving: see below **Group 1** Chips (poptato, corn, taco), Cheese puffs, Snack mix, Nuts, Regular crackers, Regular popcorn, Candy (milk chocolate, caramel, coconut)	☐	3 pts	7 pts	x 1 pts	2 pts	3 pts =	
Group 2 Air-popped or low-fat popcorn, Low-fat crackers, Hard candy, Licorice, Fruit rolls, Bread sticks, Pretzels, Fat-free chips Fruit	☐	☐	☐	☐	☐	☐	

Directions for scoring:
Multiply Weekly Consumption points (3 or 7) by Serving Size points (1, 2, 3) for Group 1 foods only except for a large serving of Group 2 meats
Example:
3 pts 7 pts 1 pts 2 pts 3 pts
3 x 7 = 21 points
Add score on page 1 and page 2 to get Final Score

Key
40 - 70   - Step I Diet
less than 40   - Step II Diet

= Foods high in fat, saturated fat, and/or cholesterol

Total _____

Score from page 1   + _____

Final Score _____

Comments: _____
(Note frequent use of foods high in fat or saturated fat, e.g. coffeee creamer, whipped topping)

APPENDIX 13–2   SAMPLE FOOD RECORD FOR STEP 1 DIET

Name _John Doe _____

Day __Monday_____   Date __8/2/99_____

Goals: 1800 Calories, 60 gm Fat, 20 gm Saturated Fat

Write ONE food on each line

Time	Amount	Food/preparation	Calories	Fat (gm)	Sat Fat (gm)
7:00	1 cup	Orange juice	110	0.6	0
	1 cup	Oatmeal	145	2.4	0.4
	½ cup	1% milk	51	1.3	0.8
	1 slice	Whole wheat toast	23	0.9	0.2
	1 tsp.	Tub margarine	34	3.8	0.7
12:30	1	Roast beef sandwich	347	13.4	4.0
	½ cup	Frozen yogurt	123	2.3	1.5
	1 cup	Cranberry juice cocktail	147	0	0
	1	Apple	81	0.5	0.1
7:00	3 oz.	Poached salmon	120	6.3	1.2
	½ cup	Brown rice	112	0.1	
	2 cups	Tossed salad	50	0.4	
	1 tbsp	Italian dressing	69	7.1	1.0
	½	Mango, raw	68	0.3	0
	11 oz.	Milkshake, vanilla, thick	350	9.5	5.9
		TOTALS	1830	48.9	15.8

APPENDIX 13–3 MEDICAL NUTRITION THERAPY ALGORITHM, PROTOCOL, AND ASSESSMENT QUESTIONNAIRE FOR THE TREATMENT OF HYPERLIPIDEMIA BY A REGISTERED DIETITIAN

HYPERLIPIDEMIA
Medical Nutrition Therapy Protocol

Session/length: #1 for 60 minutes

Session Process

Assessment

A. Obtain clinical data.
1. Laboratory values with dates (within 30 days of session): fasting cholesterol, triglycerides, LDL-C, HDL-C
2. Physician's goals for patient
3. Medical history: hyperlipidemia with CHD, cardiovascular disease, diabetes, hypertension, renal disease, risk factors, surgical history
4. Medications that affect nutrition therapy: for lipid-lowering, for hypertension, for diabetes, for food/drug interaction, other
5. Medical clearance for exercise or exercise limitations
6. Completion of self-assessment form

B. Interview patient.
1. Clinical data: current height/weight and calculate BMI
2. Nutrition history: usual food intake and pattern of intake with attention to fat intake and type of fat, weight history, frequency and choices of restaurant meals, alcohol intake, vitamin/mineral or nutrition supplement use
3. Exercise pattern: type of activity/exercise, frequency, duration, and motivation
4. Psychosocial and economic issues: living situation, cooking facilities, finances, educational background, literacy, employment, ethnic or religious belief considerations, family support, food assistance (if applicable)
5. Knowledge/readiness to learn basic food/meal planning, attitude
6. Smoking history: present pattern, cessation or participation in smoking cessation program

Intervention

A. Provide self-management training of patient on identified goals/nutrition prescription.
1. Risk factors associated with heart disease
2. Role and effect of diet, exercise, weight loss, and smoking cessation on CHD and in cholesterol management
3. Nutrition prescription
   - Calories based on individual needs; initiate plan to achieve reasonable weight.
   - Fats: restrict according to risk factors and severity of disease. Monounsaturated fat is preferred fat.
   - If no CHD and no risk factors, cholesterol > 200 mg/dL, LDL-C 130–159 mg/dL; or if Chol/HDL > 5, LDL-C > 130 mg/dL, prescribe <30% total fat, 10% monounsaturated fat, 10% saturated fat, <300 mg cholesterol diet.
   - If CHD and 2 risk factors, LDL-C > 160 mg/dL, prescribe ≤ 20% fat diet, 10% monounsaturated fat, 7% saturated fat, <200 mg cholesterol diet.

(continued)

- If triglycerides > 200 mg/dL, ensure blood glucose is under control; limit alcohol and simple sugars.
4. Meal planning and goal setting
5. How to record food record and its importance to treatment
B. Provide self-management training and materials.
1. Review education materials containing information on
- Nutrition prescription, e.g., ≤30% fat, 20% fat
- Low-fat cooking
- Food record
- Aerobic activity and impact of HDL-C on cholesterol management
- Potential food/drug interaction, if applicable
2. *Outcome Measurement*
- Meets goal(s) set with dietitian, e.g., reduce/change amount of fat used in cooking, increase walking to 15 minutes/day.
- Verbalizes potential food/drug interaction.
3. Document on Nutrition Progress Note.
C. Follow up.
1. Schedule appointment in 3–4 weeks.
2. *Expected Outcome*
- Patient completes food records.
- Evaluation of food records shows a decreased intake of fat and cholesterol.
- Increased exercise.

Communication

1. Instruct patient to call with questions/concerns.
2. Send copy of Initial Assessment and Nutrition Progress Note to referral source and place original in patient's medical record.
3. Call patient 24–48 hours prior to next appointment to confirm.

Source: Medical Nutrition Therapy Across the Continuum of Care @1996, The American Dietetic Association Developed by ADA and Morrison Health Care, Inc.

APPENDIX 13–3 *(continued)*

HYPERLIPEDIMIA
Medical Nutrition Therapy Protocol

Session/length: #2 for 30 minutes

Session Process

Assessment
Clinical data collected
- Current weight, blood pressure reading
- Food records kept by patient
- Current medication
- Current exercise pattern

Outcome Measurements: change in patient's
- Weight
- Food record
- Medication
- Exercise pattern

Intervention
A. Adjust goals/nutrition prescription.
   Review records and evaluate patient's adherence and understanding, and provide feedback on
   - % fat intake and type of fat
   - Exercise pattern
   - Smoking: packs per day
   - Alcohol intake
   - Soluble fiber intake
B. Provide self-management training and materials
   1. Change in patient's status: weight, smoking, exercise
   2. Review education materials containing information on
      - Food labeling
      - Recipe modification
      - Soluble fiber
      - Weight reduction
      - If medication changes, potential food/drug interaction
   3. *Expected Outcome*
      - Meets goal(s) set with dietitian.
      - Weight change (decrease, increase) or maintenance, as appropriate.
      - On food record, limits foods high in dietary cholesterol, total fat, and saturated fat, increases foods high in soluble fiber, and limits simple sugars and alcohol (if applicable).
      - Increases exercise.
      - Decreases smoking (if applicable).
      - Verbalizes potential food/drug interaction.
   4. Document on Nutrition Progress Note.

(continued)

C. Follow up.
   Schedule appointment in 3–4 weeks.

Communication
   1. Instruct patient to call in with questions/concerns.
   2. Send copy of Nutrition Progress Note to referral source and place original in patient's medical record.
   3. Request repeat lipid profile prior to next session.
   4. Call patient 24–48 hours prior to next appointment to confirm.

Source: Medical Nutrition Therapy Across the Continuum of Care @1996, The American Dietetic Association Developed by ADA and Morrison Health Care, Inc.

APPENDIX 13–3 *(continued)*

HYPERLIPIDEMIA
Medical Nutrition Therapy Protocol

Session/length: #3 for 30 minutes

Session Progress

Assessment

Clinical data collected

- Current weight, blood pressure reading
- Recent lab values: cholesterol, triglycerides, LDL-C, HDL-C
- Food records kept by patient
- Current exercise pattern
- Medication change, if applicable

Outcome Measurements: change in patient's

- Weight
- Lipid lab values
- Food record
- Exercise pattern
- Current medication

Intervention

A. Adjust goals/nutrition prescription.

Review records, evaluate patient's compliance and understanding, and provide feedback on

- % fat from intake and type of fat
- Exercise pattern
- Smoking: packs per day
- Alcohol intake
- Soluble fiber intake

B. Provide self-management training and materials.

1. Change in patient's status: weight, labs, medication
2. Review education materials containing information on
   - Dining out
   - If medication changes, potential food/drug interaction
3. *Expected Outcome*
   - Meets goal(s) set with dietitian.
   - Weight change (decrease, increase) or maintenance, as appropriate.
   - Decrease in blood cholesterol, LDL-C, or triglycerides lab values, as appropriate.
   - On food records, limits food high in dietary cholesterol, total fat, and saturated fat, increases foods high in soluble fiber, and limits foods high in simple sugar and alcohol (if applicable).
   - Increases exercise.
   - Decreases smoking (if applicable).
   - Verbalizes potential food/drug interaction.
4. Document on Nutrition Progress Note.

(continued)

C. Follow up.

Schedule appointment with PCP and schedule recheck of lipids in 3 months. If overweight, continue with weight reduction regimen per organization protocol.

Communication

1. Instruct patient to call in with questions/concerns.
2. Send copy of Nutrition Progress Note to referral source and place original in patient's medical record. Note includes long-term goals.

Source: Medical Nutrition Therapy Across the Continuum of Care. @1996, The American Dietetic Association Developed by ADA and Morrison Health Care, Inc.

HYPERLIPIDEMIA
Medical Nutritional Therapy Protocol

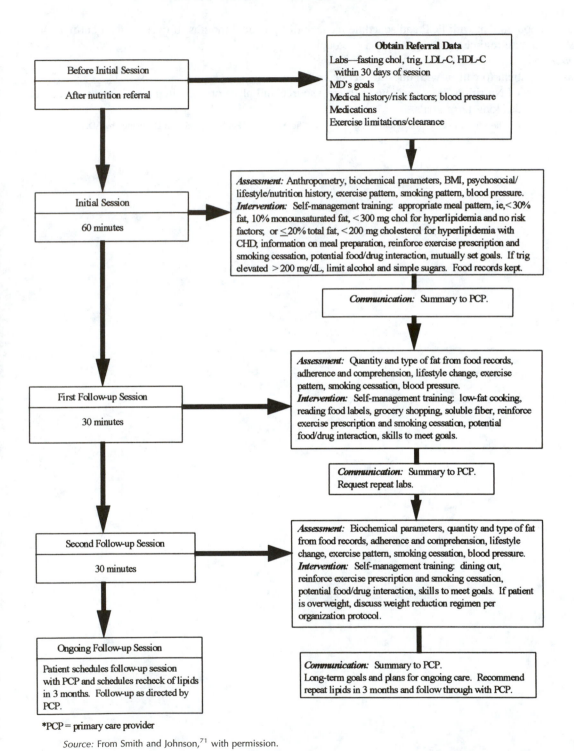

Before Initial Session

After nutrition referral

Obtain Referral Data
Labs—fasting chol, trig, LDL-C, HDL-C
  within 30 days of session
MD's goals
Medical history/risk factors; blood pressure
Medications
Exercise limitations/clearance

Initial Session

60 minutes

Assessment: Anthropometry, biochemical parameters, BMI, psychosocial/
lifestyle/nutrition history, exercise pattern, smoking pattern, blood pressure.
Intervention: Self-management training: appropriate meal pattern, ie, <30%
fat, 10% monounsaturated fat, <300 mg chol for hyperlipidemia and no risk
factors; or ≤20% total fat, <200 mg cholesterol for hyperlipidemia with
CHD; information on meal preparation, reinforce exercise prescription and
smoking cessation, potential food/drug interaction, mutually set goals. If trig
elevated >200 mg/dL, limit alcohol and simple sugars. Food records kept.

Communication: Summary to PCP.

First Follow-up Session

30 minutes

Assessment: Quantity and type of fat from food records,
adherence and comprehension, lifestyle change, exercise
pattern, smoking cessation, blood pressure.
Intervention: Self-management training: low-fat cooking,
reading food labels, grocery shopping, soluble fiber, reinforce
exercise prescription and smoking cessation, potential
food/drug interaction, skills to meet goals.

Communication: Summary to PCP.
Request repeat labs.

Second Follow-up Session

30 minutes

Assessment: Biochemical parameters, quantity and type of fat
from food records, adherence and comprehension, lifestyle
change, exercise pattern, smoking cessation, blood pressure.
Intervention: Self-management training: dining out,
reinforce exercise prescription and smoking cessation,
potential food/drug interaction, skills to meet goals. If patient
is overweight, discuss weight reduction regimen per
organization protocol.

Ongoing Follow-up Session

Patient schedules follow-up session
with PCP and schedules recheck of lipids
in 3 months. Follow-up as directed by
PCP.

Communication: Summary to PCP.
Long-term goals and plans for ongoing care. Recommend
repeat lipids in 3 months and follow through with PCP.

*PCP = primary care provider

Source: From Smith and Johnson,[71] with permission.

HYPERLIPIDEMIA
Medical Nutrition Therapy Protocol

Setting: Ambulatory Care (Adult 18+ years old)
Number of sessions: 3

No. of interventions	Length of contact	Time between interventions	Cost/charge
1	60 minutes	3-4 weeks	
2	30 minutes	3-4 weeks	
3	30 minutes	as prescribed by PCP; recheck lab in 3 months	

Expected Outcomes of Medical Nutrition Therapy

Outcome assessment factors	Base-line Intervention 1	Evaluation of Intervention 2	Intervention 3	Expected outcome	Ideal/goal value
Clinical Outcomes • Biochemical parameters (measure < 30 days prior to nutrition session) Lipid profile (blood chol, trig, LDL-C, HDL-C)	✔		✔	Chol ↓ 20% Trig ↓ or no change LDL-C ↓ HDL-C ↑ or no change Ratio TC/HDL ↓ or no change	Chol < 200 mg/dL Fasting trig < 250 mg/dL LDL-C < 130 mg/dL (non CHD) LDL-C < 100 mg/dL (w/CHD) HDL-C > 35 mg/dL Ratio TC/HDL < 4.5
• Anthropometrics Weight, height, & BMI • Clinical signs and symptoms	✔ ✔	✔	✔ ✔	↓, ↑, or maintain as appropriate As appropriate: ↓ in retinal deposit ↓ shortness of breath ↓ in angina	Within reasonable body weight
Behavioral Outcomes* • Food/meal planning	✔	✔	✔	• Limits foods ↑ in chol, total fat, & saturated fat • Uses monounsaturated fat as preferred fat	MNT Goal Fat and cholesterol consumed follow nutrition prescription, eg, < 20% total fat, 10% MUSF
• Food label reading • Knowledge of soluble fiber			✔ ✔	• Accurately reads food label • Increases intake of foods ↑ in soluble fiber	
• Recipe modification			✔	• Modifies recipes to ↓ total fat/saturated fat	
• Food preparation			✔	• Uses low-fat cooking techniques	
• Dining out		✔	✔	• Selects appropriately from restaurant menu	
• Simple sugar and alcohol intake	✔	✔	✔	• Limits per nutrition perscrip-tion, if applicable	
• Exercise pattern	✔	✔	✔	• Participates in aerobic activity 3x/wk, 45-min sessions	
• Smoking	✔	✔	✔	• Verbalizes importance of smoking cessation	
• Potential food/drug interactions	✔	✔	✔	• Verbalizes potential food/drug interaction	

*Session in which behavorial topics are covered may vary according to patient's readiness, skills, resources, and need for lifestyle changes.

APPENDIX 13–4 MEDICAL NUTRITION THERAPY ALGORITHM, PROTOCOL, AND ASSESSMENT QUESTIONNAIRE FOR THE TREATMENT OF HYPERTENSION

HYPERTENSION
Medical Nutrition Therapy Protocol

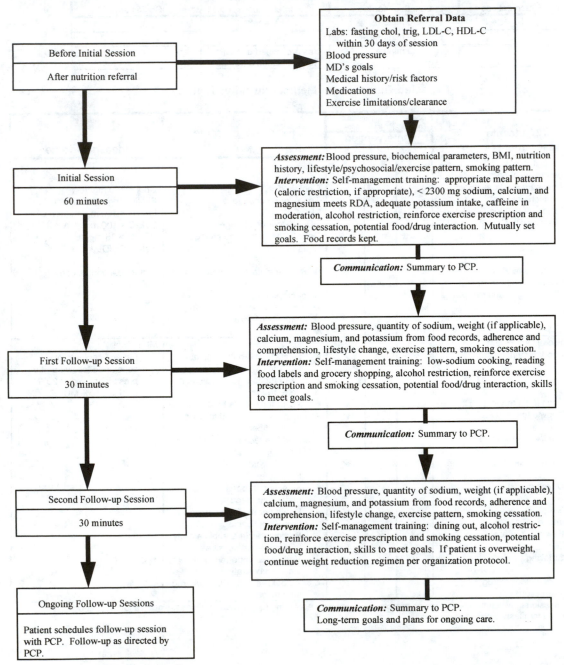

Before Initial Session

After nutrition referral

Obtain Referral Data
Labs: fasting chol, trig, LDL-C, HDL-C
    within 30 days of session
Blood pressure
MD's goals
Medical history/risk factors
Medications
Exercise limitations/clearance

Initial Session

60 minutes

Assessment: Blood pressure, biochemical parameters, BMI, nutrition history, lifestyle/psychosocial/exercise pattern, smoking pattern.
Intervention: Self-management training: appropriate meal pattern (caloric restriction, if appropriate), < 2300 mg sodium, calcium, and magnesium meets RDA, adequate potassium intake, caffeine in moderation, alcohol restriction, reinforce exercise prescription and smoking cessation, potential food/drug interaction. Mutually set goals. Food records kept.

Communication: Summary to PCP.

First Follow-up Session

30 minutes

Assessment: Blood pressure, quantity of sodium, weight (if applicable), calcium, magnesium, and potassium from food records, adherence and comprehension, lifestyle change, exercise pattern, smoking cessation.
Intervention: Self-management training: low-sodium cooking, reading food labels and grocery shopping, alcohol restriction, reinforce exercise prescription and smoking cessation, potential food/drug interaction, skills to meet goals.

Communication: Summary to PCP.

Second Follow-up Session

30 minutes

Assessment: Blood pressure, quantity of sodium, weight (if applicable), calcium, magnesium, and potassium from food records, adherence and comprehension, lifestyle change, exercise pattern, smoking cessation.
Intervention: Self-management training: dining out, alcohol restriction, reinforce exercise prescription and smoking cessation, potential food/drug interaction, skills to meet goals. If patient is overweight, continue weight reduction regimen per organization protocol.

Ongoing Follow-up Sessions

Patient schedules follow-up session with PCP. Follow-up as directed by PCP.

Communication: Summary to PCP.
Long-term goals and plans for ongoing care.

Source: From Smith and Johnson,[71] with permission.

HYPERTENSION
Medical Nutrition Therapy Protocol

Setting: Ambulatory Care (Adult 18+ years old)
Number of sessions: 3

No. of interventions	Length of contact	Time between interventions	Cost/charge
1	60 minutes	3-4 weeks	
2	30 minutes	3-4 weeks	
3	30 minutes		

Expected Outcomes of Medical Nutrition Therapy

Outcome assessment factors	Base-line Intervention 1	Evaluation of Intervention 2	Intervention 3	Expected outcome	Ideal/goal value
Clinical Outcomes					
• Biochemical parameters (measure < 30 days prior to nutrition session) Blood pressure Lipid profile (blood chol, trig, LDL-C, HDL-C)	✔ ✔	✔	✔	Blood pressure within normal limit If patient on medication, decrease or eliminate medication dosage Recheck lipid profile (session 3), if elevated	Blood pressure: Systolic < 140 mm Hg Diastolic < 90 mm Hg Chol < 200 mg/dL Fasting trig < 250 mg/dL LDL-C < 130 mg/dL (no CHD) LDL-C < 100 mg/dL HDL-C > 35 mg/dL
• Anthropometrics Weight, height & BMI • Clinical signs and symptoms	✔ ✔	✔ ✔	✔ ✔	↓, ↑, or maintain weight as appropriate As appropriate: ↓ angina ↓ shortness of breath ↓ edema ↓ headaches ↓ palpitations	Within reasonable body weight or 10 lb weight loss
Behavioral Outcomes* • Food/ meal planning	✔	✔	✔	• Restricts calories, as appropriate • Limits foods ↑ in sodium • Consumes RDA of calcium and magnesium • Maintains/increases intake of foods ↑ in potassium, if applicable	**MNT Goal** Follow nutrition prescription, eg, appropriate meal pattern (caloric restriction if appropriate), < 2300 mg sodium, calcium,
• Alcohol intake	✔	✔	✔	• Limits alcohol to 2 drinks/day	and magnesium to
• Food label reading		✔	✔	• Accurately reads food labels	meet RDA, adequate
• Recipe modification		✔	✔	• Modifies recipes to ↓ salt, sodium, and fat	potassium intake, if appropriate
• Food preparation		✔	✔	• Uses low-sodium and low-fat cooking techniques	
• Dining out	✔	✔	✔	• Selects appropriately from restaurant menu	
• Knowledge of potential food/drug interaction	✔	✔	✔	• Verbalizes potential food/drug interaction	
• Exercise	✔	✔	✔	• Participates in aerobic activity 3x/wk, 45-min sessions	
• Smoking	✔	✔	✔	• Verbalizes importance of smoking cessation	

*Session in which behavioral topic are covered may vary according to patient's readiness, skills, resources, and need for lifestyle changes.

NUTRITION PROGRESS NOTES
Hypertension

Other Diagnosis:_____

Patient's Name:_____
Medical Record#:_____
DOB:_____ Gender:_____
Ethnic Background (Optional):_____
Referring Physician:_____

Outcomes of Medical Nutrition Therapy (MNT)

Expected outcome	Intervention provided to meet goal Intervention = self management training plus patient verbalizes/ demonstrates			Goal reached Check indicates goal reached		
Date Session	1 (60 min)	2 (30 min)	3 (30 min)	1	2	3
Clinical Outcomes Blood pressure Cholesterol LDL-C HDL-C Triglycerides Height ____Weight BMI ____ As appropriate: ↓ angina ↓ shortness of breath ↓ edema ↓ headaches ↓ palpitations				Value __/___ ___mg/dL ___mg/dL ___mg/dL ___mg/dL _____lb	Value __/___ ___mg/dL ___mg/dL ___mg/dL ___mg/dL _____lb	Value __/___ ___mg/dL ___mg/dL ___mg/dL ___mg/dL _____lb
MNT Goal Follows nutrition prescription eg, appropriate meal pattern (caloric restriction if appropriate), < 2300 mg sodium, calcium and magnesium to meet RDA, adequate potassium intake, if appropriate				___Cal ___mg Na ___mg Ca ___mg K	___Cal ___mg Na ___mg Ca ___mg K	___Cal ___mg Na ___mg Ca ___mg K
Behavioral Outcomes • Restricts calories, as appropriate • Limits foods ↑ in sodium • Consumes RDA of calcium and magnesium • Maintains/increases intake of foods ↑ in potassium, if applicable • Limits alcohol to 2 drinks/day • Accurately reads food labels • Modifies recipes to ↓ salt, sodium, fat • Uses ↓ sodium, ↓fat cooking techniques • Selects appropriately from restaurant menu • Participates in aerobic activity 3x/wk, 45-min sessions • Verbalizes importance of smoking cessation • Verbalizes potential food/drug interaction Drug _____ _____ _____				__svg/day _____x/wk _____min _____ppd _____dose _____dose _____dose	__svg/day _____x/wk _____min _____ppd _____dose _____dose _____dose	__svg/day _____x/wk _____min _____ppd _____dose _____dose _____dose
Overall Compliance Potential • Comprehension • Receptivity • Adherence				E G P E G P E G P	E G P E G P E G P	E G P E G P E G P

AMBULATORY CARE SERVICES
INITIAL ASSESSMENT

PT NAME:_____

DATE:_____RECORD#:_____

DOB:_____ GENDER:_____

ETHNIC BACKGROUND (OPTIONAL):_____

REFERRING PHYSICIAN:_____

PROBLEMS: 1)   2)   3)

OCCUPATION:

HOUSEHOLD MEMBERS' AGES AND HEALTH:

COUNTRY OF ORIG: YRS IN US: YRS IN SCHOOL: LANG: INTERP:

MEDICAL HX: Onset of disease:____ (mo/yr)
              Type of treatment:

              _____
              _____

              Previous MNT   Yes ❖ No ❖   If yes, when:_____
              Other diagnoses:_____

PRESENT WEIGHT: ADULT HIGHEST WEIGHT: ADULT LOWEST WEIGHT:

ACTIVITY: TYPE   DURATION/FREQ

MEDS/DOSAGES AND
INTERACTIONS:_____

OTHER RELEVANT DATA (FOOD ALLERGIES/AVERSIONS):

VITAMIN/MINERAL INTAKE

FAMILY HX

DISEASE	**FAMILY MEMBER**		
o CAD	_____	o CVA	_____
o ATHERO	_____	o OB (high risk)	_____
o HTN	_____	o CA	_____
o CHOL	_____	o OTHER:	_____
o DM	_____		

RELIGIOUS, ETHNIC, ECON: FOOD ASSIST:

PSYCHOSOCIAL FACTORS: SMOKES: PPD

Comments_____
_____

_____RD

AMBULATORY CARE SERVICES

MEDICAL NUTRITION THERAPY CARE PLAN

PATIENT'S NAME_____ #_____

REFERRING PHYSICIAN_____

The attached protocol for patients with _____
delineates the expected outcomes, frequency of sessions, and length of treatment. This protocol is
followed and individualized for each of our patients.

_____   This patient has only the primary diagnosis and few if any barriers to complying with
therapy; the minimum of _____ sessions (total) should be adequate to reach metabolic
control.

_____   This patient has extenuating circumstances that require a minimum of _____ sessions to
attain adequate control (see Comments).

Comments:

_____
_____
_____

_____   This patient has additional diseases that would benefit from specific medical nutrition
therapy and because of this higher acuity requires an additional _____ sessions per
diagnosis.

Diagnoses (additional protocols attached):

_____
_____
_____

General comments:

_____
_____
_____

_____ Total sessions required

_____ Number sessions already authorized

_____ Additional requested: Charge _____

Medical Nutrition Therapist: _____RD

Date: _____

NUTRITION HISTORY FORM

NAME _____ DATE _____

OCCUPATION _____

HEIGHT _____,_____"
PRESENT WEIGHT`_____

┌─────────────────────────────────────┐
To be completed by dietitian
GOAL WEIGHT _____ BMI ____
└─────────────────────────────────────┘

1. How would you generally describe your eating habits? Good ❏ Fair ❏ Poor ❏

2. Has your appetite changed recently? Yes❏ No❏

3. How many times a day do you eat? _____

4. How long does it usually take to complete a meal? _____

5. When you chew your food, do you   _____ take your time?

   _____ chew a few times, then swallow?

6. Do you use a straw to drink beverages? Yes❏ No❏

7. Do you chew gum? Yes❏ No❏   How often? _____

8. Number of carbonated beverages daily _____

9. Number of caffeine beverages daily (coffee, regular colas, tea)
   _____ cups of coffee (regular)
   _____ cans of cola (regular, diet, Mellow Yellow, Mountain Dew)
   _____ cups of tea (regular)

10. Do you have dentures? Yes❏ No❏
    If so , do you wear them at mealtime? Yes❏ No❏

11. Do you have any problems chewing? Yes❏ No❏

12. Do you take any vitamin/mineral supplements? _____

13. List any foods that you do **NOT** tolerate: _____

14. Are you now or have you ever followed any special diet?_____
    If so, what type of diet?_____

15. How often do you eat out? ___ times per week. What types of restaurants?_____

FOOD INTAKE RECORD

Please indicate which foods you eat.

	Less than once a week	Not daily but at least once a week	Daily
Milk, yogurt			
Cheese			
Red meat			
Poultry			
Fish			
Eggs			
Mixed dishes			
Dried beans, legumes			
Peanut butter			
Nuts			
Breads, cereal			
Potatoes, pasta, rice			
Fruits, juices			
Vegetables			
Margarine, butter			
Cooking oil			
Sour cream, salad dressing			
Ice cream			
Cookies, cake, pie			
Candy			
Soft drink			
Coffee			
Tea, iced tea			
Alcohol			

Describe your usual daily eating pattern (include amount eaten).

Time	Meal	Food/method of preparation	Amount eaten	Calculations (for RD)
	Breakfast			
	Snack			
	Lunch			
	Dinner			
	Snack			

APPENDIX 13–5 MAXIMUM DAILY INTAKE OF FAT AND SATURATED FATTY ACIDS TO ACHIEVE THE STEP 1 AND 2 DIETS*

	Total Calorie Level							
	1600	1800	2000	2200	2400	2600	2800	3000
Total fat, g†	53	60	67	73	80	87	93	100
Saturated fat (Step 1, g)†	18	20	22	24	27	29	31	33
Saturated fat (Step 2, g)‡	12	14	16	17	19	20	22	23

*The average daily energy intake for women is about 1800 calories; for men it is about 2500 calories.

†Total fat of both diets = 30 percent of calories (estimated by multiplying calorie level by 0.3 and dividing the product by 9 calories per gram).

‡The recommended intake of saturated fat on the Step 1 Diet should be 8 to 10 percent, and less than 7 percent for the Step 2 Diet.

APPENDIX 13–6 STEP 1 SAMPLE MENUS. TRADITIONAL AMERICAN CUISINE, MALES 25 TO 49 YEARS

Breakfast

> Bagel, plain (1 medium)
> > **Cream Cheese, low-fat** (2 tsp)
> Cereal, shreaded wheat (1 1/2 cups)
> Banana (1 small)
> Milk, 1% (1 cup)
> Orange Juice (3/4 cup)
> Coffee (1 cup)
> > Milk, 1% (1 oz)

Lunch

> Minestrone Soup, canned, low sodium (1 cup)
> Roast Beef Sandwich
> > Whole Wheat Bread (2 slices)
> > *Lean Roast Beef, unseasoned (3 oz)
> > American Cheese, low-fat and low sodium (3/4 oz)
> > Lettuce (1 leaf)
> > Tomato (3 slices)
> > **Mayonnaise,** low-fat and low sodium (2 tsp)
> Fruit and Cottage Cheese Salad
> > Cottage Cheese, 2% and low sodium (1/2 cup)
> > Peaches, canned in juice (1/2 cup)
> Apple Juice, unsweetened (1 cup)

Dinner

> ***Salmon** (3 oz)
> > Vegetable Oil (1 tsp)
> *Baked Potato (1 medium)
> > Margarine (2 tsp)
> *Green Beans (1/2 cup), seasoned with margarine
> > (1/2 tsp)
> *Carrots (1/2 cup), seasoned with margarine
> > (1/2 tsp)
> White Dinner Rolls (1 medium)
> > Margarine (1 tsp)
> **Ice Milk** (1 cup)
> Iced Tea, unsweetened (1 cup)

Snack

> *Popcorn (3 cups)
> > Margarine (1 T)

Calories	2,518	Total Carb, % kcals:	53
Total Fat, % kcals:	29	Simple Carb, % Carb:	36
SFA, % kcals:	8.6	Complex Carb, % Carb:	64

(*continued*)

Cholesterol, mg: 181   *Sodium, mg: 1,821
Protein, % kcals: 18

100% RDA met for all nutrients except: zinc 90%

Boldface food items represent differences between the Step 1 and Step 2 Diets. See companion menu.

*No salt is added in recipe preparation or as seasoning. All margarine is low sodium.

Source: National Cholesterol Education Program. Second Report of the Expert Panel on Detection, Evaluation, and Treatment of High Blood Cholesterol in Adults (ATPII), National Institutes of Health, 1993.

APPENDIX 13–7 STEP 2 SAMPLE MENUS, TRADITIONAL AMERICAN CUISINE, FEMALES 25 TO 49 YEARS

Breakfast

Bagel, plain (1/2 medium)
Margarine (1 tsp)
Jelly (1 tsp)
Cereal, shredded wheat (1 cup)
Banana (1 small)
Milk, **skim** (1 cup)
Orange Juice (**1 cup**)
Coffee (1 cup)
Milk, **skim** (1 oz)

Lunch

Minestrone Soup, canned, low sodium (1/2 cup)
Roast Beef Sandwich
Whole Wheat Bread (2 slices)
*Lean Roast Beef, unseasoned (**2 oz**)
American Cheese, low-fat and low sodium (3/4 oz)
Lettuce (1 leaf)
Tomato (3 slices)
Margarine (2 tsp)
Apple (1 medium)
Water (1 cup)

Dinner

***Flounder** (3 oz)
Vegetable Oil (1 tsp)
*Baked Potato (1/2 medium)
Margarine (1 tsp)
*Green Beans (1/2 cup), seasoned with margarine
(1/2 tsp)
*Carrots (1/2 cup), seasoned with margarine
(1/2 tsp)
White Dinner Roll (1 medium)
Margarine (1 tsp)
Frozen Yogurt (1/2 cup)
Iced Tea, unsweetened (1 cup)

Snack

*Popcorn (3 cups)
Margarine (**2 tsp**)

Calories	1,867	Total Carb, % kcals:	55
Total Fat, % kcals:	29	Simple Carb, % Carb:	38

(*continued*)

SFA, % kcals:	6.8	Complex Carb, % Carb:	62
Cholesterol, mg:	134	*Sodium, mg:	1,417
Protein, % kcals:	16		

100% RDA met for all nutrients except: zinc 90%

Boldface food items represent differences between the Step I and Step II Diets. See companion menu.

*No salt is added in recipe preparation or as seasoning. All margarine is low sodium.

Source: National Cholesterol Education Program. Second Report of the Expert Panel on Detection, Evaluation, and Treatment of High Blood Cholesterol in Adults (ATPII), National Institutes of Health, 1993.

APPENDIX 13–8 SUMMARY OF DIETARY MODIFICATION INTERVENTION SESSIONS IN THE WOMEN'S HEALTH INITIATIVE (WHI)

Session Number	Session Objectives	Nutrition Topics	Behavior Topics
	Weekly		
1	Review goals and objectives of the WHI trial. Discuss the benefits and responsibilities of being a participant. Identify lower-fat food choices, especially fruits, vegetables and grains. Identify the amount of fat in foods.	Awareness of fat in foods. Awareness of fruits, vegetables, and grains.	Awareness of costs/benefits of trial participants. Social support in group and home setting. Communication skills.
2	Discuss ways to reduce added fats. Use Fat Counter to calculate fat score. Use self-monitoring to evaluate dietary changes.	Awareness of current fat intake. Method to record fat intake.	Self-monitoring of dietary behavior.
3	Identify high-fat dairy foods currently used. Discuss skills for selection and use of low-fat dairy foods. Identify reasons for goal-setting as a component of behavior change. Set goals using Guidelines for Goal Setting.	High-fat dairy foods. Low-fat substitutes Low-fat calcium sources.	Definition of problem behavior. Setting goals for behavior change.
4	Identify how other people influence their eating patterns. Read and interpret nutrition labels and marketing techniques.	Nutrition label reading. Shopping skills. Food availability.	Social influences on eating. Self-control skills.
5	Identify high-fat entrees. Discuss skills for selection and preparation of low-fat entrees. Practice modification of entree recipes. Identify strategies to accommodate family and friends in the low-fat eating plan.	Low-fat entree substitutes. Vegetarian entrees. Entree recipe modification.	Support from home-eating partners. Problem solving skills. Communication skills.
6	Discuss skills and strategies for eating in social situations. Learn the skill of fat budgeting. List strategies for low-fat restaurant eating. Practice menu selection using local restaurant menus.	Fat budgeting skills. Evaluation of restaurant menus. Low-fat dining options.	Problem-solving skills. Communication skills.

APPENDIX 13–9 SELECTED SOURCES AND AMOUNTS OF DIETARY FIBER

Food	Amount	Soluble Fiber, grams	Total Fiber, grams
Legumes (cooked)			
Kidney beans	1/2 cup	2.0	6.7
Pinto beans	1/2 cup	2.0	6.7
Vegetable (cooked)			
Brussel sprouts	1/2 cup	2.0	3.8
Broccoli	1/2 cup	1.1	2.6
Spinach	1/2 cup	0.5	2.1
Zucchini	1/2 cup	0.2	1.6
Fruits (raw)			
Apple	1 medium	1.2	3.6
Orange	1 medium	1.8	2.9
Grapefruit	1/2 medium	1.1	1.8
Grapes	1 cup	0.3	1.1
Prunes	6 medium	3.0	8.0
Grains			
Oatmeal (dry)	1/3 cup	1.3	2.8
Oat bran (dry)	1/3 cup	2.0	4.4
Corn flakes	1 ounce	0.1	0.3
Brown rice (cooked)	1/2 cup	0.4	5.3
Whole-wheat bread	1 slice	0.4	2.1
White bread	1 slice	0.2	0.4

References

1. Holme I: Relation of coronary heart disease incidence and total mortality to plasma cholesterol reduction in randomised trials: use of meta-analysis. *Br Heart J* 1993; 69(suppl):S42–S47.

2. Downs JR, Clearfield M, Weis S, Whitney E, et al: Primary prevention of acute coronary events with lovastatin in men and women with average cholesterol levels. *JAMA* 1998; 279:1615–1622.

3. ATP-II Treatment Panel: Summary of the second report of the National Cholesterol Education Program (NCEP) Expert Panel on Detection, Evaluation, and Treatment of High Blood Cholesterol in Adults. *JAMA* 1993; 269:3015–3023.

4. Keys A: *Coronary Heart Disease in Seven Countries.* American Heart Association Monograph No. 29. New York, American Heart Association, 1970.

5. Clarke R, Frost C, Collins R, et al: Dietary lipids and blood cholesterol: quantitative meta-analysis of metabolic ward studies. *BMJ* 1997; 314:112–117.

6. Yu-Poth S, Zhao G, Etherton TD, et al: Effects of the National Cholesterol Education Program's Step I and Step II dietary intervention programs on cardiovascular disease risk factors: a meta-analysis. *Am J Clin Nutr* 1999; 69:632–646.

7. Hegsted DM, McGandy RB, Myers ML, Stare FJ: Quantitative effects of dietary fat on serum cholesterol in man. *Am J Clin Nutr* 1965; 17:281–295.

8. Dattilo AM, Kris-Etherton PM: Effects of weight reduction on blood lipids and lipoproteins: a meta-analysis. *Am J Clin Nutr* 1992; 56:320–328.

9. Weksler BB: ω3 fatty acids have multiple antithrombotic effects, in Galli C, Simopoulos AP, Tremoli E (eds): *Effects of Fatty Acids and Lipids in Health and Disease.* New York, Basel Publisher, 1994.

10. Leaf A: Some effects of ω3 fatty acids on coronary heart disease. in Galli C, Simopoulos AP, Tremoli E (eds): *Effects of Fatty Acids and Lipids in Health and Disease.* New York, Basel Publisher, 1994.

11. Harris WS: n-3 fatty acids and serum lipoproteins: human studies. *Am J Clin Nutr* 1997; 65(5 suppl):1645S–1654S.

12. Bang HO, Dyerberg J: Plasma lipids and lipoproteins in Greenlandic West Coast Eskimos. *Acta Med Scand* 1972; 192:85–94.

13. Dyerberg J, Bang HO, Stofferson E, et al: Eicosapentaenoic acid and prevention of thrombosis and atherosclerosis. *Lancet* 1978; 2:117–119.

14. Hirai A, Hamazaki T, Terano T: Eicosapentaenoic acid and platelet function in Japanese. *Lancet* 1980; 2:1132–1133.

15. Kromhout D, Bosschieter EB, Coulander CL: The inverse relation between fish consumption and 20-year mortality from coronary heart disease. *N Engl J Med* 1985; 312:1205–1216.

16. Burr ML, Gilbert JF, Holliday RM, et al: Effects of changes in fat, fish and fibre intakes on death and myocardial infarction: Diet and Reinfarction Trial (DART). *Lancet* 1989: 2:757–761.

17. Nordoy A, Goodnight SH: Dietary lipids and thrombosis: relationships to atherosclerosis. *Arteriosclerosis* 1990; 10:149–163.

18. de Lorgeril M, Renaud S, Mamelle N, et al: Mediterranean alpha-linolenic acid-rich diet in secondary prevention of coronary heart disease. *Lancet* 1994; 343:1454–1459.

19. Stone NJ: Fish consumption, fish oil, lipids and coronary heart disease. *Circulation* 1996; 94:2337–2340.

20. Krauss RM, Deckelbaum RJ, Ernst N, et al: Dietary guidelines for healthy American adults: A statement for health professionals from the Nutrition Committee, American Heart Association. *Circulation* 1996; 94:1795–1800.

21. Alaimo K, McDowell M, Briefel R, et al: Dietary intake: vitamins, minerals and fiber of persons age two months and over in the United States: Third National Health and Nutrition Examination Survey: Phase 1, 1988–91. *Advance Data* 1994; 258:1–28.

22. Khaw KT, Barrett-Connor E: Dietary fiber and reduced ischemic heart disease mortality rates in men and women: a 12-year prospective study. *Am J Epidemiol* 1987; 126:1093–1102.

23. Kromhout D, Bosschieter EB, de Lezenne Coulander C: Dietary fibre and 10-year mortality from coronary heart disease, cancer, and all causes: the Zutphen Study. *Lancet* 1982; 1:518–522.

24. Kushi LH, Lew RA, Stare FJ, et al: Diet and 20-year mortality from coronary heart disease: the Ireland-Boston Diet-Heart Study. *N Engl J Med* 1985; 312:811–818.

25. Rimm EB, Ascherio A, Giovannucci E, et al: Vegetable, fruit, and cereal fiber intake and risk of coronary heart disease among men. *JAMA* 1996; 275:447–451.

26. Van Horn L: Fiber, lipids and coronary heart disease: a statement for health care professionals from the Nutrition Committee, American Heart Association. *Circulation* 1997; 95:2701–2704.

27. Ripsin CM, Keenan JM, Jacobs DR Jr, et al: Oat products and lipid lowering. A meta-analysis. *JAMA* 1992; 267:3317–3325.

28. Reaven PD, Khouw A, Beltz WF, et al: Effect of dietary antioxidant combinations in humans: protection of LDL by vitamin E but not by beta-carotene. *Arterioscler Thromb* 1993; 13:590–600.

29. Stampfer MJ, Hennekens CH, Manson JE, et al: Vitamin E consumption and risk of coronary heart disease in women. *N Engl J Med* 1993; 328:1444–1449.

30. Gaziano JM, Steinberg D: Natural antioxidants, in Manson JE, Ridker PM, Gaziano JM, Hennekens CH (eds): *Prevention of Myocardial Infarction.* New York, Oxford University Press, 1996.

31. Rimm EB, Stampfer MJ, Ascherio A, et al: Vitamin E consumption and the risk of coronary heart disease in men. *N Engl J Med* 1993; 328:1450–1456.

32. The Alpha-Tocopherol, Beta-Carotene Cancer Prevention Study Group: The effect of vitamin E and beta-carotene on the incidence of lung cancer and other cancers in male smokers. *N Engl J Med* 1994; 330:1029–1035.

33. Hennekens CH, Buring JE, Manson JE, et al: Lack of effect of long term supplementation with beta-carotene on the incidence of malignant neoplasms and cardiovascular disease. *N Engl J Med* 1996; 334:1145–1149.

34. Stephens NG, Parsons A, Schofield PM, et al: Randomised controlled trial of vitamin E in patients with coronary disease: Cambridge Heart Antioxidant Study (CHAOS). *Lancet* 1996; 347:781–786.

35. Rapola JM, Virtamo J, Ripatti S, et al: Randomised trial of α-tocopherol and β-carotene supplements on incidence of major coronary events in men with previous myocardial infarction. *Lancet* 1997; 349:1715–1720.

36. Tribble DL, for the Nutrition Committee: AHA Science Advisory—antioxidant consumption and risk of coronary heart disease: emphasis on vitamin C, vitamin E, and beta-carotene: a statement for healthcare professionals from the American Heart Association. *Circulation* 1999; 99:591–595.

37. Boushey CJ, Beresford SA, Omen GS, Motulsky AG: A quantitative assessment of plasma homocysteine as a risk factor for vascular disease. *JAMA* 1995; 274:1049–1057.

38. Ridker PM, Manson JE, Buring JE, et al: Homocysteine and risk of cardiovascular disease among postmenopausal women. *JAMA* 1999; 281:1817–1821.

39. Duell PB, Malinow MR: Homocyst(e)ine: an important risk factor for atherosclerotic vascular disease. *Curr Opin Lipidol* 1997; 8:28–34.

40. Shimakawa T, Nieto FJ, Malinow MR, et al: Vitamin intake: a possible determinant of plasma homocyst(e)ine among middle-aged adults. *Ann Epidemiol* 1997; 7:285–293.

41. Selhub J, Jacques PF, Wilson PWF, et al: Vitamin status and intake as primary determinants of homocysteinemia in an elderly population. *JAMA* 1993; 270:2693–2698.

42. Malinow MR, Bostom AG, Krauss RM: AHA Science Advisory—homocysteine, diet, and cardiovascular diseases: a statement for healthcare professionals from the Nutrition Committee, American Heart Association. *Circulation* 1999; 99:178–182.

43. Klatsky AL, Armstrong MA, Griedman GD: Alcohol and mortality. *Ann Intern Med* 1992; 117:646–654.

44. Bradley KA, Donovan DM, Larson EB: How much is too much? Advising patients about safe levels of alcohol consumption. *Arch Intern Med* 1993; 153:2734–2740.

45. Klatsky AL, Friedman GD, Siegelaub AB, Gerard MJ: Alcohol consumption and blood pressure: Kaiser Permanente Multiphasic Health Examination data. *N Engl J Med* 1977; 296:1194–1200.

46. Stampfer MJ, Colditz GA, Willett WC, et al: A prospective study of moderate alcohol consumption and the risk of coronary disease and stroke in women. *N Engl J Med* 1988; 319:267–273.

47. Gaziano JM, Buring JE, Breslow JL, et al: Moderate alcohol intake, increased levels of high density lipoprotein and its subgractions, and decreased risk of myocardial infarction. *N Engl J Med* 1993; 329:1829–1834.

48. Gordon T, Ernst N, Fisher M, Rifkind BM: Alcohol and high-density lipoprotein cholesterol. *Circulation* 1981; 64 (suppl III):III-63–III-67.

49. Hulley SB, Gordon S: Alcohol and high-density lipoprotein cholesterol: causal inference from diverse study designs. *Circulation* 1981; 64 (suppl III):III-57–III-63.

50. Ridker PM, Vaughan DE, Stampfer MJ, et al: Association of moderate alcohol consumption and plasma concentration of endogenous tissue-type plasminogen activator. *JAMA* 1994; 272:929–933.

52. Klatsky AL, Armstrong MA, Friedman GD: Red wine, white wine, liquor, beer, and risk for coronary artery disease hospitalization. *Am J Cardiol* 1997; 80:416–420.

53. Pearson TA: Alcohol and heart disease: AHA Medical/Scientific Statement. *Circulation* 1996; 94:3023–3025.

53. Hu FB, Stampfer MJ, Manson JE, et al: Frequent nut consumption and risk of coronary heart disease in women: prospective cohort study. *BMJ* 1998; 317:1341–1345.

54. Fraser GE, Sabate J, Beeson WL, Strahan TM: A possible protective effect of nut consumption on risk of coronary heart disease: the Adventist Health Study. *Arch Intern Med* 1992; 152:1416–1424.

55. Kushi LH, Folsom AR, Prineas RJ, et al: Dietary antioxidant vitamins and death from coronary heart disease in postmenopausal women. *N Engl J Med* 1996; 334:1156–1162.

56. Anderson JW, Johnstone BM, Cook-Newell ME: Meta-analysis of the effects of soy protein intake on serum lipids. *N Engl J Med* 1995; 333:276–282.

57. Potter SM, Baum JA, Teng H, et al: Soy protein and isoflavones: their effects on blood lipids and bone density in postmenopausal women. *Am J Clin Nutr* 1998; 68(suppl):1375S–1379S.

58. Raines EW, Ross R: Biology of atherosclerotic plaque formation: possible role of growth factors in lesion development and the potential impact of soy. *J Nutr* 1995; 125:624S–630S.

59. Wilcox JN, Blumenthal BF: Thrombotic mechanisms in atherosclerosis: potential impact of soy proteins. *J Nutr* 1995; 631S–638S.

60. Pelletier X, Belbraouet S, Mirabel D, et al: A diet moderately enriched in phytosterols lowers plasma cholesterol concentrations in normocholesterolemic humans. *Ann Nutr Metab.* 1995; 39:291–295.

61. Miettinen TA, Puska P, Gylling H, et al: Reduction of serum cholesterol with sitostanol-ester margarine in a mildly hypercholesterolemic population. *N Engl J Med* 1995; 333:1308–1312.

62. Lawson LD: Garlic: a review of its medicinal effects and indicated active compounds, in Lawson LD, Bauer R (eds): *Phytomedicines of Europe: Chemistry and Biologi-*

cal Activity. ACS Symposium Series 691. Washington DC: American Chemical Society, 1998, pp 176–209.

63. Berthold HK, Sudhop T, Bergmann KV: Effect of garlic on serum lipids (letter). *JAMA* 1998; 280:1568.

64. Warshafsky S, Kamer RS, Sivak SL. Effect of garlic on total serum cholesterol: a meta-analysis. *Ann Intern Med* 1993; 119:599–605.

65. Stone NJ, Nicolosi RJ, Kris-Etherton P, et al: Summary of the scientific conference on the efficacy of hypocholesterolemic dietary interventions. *Circulation* 1996; 94:3388–3391.

66. Schaefer EJ, Lamon-Fava S, Ausman LM, et al: Individual variability in lipoprotein cholesterol response to National Cholesterol Education Program Step 2 Diets. *Am J Clin Nutr* 1997; 65:823–830.

67. Lowering Blood Cholesterol to Prevent Heart Disease: National Institutes of Health Consensus Conference on Blood Cholesterol. *JAMA* 1985; 253:2080–2091.

68. Sikand G, Lee E, Downey NA, et al: Low use of medical nutrition therapy in hyperlipidemic patients with coronary artery disease. *J Am Diet Assoc* 1997; 9(suppl) 9:A-32.

69. Snetselaar LG (ed): *Overview of Nutrition Counseling in Nutritional Counseling Skills for Medical Nutrition Therapy.* Gaithersburg MD, Aspen, 1997, pp 3–20.

70. Krummel D, Berry M, Moriarity K: Medical nutrition therapy for cardiovascular disease and associated risk factors: specific diets for prevention and treatment in cardiovascular nutrition, in Kris-Etherton PM, Burns JH (eds): *Cardiovascular Nutrition: Strategies and Tools for Disease Management and Prevention.* Chicago, American Dietetic Association, 1998, pp 85–104.

71. Smith KG, Johnson EQ (eds): *Medical Nutrition Therapy Across the Continuum of Care: Patient Protocols.* Chicago, American Dietetic Association, 1996.

72. American Heart Association: *Comprehensive Risk Reduction in Patients with Coronary and other Vascular Disease.* Dallas, TX, AHA, 1996.

73. Grundy SM, Balady GJ, Criqui MH, et al: When to start cholesterol-lowering therapy in patients with coronary heart disease—a statement for health-care professionals from the American Heart Association Task Force on Risk Disease. *Circulation* 1997: 95;1683–1685.

74. McGehee MM, Johnson EQ, Rasmussen HM, et al: Benefits and costs of medical nutrition therapy by registered dietitians for patients with hypercholesterolemia. *J Am Diet Assoc* 1995; 95:1041–1043.

75. Sikand G, Kashyap ML, Yang I. Beneficial outcome and cost savings of medical nutrition therapy in hyper-cholesterolemia. *J Am Diet Assoc* 1998; 98:889–894.

76. Denke MA, Grundy SM: Individual responses to a cholesterol-lowering diet in 50 men with moderate hypercholesterolemia. *Arch Intern Med* 1994; 154:317–325.

77. Blankenhorn DH, Johnson RL, Mack WJ, et al: The influence of diet on the appearance of new lesions in human coronary arteries. *JAMA* 1990; 263:1646–1652.

78. Huninghake DB, Stein EA, Dujovne CA, et al: The efficacy of intensive dietary therapy alone or combined with lovastatin in outpatients with hypercholesterolemia. *N Engl J Med* 1993; 328:1213–1219.

79. Dallongeville J, Leboeuf N, Chantal B, et al: Short-term response to dietary counseling of hyperlipidemic outpatients of a lipid clinic. *J Am Diet Assoc* 1994; 94:616–621.

80. Rhodes KS, Bookstein LC, Aaronson LS, et al: Intensive nutrition counseling enhances outcomes of National Cholesterol Education Program dietary therapy. *J Am Diet Assoc* 1996; 96:1003–1010.

81. Geil PB, Anderson JW, Gustafson NJ: Women and men with hypercholesterolemia respond similarly to an American Heart Association Step 1 Diet. *J Am Diet Assoc* 1995; 95:436–441.

82. Krauss RN, Deckelbaum RJ, Ernst N, et al: Dietary Guidelines for Healthy American Adults: a statement for health professionals from the Nutrition Committee, American Heart Association. American Heart Association Medical/Scientific Statement. *Circulation* 1996; 94:1795–1800.

83. *Nutrition and Your Health—Dietary Guidelines for Americans.* USDA-DHHS Home and Garden Bulletin No. 232, 4th ed. Washington, DC, Department of Health and Human Services, 1995.

84. Chait A, Brunzell JD, Denke MA, et al: Rationale of the diet heart statement of the American Heart Association. Report of the Nutrition Committee. *Circulation* 1993; 88:3008–3029.

85. Denke MA, Sempos CT, Grundy SM. Excess body weight: an underrecognized contributor to high blood cholesterol levels in white American men. *Arch Intern Med* 1993; 153:1093–1103.

86. National Institutes of Health: *Clinical Guidelines on the Identification, Evaluation, and Treatment of Overweight and Obesity in Adults: The Evidence Report.* Bethesda, MD. National Institutes of Health, 1998.

87. St Jeor ST: New trends in weight management. *J Amer Diet Assoc* 1997: 97:1096–1098.

88. Wadden TA: Treatment of obesity by moderate and severe caloric restriction: results of clinical research trials. *Ann Intern Med* 1993; 119:688–693.

89. Brownell KD, Rodin J: The Dieting maelstorm: is it possible and advisable to lose weight? *Am Psychol* 1994; 49:781–791.

90. Lissner L, Odell PM, D'Agostino RB, et al: Variability of body weight and health outcomes in the Framingham population. *N Engl J Med* 1991; 324:1839–1844.

91. Manson JE, Willett WC, Stampfer MJ, et al: Body weight and mortality among women. *N Engl J Med* 1995; 333:677–685.

92. Andersen RE, Wadden TA, Bartlett SJ, et al: Relation of weight loss to changes in serum lipids and liporoteins in obese women. *Am J Clin Nutr* 1995; 62:350–357.

93. Datttilo AM, Kris-Etherton PM: Effects of weight reduction on blood lipids and lipoproteins: a meta-analysis. *Am J Clin Nutr* 1992; 56:320–328.

94. Caggiula AW, Christake G, Farrand M, et al: The Multiple Risk Factor Intervention Trial (MRFIT). 1981; 10:443–475.

95. Dolecek TA, Milas NC, Van Horn LV, et al: A long term nutrition intervention experience: lipid responses and dietary adherence patterns in the Multiple Risk Factor Intervention Trial. *J Am Diet Assoc* 1986; 86:752–758.

96. National Diet-Heart Study Research Group: The national diet-heart study final report. *Circulation* 1968; 37 (suppl 1):1–428.

97. Gordon DJ, Salz KM, Roggenkamp KJ, et al: Dietary determinants of plasma cholesterol change in the recruitment phase of the Lipid Research Clinics Primary Prevention Trial. *Arteriosclerosis* 1982; 2:537–548.

98. Wood PD, Stefanick ML, Williams PT, et al: The effects of plasma lipoproteins of a prudent weight reducing diet, with or without exercise in overweight men and women. *N Engl J Med* 1991; 325:461–466.

99. Wood PD, Stefanick ML, Dreon DM, et al: Changes in plasma lipids and lipoproteins in overweight men during weight loss through dieting as compared with exercise. *N Engl J Med* 1988; 319:1173–1179.

100. Ehnholm C, Huttunen JK, Pietinen P, et al: Effect of diet on serum lipoproteins in a population with a high risk of coronary heart disease. *N Engl J Med* 1982; 307:850–855.

101. Mennotti A, Keys A, Kromhout D, et al: Intercohort differences in coronary heart disease mortality in the 25-year follow-up of the Seven Countries Study. *Eur J Epidemiol* 1993; 9:527–536.

102. Lichtenstein AH, Van Horn L: Very Low Fat Diets: American Heart Association Scientific Advisory Nutrition Committee. *Circulation* 1998; 98:935–939.

103. Blankenhorn DH, Johnson RL, Mack WJ: The influence of diet on the appearance of new lesions in human coronary arteries. *JAMA* 1990; 263:1646–1652.

104. Schuler G, HamBrecht R, Schlierf G, et al: Regular physical exercise and low fat diet: effects on progression of coronary artery disease. *Circulation* 1992; 86:1–11.

105. Ornish D, Scherwitz LW, Billings JH, et al: Intensive lifestyle changes for reversal of coronary heart disease. *JAMA* 1998; 280:2001–2007.

106. Ornish D, Brown SE, Scherwitz LW, et al: Can lifestyle changes reverse coronary heart disease? *Lancet* 1990; 336:129–133.

107. Chen YD, Coulston AM, Zhou MY: Why do low-fat-high-carbohydrate diets accentuate post-prandial lipemia in patients with NIDDM? *Diabetes Care* 1995; 18:10–16.

108. The Women's Health Initiative Study Group: Design paper: design of the Women's Health Initiative Clinical Trial and Observational Study. *Contr Clin Trials* 1998; 19:61–109.

109. Mensink RP: Dietary monounsaturated fatty acids and serum lipoprotein levels in healthy subjects. *Atherosclerosis* 1994; 110:65–68.

110. Keys A: Coronary heart disease in seven countries. *Circulation* 1970; 41:1–211.

111. Carroll KK, Khor HT: Effects of level and type of dietary fat on incidence of mammary tumors induced in female Sprague-Dawley rats by 7,12-dimethylbenz (alpha) anthracene. *Lipids* 1971; 6:415–420.

112. Reddy BS: Amount and type of dietary fat and colon cancer: animal model studies. *Prog Clin Biol Res* 1986; 222:295–309.

113. Reaven PD, Parthasarathy S, Grasse BJ, et al: Feasibility of using an oleate-rich diet to reduce the susceptibility of low-density lipoprotein to oxidative modification in humans. *Am J Clin Nutr* 1991; 54:701–706.

114. Bonanome A, Pagnan A, Biffanti S, et al: Effect of dietary monounsaturated and polyunsaturated fatty acids on the susceptibility of plasma low-density lipoproteins to oxidative modification. *Arterioscler Thromb* 1992; 12:529–533.

115. Sarkkinen ES, Uusitupaet MIJ, Pirjo P, et al: Long-term effects of three fat-modified diets in hypercholesterolemic subjects. *Atherosclerosis* 1994; 105:9–23.

116. Oliver MF: It is more important to increase the intake of unsaturated fats than to decrease the intake of saturated fats: evidence from clinical trials relating to ischemic heart disease. *Am J Clin Nutr* 1997; 66(suppl):980S–986S.

117. Berry EM: Dietary fatty acids in the management of diabetes mellitus. *Am J Clin Nutr* 1997; 66(suppl):991S–997S.

118. Anderson JW, Smith BM, Gustafson NJ: Health benefits and practical aspects of high-fiber diets. *Am J Clin Nutr* 1994; 59:1242S–1247S.

119. Van Horn L: Fiber lipids and coronary heart disease—AHA Medical Scientific Statement. *Circulation* 1997; 95:2701–2704.

120. Bell LP, Hectorn KJ, Reynolds H, et al: Cholesterol-lowering effects of soluble fiber cereals as part of a prudent diet for patients with mild to moderate hypercholesterolemia. *Am J Clin Nutr* 1990; 52:1020–1026.

121. Glore SR, Van Treeck D, Knehans AW, et al: Soluble fiber and serum lipids: a literature review. *J Am Diet Assoc* 1994; 94:425–436.

122. Hosobuchi C, Lapa R, Bassin SL, et al: Efficacy of acacia, pectin, and guar gum-based fiber supplementation in the control of hypercholesterolemia. *Nutr Res* 1999.

123. Bell LP, Hectorne K, Reynolds H, et al: Cholesterol lowering effects of psyllium hydrophillic mucilloid. *JAMA* 1989; 261:3419–3423.

124. Rimm E, Ascherio A, Giovannucci E, et al: Vegetable, fruit and cereal intake and risk of coronary heart disease among men. *JAMA* 1996; 275:447–451.

125. Ripsin CM, Keenan JM, Jacobs DR, et al: Oat products and lipid lowering: a meta-analysis. *JAMA* 1992; 267:3317–3325.

126. Whitten C: Vegetarian diets and ischemic heart disease. *Top Clin Nutr* 1995; 10:27–33.

127. Barnard ND, Akhtar A, Nicholson A: Factors that facilitate compliance to lower fat intake. *Arch Fam Med* 1995; 4:153–158.

128. Johnston PK: Vegetarians among us: implications for health professionals. *Top Clin Nutr* 1995; 10:1–6.

129. Messina M, Messina V: *The Dietitian's Guide to Vegetarian Diets.* Gaithersburg, MD, Aspen, 1996.

130. Anderson JW, Garrity TF, Wood CL, et al: Prospective, randomized, controlled comparison of the effects of low fat and low fat plus high fiber diets on serum lipid concentrations. *Am J Clin Nutr* 1992; 56:887–894.

131. Havala S, Dwyer JT: Position of the American Dietetic Association: vegetarian diets. *J Am Diet Assoc* 1993; 93:1317–1319.

132. Whitten C: Vegetarian diets and ischemic heart disease. *Top Clin Nutr* 1995; 10:27–33.

133. Haddad EH: Development of a vegetarian food guide. *Am J Clin Nutr* 1995; 59:1248S–1254S.

134. Ornish D: *Eat More, Weigh Less.* New York, Harper Collins, 1994.

135. Dwyer JT: Vegetarianism for women, in Krummel DA, Kris-Etherton PM (eds): *Nutrition in Women's Health.* Gaithersburg, MD, Aspen, 1996, pp 232–262.

136. Stern JS: Perspectives on sodium. *Perspect Appl Nutr* 1995; 3:127–129.

137. McCarron DA: The role of adequate dietary calcium intake in the prevention and management of salt-sensitive hypertension. *Am J Clin Nutr* 1997; 65 (suppl 2):712S–716S.

138. Krummel DA: Nutritional care in heart failure and transplant, in Mahan LK, Escott-Stump S (eds): *Food and Nutrition and Diet Therapy.* Philadelphia, Saunders, 1996, pp 737–750.

139. Appel LJ, Moore TJ, Obarzanek E, et al: A clinical trial of the effects of dietary patterns on blood pressure. *N Engl J Med* 1997; 336:1117–1124.

140. Sikand G, Kashyap ML, Wong ND, et al: Dietitian intervention improves lipids and saves medication costs in niacin failures with combined hyperlipidemia. *J Am Dietetic Assoc* (in press).

141. Sikand G, Downey NA, Kashyap ML: Beneficial effect of medical nutrition therapy by a registered dietitian in the weight management outcome of dyslipidemic patients. *J Am Diet Assoc* 1995; 95(suppl 9):A-78.

142. Oster G, Thompson D: Estimated effects of reducing dietary saturated fat intake on the incidence and costs of coronary heart disease in the United States. *J Am Diet Assoc* 1996; 96:127–131.

143. Leventhal H: A self-regulation perspective, in Gentry WD (ed): *Handbook of Behavioral Medicine.* New York, Guilford Press, 1984, pp 369–436.

144. Glantz K: "Dietitians effectiveness and patient compliance with dietary regimens. *J Am Diet Assoc* 1979; 3:631.

145. DiClemente C, McConnaughty E, Norcross J, et al: Integrative dimensions for psychotherapy. *Int J Eclec Psychother* 1996; 5:256–274.

146. Marcus B, Simkin K, Rossi J, et al: Longitudinal shifts in employees' stages and process of exercise behavior change. *Am J Public Health* 1996; 10:195–200.

147. Prochaska, JO: A transtheoretical model of behavior change: Implications for diet interventions, in Henderson MM, Bowen DJ, DeRoo KK (eds): *Proceedings of the Conference on Promoting Dietary Change in Communities: Applying Existing Models of Dietary Change to Population-Based Interventions.* Seattle, Fred Hutchinson Cancer Center, 1992, pp 37–49.

148. Greene GW, Rossi SR: Stages of Change for reducing dietary fat intake over 18 months. *J Am Diet Assoc* 1998; 98:529–534.

149. Molina CW, Aguirre-Molina M (eds): *Latino Health in the US: A Growing Challenge.* Washington, DC, American Public Health Association, 1994.

150. Thernstorm S: *Harvard Encyclopedia of American Ethnic Groups.* Cambridge, MA, Harvard University Press, 1980.

151. Zola IK: Culture and symptoms-an analysis of patients presenting complaints. *Am Soc Rev* 1966; 31:615–630.

152. Higginbotham JC, Trevino FM, Ray LA: Utilization of curanderos by Mexican-Americans: prevalence and predictors findings from HHANES 1982–84. *Am J Public Health* 1990; 80(suppl):32–35.

153. Kanfer FH, Schefft, BK: *Guiding the Process of Therapeutic Change.* Champaign, IL, Research Press, 1988.

154. Rogers CR: *Client-Centered Therapy.* Boston, Houghton Mifflin, 1951, p 487.

155. Pietrofesa JJ (ed): *Counseling: Therapy Research and Practice.* Chicago, Rand McNally, 1978, pp 71–77.

156. Ivey AE (ed): *Counseling and Psychotherapy: Integrating Skills Theory and Practice,* 2d ed. Englewood Cliffs, NJ, Prentice Hall, 1987, pp 429–430.

157. Bowen M: *Family Therapy in Clinical Practice.* New York, Aronson, 1978, pp 102–104.

158. Leventhal H, Cameron L: Behavioral theories and the problem of compliance. *Patient Educ Counsel* 1987; 10:117–138.

159. Glanz K: Nutrition education for risk factor reduction and patient education: a review. *Prev Med* 1985; 14:721–745.

160. Brown SL, Pope JF, Hunt AE, Tolman NM: Motivational strategies used by dietitians to counsel individuals with diabetes. *Diabetes Educ* 1998; 24(3):313–318.

161. American Heart Association: *Dietary Treatment of Hypercholesterolemia: A Manual for Patients.* Dallas, AHA, 1988.

CHAPTER 14

Psychosocial Factors

Alice G. Luten
Lynda H. Powell

necdotal observations of the importance of psychosocial factors in the development of coronary heart disease (CHD) have been recorded throughout time. In 1892, William Osler observed: "In the worry and strain of modern life, arterial degeneration is not only very common but develops often at a relatively early age. For this, I believe that the high pressure at which men live and the habit of working the machine to its maximum capacity are responsible rather than excesses in eating and drinking."[1]

It was not until the 1950s that the concept of "coronary-prone behavior" was formalized, suggesting that certain behaviors are associated with the development of CHD. For the past 40 years, psychosocial epidemiologists and health psychologists have focused on identifying the psychosocial factors that influence CHD, with a recent emphasis on identifying coronary-prone *emotions* rather than behaviors (Table 14–1). In this chapter, we provide an overview of the literature on the association between psychosocial factors (type A behavior, hostility, anger, low social support, depression, anxiety, and distress) and CHD. Second, we describe psychosocial treatment strategies for reducing several coronary-prone emotions (depression, anxiety, anger) and an environmental risk factor (low social support). Finally, we outline how these treatment strategies may be used to improve compliance with lifestyle modification.

Psychosocial Factors and Coronary Heart Disease Risk

The Type A Behavior Pattern: The First Psychosocial Factor Recognized as Coronary-Prone

The *type A behavior pattern* (TABP), a term coined by cardiologists Meyer Friedman and Ray Rosenman, describes individuals who, in Osler's words, were "working the machine to its maximum capacity." Type A individuals are characterized by two central characteristics: excessive time urgency and free-floating hostility.[2] Although a number of questionnaires were developed to assess this behavior pattern, the "gold standard" was a structured interview[3,4] where specific speech and motor characteristics reflecting time urgency and hostility were unobtrusively recorded. An early large-scale epidemiologic study ($N = 3524$) demonstrated, over $8\frac{1}{2}$ years of follow-up, that healthy type A men were at approximately twice the risk of developing CHD as their type B (i.e., non-type A) counterparts. In subjects whose age at intake was 50 to 59 years, the relative risk (RR) was 1.98 ($p < .019$) after adjustment for confounders; in subjects whose age at intake was 39 to 49 years, the adjusted RR was 1.87 ($p < .003$).[5] Another early large-scale study found that healthy type A men and women were twice as likely to develop CHD.[6] These findings stimulated hundreds of studies aimed at refining the

TABLE 14–1 Overview of Studies Linking Negative Emotions to Coronary Heart Disease

Psychosocial Factor	Reference	Study Population	Relative Risk for Coronary Events after Adjustment for Confounders
Anger (toxic emotion of the type A behavior pattern)	Kawachi et al.,[32] 1996	1305 older men	RR = 2.66 (95% CI, 1.26 to 5.61) for combined total CHD (nonfatal MI, fatal CHD, and angina) over 7 years of follow-up; dose-response relationship between level of anger and overall CHD risk (p for trend = .008).
	Mittleman et al.,[35] 1995	1623 (31%) post-MI patients	Anger was present 2.3 times (95% CI, 1.7 to 3.2) more frequently in the 2 h before an MI than at the same time on a normal day
Depression	Frasure-Smith Lesperance et al.,[58] 1993	222 post-MI patients (22% women)	Adjusted hazard ratio = 4.29 (95% CI, 3.14 to 5.44) for coronary mortality over 6 months after index MI.
	Carney et al.,[62] 1988	52 patients (27% women) undergoing cardiac catheterization	RR = 2.2 ($p < .02$) for any cardiac event (MI, PTCA, CABG, and death) during 12 months after catheterization
Anxiety	Kawachi et al.,[84] 1994	33,999 male health professionals	RR = 6.08 (95% CI, 2.35 to 15.73) for sudden cardiac death over 2 years of follow-up.
	Moser and Dracup,[86] 1996	86 (26% women) hospitalized post-MI patients	Odds ratio = 4.9 (95% CI, 2.1 to 12.2) for ischemic and arrhythmic complications before discharge.
Distress	Allison et al.,[93] 1995	381 cardiac rehabilitation patients (18% women)	Odds ratio = 4.39, $p = .003$ for any cardiac recurrence (including MI, coronary death, PTCA, CABG, angina with verification of restenosis, CHF, embolic stroke or pulmonary embolus related to CAD) during 6 months after index hospitalization; 4.4 times greater hospitalization costs ($p < .0003$).
	Denollet and Brutsaert,[95] 1998	87 post-MI patients (7% women)	RR = 4.7 (95% CI, 1.9 to 11.8) for cardiac recurrence (MI or coronary mortality) over 7.9 mean years of follow-up.

Key: CHD, coronary heart disease; MI, myocardial infarction; PTCA, percutaneous transluminal coronary angioplasty; CABG, coronary artery bypass graft; CAD, coronary artery disease.

measurement of the TABP and understanding its physiologic mechanisms. A pivotal study[7] divided angiography patients by both their TABP and level of hostility[8] and found that the *hostility* scores were a better predictor of the degree of stenosis than were the type A scores. This discovery was followed closely by the results of the large-scale Multiple Risk

Factor Intervention Trial (MRFIT),[9,10] where *hostility* (RR = 1.5; $p = .032$), *but not the TABP* [RR = .87; 95 percent confidence interval (CI), .59 to 1.28], predicted coronary mortality in high-risk men after adjusting for confounding variables. Although even today there are studies showing that type A behavior predicts CHD independent of hostility and anger,[11] the weight of the evidence has shifted interest away from the global TABP and toward hostility, the component of the TABP that we now believe is its toxic core.

Hostility: The Toxic Personality Trait of the Type A Behavior Pattern

Like the type A behavior pattern, hostility is a multidimensional construct, but there is general agreement that two attitudinal sets are coronary-prone: cynical beliefs and mistrust of others.[12] Because hostility is a personality trait, its stability over time is excellent for adults with stability coefficients of approximately .85 over as long as 4 years.[13] It is most commonly assessed using the Cook-Medley Hostility Scale[8] (Table 14–2), a subscale of the Minnesota Multiphasic Personality Inventory (MMPI).[14]

Hostility may have a direct neuroendocrine effect on the heart, particularly via testosterone,[15] and/or it may exert a more indirect effect via its association with other cardiovascular risk factors such as smoking, adverse lipid profiles, high blood pressure, physical inactivity, excess alcohol consumption, and/or obesity.[16,17] To date there have been 14 longitudinal studies that have examined the role of hostility on hard CHD outcomes. Of these, 10 have found an association[10,13,17–24] and 4 have failed to find an association.[25–28] Studies have found evidence for the predictive value of hostility for both healthy individuals and those with CHD, for both men and women, and for both older and younger subjects. A

detailed metanalysis of research on hostility and physical health indicates that hostility is an independent risk factor for CHD.[29]

Anger: The Toxic Emotion of the Type A Behavior Pattern

Some investigators view anger as the emotional expression of a hostile attitudinal set. However, correlations between hostility and anger tend to average only around .30,[30] suggesting that anger has distinct dimensions. Anger, as distinct from hostility, has been conceptualized as trait anger (how angry one generally feels), state anger (how angry one feels right now), and anger coping style (when one feels anger, it is suppressed, expressed, or discussed rationally)[31] (Table 14–3).

Attention has recently shifted away from the concept of "coronary-prone behavior" and toward the general idea that there are "coronary-prone emotions," such as anger. Early data from Framingham indicated that healthy men and women who suppressed their anger were at increased risk for the development of CHD 8 years later.[16] This finding was replicated more recently in a study of 1305 older men who were at an almost threefold greater risk of total CHD [nonfatal myocardial infarction (MI), fatal CHD, and angina] 7 years later if they had difficulty controlling anger (after adjusting for cardiovascular risk factors, RR = 2.7; 95 percent CI, 1.3 to 5.6). Moreover, there was a significant dose-response

TABLE 14–2 Sample Items from the Cook-Medley Hostility Scale

I have often had to take orders from someone who did not know as much as I did.

It takes a lot of argument to convince most people of the truth.

I think most people would lie to get ahead.

Most people inwardly dislike putting themselves out to help other people.

Source: From Cook and Medley,[8] with permission.

TABLE 14–3 Sample Items from the Spielberger State-Trait Anger Expression Inventory—State Anger Scale

I am furious.

I feel angry.

I feel like breaking things.

I feel like swearing.

Source: Adapted and reproduced by special permission of the publisher, Psychological Assessment Resources, Inc., 16204 North Florida Ave., Getz, FL 33549, from the STAXI by Charles D. Spielberger, Ph.D., copyright 1979, 1986, 1988, by special permission from PAR, Inc.

relationship between level of anger and overall CHD risk (p for trend = .008).[32] Trait anger has been associated with severity of CHD as well as recurrent cardiac events after percutaneous transluminal coronary angioplasty (PTCA).[33] Suppressed anger, as judged by the subjects' wives, was associated with severity of ischemia.[34]

Considerable excitement has surrounded the concept that transitory events can trigger cardiac events in both men and women. State anger is among the potential triggers; in a case-crossover study of 1623 (501 women) post-MI patients, anger was 2.3 times more frequent (95% CI, 1.7 to 3.2) in the 2 h before an MI than at the same time on a normal day.[35] State anger has been associated with lowered threshold for ventricular fibrillation,[36] lowered ejection fraction,[37] and coronary vasoconstriction in previously narrowed arteries.[38]

Social Support: A Cushion Against CHD

The "social" part of psychosocial factors assumes that the resistance of the "host" to the "pathogenic agent" lies in environmental resources.[39] Early studies of the adverse health consequences of low social support focused on the relationship between limited social connectedness and total mortality in community-based studies. In middle-aged cohorts, the association was stronger for men than women, whereas in the elderly, the association was strong for both men and women.[40-45]

In studies of CHD mortality in middle-aged cohorts, the association with low social support was strongest in men.[46-49] In a prospective study of 13,301 men and women (the percentage of women was not reported), men with few social connections were at increased risk [odds ratio (OR) = 1.5; 95 percent CI, 1.1 to 2.1] of cardiac death after adjustment for standard risk factors.[47] In a study of 736 men, social integration (OR = 3.8; 95 percent CI, 1.1 to 13.9) and social attachment (OR = 3.1; 95 percent CI, 1.3 to 7.6) were significant predictors of new CHD events after adjustment for other risk factors.[48] In studies of patients with CHD, a number of measures of social support—living alone,[50] living alone without a confidant,[51] emotional support,[52,53] social

TABLE 14–4 Sample Items from the Perceived Social Support Scale

There is a special person who is around when I am in need.

I get the emotional help and support I need from my family.

There is a special person in my life who cares about my feelings.

I can talk about my problems with my friends.

Source: From Blumenthal et al.,[53] with permission.

isolation with life stress,[54] instrumental support,[55] social integration,[56] and availability of support[57]—were associated with new cardiovascular outcomes after adjustment for other CHD risk factors.

Because people with low social support are often depressed, a critical question in this literature is whether social support exerts an effect on CHD outcomes independently of depression. Two studies, one of post-MI patients[58,59] and another of patients with premature ventricular arrhythmias,[60] found that depression was a better predictor than social support, suggesting that social support influences cardiovascular outcomes partially via its association with depression. A limitation of the social support field is the lack of standardization in the conceptualization and measurement of support. Studies of healthy individuals suggest that the most important risk factor is absence of social ties, whereas studies of coronary patients suggest that lack of emotional support is the most important risk factor (Table 14–4).

Major Depression and Depressed Affect: Coronary-Prone Emotions That Are Independent of Poor Cardiac Function

Early studies of patients with CHD suggested that those who were depressed in the hospital had a poorer prognosis.[61] However, not only were these small studies using nonstandardized measures of depression but also they left unanswered the key question of what came first—the depression or the heart disease. Because depression is a common response to severe cardiac symptoms, it was not clear whether the severity of the disease, not the depression, led to increased risk of cardiovascular mortality.

Recent studies of depression in coronary patients have caught the attention of the medical community because they feature standardized assessments of depression (Table 14–5) and excellent controls for indices of cardiac function. In a prospective study of 222 patients (22 percent women) hospitalized for MI, patients with major depression were more than four times as likely to die over the subsequent 6 months (RR = 4.3; 95 percent CI, 3.1 to 5.4) after adjustment for Killip class and previous MI.[58] Another study of 52 patients (27 percent women) undergoing cardiac catheterization found that patients diagnosed with major depression were at twice the risk of having a cardiac event (MI, coronary revascularization, or death) over the following year (RR = 2.2; $p <$ .02) independent of the severity of CHD, left ventricular ejection fraction (LVEF), and smoking status.[62] Studies have also shown that, in patients with CHD, minor depression is associated with a poorer prognosis independent of cardiac function.[59,60,63–65] A smaller number of studies fail to find this association.[66,67] Although most of these studies had predominantly male samples, a more recent investigation found that depression predicted cardiac mortality equally well in both males and females.[63] Furthermore, a literature is now accumulating in healthy community samples that depression increases risk of MI.[68,69] In elderly cohorts, there is inconsistency in whether it predicts CHD for men only[70,71] or for women only.[72,73]

A recent metanalysis of the relationship between depression and mortality uncovered 28 studies that focused on cardiovascular death. Of these, 15 found a positive association, 8 failed to find an association, 4 found the association in men only, and 1 found the association in women only.[74,75] Because the majority of the studies in this area have found a positive association, there is a call to delineate the mechanisms by which such an association might exist. One convincing possibility is that depression is associated with neuroendocrine shifts, including excess secretion of cortisol and catecholamines, triggering increased platelet activity and heart rate variability. Another hypothesis is that depression leads to poor compliance and/or risky behaviors such as smoking and alcohol abuse.[74,76,77]

TABLE 14–5 Criteria for a Major Depressive Episode

Five (or more) of the following symptoms have been present during the same 2-week period and represent a change from previous functioning; at least one of the symptoms is either (1) depressed mood or (2) loss of interest or pleasure.

1. Depressed mood most of the day, nearly every day (as indicated by either subjective account or observation made by others)

2. Markedly diminished interest or pleasure in all, or almost all, activities most of the day, nearly every day (as indicated by either subjective account or observation made by others)

3. Significant weight loss when not dieting or weight gain, or decrease or increase in appetite nearly every day.

4. Insomnia or hypersomnia nearly every day.

5. Psychomotor agitation or retardation nearly every day

6. Fatigue or loss of energy nearly every day

7. Feelings of worthlessness or excessive or inappropriate guilt nearly every day

8. Diminished ability to think or concentrate, or indecisiveness, nearly every day (as indicated by either subjective account or observation made by others)

9. Recurrent thoughts of death (not just fear of dying), recurrent suicidal ideation without a specific plan, or a suicide attempt or a specific plan for committing suicide

---

Source: Reprinted with permission from the *Diagnostic and Statistical Manual of Mental Disorders*, Fourth Edition.[78] Copyright 1994 American Psychological Association.

TABLE 14–6 Sample Items from the Spielberger State-Trait Anxiety Inventory—State Form

I am tense.

I am presently worrying over possible misfortunes.

I feel anxious.

I am jittery.

Source: Reproduced by special permission of the Publisher, Mind Garden, Inc., 1690 Woodside Rd. #202, Redwood City, CA 94061, (650) 261-3500 from the State-Trait Anxiety Inventory[88] by Charles D. Spielberger. Copyright 1977 by Charles D. Spielberger. All rights reserved. Further reproduction is prohibited without the Distributor's written consent.

Anxiety: A Newly Identified Coronary-Prone Emotion

Early studies of both inpatients and outpatients with anxiety or panic disorders suggested that these patients, particularly the males, had an increased risk of developing heart disease.[79–82] Moreover, in a community sample of 1457 middle-aged men, the presence of phobic anxiety was related to nearly a fourfold greater risk of cardiac death (RR = 3.8; 95 percent CI, 1.6 to 8.6).[83] However, these findings did not receive much attention in the medical community until the concept of "coronary-prone emotions" gained general acceptance. Then, a large-scale study of 33,999 male health professionals found that, over 2 years of follow-up, phobic anxiety was associated with a sixfold increase in the risk of sudden cardiac death (RR = 6.1; 95 percent CI, 2.4 to 15.7) after adjustment for other risk factors.[84] A second paper that same year showed that, in another large cohort of middle-aged men, anxiety was associated with increased risk of CHD, particularly sudden cardiac death.[85] A study of 86 (26 percent women) post-MI patients found that in-hospital anxiety was associated with an almost fivefold increased risk of ischemic and arrhythmic complications before discharge (OR = 4.9; 95 percent CI, 2.1 to 12.2).[86] More recent studies have focused on elderly populations, with mixed results. In one study, worrying was associated with approximately a threefold increase in risk of total CHD in men,[87] but another study found that depression but not anxiety was associated with incidence of CHD in both men and women.[70] Although the weight of the evidence is stronger for men than it is for women, it has led researchers to suggest that anxiety is another important coronary-prone emotion (Table 14–6).

Distress: A Unifying Approach to Coronary-Prone Emotions

In a 1987 review of psychological predictors of heart disease, the picture of coronary vulnerability that emerged was of a person with one or more negative emotions.[89] Because there is now evidence that several emotions—anger, depression, and anxiety—are linked to coronary outcomes, some have attempted to find the *most* significant coronary-prone emotion. A recent study of 222 post-MI patients (22 percent of whom were women) examined the respective impact of depression, anxiety, anger coping style, and low social support on total cardiac events after one year.[90] The correlations among these psychosocial factors ranged between .25 and .30 except for depression and anxiety, which were correlated .43. Results suggested that depression and anxiety exerted independent contributions on total coronary events, and suppressed anger and depressed affect contributed to arrhythmic events.

Because of the interrelationships among the coronary-prone emotions, it is possible that the chronic experience of any kind of negative emotion is coronary-prone. This hypothesis has prompted some researchers to study general distress, rather than to limit attention to a specific type of distress (Table 14–7). An early paper of 125 post-MI patients (26 percent women) found that general distress was associated with increased

TABLE 14–7 Sample Items from the SCL-90— A General Distress Measure

Headaches

Feeling easily annoyed or irritated

Feeling blue

Feeling fearful

Feeling very self-conscious with others

Source: From Derogatis,[97] with permission.

arrhythmias over a 1-year period.[91] Another early paper of 461 post-MI men found that those who were distressed had a 2.1-fold increase in odds of cardiac mortality ($p = .018$) after adjustment for confounders.[92]

More recent studies have compared the predictive capability of distress to that of other coronary-prone emotions. In a 6-month follow-up study of 381 cardiac rehabilitation patients (18 percent women) who had been hospitalized for a cardiac event (unstable angina, MI, angioplasty, bypass surgery), those who were the most distressed had a threefold higher rate of rehospitalization (odds ratio = 3.1; $p = .013$) and a 4.4-fold higher rate of any type of recurrence (odds ratio = 4.4; $p = .003$) after adjustment for confounders. Moreover, those who were most distressed had 4.4-fold greater hospitalization costs ($p < .0003$).[93] Distress was a more important predictor than depression, anxiety, and hostility. Denollet et al.[94,95] extended the concept of general distress by coining the term *type D personality,* which denoted the tendency to experience negative emotions (including anxiety, anger, and depression) combined with a suppressed coping style. In a study of 105 post-MI men, type D was associated with increased cardiac mortality.[94] In a more recent study of 87 post-MI patients (7 percent women), type D was associated with increased incidence of cardiac recurrence (RR = 4.7; 95 percent CI, 1.9 to 11.8) after adjustment for the severity of cardiac disorder at baseline.[95] The specific emotions of anxiety, anger, depression, and life stress did not add to the predictive power of type D.[94,95] It is premature to conclude that general distress is more important than specific emotions, in absence of a clear understanding of physiological mechanisms linking any of these emotions to disease.[96] Nonetheless, the evidence that general distress is a coronary-prone emotion in post-MI men is consistent enough to warrant further study, particularly in women and healthy individuals.

Psychosocial Interventions

Clinical Trials with Cardiac Patients

In general, randomized psychosocial intervention trials have targeted general distress rather than a spe-

cific emotion, probably owing to clinical observations that these factors frequently occur together. Early psychosocial interventions for patients with CHD featured the provision of support in small group settings and showed promising results on morbidity and mortality data over 1 to 4 years of follow-up.[98–100]

The most ambitious intervention study to date was the Recurrent Coronary Prevention Project (RCCP), a large-scale clinical trial of 862 post-MI patients (9.6 percent women) aimed at testing the hypothesis that counseling to reduce type A behavior would have a salutary effect on the cardiac recurrence rate. Patients were randomized to receive either type A counseling plus cardiac education or cardiac education alone. Those randomized to the intervention met in monthly small groups for 4.5 years. After 2 years, significant reductions in the type A targets were achieved.[101] After 3 years, a significant 44 percent reduction in the cardiac recurrence rate (cardiac death plus nonfatal MI) was observed,[102] and it was maintained through 4.5 years[103] (Fig. 14–1). Cardiac mortality was reduced in the subgroup of patients with good cardiac function only.[104] In separate analyses of the limited sample of 83 women in the trial, there was little evidence that the intervention had an impact or that type A behavior protected against mortality.[105]

After the conclusion of the RCCP, it was observed that not only type A behavior but also a number of *other psychosocial factors* were improved by treatment, including hostility, anger, impatience, time urgency, self-efficacy at managing stress, depression, and well-being.[106] It was unclear whether it was the reduction in type A, reduction in specific type A components, or reduction in some other, non-type A factor that resulted in the salutary impact on cardiac recurrence rates in males.

An alternative, cost-effective approach was presented by the Ischemic Heart Disease Life Stress Monitoring Program ($N = 453$ post-MI men).[107] These researchers hypothesized that the experience of stress was associated with an increased risk of recurrence and that only the subgroup of patients who experienced distress would need help. Those randomized to the intervention (versus usual care) received monthly telephone monitoring; when distress

FIGURE 14–1 Cumulative annualized recurrence rate in section 1 (cardiac education) and section 2 (type A counseling plus cardiac education) participants calculated quarterly for 4.5 years. Note that the 95 percent confidence limits of quarterly calculated cardiac recurrence rates of the two sections no longer intersect at the end of 36 months. (Reprinted from Friedman et al.,[103] with permission.)

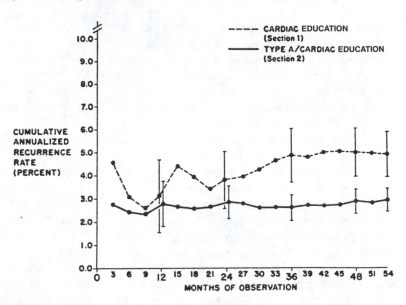

rose above a critical level, the patient received a home visit from a nurse, who provided emotional support, referrals to health care providers, and/or education about CHD. Major results indicated that this intervention lowered distress, reduced cardiac deaths by 50 percent during the program year, and lowered nonfatal MI during the 3 to 4 years after the termination of the program.[108] However, the two groups did not remain randomly equivalent but instead had more lower socioeconomic men in the control group. As such, it was unclear whether the salutary results in the intervention group were due to the treatment or to their higher socioeconomic status.[109]

To answer these methodologic concerns, a replication of the trial was conducted which included 1376 post-MI patients (34 percent women).[110] Randomization provided equal comparison groups. Results indicated that treatment had no effect on anxiety or depression, no impact on cardiac or total mortality, and, for the women, led to *greater* cardiac (9.4 versus 5.4 percent) and total (10.3 versus 5.4 percent) mortality. Thus, in the replication where women were added, the nurse-based home intervention was unsuccessful in reducing proposed psy-

chosocial targets. Not only did it have no impact on the proposed cardiac endpoints but, in the subgroup of women, it was associated with increased mortality.

Another ambitious psychosocial intervention, conducted at six centers in Wales, featured 2328 post-MI patients who were randomized to stress reduction treatment or usual-care groups.[111] Those in treatment received seven 2-h sessions (individual and group) that included education about heart disease, relaxation training, identification of stress, and development of confidence. The results after 1 year of treatment indicated that there was no difference between groups on anxiety or depression, clinical complications, clinical sequelae, or mortality. Thus, this seven-session treatment was not powerful enough to have an impact on psychosocial targets. In absence of any impact on proposed psychosocial targets, it could not be expected that it would have an impact on cardiac outcomes.

An innovative approach to patients with ischemia induced by mental stress tested the effect of two interventions (stress reduction and exercise) on cardiac events and ischemia during daily life.[112] When compared to usual care, the stress-management intervention was associated with a significant 26 percent reduction in risk of 5-year cardiac events as well as reductions in ambulatory ischemia and mental stress ischemia. Although this intervention went beyond a simple calculation of numbers of events to a systematic study of mechanisms, the nonrandom assembly of the usual-care group limited its explanatory power.

Another innovative intervention for post-MI patients featured self-help materials for cardiac risk-factor reduction and referrals for patients with elevated distress.[113] Results indicated that *both* treatment and control groups decreased their psychological distress during the 12 months after the MI, although there were isolated treatment-only decreases in the specific emotions of anxiety and anger. This intervention represents a potentially cost-effective approach to the reduction of distress, but the loss of one-third of the randomized patients due to missing data limits its explanatory power.

In summary, the most influential psychosocial intervention studies to date have produced mixed results, and it is difficult to interpret most of the studies with positive findings owing to methodologic limitations. The intervention of the longest duration—the Recurrent Coronary Prevention Project—was the most successful in reducing psychosocial endpoints and cardiac recurrence. Thus, it is possible that the more recent interventions that aim to change psychosocial endpoints in as few as five to seven contacts are simply too brief to have a psychological or cardiac impact. Psychosocial interventions in general have excluded women and, when women have been included and examined separately, they have little or even an adverse impact. More work on developing effective interventions for women with CHD is desperately needed. A new multicenter clinical trial sponsored by the National Heart, Lung, and Blood Institute (NHLBI) called ENRICHD is currently under way, with the aim of treating depression and/or low social support and determining the impact on cardiac recurrence rates. The ENRICHD study population will feature approximately 3000 participants, including 50 percent women and 50 percent minorities. As the results of this study become available, we will have more information about how to conduct psychosocial trials in general and how to conduct them for women in particular.

Strategies for Managing Emotional Distress and Improving Social Support

Distress refers to the emotional state of the patient and is distinguished from *stress,* which refers to environmental triggers. The two most important mechanisms that explain the toxic effect of emotional distress on the heart are neuroendocrine and behavioral. First, increased autonomic arousal occurs when an individual is distressed, resulting in increased blood pressure, heart rate, and platelet aggregation. The coronary arteries constrict, reducing blood flow to the heart, and there is an increased likelihood of plaque formation and cardiac arrhythmias.[114] Second, distress may be associated with adverse behaviors, particularly poor compliance with medical treatment and recommended lifestyle changes, such as quitting smoking, losing weight, and exercising.

Psychosocial treatment assumes that distress is precipitated by specific environmental events (e.g., being criticized by one's boss) and by the way one thinks (e.g., "He's out to get me") and behaves (e.g., vehemently defending oneself) in response to these events. These environmental, cognitive, and behavioral precipitants lead to emotions (i.e., depression, anxiety, anger) and behaviors (poor compliance) that have a direct impact on the heart. Experience of these emotions and behaviors then feeds back to cognitions and environmental interactions that sustain the cycle. Figure 14–2 depicts the reciprocal interaction among cognitions, environmental factors, emotions, and behaviors[115] and the two hypothesized pathways to CHD. Because these factors all influence each other, psychosocial treatment is aimed at targeting one or more of these factors as a way to break the cycle.

Problems will inevitably occur in life, and patients can benefit from learning a variety of tools for coping with these. In a sense, patients are taking a journey along the road of life and learning to negotiate the inevitable "bumps in the road."[116] When a bump is encountered, patients make a choice about how to

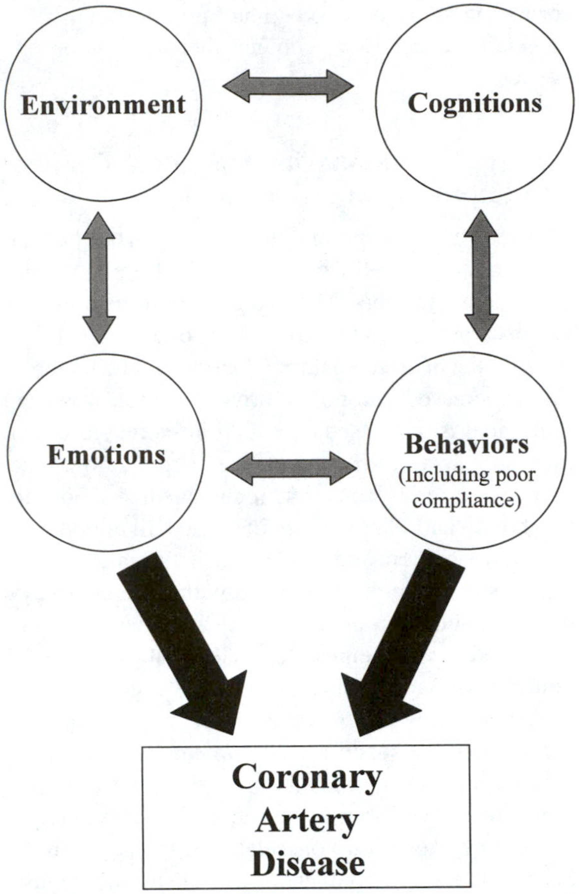

FIGURE 14-2 Reciprocal interaction among psychosocial factors and hypothesized pathways to CAD.

one presenting problem. For example, relaxation to accompany mytraining is useful for decreasing sympathetic arousal during angry as well as anxious episodes. Good communications skills not only improve social support but also decrease the isolation that is felt in depression.

Situation: Male post-MI patient thinking about moving his daughter home from college for the summer.

Automatic Thought	Emotion
"It's dreadful not to move her furniture myself."	Very depressed.

Evidence for (It is dreadful.)	Evidence against (It is not dreadful.)
I don't have the physical strength myself.	My daughter doesn't seem to be concerned.
I might not even be able daughter on her drive home from college.	My daughter will still get moved home, which is the important thing.
	My brother-in-law seems willing to help.
	My wife doesn't seem disappointed in me.
	I do help my daughter financially, and I do give her emotional support.

New Thought	New Emotion
"Getting the job done is what's important, not doing it myself."	Much less depressed.

deal with it. We do not always have a choice about what occurs in life (e.g., having had a heart attack, losing a loved one, having to retire), but we always have a choice about how to handle these events.

For the sake of clarity, we present separate sections for the different types of distress (depression, anxiety, anger) and an important environmental factor (low social support) and outline intervention strategies that are most efficacious for each. Cognitive change is discussed in every section in order to demonstrate how this general technique is tailored to each treatment target (Table 14-8). The other intervention strategies can also be applied to more than

Depression Cognitive Change. Cognitive therapy has been shown to be effective in the treatment of acute depression and in the prevention of relapse following termination of treatment.[117] Central to this approach is the development of skills in identifying and evaluating negative thoughts that trigger depressed feelings.[118,119] In depression/sadness, negative thoughts center around perceived loss and failure. Because these thoughts occur spontaneously; they are labeled "automatic." Automatic thoughts can focus on any life situation and are not limited to reactions to the patient's physical condition. If a pa-

TABLE 14-8 Some Typical Cognitive Distortions

Situation	Cognitive Distortion	Thought	Emotion	Definition	Alternatives to Consider
Going to work-related conference—can't do setup for own presentation	All-or-nothing thinking	"I'm an invalid."	Depressed	All-or-nothing thinking: you conclude everything is one extreme or another and don't consider intermediate possibilities.	Just because I can't do my own setup, that doesn't make me an invalid. After all, I'm still going to the conference and making the presentation.
	Mind reading	"They'll think I'm an invalid."	Angry	Mind reading: you arbitrarily conclude that someone is thinking negatively about you, and you don't bother to check this out.	I can't know what my colleagues think unless I ask them. They may be more sympathetic than I assume. Even if they notice I'm not doing my own set-up, that doesn't mean they view me as an invalid. And if they did think I'm an invalid, I know that's distorted thinking on their part.
	Jumping to conclusions	"I might make a fool of myself when I present."	Anxious	Jumping to conclusions: you think the worst without looking at the evidence that challenges your negative conclusion	I've never made a fool out of myself before when I've given presentations, even though they haven't always gone perfectly. Even though this is my first presentation after my heart attack, I know there are other tasks I've handled well since I've gone back to work.

tient continues to have extreme negative thoughts without challenging their accuracy, the depressed mood is intensified.

Some patients are well aware of their negative thoughts; others have such thoughts so habitually that they do not even notice them. Once negative thoughts are identified, they can then be evaluated. Patients can typically provide evidence supporting the accuracy of the negative thought without hesitation. They usually need help gathering evidence that challenges the accuracy of the negative thought. When all of the accumulated evidence on both sides of the matter is considered, a more accurate appraisal of the situation generally results. The previous example shows how this process of identification and evaluation of negative thoughts works.

Behavioral activation When they are depressed, patients often withdraw from activities that give them a sense of pleasure or accomplishment. They often have negative thoughts during periods of withdrawal and tend to interpret their inactivity as proof of their negative conclusions about themselves (e.g., "I'm useless"). As a result, mood deteriorates even further, and a vicious cycle is created (Fig. 14–3).[118] Patients should be encouraged to push themselves to participate in some of their usual activities. As they increase their activity levels, patients should be guided toward challenging their own negative thoughts about being completely weak or ineffective.

Anxiety *Cognitive change.* Cognitive therapy has been shown to be effective at reducing anxiety.[117] Negative thoughts about perceived threats trigger anxiety.[120] Identification and evaluation of the automatic thought would go something like this:

Situation: Male patient with coronary heart disease has muscle twitch in chest.

Automatic Thought	**Emotion**
"There is something wrong with my heart."	Very anxious.

Evidence for (something wrong with my heart)	*Evidence against* (nothing wrong with my heart)
I have frequent muscle twitches near where my bypass was done.	I spoke with my doctor, and she said fleeting pains (lasting less than 2 min) are not a source of concern.

New Thoughts	**New Emotion**
"The muscle twitches are harmless. I'm just noticing sensations in my chest more than I ever did before my bypass."	Much less anxious.

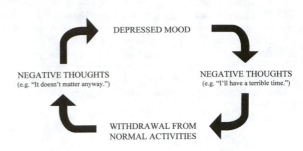

FIGURE 14–3 Vicious cycle of behavioral withdrawal and depression.

Relaxation training. Teaching patients to develop an ability to relax the body and mind is essentially teaching them to switch off the sympathetic drive and switch on parasympathetic relaxation. The more skilled a patient becomes at relaxation, the easier it becomes to use this skill response to daily stressors.

There are several different approaches to relaxation that can be used:

Diaphragmatic breathing helps patients shift from rapid, shallow breathing from the chest to slow, deep breathing from the abdomen.[121] The extent to which a patient engages in chest breathing can be made readily apparent by asking him or her to place one hand on the upper chest and the other on the abdomen and observing which hand moves while the patient inhales and exhales. During relaxation, blood is shifted away from the heart and lungs and toward the extremities. This shift in blood flow leads to vasodilation of the capillaries in the arms and legs, which is associated with a pleasant sensation of warmth or heaviness.

Progressive muscle relaxation (PMR) targets tension in all of the major muscle groups.[122] By first tensing a given muscle and then relaxing it, a greater release occurs than would occur by simply trying to relax that muscle. Make a tight fist for 10 s, then allow the hand to go limp. The limp hand is the relaxed hand, and sensations of heaviness and/or warmth are signs of that relaxation. PMR helps patients learn the subjective difference between tense and relaxed muscles and may be used to target specific areas of muscle tension.

Passive muscle relaxation involves relaxing the muscles without tensing them first.

Relaxation is maximally effective when it is practiced both daily and in response to specific situations that trigger distress, such as a deadline at work. Slow breathing and passive relaxation are noticeable to others and thus may be practiced when needed during the course of day-to-day activities. Patients may even use relaxation to help them cope with stressors *before* they occur—for example, taking a few deep breaths before making a difficult telephone call.

Anger The Three A's (Avoid, Alter, and Adapt). The mnemonic of the "three A's"[123] can be presented to help patients handle anger constructively. A patient can make a choice from three alternatives: *avoid* the situation that triggers the anger, try to *alter* the situation, or *adapt* to the situation. This set of alternatives makes it clear that anger management is the patient's responsibility; this approach is different from looking for someone to blame.

Avoidance may work in certain situations, as when a patient is able to avoid dealing with a difficult coworker. However, many patients are quick to rely solely on avoidance and need to be encouraged to include the other two strategies in their skills repertoire.

Altering the situation usually involves using good assertiveness skills to bring about a change. Assertiveness guidelines are equally important for males and females. When men try to alter difficult situations, some tend to do so in an aggressive, rather than assertive, manner. Women, especially older ones, generally hesitate to ask for change at all. In practicing assertiveness, patients are encouraged to include the following key elements:

1. Describe the facts of the situation.
2. Share your feelings briefly.
3. Request a specific change.
4. State the consequences if the change does not occur (optional).

Adapting to the situation (i.e., cognitive change) involves modifying one's negative thoughts about a difficult person or situation. Negative thoughts associated with anger involve the theme of being attacked or unfairly treated.[124] "Should" thoughts are red flags because they are frequent anger triggers. Here is an example:

Situation: Neighbor mowing lawn at 7 A.M. Saturday.

Automatic Thought	**Emotion**
"I shouldn't have to be the one to complain."	Angry.

Evidence for (I shouldn't be the one to complain.)	*Evidence against* (It makes sense for me to complain.)
Other neighbors live closer than I do.	I was woken up, so I have a right to complain.
	The squeaky wheel gets the grease.

New Thought	**New Emotion**
"I'm the one who is bothered by this so it makes sense for me to complain."	Less angry.

In the Recurrent Coronary Prevention Project (RCCP),[101–103] the metaphor of the hook was developed to decrease reactivity to daily irritants. By viewing external triggers for anger as "hooks," patients can choose not to "bite"—that is, to react angrily. "We, as fish, begin our swim for the day in clear water. Suddenly, a hook drops before us with attractive bait, and we make the decision to bite (get angry, irritated, annoyed) or to let the hook float by."[125]

Behavioral drills can be used to elicit changes in cognition. By practicing calmer, less hostile behaviors, patients may have new experiences that lead them to modify some of their hostile thoughts. Here are some examples from the RCCP[125]:

Ask a member of the family about the day's activities.

Verbalize your affection to spouse/children.

Practice smiling and look at your face carefully to see if you detect hostility or tension.

Recall memories for 10 min.

Invite someone to lunch and keep your friend talking about his/her interests—not yours.

Say "good morning" or "good afternoon" with a soft voice.

Low Social Support

Good communication skills enhance close relationships—important elements of social support—which help attenuate the emotional distress that arises when one is facing the inevitable difficulties of life. These skills include both speaking and listening.

Speaking skills Statements are more likely to be well received when the speaker uses the pronoun "I" (e.g., "I was worried when you didn't come home") rather than "you" (e.g., "You never remember to call when you're late!") Timing is critical. The best time to share one's upset feelings is after cooling down. Nonverbal cues are important, such as making eye contact and smiling when appropriate.

Listening skills Many patients complain that no one listens to them, but they do not realize that they are not listening either. Nonverbal cues, such as making good eye contact and refraining from doing something else while listening, are essential. The listener should convey that he or she has heard what is important to the speaker by restating the *content* of what has been said (e.g., "You're not able to pay your mortgage") and by reflecting the speaker's *emotions* (e.g., "It's upsetting you to be in this situation.")

Cognitive change Negative thoughts often prohibit patients from enjoying the support that is available to them. For example, a post-MI patient may interpret his wife's hesitation to have sex as a lack of caring. If he expresses his concern to his wife in a nonaccusatory manner, she may then share her fear of triggering a second heart attack. This new information can help the patient to evaluate his thought "She's no longer cares about me" and replace it with a more accurate interpretation, "She's been through a lot, and she is afraid." Such a cognitive shift may prompt the patient to continue to raise his concerns directly with his wife rather than worrying privately and prolonging feelings of alienation.

Drug Therapy

Effective pharmacological intervention can provide relatively immediate reductions in distress.

Antidepressants Selective serotonin reuptake inhibitors (SSRIs) have demonstrated efficacy and are appropriate for coronary patients because they do not cause severe adverse effects such as cardiac conduction delays and postural hypotension.[126] *Tricyclic antidepressants (TCAs) should be avoided in coronary patients, especially during the first 6 months post-MI, owing to the increased risk of cardiac arrhythmias.*

Anxiolytics Buspirone is a good choice for chronic anxiety because it is nonaddictive and does not interact with alcohol.[126] For patients with a history of substance abuse, benzodiazepines should be avoided owing to their addictive potential. If the respiratory system is compromised, benzodiazepines should be used judiciously because they can cause respiratory depression in high doses. Neuroleptic medication should not be prescribed for anxious, nonpsychotic patients because of the risk of serious adverse events such as tardive dyskinesia, neuroleptic malignant syndrome, and severe dystonias.

Beta blockers Beta blockers can be used to dampen sympathetic arousal during episodes of intense anxiety even though patients continue to report cognitive distress. Although results have been mixed, several studies have shown that beta blockers are effective for treating social phobia,[127,128] a disorder characterized by marked increases in anxiety and sympathetic arousal during social interactions. Because beta blockers were originally designed as antihypertensive drugs, they are contraindicated for those with hypotension.

Aspirin Aspirin may be used to decrease platelet aggregation in patients prone to anger. In a study linking anger to the triggering of acute MI, the increased risk of MI following an angry episode was eliminated in the subgroup who used aspirin.[35]

Compliance

Impact of depression on compliance Depression has been shown to interfere with weight loss, smoking cessation, and dietary modifications.[129,130] Depressed patients lack motivation and have difficulty taking initiative with recommended health behaviors.

Cognitive strategies can help depressed patients improve their compliance. For example, a patient might start the week resolving to follow a low-fat diet, succeed for several days, and then succumb to the temptation of eating dessert. If she has the extreme, all-or-nothing thought "I'm a failure," she is more likely to continue eating forbidden fatty foods. Because she is already a failure in her own mind, more fatty food is similar to less fatty food. However, if she thinks "Backsliding on occasion is a normal part of learning to change my habits," she is more likely to resume healthy eating right away. Patients must learn to view missteps in the process of behavior change as common, temporary occurrences and then generate a plan of action to prevent recurrence.[131]

"I can't do *anything* that I used to enjoy" is a common all-or-nothing thought in patients contemplating lifestyle modification. Although this is an understandable reaction, the patient can evaluate this thought by recalling other *continuing* sources of enjoyment, such as taking pleasure from being with family, exercising, and engaging in a favorite hobby.

A patient's self-evaluations should be assessed in order to identify potential obstacles to behavior change.[132] Specific lifestyle changes may trigger depressive feelings by challenging the patient's view of himself. For example, the patient who has consistently drawn much of her self-esteem from cooking for her family may have difficulty implementing a diet low in saturated fat.

Impact of anxiety on compliance Anxiety has an impact on a patient's tendency to cooperate with recommended behavioral changes. There is a curvilinear relationship between arousal and performance.[133,134] Too little anxiety is associated with inappropriate denial of risk, whereas excessive anxiety interferes with the ability to implement needed changes in behavior. A *moderate* level of anxiety is optimal for compliance (Fig. 14–4).

Denial It is not uncommon for post-MI patients to doubt that they had a heart attack. Denial in the hospital may serve the protective function of decreasing anxiety,[135] but denial after discharge may impede compliance with medical regimens.[136] A patient may

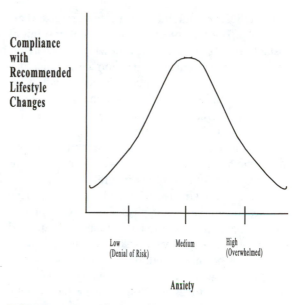

FIGURE 14–4 Relation of level of anxiety to compliance with recommended lifestyle changes.

adamantly deny that he or she has suffered an MI and, as a result, may fail to see the importance of quitting smoking and losing weight. Other post-MI patients may privately deny their own vulnerability and continue to engage in strenuous activities, such as pushing a stalled car to the closest gas station.

Breaking through denial, so that anxiety increases moderately, is a necessary challenge. Verbal persuasion can be helpful, as in the case of the fiercely independent 78-year-old woman, a post-MI patient, whose cardiologist said, "If you decide to shovel snow, call me first to say goodbye." The persuader, however, must be careful to refrain from becoming angry or critical, lest the patient become defensive and miss the message altogether. Observing peers' reactions can be another powerful stimulus for change. For example, if a patient brags about his physical invincibility in a support-group setting, the group leader may ask how many of the other members have consulted their physicians about activity restrictions. Their responses convey to the overconfident patient that he is different from his peers.

Excessive anxiety Patients' distress about their health has been shown to be negatively correlated with medication and adherence to an exercise regimen.[76,137] The fear of exertion is a common initial obstacle to lifestyle change following the heart attack.[138] Some patients may develop a panic disorder after an MI due to repeated misinterpretations of physical sensations as signs of another heart attack. Such patients may avoid cardiac rehabilitation for fear of triggering a heart attack. In such cases, treating the panic disorder (through counseling and/or anxiolytic medication) is a necessary prerequisite for a later successful trial of cardiac rehabilitation.

Patients who are overwhelmed by anxiety have trouble concentrating on physicians' recommendations. Some patients are so anxious about having had a heart attack that they insist that the words "heart attack" not be mentioned. The anxiety and associated physiologic arousal is so unpleasant to these patients that they focus only on reducing the anxiety, not on learning how to prevent recurrence. For such patients, recommendations about lifestyle change should be repeated after discharge when the shock of their brush with death has subsided.

Impact of social support on compliance The support of family and friends is associated with enhanced compliance with recommended behavioral changes such as quitting smoking,[139] adhering to medical regimens,[140] modifying diet,[141] and complying with cardiac rehabilitation programs.[142] Information support, tangible support, and emotional support[143–145] are important for enhancing compliance.

Informational support, such as guidance and education from doctors and nurses, helps the patient know what changes need to be made and what approaches are likely to be successful. Encouraging patients to write down a list of their questions prior to their appointments facilitates the delivery of information that is most relevant to each patient. Simply encouraging patients to ask all of their questions can go a long way toward dismantling inhibiting cognitions, such as "My doctor is too busy," and "I don't want to make a mountain out of a molehill."

Tangible support refers to concrete help from others, such as picking up prescription refills and doing grocery shopping. Assertiveness skills are important for obtaining tangible support. Patients must decrease their tendency to read minds (e.g., "She's too busy with her own life to help me") and increase the frequency with which they ask for what they need (e.g., "Do you have time to drive me to my doctor's appointment?"). Family members can be helpful by asking the patient what type of assistance he or she needs rather than making assumptions about what is helpful. For example, one patient might appreciate her husband's careful checking of nutrition labels while shopping, whereas another might resent his attempt to monitor her fat intake.

Emotional support refers to the encouragement and reassurance that the patient receives from others in his or her life who are willing to hear about his or her feelings. For example, a doctor or family member can be extremely helpful by listening to the patient's concerns about having a "special diet" that is different from that of the rest of the family. As with informational and tangible support, the patient must often learn to ask for emotional support rather than expecting others to know when he or she needs it (via mind reading). Patients can be reminded that everyone needs emotional support: it is not a sign of weakness or dependency. Moreover, patients sometimes forget that giving support is beneficial to the giver as well as to the receiver; they are often more willing to ask for support when they first recall times they have felt good about bolstering others. For some self-involved patients, the best way to receive more emotional support is first to start giving it to their own loved ones.

Impact of the doctor-patient relationship on compliance The doctor-patient relationship is a powerful moderator of patient adherence. An emotionally supportive manner on the part of the physician may instill hope and reduce anxiety. The art of medicine has historically involved transmitting positive expectations to the patient for his or her recovery.[146,147] Optimism on the part of the patient helps reduce anxiety and is associated with the tendency to take positive, goal-oriented action. When patients *expect* positive outcomes, they are more likely to engage in the active problem solving that is critical for reaching goals,[148] such as quitting smoking or losing weight.

A patient's lack of compliance may result from a failure to understand why certain recommendations are being made.[149] When the physician detects hesitation, she should ask the patient about any potential obstacles to compliance. For example, a post-MI patient may hesitate to follow through with cardiac rehabilitation because he does not know that his heart is a muscle. Once the patient understands that cardiac rehabilitation strengthens not only the arms and legs but also the heart, he is more likely to feel motivated to complete a full course of cardiac rehabilitation.

The physician may proactively enhance compliance by checking patients' degree of understanding. Asking patients to restate recommendations makes apparent any gaps in understanding, and actively eliciting questions helps patients feel comfortable in acknowledging their uncertainties. When physicians reported answering patients' questions thoroughly, there was greater exercise adherence at follow-up.[137] The physician's willingness to take as much time as is needed may be necessary to overcome patients' reluctance to "bother" their physicians with questions—a concern cited by many of our patients. Written recommendations further ensure that crucial information is remembered.

Conclusions

Research on the role of psychosocial factors in coronary heart disease initially focused on coronary-prone behaviors (the type A behavior pattern) and later on coronary-prone attitudes (hostility) and environmental factors (low social support). Most recently, emphasis has shifted toward identifying coronary-prone emotions. The specific emotions of anger, depression, and anxiety as well as the general experience of distress have all been linked to poor cardiac outcomes.

Results of the Recurrent Coronary Prevention Project[101–105] clearly indicated that a psychosocial intervention led to reduced recurrence of cardiac events in males. Other psychosocial intervention trials have produced mixed results, and more research is needed in this area because of the methodologic limitations of these studies.

Numerous psychosocial treatments are available for reducing distress and improving social support, including cognitive change, relaxation training, and communication skills training. Treatment of depression, anxiety, and low social support is also critical for improving patient compliance with recommended lifestyle changes. Psychosocial evaluation and treatment should be incorporated into the routine care of both at-risk patients and patients with established CHD.

Acknowledgments

We thank Charlotte Jonsson, Sara Byrne, and Gwendolyn Brown for their assistance in the preparation of this manuscript.

References

1. Osler W: *Lectures on Angina Pectoris and Allied States.* New York, Appleton, 1892.
2. Friedman M, Rosenman RH: *Type A Behavior and Your Heart.* New York, Knopf, 1974.
3. Friedman M, Powell LH: The diagnosis and quantitative assessment of type A behavior: introduction and description of the Videotaped Structured Interview. *Integr Psychiatry* 1984; 1:123–129.
4. Rosenman RH: The interview method of assessment of the coronary-prone behavior pattern, in Dembroski TM, Weiss S, Schillar J, et al (eds): *Coronary Prone Behavior.* New York, Springer-Verlag, 1978.
5. Rosenman RH, Brand RJ, Jenkins CD, et al: Coronary heart disease in the Western Collaborative Group Study: final follow-up experience of $8\frac{1}{2}$ years. *JAMA* 1975; 223:872–877.
6. Haynes SG, Feinleib M, Kannel WB: The relationship of psychosocial factors to coronary heart disease in the Framingham study: III. Eight-year incidence of coronary heart disease. *Am J Epidemiol* 1980; 111:37–58.
7. Williams RB, Haney TL, Lee KL, et al: Type A behavior, hostility, and coronary atherosclerosis. *Psychosom Med* 1980; 42:539–549.
8. Cook W, Medley D: Proposed hostility and pharasaic-virtue scales for the MMPI. *J Appl Psychol* 1954; 38:414–418.

9. Shekelle RB, Hulley SB, Neaton J: The MRFIT behavioral pattern study: II. Type A behavior pattern and risk of coronary death in MRFIT. *Am J Epidemiol* 1985; 122:559–570.

10. Dembroski TM, MacDougall TM, Costa PT, Grandits GA: Components of hostility as predictors of sudden death and myocardial infarction in the Multiple Risk Factor Intervention Trial. *Psychosom Med* 1989; 51:514–522.

11. Kawachi I, Sparrow D, Kubzansky LD, et al: Prospective study of a self-report type A scale and risk of coronary heart disease. *Circulation* 1998; 98:405–412.

12. Barefoot JC, Lipkus IM: The assessment of anger and hostility, in Siegman AW, Smith TW (eds): *Anger, Hostility, and the Heart*. Hillsdale, NJ, Erlbaum, 1994.

13. Shekelle RB, Gale M, Ostfeld AM, Oglesby P: Hostility, risk of coronary heart disease, and mortality. *Psychosom Med* 1983; 45:109–114.

14. Graham, JR: *The MMPI: A Practical Guide*. Englewood Cliffs, NJ, Prentice-Hall, 1977.

15. Williams RB Jr: Basic biological mechanisms, in Siegman, AW, Smith TW (eds): *Anger, Hostility, and the Heart*. Hillsdale, NJ, Erlbaum, 1994.

16. Siegler IC, Zonderman AB, Barefoot JC, et al: Predicting personality in adulthood from college MMPI scores: implications for follow-up studies in psychosomatic medicine. *Psychosom Med* 1990; 52:644–652.

17. Everson SA, Kauhanen J, Kaplan GA, et al: Hostility ad increased risk of mortality and acute myocardial infarction: the mediating role of behavioral risk factors. *Am J Epidemiol* 1997; 146:142–152.

18. Matthews KA, Glass DC, Rosenman RH, Bortner RW: Competitive drive, pattern A, and coronary heart disease: a further analysis of some data from the Western Collaborative Group Study. *J Chronic Dis* 1977; 30:489–498.

19. Powell LH, Thoresen CE: Behavioral and physiologic determinants of long-term prognosis after myocardial infarction. *J Chronic Dis* 1985; 38:253–263.

20. Barefoot JC, Dahlstrom WG, Williams RB: Hostility, CHD incidence and total mortality: a 25-year follow-up study of 255 physicians. *Psychosom Med* 1983; 45:59–64.

21. Barefoot JC, Dodge K, Peterson B, et al: The Cook-Medley hostility scale: item content and ability to predict survival. *Psychosom Med* 1989; 51:46–57.

22. Barefoot JC, Larsen S, von der Lieth L, Schroll M: Hostility, incidence of acute myocardial infarction, and mortality in a sample of older Danish men and women. *Am J Epidemiol* 1995; 142:477–484.

23. Hecker M, Chesney M, Black G, Frautschi N: Coronary-prone behaviors in the Western Collaborative Group Study. *Psychosom Med* 1988; 50:153–164.

24. Koskenvuo M, Kaprio J, Rose R, et al: Hostility as a risk factor for mortality and ischemic heart disease in men. *Psychosom Med* 1988; 50:330–340.

25. Hallstrom T, Lapidus L, Bengtsson C, Edstrom K: Psychosocial factors and risk of ischemic heart disease and death in women: a twelve-year follow-up of participants in the population study of women in Gothenburg, Sweden. *J Psychosom Res* 1986; 30:451–459.

26. Hearn M, Murray D, Luepker R: Hostility, coronary heart disease, and total mortality: a 33-year follow-up study of university students. *J Behav Med* 1989; 12:105–121.

27. Leon G, Finn S, Bailey J, Murray D: The inability to predict cardiovascular disease from MMPI special scales related to type A patterns. *Psychosom Med* 1987; 49:205.

28. McCranie E, Watkins L, Brandsma J, Sisson B: Hostility, coronary heart disease (CHD) incidence, and total mortality: lack of association in a 25-year follow-up study of 478 physicians. *J Behav Med* 1986; 9:119–125.

29. Miller TQ, Smith TW, Turner CW, et al: A meta-analytic review of research on hostility and physical health. *Psych Bull* 1996; 119:322–348.

30. Siegman AW: From type A to hostility to anger: reflections on the history of coronary-prone behavior, in Siegman AW, Smith TW (eds): *Anger, Hostility, and the Heart*. Hillsdale, NJ: Erlbaum, 1994.

31. Spielberger, CD: *State-Trait Anger Expression Inventory: Research Edition*. Odessa, FL, Psychological Assessment Resources, 1988.

32. Kawachi I, Sparrow D, Spiro A III, et al: A prospective study of anger and coronary heart disease: the Normative Aging Study. *Circulation* 1996; 94:2090–2095.

33. Mendes de Leon CF, Kop WJ, et al: Psychosocial characteristics and recurrent events after percutaneous transluminal coronary angioplasty. *Am J Cardiol* 1996; 77:252–255.

34. Kneip RC, Delamater AM, Ismond T, et al: Self- and spouse ratings of anger and hostility as predictors of coronary heart disease. *Health Psychol* 1993; 12:301–307.

35. Mittleman MA, Maclure M, Sherwood JB, et al: Triggering of acute myocardial infarction onset by episodes of anger. *Circulation* 1995; 92:1720–1725.

36. Verrier RL, Hagestad EL, Lown B: Delayed myocardial ischemia induced by anger. *Circulation* 1987; 75:249–254.

37. Ironson G, Taylor CB, Boltwood M, et al: Effects of anger on left ventricular ejection fraction in coronary artery disease. *Am J Cardiol* 1992; 70:281–285.

38. Boltwood MD, Taylor CB, Boutte Burke M, et al: Anger report predicts coronary artery vasomotor response to mental stress in atherosclerotic segments. *Am J Cardiol* 1993; 72:1361–1365.

39. Cassel J: The contribution of the social environment to host resistance. *Am J Epidemiol* 1976; 104:107–123.

40. Berkman LF, Syme SL: Social networks, host resistance, and mortality: a nine-year follow-up study of Alameda County residents. *Am J Epidemiol* 1979; 109:186–204.

41. House JS, Robbins C, Matzner HL: The association of social relationships and activities with mortality: prospective evidence from the Tecumseh Community Health Study. *Am J Epidemiol* 1982; 116:123–140.

42. Blazer DG: Social support and mortality in an elderly community population. *Am J Epidemiol* 1982; 115:684–694.

43. Schoenbach VJ, Kaplan BH, Fredman L, Kleinbaum DG: Social ties and mortality in Evans County, Georgia. *Am J Epidemiol* 1986; 123:577–591.

44. Welin L, Svardsudd K, Ander-Peciva S, Tibblin G et al: Prospective study of social influences on mortality: The Study of Men Born in 1913 and 1923. *Lancet* 1985; (8434):915–918.

45. Seeman TE, Berkman LF, Kohout F, et al: Intercommunity variations in the association between social ties and mortality: a comparative analysis of three communities. *Ann Epidemiol* 1993; 3:325–335.

46. Orth-Gomer K, Unden A-L, Edwards M-E: Social isolation and mortality in ischemic heart disease: a 10-year follow-up study of 150 middle-aged men. *Acta Med Scand* 1988; 224:205–215.

47. Kaplan GA, Salonen JT, Cohen RD, et al: Social connections and mortality from all causes and from cardiovascular disease: prospective evidence from Eastern Finland. *Am J Epidemiol* 1988; 128:370–380.

48. Orth-Gomer K, Rosengren A, Wilhelmsen L: Lack of social support and incidence of coronary heart disease in middle-aged Swedish men. *Psychosom Med* 1993; 55:37–43.

49. Orth-Gomer K, Johnson JV: Social network interaction and mortality: a six year follow-up study of a random sample of the Swedish population. *J Chronic Dis* 1987; 40:949–957.

50. Case RB, Moss AJ, Case N, et al. Living alone after myocardial infarction: impact on prognosis. *JAMA* 1992; 267:515–519.

51. Williams RB, Barefoot JC, Califf RM, et al: Prognostic importance of social and economic resources among medically treated patients with angiographically documented coronary artery disease. *JAMA* 1992; 267:520–524.

52. Berkman LF, Leo-Summers L, Horwitz RI: Emotional support and survival after myocardial infarction: a prospective, population-based study of the elderly. *Ann Intern Med* 1992; 117:1003–1009.

53. Blumenthal JA, Burg MM, Barefoot J, et al: Social support, type A behavior, and coronary artery disease. *Psychosom Med* 1987; 49:331–340.

54. Ruberman W, Weinblatt E, Goldberg JD, Chaudhary BS: Psychosocial influences on mortality after myocardial infarction. *N Engl J Med* 1984; 311:552–559.

55. Seeman TE, Syme SL: Social networks and coronary artery disease: a comparison of the structure and function of social relations as predictors of disease. *Psychosom Med* 1987; 49:341–354.

56. Orth-Gomer K, Horsten M, Wamala SP, et al: Social relations and extent and severity of coronary artery disease: the Stockholm Female Coronary Risk Study. *Eur Heart J* 1993; 19:1648–1656.

57. Gorkin L, Schron EB, Brooks MM, et al: Psychosocial predictors of mortality in the cardiac arrhythmia suppression trial-1 (CAST-1). *Am J Cardiol* 1993; 71:263–267.

58. Frasure-Smith N, Lesperance F, Talajic M: Depression following myocardial infarction: impact on 6-month survival. *JAMA* 1993; 270:1819–1825.

59. Frasure-Smith N, Lesperance F, Talajic M: Depression and 18-month prognosis after myocardial infarction. *Circulation* 1995; 91:999–1005.

60. Ahern DK, Gorkin L, Anderson JL, et al: Biobehavioral variables and mortality or cardiac arrest in the Cardiac Arrhythmia Pilot Study (CAPS). *Am J Cardiol* 1990; 66:59–62.

61. Silverstone PH: Depression and outcome in acute myocardial infarction. *BMJ* 1987; 294:219–220.

62. Carney RM, Rich MW, Freedland KE, et al: Major depressive disorder predicts cardiac events in patients with coronary artery disease. *Psychosom Med* 1988; 50:627–633.

63. Frasure-Smith N, Lesperance F, Juneau M, et al: Gender, depression, and one-year prognosis after myocardial infarction. *Psychosom Med* 1999; 61:26–37.

64. Ladwig KH, Kieser M, Konig J, Breithardt G: Affective disorders and survival after acute myocardial infarction: results from the Post-infarction Late Potential Study. *Eur Heart J* 1991; 12:959–964.

65. Barefoot JC, Helms MJ, Mark DB, et al: Depression and long-term mortality risk in patients with coronary artery disease. *Am J Cardiol* 1996; 78:613–617.

66. Barefoot JC, Peterson BL, Harrell FE Jr, et al: Type A behavior and survival: a follow-up study of 1,467 patients with coronary artery disease. *Am J Cardiol* 1989; 64:427–432.

67. Oxman TE, Freeman DH Jr, Manheimer ED: Lack of social participation or religious strength and comfort as risk factors for death after cardiac surgery in the elderly. *Psychosom Med* 1995; 57:5–15.

68. Barefoot JC, Schroll M: Symptoms of depression, acute myocardial infarction, and total mortality in a community sample. *Circulation* 1996; 93:1976–1980.

69. Pratt LA, Ford DE, Crum RM, et al: Depression, psychotropic medication, and risk of myocardial infarction: prospective data from the Baltimore ECA follow-up. *Circulation* 1996; 94:3123–3129.

70. Hippisley-Cox J, Fielding K, Pringle M: Depression as a risk factor for ischaemic heart disease in men: population based case-control study. *BMJ* 1998; 316:1714–1719.

71. Sesso HD, Kawachi I, Vokonas PS, Sparrow D: Depression and the risk of coronary heart disease in the Normative Aging Study. *Am J Cardiol* 1998; 82:851–856.

72. Mendes de Leon CF, Krumholz HM, Seeman TS, et al: Depression and risk for coronary heart disease in elderly men and women. *Arch Intern Med* 1998; 158:2341–2348.

73. Whooley MA, Browner WS for the Study of Osteoporotic Fractures Research Group: Association between depressive symptoms and mortality in older women. *Arch Intern Med* 1998; 158:2129–2135.

74. Wulsin LR, Vaillant GE, Wells VE: A systematic review of the mortality of depression. *Psychosom Med* 1999; 61:6–17.

75. Lesperance F, Frasure-Smith N: The seduction of death. *Psychosom Med* 1999; 61:18–20.

76. Blumenthal JA, Williams RS, Wallace AG, et al: Physiological and psychological variables predict compliance to prescribed exercise therapy in patients recovering from myocardial infarction. *Psychosom Med* 1982; 44:519–527.

77. Musselman DL, Tomer A, Manatunga AK, et al: Exaggerated platelet activity in major depression. *Am J Psychiatry* 1996; 153:1313–1317.

78. American Psychiatric Association: *Diagnostic and Statistical Manual of Mental Disorders,* 4th ed. Washington, DC, APA, 1994.

79. Coryell W, Noyes R, Clancy J: Excess mortality in panic disorder. *Arch Gen Psychiatry* 1982; 39:701–703.

80. Coryell W. Noyes R, House JD: Mortality among outpatients with anxiety disorders. *Am J Psychiatry* 1986; 143:508–510.

81. Sims A, Prior P: Arteriosclerosis related deaths in severe neurosis. *Compr Psychiatry* 1982; 23:181–185.

82. Sims A: Neurosis and mortality: investigating an association. *J Psychosom Res* 1984; 28:353–362.

83. Haines AP, Imeson JD, Meade TW: Phobic anxiety and ischaemic heart disease. *BMJ* 1987; 295:297–299.

84. Kawachi I, Colditz GA, Ascherio A, et al: Prospective study of phobic anxiety and risk of coronary heart disease in men. *Circulation* 1994; 89:1992–1997.

85. Kawachi I, Sparrow D, Vokonas PS, Weiss ST: Symptoms of anxiety and risk of coronary heart disease: the Normative Aging Study. *Circulation* 1994; 90:2225–2229.

86. Moser DK, Dracup K: Is anxiety early after myocardial infarction associated with subsequent ischemic and arrhythmic events? *Psychosom Med* 1996; 58:395–401.

87. Kubzansky LD, Kawachi I, Spiro A III, et al: Is worrying bad for your heart? A prospective study of worry and coronary heart disease in the Normative Aging Study. *Circulation* 1997; 95:818–824.

88. Spielberger, CD, Gorsuch, RL, Lushene R: *STAI Manual for the State-Trait Anxiety Inventory.* Palo Alto, CA, Consulting Psychologists Press, 1970.

89. Booth-Kewley S, Friedman HS: Psychological predictors of heart disease: a quantitative review. *Psychol Bull* 1987; 101:343–362.

90. Frasure-Smith N, Lesperance F, Talajic M: The impact of negative emotions on prognosis following myocardial infarction: is it more than depression? *Health Psychol* 1995; 14:388–398.

91. Follick MJ, Gorkin L, Capone RJ, et al: Psychological distress as a predictor of ventricular arrhythmias in a post-myocardial infarction population. *Am Heart J* 1988; 116:32–36.

92. Frasure-Smith N: In-hospital symptoms of psychological stress as predictors of long-term outcome after acute myocardial infarction in men. *Am J Cardiol* 1991; 67:121–127.

93. Allison TG, Williams DE, Miller TD, et al: Medical and economic costs of psychologic distress in patients with coronary artery disease. *Mayo Clin Proc* 1995; 70:734–742.

94. Denollet J, Sys SU, Brutsaert DL: Personality and mortality after myocardial infarction. *Psychosom Med* 1995; 57:582–591.

95. Denollet J, Brutsaert DL: Personality, disease severity, and the risk of long-term cardiac events in patients with a decreased ejection fraction after myocardial infarction. *Circulation* 1998; 97:167–173.

96. Carney RM: Psychological risk factors for cardiac events: could there be just one? *Circulation* 1998; 97:128–129.

97. Derogatis LR: *SCL-90-R: Administration, Scoring, and Procedure Manual.* Baltimore, Clinical Psychometrics Research, 1983.

98. Adsett CA, Bruhn JG: Short-term group psychotherapy for post–myocardial infarction patients and their wives. *Can Med Assoc J* 1968; 99:577–584.

99. Ibrahim MA, Feldman JG, Sultz HA, et al: Management after myocardial infarction: a controlled trial of the effect of group psychotherapy. *Int J Psychiatr Med* 1974; 5:253–254.

100. Rahe RH, Ward HW, Hayes V: Brief group therapy in myocardial infarction rehabilitation: three- to four-year follow-up of a controlled trial. *Psychosom Med* 1979; 41:229–242.

101. Powell LH, Friedman M, Thoresen CE, et al: Can the type A behavior pattern be altered after myocardial infarction? A second year report from the Recurrent Coronary Prevention Project. *Psychosom Med* 1984; 46:293–313.

102. Friedman M, Thoresen CE, Gill JJ, et al: Alteration of type A behavior and reduction in cardiac recurrences in post myocardial infarction patients. *Am Heart J* 1984; 108:237–248.

103. Friedman M, Thoresen CE, Gill JJ, et al: Alteration of type A behavior and its effect upon cardiac recurrences in post–myocardial infarction patients: summary results of the Recurrent Coronary Prevention Project. *Am Heart J* 1986; 112:653–665.

104. Powell LH, Thoresen CE: Effects of type A behavioral counseling and severity of prior acute myocardial infarction on survival. *Am J Cardiol* 1988; 62:1159–1163.

105. Powell LH, Shaker LS, Jones BA, et al: Psychosocial predictors of mortality in 83 women with premature acute myocardial infarction. *Psychosom Med* 1993; 55:426–433.

106. Mendes de Leon CE, Powell LH, Kaplan BH: Change in coronary-prone behaviors in the Recurrent Coronary Prevention Project. *Psychosom Med* 1991; 53:407–419.

107. Frasure-Smith N, Prince R: The Ischemic Heart Disease Life Stress Monitoring Program: impact on mortality. *Psychosom Med* 1985; 47:431–445.

108. Frasure-Smith N, Prince R: Long-term follow-up of the Ischemic Heart Disease Life Stress Monitoring Program. *Psychosom Med* 1989; 51:485–513.

109. Powell LH: Unanswered questions: the Ischemic Heart Disease Life Stress Monitoring Program. *Psychosom Med* 1989; 51:479–484.

110. Frasure-Smith N, Lesperance F, Prince RH, et al: Randomised trial of home-based psychosocial nursing intervention for patients recovering from myocardial infarction. *Lancet* 1997; 350:473–479.

111. Jones DA, West RR: Psychological rehabilitation after myocardial infarction: multicentre randomized controlled trial. *BMJ* 1996; 313:1517–1521.

112. Blumenthal JA, Jiang W, Babyak MA, et al: Stress management and exercise training in cardiac patients with myocardial ischemia: effects on prognosis and evaluation of mechanisms. *Arch Intern Med* 1997; 157:2213–2223.

113. Taylor CB, Houston Miller N, Smith PM, DeBusk R: The effect of a home-based, case-managed multifactorial risk-reduction program on reducing psychological distress in patients with cardiovascular disease. *J Cardiopulm Rehab* 1997; 17:157–162.

114. Allan R, Scheidt S: Empirical basis for cardiac psychology, in Allan R, Scheidt S (eds): *Heart and Mind: The Practice at Cardiac Psychology*. Washington DC, American Psychological Association, 1996, pp 63–123.

115. Bandura A. *Social Foundations of Thought and Action: A Social Cognitive Theory*. Englewood Cliffs, NJ, Prentice-Hall, 1986.

116. Enriched Steering Committee, National Institute of Health: *Enhancing Recovery in Coronary Heart Disease: Patient's Manual of Operations: Vol. 2, Intervention,* National Institute of Health, Bethesda, MD, 1998.

117. Hollon, SD, Beck, AT: Cognitive and cognitive-behavioral therapies, in Bergin, AE, Garfield, SL (eds): *Handbook of Psychotherapy and Behavior Change,* 4th ed. New York, Wiley, 1994, pp 428–466.

118. Beck AT, Rush AJ, Shaw BF, Emergy G: *Cognitive Therapy of Depression*. New York, Guilford Press, 1979.

119. Beck, Judith S: *Cognitive Therapy: Basics and Beyond*. New York: Guilford Press, 1995.

120. Finlay-Jones R, Brown GW: Types of stressful life events and the onset of anxiety and depressives disorders. *Psychol Med* 1981; 11:803–815.

121. Rapee, RM, Barlow, DH: The cognitive-behavioral treatment of panic attacks and agoraphobic avoidance, in Walker, JR, Norton, GR, Ross, CA (eds): *Panic Disorder and Agoraphobia: A Comprehensive Guide for the Practitioner.* Pacific Grove, CA: Brooks/Cole, 1991, pp 252–305.

122. Barlow, DH, Cerny, JA: *Psychological Treatment of Panic.* New York, Guilford Press, 1988.

123. Berra K, Breitrose P, Clark M, et al: *An Active Partnership for the Health of Your Heart.* Dallas, TX, American Heart Association, 1990.

124. Powell LH: The cognitive underpinnings of coronary-prone behaviors. *Cogn Ther Res* 1992; 16:123–142.

125. Powell, LH, Thoresen, CE: Modifying the type A behavior pattern: a small group treatment approach, in Blumenthal, JA, McKee, DC (eds): *Applications in Behavioral Medicine and Health Psychology: A Clinician's Source Book.* Sarasota, FL, Professional Resource Exchange, 1987, pp 171–207.

126. Janicak, PG, Davis, JM, Preskorn, SH, Ayd, FJ: *Principles and Practice of Psychopharmacotherapy.* Baltimore, Williams & Wilkins, 1997.

127. Gorman, JM, Liebowitz, MR, Fyer, AJ, et al: Treatment of social phobia with atenolol. *J Clin Psychopharmacol* 1985; 5:298–301.

128. Liebowitz, MR, Schneier FR, Hollander E, et al: Treatment of social phobia with drugs other than benzodiazepines. *J Clin Psychiatry* 1991; 52:10–15.

129. Guiry E, Conroy RM, Hickey N, Mulcahy R: Psychological response to an acute coronary event and its effect on subsequent rehabilitation and lifestyle change. *Clin Cardiol* 1987; 10:256–260.

130. Carney RM, Freedland KE, Rich MW, Jaffe AS: Depression as a risk factor for cardiac events in established coronary heart disease: a review of possible mechanisms. *Ann Behav Med* 1995; 17:142–149.

131. Marlatt, GA, Gordon, J: *Relapse Prevention: Maintenance Strategies in Addictive Behavior Change.* New York, Guilford Press, 1985.

132. Ewart CK: A social problem-solving approach to behavior change in coronary heart disease, in Shumaker SA, Schron EB, Ockene JK (eds): *The Handbook of Health Behavior Change.* New York, Springer-Verlag, 1990, pp 153–190.

133. Hebb DO: Drives and the CNS (conceptual nervous system). *Psychol Rev* 1955; 62:243–254.

134. Yerkes RM, Dodson JD: The relation of strength of stimulus to rapidity of habit-formation. *J Comp Neurol Psychol* 1908; 18:459–482.

135. Cassem NH, Hackett TP: Psychiatric consultation in a coronary care unit. *Ann Intern Med* 1971; 75:9–14.

136. Croog SH, Shapiro DS, Levine S: Denial among male heart patients. *Psychosom Med* 1971; 33:385–397.

137. DiMatteo MR, Sherbourne CD, Hays RD, et al: Physicians' characteristics influence patients' adherence to medical treatment: results from the medical outcomes study. *Health Psychol* 1993; 12:93–102.

138. Oldridge NB: Compliance and exercise in primary and secondary prevention of coronary heart disease: a review. *Prev Med* 1982; 11:56–70.

139. Gianetti VJ, Reynolds J, Rign T: Factors which differentiate smokers from ex-smokers among cardiovascular patients: a discriminant analysis. *Soc Sci Med* 1985; 20:241–245.

140. Brownell A, Shumaker SA: Social support: an introduction to a complex phenomenon. *J Soc Issues* 1984; 40:1–9.

141. Johnson ML, Vickery CE: Dietary practices, nutrition knowledge and attitudes of coronary heart disease patients. *Health Values* 1990; 14:3–8.

142. Andrew GM, Oldridge NB, Parker JO, et al: Reasons for dropout from exercise programs in post-coronary patients. *Med Sci Sports Exerc* 1979; 11:376–378.

143. Cobb S: Social support as a moderator of life stress—presidential address. *Psychosom Med* 1976; 38:300–314.

144. Berkman LE: Assessing the physical health effects of social networks and social support. *Ann Rev Public Health* 1984; 5:413–432.

145. Cohen S, Syme SL (eds): *Social Support and Health*. New York, Academic Press, 1985.

146. Shapiro AK: A contribution to a history of the placebo effect. *Behav Sci* 1960; 5:109–135.

147. Shapiro AK: Placebo effects in medicine, psychotherapy, and psychoanalysis, in Bergin AE, Garfield SL (eds): *Handbook of Psychotherapy and Behavior Change*: *An Empirical Analysis*. New York, Wiley, 1971, pp 439–473.

148. Shepperd JA, Maroto JJ, Pbert LA: Dispositional optimism as a predictor of health changes among cardiac patients. *J Res Personality* 1996; 30:517–534.

149. Hulka BS: Patient-clinician interactions and compliance, in Haynes RB, Taylor DW, Sackett DL (eds): *Compliance in Health Care*. Baltimore, Johns Hopkins University Press, 1979, pp 63–77.

Part IV

Preventing Heart Disease in Special Populations

CHAPTER 15

Cardiovascular Risk Reduction in Women

Marian C. Limacher

ardiovascular disease (CVD) remains the leading cause of death in women as well as in men. With more women surviving to older age, the absolute number of women dying from CVDs, especially coronary heart disease (CHD) and stroke, exceeds the number of men.[1] Yet many women do not recognize the significance of this problem. Recent surveys have demonstrated that women believe breast cancer to be their major serious health risk, when, in fact, women are 8 to 10 times more likely to die of CVD than of breast cancer.[2] Recent directives have been developed to heighten awareness of CVD as a major cause of morbidity and mortality in women and to focus efforts on improving outcomes of women with heart disease.[3,4] Reducing cardiovascular risk factors and improving healthy behaviors throughout the life span should be a goal for practitioners and the public alike. This chapter reviews some of the important findings that affect our approach to the diagnosis and treatment of women at risk for CVD and those who have CVD. Practical suggestions for the approach to risk evaluation and management are included.

Incidence and Prognosis

The first manifestations of CHD typically occur more than 10 years later in women than in men. Thus, CHD has its biggest impact in elderly women, while men experience an increase in risk during middle age. One of the consequences of the burden of CHD in the elderly is that studies have consistently reported that women, as compared with men, have an increased morbidity and mortality from recurrent myocardial infarction during the first year following infarction.[5–9] Interestingly, women have less than half the risk of men for dying suddenly (within 1 h of symptoms) from CHD.[10] One study has reported that women experience a higher frequency of hypotension and bradycardia with acute coronary occlusion during angioplasty, possibly related to more intense vagal activation, which may have antifibrillatory protective properties.[11] Others suggest that the apparent higher fatality rate after an acute cardiac event in women is largely balanced by their lower fatality rate before admission (i.e., by a lower sudden death rate as well as the differences in potentially confounding variables).[12] Many studies demonstrate that women with an acute coronary event are older, more likely to be living alone, of lower income, and less frequently receiving aspirin; but they are more likely receiving nitrates and diuretics than men[13] (Figs. 15–1 and 15–2). When the odds ratios for mortality are adjusted by these and other factors, such as smoking and use of other treatments, the risk for women of dying from their acute event is only slightly higher than that for men.[12] Data from the Framingham Heart Study show, in survivors of myocardial infarction, that after adjusting for cholesterol levels, systolic blood pressure, and diabetes (all of which are higher or more common in women post-myocardial infarction), women actually have a lower long-term risk of recurrent events or mortality than do men.[14]

Another observation confirmed in multiple reports is that women report more symptoms of congestive heart failure despite higher left ventricular ejection

FIGURE 15–1 Characteristics of women and men following myocardial infarction. Bars reflect mean age *(far left)* and percent of women and men at lower income levels, married, and living alone. (Modified from Schwartz et al.,[13] with permission.)

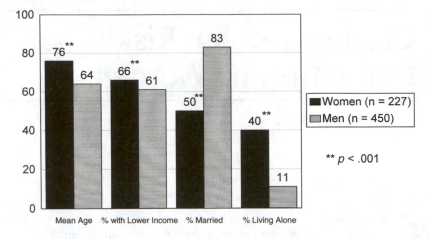

FIGURE 15–2 Percent of women and men receiving aspirin, beta blockers, nitrates, and diuretics after myocardial infarction. (Modified from Schwartz et al.,[13] with permission.)

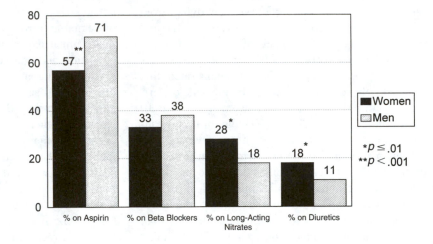

fractions following myocardial infarction.[15–17] At catheterization, women have been found to have a higher mean left ventricular ejection fraction but smaller end-diastolic volume index in the presence of higher left ventricular end-diastolic pressure, supporting the hypothesis that diastolic dysfunction contributes to the discordance between heart failure symptoms and higher left ventricular ejection fraction seen in women.[18] These findings may be related to the higher prevalence of hypertension and diabetes in women, although gender is an independent predictor of heart failure after adjusting for these covariables.[18]

Women and elderly patients are likely to delay presentation to the hospital when having an acute myocardial infarction. Delays are greatest when symptoms occurred during the evening and early morning hours and were also related to the absence of a spouse or living companion.[19] Once evaluated in the emergency department, women are less likely to receive thrombolytic therapy even when deemed eligible by standard criteria[20] (Fig. 15–3). Women are also less likely than men to undergo other interventional procedures, including coronary angiography and bypass graft surgery, following myocardial infarction.[21,22] It has been questioned whether

FIGURE 15–3 Percent of eligible women and men who received thrombolytic therapy for acute myocardial infarction in the Myocardial Intervention and Treatment Intervention trial. (Modified from Maynard et al.,[20] with permission).

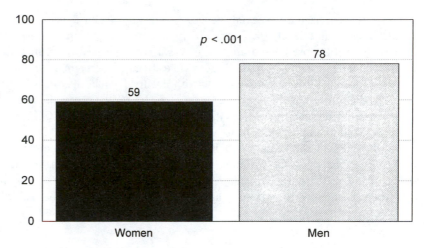

women were less likely to agree to additional procedures or whether they were not being offered such procedures as often as men. In one analysis, the following factors were associated a coronary-care-unit patient's disagreement with a physician's recommendation for undergoing cardiac catheterization: education below college level, poor cardiac function, no previous cardiac catheterization, hospitalization in a nonreferral community hospital, and current smoking. Neither gender nor race explained the lower rates of cardiac procedures in women in this study, although women and minority patients were more likely to have these characteristics.[23] There was also wide variation in patient attitudes about invasive procedures between two types of hospitals, community-based and tertiary referral.[23] On the other hand, another recent study of internists and family physicians has revealed that patient race and sex independently influence how physicians manage chest pain.[24] Physician bias continues to be a consideration in the treatment decisions of women with CHD. Patient characteristics and behaviors must also be evaluated.

If improvements in the time delay to seeking assistance are to be realized, a broad public health message about the importance of seeking medical attention rapidly must be clearly addressed to women and the elderly. It has also been suggested that primary prevention may well be the most practical solution to the epidemic of CVD in women—i.e., to prevent the onset of clinical CVD for as long as possible to avoid the difficulties inherent in the management of manifest disease.[3]

Gender Differences in Diagnosis and Assessment of Cardiovascular Disease

Diagnosis

The presence of chest pain has been an unreliable indicator of CHD in many studies. In the Framingham study, women with chest discomfort that was considered to have anginal qualities were less likely than men to have cardiovascular events in follow-up.[25] Women screened for the Coronary Artery Surgery Study (CASS), all of whom were under age 65 by study design, were less likely than men to have obstructive CHD at catheterization.[26] These observations have led to widespread interpretations that women with chest pain are unlikely to have CHD and that CHD is not a significant source of morbidity and mortality for women. Yet, even in the Framingham study, women over age 65 with chest pain actually have rates of cardiovascular events and mortality comparable with those of men one decade younger.[27] Thus, the evaluation of a woman with chest discomfort must include a full assessment of her level of risk, starting with her age.

Since women have a lower prevalence of CHD at virtually every age level, Bayesian principles hold that testing for the presence of disease is less useful in women than in men.[28] Treadmill exercise testing, for example, has a lower positive predictive value for women than for men in the diagnosis of CHD. Younger women typically exercise for a shorter time than men and to a lower peak heart rate, resulting in a lower workload achieved, although older women may exceed the workload for men of similar age[29] (Figs. 15–4 and 15–5). Most comparative studies have been completed in women at ages comparable with those of the men in the study, resulting in a study population of women at lower risk for disease.[30–32] Other studies, when stratified by quality of anginal symptoms, have demonstrated that maximal electrocardiographic (ECG) treadmill testing can be especially useful if negative. Women with normal exercise ECG tests are very unlikely to have significant CHD.[33]

Radionuclide scintigraphy is also reported to have limitations for the diagnosis of CHD in women, in many cases owing to attenuation artifact from breast tissue or the inability to achieve adequate stress lev-

FIGURE 15–4 Peak exercise performance for women and men under age 65. (Modified from Shaw et al.,[29] with permission).

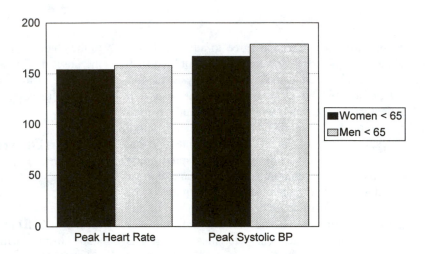

FIGURE 15–5 Peak exercise performance for women and men over age 65. (Modified from Shaw et al.,[29] with permission).

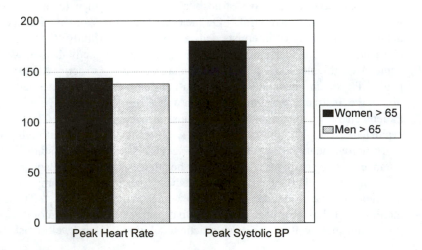

els.[34] Use of higher-energy radionuclides and ECG-gated single-photon emission computed tomography (SPECT) may improve test accuracy.[35] Radionuclide angiography, which is now less commonly performed as a diagnostic test modality, may yield misleading results because it detects intrinsic differences in ventricular mechanics between women and men.[36–38] Other techniques, such as three-dimensional magnetic resonance imaging or positron emission tomography, may prove valuable for diagnostic testing in women but are limited by availability and cost.[39]

In recent years, exercise echocardiography has been promoted as an accurate and cost-effective technique for testing women suspected of having CHD.[40–42] Most studies, however, analyze findings for a cohort of women only or in women selected to undergo angiographic referrals. When testing methods are evaluated in less selected populations, the reported sensitivity and specificity rates prove an overestimation compared with more common practice settings of less segregated types of patients.[43] Roger et al.[44] have conducted a study in a large number of unselected men and women who underwent exercise echocardiography. They found that the observed sensitivity and specificity was 78 and 44 percent for men and 79 and 37 percent for women without adjustment. After adjusting for test verification bias (defined as the tendency to perform angiography in those with positive tests), the sensitivity fell to 32 percent for women and 42 percent for men. The overall positive predictive value was lower in women compared with men (66 versus 84 percent).[44]

Dobutamine stress echocardiography is also promoted as a safe and accurate technique for diagnosing CHD in women who have chest pain and limited exercise capacity. Sensitivity, specificity, and overall accuracy has been reported to be higher for women than for men, possibly related to better image quality due to a thinner chest wall in women[45] (Table 15–1).

Although myocardial ischemia can be provoked by exercise or pharmacologic stress, exercise appears to provide a greater hemodynamic burden. Exercise and dobutamine stress echocardiography were com-

TABLE 15–1 Characteristics of Dobutamine Echocardiography for Women and Men

	Women, n = 96	Men, n = 210
Percent with CAD	65%	81%
Percent with multivessel CAD	27%	55%
Overall sensitivity	76%	73%
Overall specificity	94%	77%
Overall accuracy	82%	74%
Accuracy for multivessel CAD	83%	70%
Accuracy for LCx disease	89%	78%
Accuracy for RCA disease	84%	73%
Accuracy in all arteries combined	84%	75%

Key: CAD, coronary artery disease; L, left; Cx, circumflex; RCA, right coronary artery.

Source: Modified from Elhendy et al.,[45] with permission.

pared in a population of 85 patients with stable coronary artery disease (85 percent men). Dobutamine infusions (combined with atropine up to 1.8 mg if heart rate at peak dose did not achieve 85 percent of the predicted maximum) produced faster heart rates than treadmill exercise, while peak exercise achieved higher blood pressures and higher rate-pressure products. Only one patient became hypotensive with exercise, while 26 percent were hypotensive during the dobutamine infusions. All 53 patients (62 percent) who had positive results on dobutamine studies also had positive results on exercise testing, although 33 of the 53 (62 percent) had higher wall motion scores, indicating greater myocardial ischemia with exercise, and only 4 percent had higher wall motion scores with dobutamine. Overall, the positive predictive value for exercise echo was 73 percent compared with 62 percent with dobutamine.[46] However, women may not exercise as long or achieve as high a heart rate or blood pressure response as men. In women who are deconditioned or older, it may be more appropriate to use dobutamine stress for echocardiographic imaging studies.

In another study, treadmill exercise ECG testing, treadmill exercise thallium scintigraphy, transesophageal dobutamine stress echocardiography, and coronary angiography were performed on 84 women. Twenty-six percent had significant CHD defined by coronary angiography. The transesophageal approach resulted in 82 percent sensitivity, but 100 percent specificity for detecting new or worsening regional wall motion abnormalities as the indication of CHD. Optimal image quality, obtained by the transesophageal approach, likely contributed to the improved overall accuracy compared with the less invasive techniques.[47] However, the invasive nature of transesophageal echocardiography limits its applicability as a first-line diagnostic test.

Although diagnostic tests cannot be completely accurate in detecting disease, it has been shown that the overall cardiac risk for patients who have normal findings with exercise echocardiography is low over an average follow-up period of 2 years. For 1325 patients (52 percent women) with normal findings, the cardiac event–free survival rates were 99.2 percent at 1 year, 97.8 percent at 2 years, and 97.4 percent at 3 years. Only three died of cardiac causes, compared with 14 dying of noncardiac causes; 10 had nonfatal myocardial infarctions and 20 underwent coronary revascularization procedures. The authors identified four independent predictors of cardiac events:

• Development of angina during exercise
• Maximal workload achieved less than 7 metabolic equivalents (METs) for men or 5 METs for women
• Echo evidence for left ventricular hypertrophy (LVH)
• Older age

A risk score for patients could be calculated as follows:

$$\text{Score} = (\text{age} \times 0.04) + (1.17 \text{ if workload was low})$$
$$+ (0.97 \text{ if LVH present})$$
$$+ (1.42 \text{ if angina developed})$$

A risk score of 4 or less predicted a cardiac event rate of 0.6 percent per person-year of follow-up, while a higher score resulted in an event rate of 4.8 percent per person-year of follow-up.[48]

Newer modalities, such as electron beam computed tomography, hold promise but require larger and more rigorous comparisons to assign a place in the recommendations for diagnostic testing.[49,50] Chapters 3 and 4 extensively review newer techniques for subclinical CVD assessment.

Assessment

The sobering analysis of the diagnostic value of a single test emphasizes the need to individualize the assessment for women. For CHD, several strategies have been proposed over recent years, taking into account that the accuracy of testing is related to the lower prevalence of disease and of multivessel disease in women compared with men, possible sex-related differences in the pathophysiology of CHD, impact of risk factors, altered referral patterns for testing and for angiography, and features related to a specific test.[51] Douglas and Ginsburg recommend a stratified approach to diagnosing CHD in women utilizing risk-factor assessment and weighting followed by appropriate diagnostic testing[52] (Table 15–2). After the level of clinical risk for CHD is determined by categorizing risk factors and symptoms, a rational testing strategy can be followed based on the determination of low-, intermediate-, or high-risk status from Table 15–3. The risk status determines which testing strategy to follow, as outlined in Figs. 15–6, 15–7, and 15–8, for low-, intermediate-, and high-risk women, respectively. It is important to carefully evaluate all available information and individualize the diagnostic strategy for every patient, since all tests are imperfect. The strategies proposed here take advantage of the lower-cost exercise ECG test for women able to exercise, recognizing that any abnormal result will require an additional study. Others have proposed imaging stress studies, particularly echocardiography, as first-line testing, finding it cost-effective to avoid confirmatory testing for abnormal exercise ECG tests.[42] However, clinicians should select the strategy that best suits the patient's characteristics, test availability, and funding resources, recognizing that additional tests may be necessary.

TABLE 15–2 Classification of Risks for Coronary Artery Disease in Women

Major	Intermediate	Minor
Known coronary artery disease or peripheral vascular disease	Hypertension	Age ≥ 55
Typical angina pectoris	Cigarette smoking	Obesity, especially central obesity
Diabetes mellitus	Abnormal lipids, especially low HDL-C < 45 mg/dL, LDL-C ≥ 160 mg/dL, triglycerides ≥ 400 mg/dL	Sedentary lifestyle
		Family history of coronary artery disease
		Psychosocial factors, such as poor social support, high stress with low situational control
		Hemostatic risk factors such as elevated fibrinogen or plasminogen-activated inhibitor type 1
		Elevated homocysteine

Key: HDL-C, high-density-lipoprotein cholesterol; LDL-C, low-density-lipoprotein cholesterol.
Source: Modified from Douglas and Ginsburg[52] and Mosca et al.,[3] with permission.

TABLE 15–3 Categories of Global Risk to Determine Testing Strategies in Women

Low, <20%	Intermediate, 20–80%	High, >80%
No major risk factors and/or ≤2 minor and/or ≤1 intermediate risk factor with chest discomfort not typical for angina	One major risk factor or ≥2 intermediate and minor risk factors with chest discomfort not typical for angina	Typical angina and ≥2 major risk factors or 1 major plus ≥1 intermediate and minor risk factors

Source: Modified from Douglas and Ginsburg,[52] with permission.

Gender Differences in Referral for Interventions and Outcomes

A number of studies have reported differences in the referral patterns to coronary angiography and further intervention, even after positive results on stress testing or after a cardiac ischemic event.[24,53–56] Others have detected no referral bias toward women but concluded that differences in management were the result of clinical differences in patients.[57–59] One of the largest series reported to date has found that women were only slightly less likely to be referred for cardiac catheterization after exercise treadmill testing but that they were much less likely to be referred directly to coronary angiography. Women had lower exercise capacity, were less likely to develop ischemic ST-segment changes or to achieve at least 85 percent of the predicted maximal heart rate response, but were more likely to report anginal chest pain. When only ischemic ST changes were considered, there was no difference in referral for catheterization or additional testing.[60] Recommendations for clinical practice are to weigh the pretest likelihood of CHD based on risk factors (Tables 15–2 and 15–3), determine the severity of symptoms, and then to decide on the most appropriate test for an individual patient at a given institution. For a woman with stable typical or atypical symptoms who is able to exercise and has an interpretable ECG, it may be

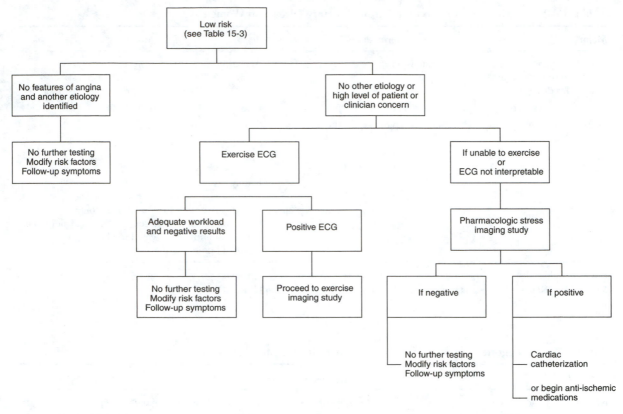

FIGURE 15–6 Testing algorithm for low-risk women with chest discomfort. (Modified from Douglas and Ginsburg,[52] with permission).

appropriate to first use the treadmill ECG test. If no ischemic changes are found after adequate exertion, no further workup is needed and risk-factor modification and follow-up is indicated. For the woman with ischemic changes induced on treadmill ECG testing, the severity of findings and magnitude of pretest risk should determine whether the next step should be a confirmatory imaging study (echocardiography or radionuclide scintigraphy) or direct referral for coronary angiography. The specific selection of testing modality should be based on local availability and expertise.

Treatment interventions may have different outcomes for women than for men. O'Keefe et al.[61] have recently reported that women receiving estrogen replacement therapy at the time of percutaneous transluminal coronary angioplasty had a substantial de-

crease in risk of cardiac death and all-cause mortality for 7 years following angioplasty. Subsequent revascularization rates, however, were not different.[61] There has been long-standing controversy surrounding the risk for women undergoing coronary artery bypass graft (CABG) surgery. Many studies report higher mortality rates for women undergoing CABG and suggest that female gender and body size may confer an independent risk for surgical morbidity and mortality.[15,62,63] Others, however, suggest that women are at higher risk because of increased age and number of comorbid conditions, these being the primary reasons for higher risk, rather than female gender or relatively smaller size of the coronary arteries.[64] The relatively lower rate of use of the internal mammary artery for bypass surgery in

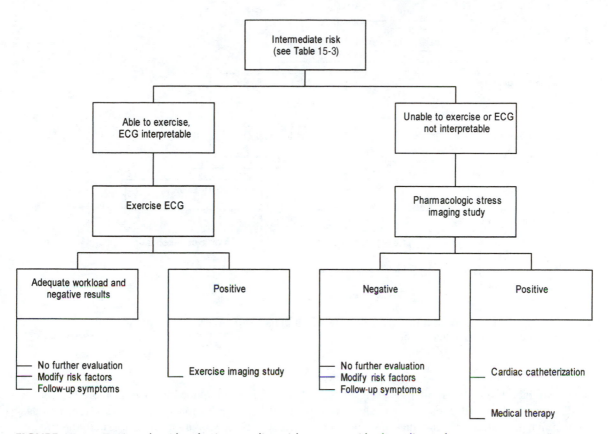

FIGURE 15–7 Testing algorithm for intermediate-risk women with chest discomfort. (Modified from Douglas and Ginsburg,[52] with permission).

women has also been implicated as a reason for higher mortality rates.[62,65] Although the disparity in operative mortality between men and women persists, regardless of the explanation, the long-term results for women undergoing coronary bypass surgery show symptom control and similar survival benefit.[66]

Cardiovascular Risk Factors in Women and Evidence of Benefit from Risk-Factor Control

One of the important lessons to be learned from studying CVD in women is that there is a profound interaction with aging. The prevalence of myocardial infarction in the Cardiovascular Health Study was

9.7 percent for women between age 65 and 69 and 17.9 percent for those age 85 and older.[3] Thus, the highest-risk women are those who are oldest and who have concomitant illnesses and concerns that will likely influence diagnosis, treatment, and intervention recommendations.

The American Heart Association and the American College of Cardiology recently released a consensus panel statement of recommendations for screening and risk reduction, "Guide to Preventive Cardiology for Women" (Appendix 15–1).

Lipids

Although women have lower levels of total and low-density-lipoprotein cholesterol (LDL-C) prior to

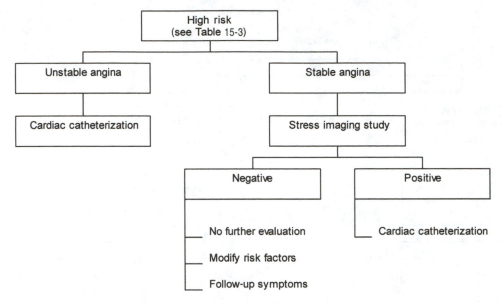

FIGURE 15–8 Testing algorithm for high-risk women with chest discomfort. (Modified from Douglas and Ginsburg,[52] with permission).

menopause than do men of similar age, this advantage disappears afterward. Increased prevalences of dyslipidemia, hypertension, and diabetes are seen after menopause. Of women over the age of 55, over 50 percent have cholesterol levels of 240 mg/dL or higher.[67] Nearly all reported observational studies show a relation of increased total cholesterol levels to CHD risk in women, and high-density-lipoprotein cholesterol (HDL-C) bears a particularly strong inverse relation to CHD risk.[68] Although the relation of total cholesterol to CHD mortality tends to be weaker in older women,[69] low HDL-C and elevated triglycerides retain their importance as risk factors in middle-aged and older women.[70]

Reduction in mortality and in recurrent cardiovascular events has been demonstrated in women treated with HMG-CoA reductase inhibitors after myocardial infarction. In the Scandinavian Simvastatin Survival Study, major coronary events in the treated group (relative to the control group) were reduced significantly by 35 percent in women, similar to the 34 percent reduction in risk in men. There was, however, no reduction in total mortality, contrary to

the 34 percent reduction in total mortality seen in men.[71] The reduction in risk of recurrent coronary events among women in the Cholesterol and Recurrent Events (CARE) study was more than twice that observed in men (46 versus 20 percent).[72] Previous studies on the primary prevention of CHD have enrolled mostly men, leaving unanswered the question of whether women would benefit from cholesterol lowering to reduce the risk of a first cardiac event. The Air Force/Texas Coronary Atherosclerosis Prevention Study (AFCAPS/TexCAPS) primary prevention trial of lovastatin in men and women without previous cardiac events has now demonstrated a reduction in initial CHD events in both men and women; the decrease was more marked in women (42 percent risk reduction in women versus 37 percent in men)[73] (see also Chap. 7).

Hypertension

Among women aged 20 years and over, the estimated prevalence of hypertension is 19 percent for non-Hispanic whites, 34 percent for non-Hispanic blacks, and 22 percent for Mexican Americans. An estimated 8 percent of Asian/Pacific Islander women and 28 precent of Native American women also have hypertension.[1] A strong relation between elevated blood pressure and CHD in women has been observed in numerous observational studies, and the benefits of treating hypertension in both men and women are well documented, with approximately a 9 to 30 percent reduction in cardiovascular events, although the reduction in CHD events has been less conclusive.[68] The reduction in stroke rates has been more dramatic, with a mean decrease of 6 mmHg diastolic pressure, resulting in a lowering of fatal and nonfatal stroke by 42 percent.[74] Of particular concern are the approximately 30 percent of older women who have isolated systolic hypertension ($\geq$140 mmHg systolic and <90 mmHg diastolic).[75] Of note is that a meta-analysis of antihypertensive therapy showed beta blockers and diuretics to be beneficial in preventing stroke and major cardiovascular events in women.[76] Clinical trials of hypertension treatment that have included both men and women have demonstrated similar efficacy of blood pressure control on outcomes. With a few exceptions, a similar approach to treatment is generally recommended for both men and women. Oral contraceptives are noted to increase the risk of hypertension and should be discontinued if a significant rise in blood pressure occurs; in most cases, blood pressure will then normalize. When hypertension occurs during pregnancy, these risks should be reduced while avoiding therapy that may be harmful to the fetus, such as angiotensin-converting enzyme inhibitors and angiotensin II receptor blockers[77] (see also Chap. 6).

Diabetes

Diabetes is a more important risk factor in women than in men; it is associated with a two- to fourfold greater risk of CHD in men but a three- to sevenfold greater risk in women.[78] Efforts to identify and control diabetes in women, including concomitant risk factors such as dyslipidemia or hypertension, are critical to preventing CVD morbidity and mortality. Although women with diabetes are known to have higher rates of cardiovascular events, there are no data available suggesting that treatment goals and results should differ for women versus men.

Gestational diabetes develops in about 3 percent of pregnant women in the United States and may be related to an increased risk of CHD, with some follow-up studies showing more than one-third of those with gestational diabetes subsequently developing non-insulin-dependent diabetes mellitus, compared with only 5 percent of those with normal pregnancies. A higher incidence of insulin resistance, hypertension, and dyslipidemia is also seen later in those with versus those without gestational diabetes, thus warranting early preventive efforts in this group.[68]

Insulin resistance is an independent risk factor for CHD and may promote atherosclerosis by stimulating the proliferation and migration of arterial smooth muscle cells and cholesterol synthesis. Other risk factors are also commonly associated with insulin resistance. Relatively low insulin levels in the presence of elevated glucose lead to high very low density lipoprotein (VLDL) levels and triglycerides and low HDL-C levels. Sodium retention, obesity and hypertension are frequently seen. The term *syndrome X* was originally applied by Reaven to the group of conditions listed in Table 15–4.[79] It is also described as *insulin-resistance syndrome* or *multiple metabolic*

TABLE 15–4   Features of the Insulin-Resistance Syndrome

Hyperinsulinemia
Obesity
Type 2 diabetes mellitus
Microalbuminuria
Hypertension
Salt sensitivity
Hyperlipidemia
Hyperuricemia
Elevated plasminogen activator inhibitor 1
Elevated lipoprotein(a)
Coronary artery disease

Source: From Reaven,[79] with permission.

syndrome and includes many of the major risk factors for CHD. Likewise, although the insulin-resistance syndrome may be more prevalent in women than in men, particularly younger women and those who are obese or have diabetes, there is no information to date supporting different recommendations for its management in women versus men (see also Chap. 8).

Cigarette Smoking

Women who smoke 1 pack of cigarettes or more per day are at a two- to fourfold greater risk of CHD than those who do not smoke, and there is a clear dose-response relation, such that even light smokers run a twofold increased risk.[68] Recent national statistics indicate that 23 percent of women in the United States smoke cigarettes, although this varies widely by race, from 4.3 percent among Asian/Pacific Islanders to 35.4 percent among Native Americans.[1] Unfortunately, more young women than men begin smoking. Smoking lowers the age of first myocardial infarction more for women than for men and also adversely affects other cardiovascular risk factors, lowering HDL-C levels, raising fibrinogen levels, and increasing platelet aggregability.[80] Smokers (as compared with nonsmokers) who use oral contraceptives have also been reported to have higher risks of myocardial infarction and stroke.[3] Although it is important to inform women who smoke of their greatly increased risk of cardiac disease, it is also important to emphasize how effective smoking cessation is in lowering cardiac risk. Within 3 to 5 years of stopping cigarette smoking, a woman's risk for CHD events is at the level of a woman who has never smoked.[81] Since women may smoke cigarettes as a weight-control measure, smoking-cessation efforts for women should include advice on weight management (see also Chap. 9).

Physical Activity

Most Americans do not engage in regular physical activity, and women are less likely to exercise than men and less likely to keep active as they age. Only 38 percent of women over age 80 report even minimal regular leisure-time physical activity.[82] Results from observational studies show between a 60 and 75 percent lower risk of CHD in physically active women than in sedentary women.[68] Physical activity also reduces risks for cardiovascular and all-cause mortality, with the lowest death rates seen in the most fit women. An 8-year follow-up of more than 3000 healthy women showed level of fitness as assessed by treadmill testing to be inversely related to CVD mortality, with age-adjusted rates of 0.8 per 10,000 person-years in the most fit women compared with 7.4 per 10,000 person-years in the least fit.[83] In the Postmenopausal Estrogens/Progestins Intervention (PEPI) study, postmenopausal women with higher levels of physical activity had higher HDL-C levels and lower levels of insulin and fibrinogen.[84] Women should be encouraged to increase their level of physical activity to 30 min or more of moderately intense physical activity on most and preferably all days of the week.[85] Activities do not have to be continuous but can accumulate through the day to the 30-min goal. Activities should obviously be tailored to the interests, capabilities, and risk levels of the individual, with selection of low-impact activities for older women. Muscle strengthening and stretching activities should also be incorporated into a complete physical activity program. Further recommendations for physical activity are described in Chap. 12.

Obesity

Obesity (particularly abdominal obesity) remains an important problem of increasingly greater magnitude, and numerous prospective cohort studies have shown direct positive associations between obesity and the risk of CHD.[68] In a study of more than 120,000 middle-aged women, a nearly twofold risk was seen among those moderately overweight (body mass index of 25 to 28.9), and more than a threefold greater risk among those with a body mass index of 29 or higher, as compared to less than 21.[86] The American Heart Association recently reclassified obesity as a major modifiable risk factor for CHD, calling for an increased emphasis on calorie restriction and increased physical activity.[87] Chapter 10 provides recommendations for the prevention and control of obesity.

Homocysteine and Folic Acid

A recent case-control study has demonstrated that both men and women with elevated plasma homocysteine levels in the top quintile of distribution (generally greater than 12 μmol/L) have a twofold increase in vascular disease risk as compared with the remaining four-fifths. The increase in risk was equivalent to that of elevated cholesterol levels or for smoking. The investigators also noted a multiplicative indication of increased risk when both fasting and post-methionine-load homocysteine levels were analyzed. The relative risk for each 5 μmol/L increment in fasting homocysteine level was 1.42 (95 percent CI = 0.99 to 2.05) for women compared with 1.35 (95 percent CI = 1.1 to 1.6) for men.[88] Other estimates have suggested an odds ratio for CHD for a 5-μmol/L increment in plasma homocysteine level is 1.6 (95 percent CI = 1.4 to 1.7) for men and 1.8 (95 percent CI = 1.3 to 1.9) for women.[89] Graham et al. also note that there was a stronger interaction between elevated fasting homocysteine level and hypertension in women than in men[88] (Fig. 15–9).

Although increased supplements of folic acid in the food supply will probably provide the required amounts for preventing neural tube defects, some ex-

perts have recommended intakes of 400 μg/day in order to help prevent CVD. However, there have been no published clinical trials of folic acid supplementation to examine an effect on coronary events, and there currently exist no recommendations by a consensus panel supporting supplemental intake of folic acid for CVD prevention (see also Chap. 13).

Alcohol, Aspirin, and Antioxidants

Studies show that low-to-moderate daily consumption of alcohol is related to a 30 to 70 percent reduction in the risk of CHD, regardless of the type of alcoholic beverage consumed. But moderate alcohol consumption has also been linked to hypertension and a possible increase in the risk of breast cancer, and heavy consumption is the second leading preventable cause of death in the United States. Given the relatively lower risk of heart disease in women as compared with men, the overall benefit, given other risks, may be even less clear in women. Therefore, a public health recommendation that women or men even drink moderate amounts of alcohol is not warranted.[68]

Recent observational studies show lower risks of CHD among women who take prophylactic aspirin. In men over the age of 40 at sufficiently high risk of myocardial infarction, aspirin is recommended for primary prevention of myocardial infarction. As primary prevention trials in women have not been

FIGURE 15–9 Relative risk for cardiovascular disease in men and women with elevated fasting homocysteine (defined as ≥12 μmol/L) in the presence of other risk factors (adjusted for age, sex, and study center). Women with hypertension and elevated fasting homocysteine were at particularly increased risk compared with men and and with men and women with other risk factors. (Modified from Graham et al.,[88] with permission).

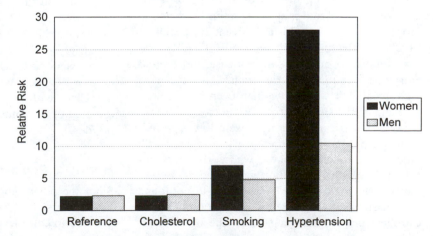

completed, there is no similar recommendation in women; however, the ongoing Women's Health Study involving low-dose aspirin in 40,000 healthy female professionals will provide these critically needed data[68] (see also Chap. 11).

Data from observational studies support a protective effect from both vitamin E and betacarotene in women, with the highest intakes associated with approximately a 25 percent reduction in risk for CHD.[68] Recent results from carefully conducted clinical trials, although done in men, cast doubt on any protective effect for betacarotene. Most observational studies show a protective effect from vitamin E dosages of 60 to 200 U/day consumption. These results are promising, but they will have to be confirmed by clinical trials, and the American Heart Association does not at this time recommend antioxidant supplementation. Instead it promotes guidelines for a well-balanced diet high in fresh vegetables and fruits (see also Chap. 13).

Hormone Protection and Influence of Postmenopausal Hormone Replacement Therapy

Oral Contraceptives

CHD events are very rare in premenopausal women. Although the use of oral contraceptives has been reported to be associated with an increased risk of myocardial infarction and stroke, current formulations contain one-quarter to one-half the original dose of estradiol and may contain third-generation progestins, which may lower LDL and raise HDL.[90] The World Health Organization (WHO) Collaborative Study of Cardiovascular Disease and Steroid Hormone Contraception determined that the most significant risk was for women over age 35 who smoked.[91] Risks for younger nonsmokers were increased, but the absolute risks were low: approximately 3 per million woman-years, compared with older women who smoked, whose risk was approximately 400 per million woman-years. Importantly, risk for myocardial infarction was not found to be associated with the dose or duration of use of estrogen and did not persist after the oral contra-

ceptives were discontinued.[92] Another study concluded that oral contraceptives do not increase the risk of infarction for women who do not have risk factors for heart disease.[93] A recent extensive review confirmed that all available evidence indicates that CVD among oral contraceptive users occurs predominantly in smokers and women with cardiovascular risk factors.[94] Recommendations for a choice of contraceptive, therefore, require an assessment of cardiac risk factors prior to prescribing hormonal contraceptives and avoidance of oral contraceptives for women who are current or recent smokers, at high risk by their risk profile, or over the age of 35.

Another issue related to oral contraceptive use is whether past use, perhaps by adversely affecting risk factors during the years of use, results in increased rates of CVD later in life. A meta-analysis of past use of oral contraceptives estimates that past users had a pooled relative risk of 1.01 (CI = 0.91 to 1.13) for myocardial infarction.[95] Thus, the risk for myocardial infarction appears primarily due to the acute impact of oral contraceptives on thrombotic mechanisms for infarction, especially because of the interaction with cigarette smoking.

It has also been noted that women with polycystic ovaries have a higher risk for CHD.[96] Many of the clinical features associated with polycystic ovaries are also features of the insulin-resistance syndrome. In a recent study of women under age 60 undergoing coronary angiography for the evaluation of chest pain, ultrasonography demonstrated polycystic ovaries in 42 percent. Women with polycystic ovaries had higher free testosterone, C-reactive protein, triglycerides, and lower HDL-C. They also had more extensive CHD.[96] Thus women with polycystic ovaries appear to be at increased risk for premature CHD, with clinical features appearing at an age (before 60) not common for women with lower-risk profiles.

Hormone Replacement Therapy

Since the postmenopausal years mark the onset of increased risk for CHD in women, it is a logical progression to consider the role of estrogen on cardiac disease. Observational studies have consistently demonstrated that cardiovascular mortality is lower for women who have received estrogen replacement therapy than for those who have not.[97,98] It has also been observed that all-cause mortality is lower for women on estrogen replacement therapy.[99,100] Estimated rates of reduction in event rates with postmenopausal hormone replacement are substantial.[101–104] A meta-analysis of 31 observational studies showed a 44 percent reduction in risk for CHD associated with estrogen use only.[98] Those on combined estrogen-progestin therapy appear to have at least as much reduction in risk for CHD. The Nurses' Health Study recently reported a 61 percent lower risk of CHD in those on combined estrogen-progestin therapy as compared with a 40 percent risk reduction in those on estrogen alone.[105] For women with CHD, retrospective studies have suggested that estrogen replacement provides even greater benefit, with a reduction of up to 89 percent in relative risk.[106]

Estrogen has many biological effects that potentially explain the benefits observed for premenopausal and postmenopausal women on hormone replacement therapy. Estrogen produces favorable changes in the lipid profile, with reductions in LDL-C and total cholesterol and an increase in HDL-C, despite modest increases in triglycerides.[107,108] Estrogen use also reduces lipoprotein(a) and fibrinogen levels and increases apolipoprotein A-1 levels.[107,108] Estrogen has also been shown to improve the vascular reactivity of coronary arteries and prevent the progression of coronary artery atherosclerosis in nonhuman primates, but not when combined with medroxyprogesterone acetate.[109,110] Other actions of estrogen improve endothelial function, fibrinolytic potential, and the antioxidant activity of arteries.[111–116]

Yet because these estimates of benefit have been derived from observational studies, there may be considerable bias for the women choosing to receive estrogen compared with those who do not. Women who are healthier, better educated, wealthier, and practice better health maintenance self-care are more likely to have estrogen prescribed and more likely to take estrogen.[105,117,118] A randomized multicenter clinical trial (the Women's Health Initiative) that will determine the benefits and risks of estrogen, or estrogen plus progesterone therapy in postmenopausal women is finally under way, with results anticipated in 2005.[119,120] The population studied (postmenopausal and aged 50 to 79 years) is predominantly without evidence for CHD at baseline and will permit the assessment of the value of hormone therapy as a primary preventive measure over an average follow-up of 9 years. Another important reason to complete large-scale clinical trials on hormone replacement therapy is that there is concern regarding the risk of breast cancer with long-term use.[121] In fact, women themselves cite concern about breast cancer as the leading factor in their decision on whether or not to take postmenopausal hormone replacement therapy.[122]

The most significant recent development in efforts to delineate the risk/benefit ratio for use of postmenopausal hormone replacement therapy has been the recent report from the Heart and Estrogen/Progestin Replacement Study (HERS). This was a secondary prevention study of postmenopausal women with CHD who had an intact uterus. A total of 2763 women were randomized to receive 0.625 mg conjugated equine estrogens plus 2.5 mg medroxyprogesterone in one daily tablet or a matching placebo. After an average follow-up of 4.1 years, there was no difference in the occurrence of the primary cardiovascular outcome (nonfatal myocardial infarction or CHD death) or of any of the secondary cardiovascular outcomes despite beneficial changes in lipids.[123] An analysis of the endpoint data suggests that there is actually an increase in events within the first 2 to 3 years for women receiving estrogen-progestin compared with those on placebo. After 3 years, the incidence of myocardial infarction falls for women receiving hormones, with a significant trend toward improved benefit over time, for women on hormone treatment compared with placebo throughout the study period.[123] The possibility of an early prothrombotic effect, gradually replaced by an antiatherosclerotic benefit, was raised by the authors.

There are a number of considerations that require clarification before practitioners can know how to implement the results of HERS into clinical practice. The report did not reveal the date of preceding cardiovascular event or diagnosis for women entering the study, although myocardial infarction or revascularization must have occurred more than 6 months prior to randomization. Thus, if initiation of hormone therapy produces an unstable (e.g., prothrombotic, proarrhythmic, or proischemic) environment, there may be a differential effect for women who have been recently symptomatic compared with those whose events occurred in the distant past. It is also important to remember that all women randomized to active treatment were receiving a combination hormone therapy of estrogen plus progestin. There was no estrogen-only treatment arm and no women with previous hysterectomy. The discrepant results from the clinical trial compared to preceding observational studies may reflect the interaction of both hormones on cardiovascular outcomes as opposed to a potential beneficial effect with estrogen alone. Finally, it is important to point out that fewer women randomized to hormone treatment adhered to the prescribed number of pills than those receiving placebo, which may have tempered the reported findings.

Although additional analyses are needed, HERS has demonstrated the importance of testing promising treatments with a randomized clinical trial. Reliance on observational data may be misleading. This study has questioned whether there is cardiovascular benefit for women with evidence of CHD, as defined by HERS entry criteria, with 4 years of treatment with combination estrogen-progestin (using combined conjugated equine estrogens and medroxyprogesterone). The results do not apply to the primary prevention setting, where therapy could be potentially beneficial for preventing CHD events. Whether therapy is beneficial in secondary prevention when used for longer periods or using different hormone preparations or combinations is a subject for further investigation. However, until the results of ongoing long-term clinical trials are completed,[120] health care providers will need to continue to discuss the individualized risks and benefits of hormone replacement therapy with women. There is still no easy answer for the present.[124]

Summary

Women are at substantial risk for CHD and its consequences. Risk increases with levels of established cardiovascular risk factors and with increasing age. There is established evidence for the effectiveness of risk-factor intervention in women for secondary prevention of cardiac events as well as for primary prevention. Based on the evidence from observational studies and clinical trials, control of each of the major risk factors could be expected to reduce the risk of coronary heart disease by 20 percent to more than 50 percent (Table 15–5).[80] Collectively, even greater risk-reduction could be realized by multiple risk factor management.[68] Although estimates from observational studies suggest that hormone replacement therapy may reduce risk by as much as 50 percent or even more, the HERS results have tempered enthusiasm for universal promotion of hormone use to prevent CVD, particularly in those with existing CHD, and universal guidelines must await the completion of other studies. Although secondary prevention may afford the most cost-effective and clinically efficacious public health approach to CHD,[125] the importance of encouraging healthy lifestyles and other primary prevention practices beginning in youth cannot be overemphasized. The diagnosis of CHD in women has been considered problematic in that the pretest probability of disease and test results appear less reliable for women than for men. Nonetheless, with appropriate screening and risk stratification, a rational testing strategy can be employed for the evaluation of women with risk factors or symptoms of CHD. The goal of systematic risk-factor assessment and modification along with early, appropriate diagnosis of disease is to reduce the threat of cardiovascular morbidity and mortality in women.

TABLE 15–5 Projected Reductions in the Risk of Coronary Heart Disease (CHD) among Women According to Type of Intervention

Intervention	Source of Data	Estimated Risk Reduction
Smoking cessation	Observational studies	50–80% within 3–5 years
Cholesterol reduction	Trials including men and women (one primary prevention, two secondary)	46% in primary prevention; up to 46% from secondary prevention trials[71,72]
Hypertension treatment	Meta-analysis of randomized drug trials (50% women)	16% after 3–6 years of treatment
Treatment of isolated systolic hypertenstion	One randomized trial (57% women)	25%
Glycemic control in diabetics	Trials in progress	Insufficient data
Maintenance of ideal body weight	Observational studies	35–60% in those at ideal body weight versus obese
Physical activity	Observational studies	50–60% for active versus sedentary women
Small to moderate alcohol intake	Observational studies	50% lower risk in drinkers versus nondrinkers
Prophylactic low-dose aspirin	Observational studies	Inconsistent results
Antioxidant vitamin supplementation	Observational studies	Insufficient data
Estrogen replacement therapy	Observational studies	44% from estrogen alone; 61% estrogen-progestin[105]
	Two randomized trials	Beneficial risk factor changes
		No reduction in recurrent CHD events in secondary prevention[123]

Source: Modified from Rich-Edwards et al.,[68] with permission.

APPENDIX 15–1 GUIDE TO PREVENTIVE CARDIOLOGY FOR WOMEN

Lifestyle Factors	Goal(s)	Screening	Recommendations
Cigarette smoking	1. Complete cessation. 2. Avoid passive cigarette smoke.	1. Ask about current smoking status and exposure to others' cigarette smoke as part of routine evaluation. 2. Assess total exposure to cigarette smoke (pack-years) and prior attempts at quitting. 3. Evaluate readiness to stop smoking.	1. At each visit, strongly encourage patient and family to stop smoking. If complete cessation is not achievable, a reduction in intake is beneficial as a step toward cessation. 2. Reinforce nonsmoking status. 3. Provide counseling, nicotine replacement, and other pharmacotherapy as indicated in conjunction with behavioral therapy or a formal cessation program.
Physical activity stairs).	1. Accumulate $\geq$30 min of moderate-intensity physical activity on most, or preferably all, days of the week. 2. Women who have had recent cardiovascular events or procedures should participate in cardiac rehabilitation, a physician-guided home exercise program, or a comprehensive secondary prevention program.	1. Ask about physical activity (household work as well as occupational and leisure-time physical activity) as part of routine evaluation. 2. In women with symptoms that suggest CVD or in previously sedentary women >50 y old with $\geq$2 risk factors for CVD, consider a stress test* to establish safety of exercise and to guide the exercise prescription.	1. Encourage a minimum of 30 min of moderate-intensity dynamic exercise (e.g., brisk walking) daily. This may be performed in intermittent or shorter bouts ($\geq$10 min) of activity throughout the day. 2. Women who already meet minimum standards may be encouraged to become more physically active or to include more vigorous activities. 3. Incorporate physical activity in daily activities (e.g., using 4. Muscle strengthening and stretching exercises should be recommended as part of an overall activity program. 5. Recommend medically supervised programs for women who have had a recent MI or revascularization procedure.
Nutrition	1. AHA Step 1 Diet in healthy women ($\leq$30% fat, 8–10% saturated fat, and <300 mg/d cholesterol). 2. AHA Step 2 Diet in women with CVD or if a further reduction in cholesterol is needed ($\leq$30% fat, <7% saturated fat, and <200 mg/d cholesterol). 3. Limit sodium chloride (salt) intake to 6 g/d.	1. Assess nutritional habits as part of a routine evaluation in all women. 2. Consider formal dietary assessment in women with hyperlipidemia, diabetes, obesity, and hypertension.	1. Encourage a well-balanced and diversified diet that is low in saturated fat and high in fiber. 2. Use skim milk instead of milk with a higher fat content. 3. Diets rich in antioxidant (e.g., vitamin C, E, and betacarotene) and folate are preferred over nutritional supplements. Note: Daily supplements of 0.4 mg of folic acid are recommended for women of child-bearing age to help prevent neural tube defects.

	Women with high blood pressure may require further restriction. 4. Total dietary fiber intake of 25–30 g/d from foods. 5. Consume ≥5 servings of fruits and vegetables per day.		4. Limit alcohol intake to ≤1 glass of alcohol per day. (1 glass = 4 oz wine, 12 oz beer, or 1½ oz 80-proof spirits.) Pregnant women should abstain from drinking alcohol.
Weight management	1. Achieve and maintain desirable weight. 2. Target BMI (weight in kilograms divided by height in meters squared) between 18.5 and 24.9 kg/m² (BMI of 25 kg/m² = 110% of desirable body weight). 3. Desirable waist circumference <88 cm (<35 inches) in women with a BMI of 25–34.9 kg/m².	Measure patient's weight and height, calculate BMI, and measure waist circumference as part of a periodic evaluation. Note: BMI and waist circumference are used for diagnosis, and measurement of height and weight are used for follow-up.	1. Encourage gradual and sustained weight loss in persons whose weight exceeds the ideal weight for their height. 2. Formal nutritional counseling is encouraged for women with hypertension, hyperlipidemia, or elevated glucose levels associated with overweight. 3. The recommended weight gain during pregnancy is 25–35 lb if the patient's prepregnancy weight is normal. Adjust for multiple gestation and prepregnancy weight (e.g., overweight women should gain 15–25 lb, obese women, <15 lb).
Psychosocial factors	1. Positive adaptation to to stressful situations. 2. Improved quality of life. 3. Maintain or establish social connections.	1. Assess presence of stressful situations and response to stress as part of a routine evaluation. 2. Evaluate for depression, especially in women with recent cardiovascular events. 3. Assess social support system and evalute for social isolation.	1. Encourage positive coping mechanisms for stress (e.g., substitute physical activity for overeating or excessive smoking in response to stress). 2. Encourage adequate rest and relief for women who are caretakers of others. 3. Consider treatment of depression and anxiety when appropriate. 4. Encourage participation in social activities or volunteer work for socially isolated women.

Risk Factors	Goals	Screening	Recommendations
Blood pressure	1. Achieve and maintain blood pressure <140/90 mmHg and lower if tolorated (optimal <120/80). 2. In pregnant women with hypertension, the goal of treatment is to minimize short-term risk of elevated blood pressure in the mother while avoiding therapy that	1. Measure blood pressure as part of a routine evaluation. 2. Follow-up is based on initial measurement as follows: SBP, DBP, mmHg mmHg Follow-up <130 <85 Recheck in 2 y 130–139 85–89 Recheck in 1 y	1. Promote the lifestyle behaviors described above (weight control, physical activity, moderation in alcohol intake) and moderate sodium restriction. 2. If blood pressure remains ≥140/90 mmHg after 3 months of lifestyle modification or if initial level is >160 mmHg systolic or 100 mmHg diastolic, then initiate and individualize pharmacotherapy based on the

Risk Factors	Goals	Screening	Recommendations
	may compromise the well-being of the fetus.	140–159 90–99 Confirm in 2 mo 160–179 100–109 Evaluate in 1 mo ≥180 ≥110 Evaluate in 1 wk (Follow-up screening may be modified on the basis of prior history, symptoms, presence of other risk factors, and end-organ damage.) 3. In pregnant women with hypertension, evaluate for preeclampsia.	patient's characteristics. 3. In pregnant women with hypertension, reduction of diastolic blood pressure to 90–100 mmHg is recommended.
Lipids, lipoproteins	Primary goal: Women without CVD Lower risk (<2 risk factors) LDL goal <160 mg/dL (optimal <130 mg/dL) Higher risk (≥2 risk factors) LDL goal <130 mg/dL Women with CVD LDL ≤100 mg/dL Secondary goals: HDL >35 mg/dL Triglycerides <200 mg/dL Note: In women, the optimal level of triglycerides may be lower (≤150 mg/dL) and the HDL higher (≥45 mg/dL).	Women without CVD† Measure nonfasting total and HDL cholesterol and assess nonlipid risk factors. Follow-up is based on the following initial measurements: TC <200, HDL ≥45, follow-up in 5 y TC <200, HDL <45, follow-up with fasting lipoprotein analysis. TC 200–239, HDL ≥45, and <2 risk factors, follow-up in 1–2 years. TC 200–239, HDL <45 or ≥2 risk factors, follow-up with fasting lipoprotein analysis. TC ≥240, follow-up with fasting lipoprotein analysis. (All cholesterol values in mg/dL.) Women with CVD Fasting lipoprotein analysis (may take 4–6 wk to stabilize after cardiovascular event or bypass surgery).	1. Promote lifestyle approach in all women (diet, weight management, smoking avoidance, and exercise as described above). Rule out other secondary causes of dyslipidemia. 2. Suggested drug therapy for high LDL levels (defined as [a] ≥220 mg/dL in low-risk, premenopausal women, [b] ≥190 mg/dL in postmenopausal women with <2 risk factors, and [c] ≥160 mg/dL with ≥2 risk factors) is based on triglyceride level as follows: TG <200 mg/dL statin, resin, niacin Note: ERT is an option for postmenopausal women, but treatment should be individualized and considered with other health risks. TG 200–400 mg/dL statin, niacin TG >400 mg/dL Consider monotherapy with statin, niacin, fibrate, or a combination of the above.
Diabetes	For patients with diabetes: 1. Maintain blood glucose: preprandial = 80–120 mg/dL bedtime = 100–140 mg/dL. 2. Maintain Hb A1$_c$ <7%. 3. LDL <130 mg/dL (<100 mg/dL if established	1. Monitor glucose and hemoglobin A1$_c$ as part of a routine periodic evaluation in women with diabetes. 2. Screen for diabetes (fasting glucose >125 mg/dL or >200 mg/dL 2 h after	1. Encourage adoption of American Diabetes Association Diet (<30% fat, <10% saturated fat, 6–8% polyunsaturated fat, cholesterol <300 mg/d). 2. A low-calorie diet may be recommended for weight loss.

CVD). Note: Many authorities believe that LDL should be <100 mg/dL in all patients with diabetes.
4. Triglycerides <150 mg/dL.
5. Control blood pressure.

75 g glucose) as part of a periodic examination in women with risk factors for diabetes, such as obesity.

3. Encourage regular physical activity.
4. Pharmacotherapy with oral agents or insulin should be used when indicated.

Pharmacological Interventions	Goal(s)	Screening	Recommendations
Hormone replacement therapy	1. Initiation or continuation of therapy in women for whom the potential benefits may exceed the potential risks of therapy. (Short-term therapy is indicated for treatment of menopausal symptoms.) 2. Minimize risk of adverse side effects through careful patient selection and appropriate choice of therapy.	1. Review menstrual status of women >40 y old. 2. If menopausal status is unclear, measure FSH level.	1. Counsel all women about the potential benefits and risks of HRT, beginning at age 40 or as requested. 2. Individualize decision based on prior history and risk factors for CVD as well as risks of thromboembolic disease, gallbladder disease, osteoporosis, breast cancer, and other health risks. 3. Combination therapy with a progestin is usually indicated to prevent endometrial hyperplasia in a woman with an intact uterus and prescribed estrogen. The choice of agent should be made on an individual basis.
Oral contraceptives	1. Minimize risk of adverse cardiovascular effects while preventing pregnancy. 2. Use the lowest effective dose of estrogen/progestin.	Determine contraindications and cardiovascular risk factor status of women who are considering using oral contraceptives.	1. Use of oral contraceptives is relatively contraindicated in women ≥35 y old who smoke. 2. Women with a family history of premature heart disease should have lipid analysis before taking oral contraceptives. 3. Women with significant risk factors for diabetes should have glucose testing before taking oral contraceptives. 4. If a woman develops hypertension while using oral contraceptives, she should be advised to stop taking them.
Antiplatelet agents/anticoagulants	Prevention of clinical thrombotic and embolic events in women with established CVD.	1. Determine if contra-indications to therapy exist at the time of the initial cardiovascular event. 2. Evaluate ongoing compliance, risk, and side effects as part of a routine follow-up evaluation.	1. If no contraindications, women with atherosclerotic CVD should use aspirin 80–325 mg/d. 2. Other antiplatelet agents, such as newer thiopyridine derivatives, may be used to prevent vascular events in women who cannot take aspirin.
β blockers	To reduce the reinfarction rate, incidence of sudden	1. Determine if contra-indications to therapy exist	Start within hours of hospitalization in women with an evolving MI

Pharmacological Interventions	Goal(s)	Screening	Recommendations
	death, and overall mortality in women after MI.	at the time of the initial cardiovascular event. 2. Evaluate ongoing compliance, risk, and side effects as part of a routine follow-up evaluation.	without contraindications. If not started acutely, treatment should begin withn a few days of the event and continue indefinitely.
ACE inhibitors	To reduce morbidity and mortality among MI survivors and patients with LV dysfunction.	1. Determine if contra-indications to therapy exist at the time of the initial cardiovascular event. 2. Evaluate ongoing compliance, risk, and side effects as part of a routine effects as part of a routine follow-up evaluation.	1. Start early during hospitalization for MI unless hypotension or other contraindications exist. Continue indefinitely for all with LV dysfunction (ejection fraction ≤40%) or symptoms of congestive heart failure; otherwise, ACE inhibitors may be stopped at 6 wk. 2. Discontinue ACE inhibitors if a woman becomes pregnant.

CVD indicates cardiovascular disease; BMI, body mass index; SBP, systolic blood pressure; DBP, diastolic blood pressure; TC, total cholesterol; TG, triglycerides; HRT, hormone replacement therapy; and FSH, follicle-stimulating hormone.

*The choice of test modality should be based on the resting ECG, physical ability to exercise, and local expertise and technologies.

†The ACC and the AHA recommend cholesterol screening guidelines as outlined by the National Cholesterol Education Panel (measure total and HDL cholesterol at least once every 5 years in all adults ≥20 y old). The consensus panel recognizes that some organizations use other guidelines, such as the US Preventive Services Task Force, which recommends that cholesterol screening in women without risk factors begin at age 45 y.

Source: AHA/ACC Scientific Statement: Consensus Panel Statement, Guide to Preventive Cardiology for Women. Reproduced with permission from Mosca et al.[4]

References

1. American Heart Association: *1998 Heart and Stroke Facts: Statistical Update.* Dallas, American Heart Association, 1997.

2. Pilote L, Hlatky MA: Attitudes of women toward hormone therapy and prevention of heart disease. *Am Heart J* 1995; 129:1237–1238.

3. Mosca L, Manson JE, Sutherland SE, et al: Cardiovascular disease in women: a statement for healthcare professionals from the American Heart Association. *Circulation* 1997; 96:2468–2482.

4. Mosca L, Grundy SM, Judelson D, et al: American Heart Association/American College of Cardiology Medical/Scientific Consensus Panel Statement: a guide to preventive cardiology for women. *Circulation* 1999; 33:1751–1755.

5. Kannel WB, Sorlie P, McNamara PM: Prognosis after initial myocardial infarction: the Framingham study. *Am J Cardiol* 1979; 44:53–59.

6. Tofler GH, Stone PH, Muller JE, et al: Effects of gender and race on prognosis after myocardial infarction: ad-

verse prognosis for women, particularly black women. *J Am Coll Cardiol* 1987; 9:473–482.

7. Greenland P, Reicher-Reiss H, Goldbourt U, et al: In-hospital and 1-year mortality in 124 women after myocardial infarction: comparison with 4315 men. *Circulation* 1991; 83:484–491.

8. The GUSTO Investigators: An international randomized trial comparing four thrombolytic strategies for acute myocardial infarction. *N Engl J Med* 1993; 329:673–682.

9. Fibrinolytic Therapy Trialists (FTT) Collaborative Group: Indications for fibrinolytic therapy in suspected acute myocardial infarction: collaborative overview of early mortality and major morbidity results from all randomized trials of more than 1000 patients. *Lancet* 1994; 343:311–322.

10. Escobedo LG, Zack MM: Comparison of sudden and nonsudden coronary deaths in the United States. *Circulation* 1996; 93:2033–2036.

11. Airaksinen KEJ, Ikaheimo MJ, Linnaluoto M, et al: Gender difference in autonomic and hemodynamic reactions to abrupt coronary occlusion. *J Am Coll Cardiol* 1998; 31:301–306.

12. Sonke GS, Beaglehole R, Stewart AW, et al: Sex differences in case fatality before and after admission to hospital after acute cardiac events: analysis of community based coronary heart disease register. *BMJ* 1996; 313:853–855.

13. Schwartz LM, Fisher ES, Tosteson ANA, et al: Treatment and health outcomes of women and men in a cohort with coronary artery disease. *Arch Intern Med* 1997; 157:1545–1551.

14. Wong ND, Cupples LA, Ostfeld AM, Levy D, Kannel WB: Risk factors for long-term coronary prognosis following initial myocardial infarction: the Framingham study. *Am J Epidemiol* 1989; 130:469–480.

15. Fisher LD, Kennedy JW, Davis KB, et al, and the participating CASS Clinics: Association of sex, physical size, and operative mortality after coronary artery bypass in the Coronary Artery Surgery Study (CASS). *J Thorac Cardiovasc Surg* 1982; 84:334–341.

16. Kennedy JW, Kaiser GC, Fisher LD, et al: Clinical and angiographic predictors of operative mortality from the Collborative Study in Coronary Artery Surgery (CASS). *Circulation* 1981; 63:793–802.

17. Kelsey SF, James M, Holubkov AL, et al, and Investigators from the National Heart, Lung, and Blood Institutes Percutaneous Coronary Angioplasty Registry: Results of percutaneous transluminal coronary angioplasty in women. 1985–1986 National Heart, Lung, and Blood Institute's Coronary Angioplasty Registry. *Circulation* 1993; 87:720–727.

18. Mendes LA, Davidoff R, Cupples LA, et al: Congestive heart failure in patients with coronary artery disease: the gender paradox. *Am Heart J* 1997; 134:207–212.

19. Gurwitz JH, McLaughlin TJ, Willison DJ, et al: Delayed hospital presentation in patients who have had acute myocardial infarction. *Ann Intern Med* 1997; 126:593–599.

20. Maynard C, Althouse R, Cerqueira M, et al: Underutilization of thrombolytic therapy in eligible women with acute myocardial infarction. *Am J Cardiol* 1991; 68:529–530.

21. Kudenchuk P, Maynard C, Martin J, et al: Comparison of presentation, treatment and outcome of acute myocardial infarction in men versus women (the Myocardial Infarction Triage and Intervention Registry). *Am J Cardiol* 1996; 78:9–14.

22. Weitzman S, Cooper L, Chambless L, et al: Gender, racial and geographic differences in the performance of cardiac diagnostic and therapeutic procedures for hospitalized acute myocardial infarction in four states. *Am J Cardiol* 1997; 79:722–726.

23. Schecter AD, Goldschmidt-Clermont PJ, McKee G, et al: Influence of gender, race, and education on patient preferences and receipt of cardiac catheterizations among coronary care unitpatients. *Am J Cardiol* 1996; 78:996–1001.

24. Schulman KA, Berlin JA, Harless W, et al: The effect of race and sex on physicians' recommendations for cardiac catheterization. *N Engl J Med* 1999; 340:618–626.

25. Lerner DJ, Kannel WB: Patterns of coronary heart disease morbidity and mortality in the sexes: a 26-year follow-up of the Framingham population. *Am Heart J* 1986; 111:383–390.

26. Kennedy JW, Killip T, Fisher LD, et al: The clinical spectrum of coronary artery disease and its surgical and medical management. The Coronary Artery Surgery Study. *Circulation* 1982; 66:16–23.

27. Kannel WB, Feinleib M: Natural history of angina pectoris in the Framingham study: prognosis and survival. *Am J Cardiol* 1972; 29:154–163.

28. Diamond GA, Forrester JS: Analysis of probability as an aid in the clinical diagnosis of coronary artery disease. *N Engl J Med* 1979; 300:1350–1358.

29. Shaw LJ, Miller DD, Romeis MJ, et al: Prognostic value of noninvasive risk stratification in younger and older patients referred for evaluation of suspected coronary artery disease. *J Am Geriatr Soc* 1996; 44:1190–1197.

30. Sketch MH, Mohiuddin SM, Lynch JD, et al: Significant sex differences in the correlation of electrocardiographic exercise testing and coronary arteriograms. *Am J Cardiol* 1975; 36:169–172.

31. Barolsky SM, Gilbert CA, Faruqui A, et al: Differences in electrocardiographic response to exercise of women and men: a non-Bayesian factor. *Circulation* 1979; 60:1021–1027.

32. Tavel ME: Specificity of electrocardiographic stress test in women versus men. *Am J Cardiol* 1992; 70:545–547.

33. Hung J, Chaitman BR, Lam J, et al: Noninvasive diagnostic test choices for the evaluation of coronary artery disease in women: a multivariate comparison of cardiac fluoroscopy, exercise electrocardiography and exercise thallium myocardial perfusion scintigraphy. *J Am Coll Cardiol* 1984; 4:8–16.

34. Friedman T, Greene A, Iskandrian A, et al: Exercise thallium-201 myocardial scintigraphy in women: correlation with coronary angiography. *Am J Cardiol* 1982; 49:1632–1637.

35. Taillefer R, dePuey G, Udelson J, et al: Comparative diagnostic accuracy of Tl-201 and Tc99m Sestamibi SPECT imaging (perfusion and ECG-gated SPECT) in detecting coronary artery disease in women. *J Am Coll Cardiol* 1997; 29:69–77.

36. Higginbotham MB, Morris KG, Coleman RE, et al: Sex-related differences in the normal cardiac response to upright exercise. *Circulation* 1984; 70:357–366.

37. Hanley PC, Zinsmeister AR, Clements IP, et al: Gender-related differences in cardiac response to supine exercise assessed by radionuclide angiography. *J Am Coll Cardiol* 1989; 13:624–629.

38. Moriel M, Rozanski A, Klein J, et al: The limited efficacy of exercise radionuclide ventriculography in assessing prognosis of women with coronary artery disease. *Am J Cardiol* 1995; 76:1030–1035.

39. Patterson RE, Churchwell KB, Eisner RL: Diagnosis of coronary artery disease in women: roles of three dimensional imaging with magnetic resonance or positron emission tomography. *Am J Cardiac Imaging* 1996; 10:78–88.

40. Sawada SG, Ryan T, Fineberg NS, et al: Exercise echocardiographic detection of coronary artery disease in women. *J Am Coll Cardiol* 1989; 14:1440–1447.

41. Williams MJ, Marwick TH, O'Gorman D, et al: Comparison of exercise echocardiography with an exercise score to diagnose coronary artery disease in women. *Am J Cardiol* 1994; 74:435–438.

42. Marwick TH, Anderson T, Williams MJ, et al: Exercise echocardiography is an accurate and cost efficient technique for detection of coronary artery disease in women. *J Am Coll Cardiol* 1995; 26:335–341.

43. Rozanski A, Diamond GA, Berman D, et al: The declining specificity of exercise radionuclide ventriculography. *N Engl J Med* 1983; 309:518–522.

44. Roger VL, Pellikka PA, Bell MR, et al: Sex and test verification bias: impact on the diagnostic value of exercise echocardiography. *Circulation* 1997; 95:405–410.

45. Elhendy A, Geleijnse ML, Van Domburg RT, et al: Gender differences in the accuracy of dobutamine stress echocardiography for the diagnosis of coronary artery disease. *Am J Cardiol* 1997; 80:1414–1418.

46. Rallidis L, Cokkinos P, Tousoulis D, et al: Comparison of dobutamine and treadmill exercise echocardiography in inducing ischemia in patients with coronary artery disease. *J Am Coll Cardiol* 1997; 30:1660–1668.

47. Laurienzo JM, Cannon RO III, Quyyumi AA, et al: Improved specificity of transesophageal dobutamine stress echocardiography compared to standard tests for evaluation of coronary artery disease in women presenting with chest pain. *Am J Cardiol* 1997; 80:1402–1407.

48. McCully RB, Roger VL, Mahoney DW, et al: Outcome after normal exercise echocardiography and predictors of subsequent cardiac events: follow-up of 1,325 patients. *J Am Coll Cardiol* 1998; 31:144–149.

49. Wexler L, Brundage B, Crouse J, et al: Coronary artery calcification: pathophysiology, epidemiology, imaging methods and clinical implications: a statement for health professionals from the American Heart Association. *Circulation* 1996; 94:1175–1192.

50. Kung S, Detrano RC: Are there gender differences regarding coronary artery calcification? *Am J Cardiac Imaging* 1996; 10:72–77.

51. Cerqueria MD: Diagnostic testing strategies for coronary artery disease: special issues related to gender. *Am J Cardiol* 1995; 75:52D–60D.

52. Douglas PS, Ginsburg GS: The evaluation of chest pain in women. *N Engl J Med* 1996; 344:1311–1315.

53. Tobin JN, Wassertheil-Smoller S, Wexler JP, et al: Sex bias in considering coronary bypass surgery. *Ann Intern Med* 1987; 107:19–25.

54. Ayanian JZ, Epstein AM: Differences in the use of procedures between women and men hospitalized for coronary artery disease. *N Engl J Med* 1991; 325:221–225.

55. Shaw LJ, Miller DD, Romeis JC, et al: Gender differences in the noninvasive evaluation and management of patients with suspected coronary artery disease. *Ann Intern Med* 1994; 120:559–566.

56. Steingart RM, Packer M, Hamm P, et al: Sex differences in the management of coronary heart disease. *N Engl J Med* 1991; 324:226–230.

57. Krumholz HM, Douglas PS, Lauer MS, et al: Selection of patients for coronary angiography early after myocardial infarction: is there evidence for a gender bias? *Ann Intern Med* 1992; 116:785–790.

58. Bickell NA, Pieper KS, Lee KL, et al: Referral patterns for coronary artery disease treatment: gender bias or good clinical judgement? *Ann Intern Med* 1992; 116:791–797.

59. Mark DB, Shaw LK, DeLong ER, et al: Absence of sex bias in the referral of patients for cardiac catheterization. *N Engl J Med* 1994; 330:1101–1106.

60. Lauer MS, Pashkow FJ, Snader CE, et al: Sex and diagnostic evaluation of possible coronary artery disease after exercise treadmill testing at one academic teaching center. *Am Heart J* 1997; 134:807–813.

61. O'Keefe JH, Kim SC, Hall RR, et al: Estrogen replacement therapy after coronary angioplasty in women. *J Am Coll Cardiol* 1997; 29:1–5.

62. O'Connor GT, Morton JR, Diehl MJ, et al: Differences between men and women in hospital mortality associated with coronary artery bypass graft surgery. *Circulation* 1993; 88(part 1):2104–2110.

63. Edwards FH, Carey JS, Grover FL, et al: Impact of gender on coronary bypass operative mortality. *Ann Thorac Surg* 1998; 66:125–131.

64. Khan SS, Nessim S, Gray R, et al: Increased mortality of women in coronary artery bypass surgery: evidence for referral bias. *Ann Intern Med* 1990; 112:561–567.

65. Mickleborough LL, Takagi Y, Maruyama H, et al: Is sex a factor in determining operative risk for aortocoronary bypass graft surgery? *Circulation* 1995; 92(suppl 2):80–84.

66. Carey JS, Cukingnan RA, Singer LKM: Health status after myocardial revascularization; inferior status in women. *Ann Thorac Surg* 1995; 59:112–117.

67. Sempos CT, Cleeman JI, Carroll MD, et al: Prevalence of high blood cholesterol among U.S. adults: an update based on guidelines from the Second Report of the National Cholesterol Education Program Adult Treatment Panel. *JAMA* 1993; 269:3009–3014.

68. Rich-Edwards JW, Manson JE, Henekens CH, Buring JE: The primary prevention of coronary heart disease in women. *N Engl J Med* 1995; 332:1758–1766.

69. Krumholz HM, Seeman TE, Merrill SS, et al: Lack of association between cholesterol and coronary heart disease

mortality and morbidity and all-cause mortality in persons older than 70 years. *JAMA* 1994; 272:1335–1340.

70. LaRosa JC: Triglycerides and coronary risk in women and the elderly. *Arch Intern Med* 1997; 157:961–968.

71. Scandinavian Simvastatin Survival Study Group: Randomised trial of cholesterol lowering in 4444 patients with coronary heart disease: the Scandinavian Simvastatin Survival Study (4S). *Lancet* 1994; 344:1383–1389.

72. Lewis SJ, Sacks FM, Mitchell JS, et al: Effect of pravastatin on cardiovascular events in women after myocardial infarction: the Cholesterol and Recurrent Events (CARE) trial: *J Am Coll Cardiol* 1998; 32:140–146.

73. Downs JR, Clearfield M, Weis S, et al, for the AFCAPS/TexCAPS Research Group: Primary prevention of acute coronary events with lovastatin in men and women with average cholesterol levels. *JAMA* 1998; 279:1615–1622.

74. Collins R, Peto R, MacMahon W, et al: Blood pressure, stroke and coronary heart disease: 2. Short-term reductions in blood pressure: overview of randomized drug trials in their epidemiological context. *Lancet* 1990; 335:827–829.

75. National High Blood Pressure Education Program Working Group: National High Blood Pressure working group report on hypertension in the elderly. *Hypertension* 1994; 23:275–285.

76. Gueyffier F, Boutitie F, Boissel JP, et al: Effect of antihypertensive drug treatment on cardiovascular outcomes in women and men: a meta-analysis of individual patient data from randomized controlled trials. *Ann Intern Med* 1997; 126:761–767.

77. Joint National Committee on Prevention, Detection, Evaluation, and Treatment of High Blood Pressure: The Sixth Report of the Joint National Committee on Prevention, Detection, Evaluation, and Treatment of High Blood Pressure. *Arch Intern Med* 1997; 157:2413.

78. Wyngard DL, Barrett-Connor E: Heart disease and diabetes. In: *Diabetes in America,* 2d ed. NIDDK, NIH Pub. No. 95-1468. Bethesda, MD, National Institutes of Health, 1995.

79. Reaven GM: Banting lecture 1988: role of insulin resistance in human disease. *Diabetes* 1988; 112:432–437.

80. Wenger NK: Addressing coronary heart disease risk in women. *Cleve Clin J Med* 1998; 65:464–469.

81. Kawachi I, Colditz GA, Stampfer MJ, et al: Smoking cessation in relation to total mortality rates in women: a prospective cohort study. *Ann Intern Med* 1993; 119:992–1000.

82. Crespo CJ, Keteyian SJ, Heath GW, et al: Leisure-time physical activity among U.S. adults. Results from the Third National Health and Nutrition Examination Survey. *Arch Intern Med* 1996; 156:93–98.

83. Blair SN, Kohl HW, Paffenbarger RS, et al: Physical fitness and all-cause mortality: a prospective study of healthy men and women. *JAMA* 1989; 262:2395–2401.

84. Greendale GA, Bodin-Dunn L, Ingles S, et al: Leisure, home and occupational physical activity and cardiovascular risk factors in postmenopausal women: the Postmenopausal Estrogens/Progestins Intervention (PEPI) study. *Arch Intern Med* 1996; 156:418–424.

85. Pate RR, Pratt M, Blair SN, et al: Physical activity and public health: a recommendation from the Centers for Disease Control and Prevention and the American College of Sports Medicine. *JAMA* 1995; 273:402–407.

86. Manson JE, Colditz GA, Stampfer MJ, et al: A prospective study of obesity and risk of coronary heart disease in women. *N Engl J Med* 1990; 322:882–889.

87. Eckel RJ, Krauss RM for the AHA Nutrition Committee: American Heart Association call to action: obesity as a major risk factor for coronary heart disease. *Circulation* 1998; 97:2099–2100.

88. Graham IM, Daly LE, Refsum HM, et al: Plasma homocysteine as a risk factor for vascular disease: the European Concerted Action Project. *JAMA* 1997; 277:1775–1781.

89. Boushey CJ, Beresford SAA, Omenn GS, et al: A quantitative assessment of plasma homocysteine as a risk factor for vascular disease: probable benefits of increasing folic acid intakes. *JAMA* 1995; 274:1049–1057.

90. Glodsland IF, Crook D, Simpson R, et al: The effects of different formulations of oral contraceptive agents on lipid and carbohydrate metabolism. *N Engl J Med* 1990; 323:1375–1381.

91. World Health Organization Collaborative Study of Cardiovascular Disease and Steroid Hormone Contraception: Acute myocardial infarction and combined oral contraceptives: results of an international multicentre case-control study. *Lancet* 1997; 349:1202–1209.

92. Bush TL, Barrett-Connor E, Cowan LD, et al: Cardiovascular mortality and noncontraceptive use of estrogen in women: results from Lipid Research Clinics Program follow-up study. *Circulation* 1987; 75:1102–1109.

93. Sidney S, Petitti DB, Quesenberry CP Jr, et al: Myocardial infarction in users of low-dose oral contraceptives. *Obstet Gynecol* 1996; 88:939–944.

94. Chasan-Taber L, Stampfer MJ: Epidemiology of oral contraceptives and cardiovascular disease. *Ann Intern Med* 1998; 128:467–477.

95. Stampfer MJ, Willett WC, Colditz GA, et al: Past use of oral contraceptives and cardiovascular disease: a meta-analysis in the context of the Nurses' Health Study. *Am J Obstet Gynecol* 1990; 163:285–291.

96. Birdsall MA, Farquhar CM, White HD: Association between polycystic ovaries and extent of coronary artery disease in women having cardiac catheterization. *Ann Intern Med* 1997; 126:32–35.

97. Stampfer MJ, Colditz GA, Willett WC, et al: Postmenopausal estrogen therapy and cardiovascular disease. *N Engl J Med* 1991; 325:756–762.

98. Stampfer MJ, Colditz GA: Estrogen replacement therapy

and coronary heart disease: a quantitative assessment of the epidemiologic evidence. *Prev Med* 1991; 20:47–63.

99. Henderson BE, Paganini-Hill A, Ross RK: Decreased mortality in users of estrogen replacement therapy. *Arch Intern Med* 1991; 151:75–77.

100. Grodstein F, Stampfer MJ, Colditz GA, et al: Post-menopausal hormone therapy and mortality. *N Engl J Med* 1997; 336:1769–1775.

101. Sullivan JM, Vander Zwaag R, Lemp GF, et al: A review of the association of estrogens and progestins with cardiovascular disease in postmenopausal women. *Arch Intern Med* 1990; 150:2557–2562.

102. Bush TL, Barrett-Connor E, Cowan LD, et al: Cardiovascular mortality and noncontraceptive use of estrogen in women: results from Lipid Research Clinics Program follow-up study. *Circulation* 1987; 75:1102–1109.

103. Forrester JS, Merz CNB, Bush TL, et al: Task Force 4: efficacy of risk factor management. *J Am Coll Cardiol* 1996; 27:991–1006.

104. Sullivan JM, Vander Zwaag R, Lemp GF, et al: Post-menopausal estrogen use and coronary atherosclerosis. *Ann Intern Med* 1988; 108:358–363.

105. Grodstein F, Stampfer MJ, Manson JE, et al: Post-menopausal estrogen and progestin use and the risk of cardiovascular disease. *N Engl J Med* 1996; 335:453–461.

106. Sullivan JM, Vander Zwaag R, Hughes JP et al: Estrogen replacement and coronary artery diease: effect on survival in postmenopausal women. *Arch Intern Med* 1990; 150:2557–2562.

107. Walsh BW, Schiff I, Rosner B, et al: Effects of post-menopausal estrogen replacement on the concentrations and metabolism of plasma lipoproteins. *N Engl J Med* 1991; 325:1196–1204.

108. The Writing Group for PEPI: Effects of estrogen or estrogen/progestin regimens on heart disease risk factors in postmenopausal women. *JAMA* 1995; 273:199–208.

109. Williams JK, Anthony MS, Nonor EK, et al: Regression of atherosclerosis in female monkeys. *Arterioscler Thromb Vasc Biol* 1995; 15:827–836.

110. Adams MR, Register TC, Golden DL, et al: Medroxy-progesterone acetate antagonizes inhibitor effects of conjugated equine estrogens on coronary artery atherosclerosis. *Arterioscler Thromb Vasc Biol* 1997; 17:217–221.

111. Gebara OC, Mittleman MA, Sutherland P, et al: Association between increased estrogen status and increased fibrinolytic potential in the Framingham Offspring Study. *Circulation* 1995; 91:1952–1958.

112. Knopp JR, Zhu X, Bonet B: Effects of estrogen on lipoprotein metabolism and cardiovascular disease in women. Atherosclerosis 1994; 110(suppl):S83–S91.

113. Samaan SA, Crawford MH: Estrogen and cardiovascular function after menopause. *J Am Coll Cardiol* 1995; 26:1403–1410.

114. Collins P, Rosano G, Sarrel PJ, et al: 17β-Estradiol attenuates acetylcholine-induced coronary arterial constriction in women but not men with coronary artery disease. *Circulation* 1995; 92:24–30.

115. Wilson PWF, Garrison RJ, Castelli WP: Postmenopausal estrogen use, cigarette smoking and cardiovascular morbidity in women over 50: the Framingham study. *N Engl J Med* 1985; 313:1038–1043.

116. Guetta V, Cannon RO III: Cardiovascular effects of estrogen and lipid-lowering therapies in postmenopausal women. *Circulation* 1996; 93:1928–1937.

117. Matthews KA, Kuller LH, Wing RR, et al: Prior to use of estrogen replacement therapy, are users healthier than nonusers? *Am J Epidemiol* 1996; 143:971–978.

119. Rossouw JE, Finnegan CP, Harlan WR, et al: The evolution of the Women's Health Initiative: perspectives from the NIH. *J Am Med Women's Assoc* 1995; 50:50–55.

120. The Women's Health Initiative Study Group: Design of the Women's Health Initiative Clinical Trial and Observational Study. *Control Clin Trials* 1998; 19:61–109.

121. Collaborative Group on Hormonal Factors in Breast Cancer: Breast cancer and hormone replacement therapy: collaborative reanalysis of data from 51 epidemiologic studies of 52,705 women with breast cancer and 108,411 women without breast cancer. *Lancet* 1997; 350:1047–1059.

122. Salamone LM, Pressman AR, Seeley DG, et al: Estrogen replacement therapy: a survey of older women's attitudes. *Arch Intern Med* 1996; 156:1293–1297.

123. Hulley S, Grady D, Bush T, et al, for the Heart and Estrogen/Progestin Replacement Study (HERS) Research Group: Randomized trial of estrogen plus progestin for secondary prevention of coronary heart disease in postmenopausal women. *JAMA* 1998; 280:605–613.

124. Petitti DB: Hormone replacement therapy and heart disease prevention: experimentation trumps observation. *JAMA* 1998; 280:650–652.

125. Fuster V, Pearson TA: 27th Bethesda Conference: matching the intensity of risk factor management with the hazard for coronary artery disease events. *J Am Coll Cardiol* 1996; 27:957–1047.

CHAPTER 16

Children and Adolescents

Dennis M. Davidson
Cynthia Iftner Traum
Elaine J. Stone
Nathan D. Wong

In the past five decades, considerable evidence has accumulated to support the contention that atherosclerosis may begin early in life and can progress to an advanced stage by young adulthood.[1] Korean War autopsy studies showed significant evidence of coronary heart disease (CHD) in 77 percent of soldiers averaging only 22 years old.[2] These results were confirmed later in men dying in Vietnam.[3] Postmortem examination of American and Finnish schoolchildren revealed fatty streaks and intimal thickening in youth.[4,5] In a large analysis of 4737 subjects aged 10 to 39, coronary fatty streaks were found to develop beginning in the 10 to 14 year-old age group; they were present in all those over age 20 in New Orleans and by age 30 in most persons from other populations.[6] Subsequent studies found evidence that such lesions progressed to fibrous plaques.[7,8]

In adults, CHD has been clearly associated with a number of risk factors. These include modifiable factors such as cigarette smoking, dyslipidemias [high levels of low-density-lipoprotein cholesterol (LDL-C) and low levels of high-density-lipoprotein cholesterol (HDL-C)], high blood pressure, physical inactivity, obesity, and diabetes as well as those factors that are not amenable to change, such as age and a premature family history of CHD.[9]

Logically, one would next look for evidence that elevated levels of risk factors in children are closely correlated with high levels of the same indicators in adults who develop CHD. Such investigations examine the reliability and reproducibility of risk factor measurements as well as their consistency to indicate high risk (to "track") over time. During the past 25 years, several investigations have systematically examined smoking, dyslipidemias, high blood pressure, physical inactivity, obesity, and glucose intolerance in children (Table 16–1); some of these studies have followed their subjects into adulthood.[10]

If certain risk factors (in childhood) are predictive of subsequent development of CHD in adult life, the following questions arise: Do we currently have

TABLE 16–1 Coronary Artery Disease Risk Indicators in Children

High LDL cholesterol
Low HDL cholesterol
High blood pressure
Obesity
Physical inactivity
Diabetes/glucose intolerance
Smoking
Family history of above risk indicators and/or CAD events at an early age

Key: LDL, low-density-lipoprotein; HDL, high-density lipoprotein; CAD, cardiovascular disease.

interventions that can successfully modify these risk indicators? Can we lower LDL cholesterol and blood pressure? Can we induce young persons to be more physically active and to avoid cigarette smoking?

An important goal of preventive cardiology is to develop interventions to lower risk during childhood and adolescence that will persist into adulthood, thereby preventing or postponing CHD events such as myocardial infarction, coronary angioplasty, and bypass surgery. Confirmation of such long-term success will require several more decades of follow-up. However, evidence accumulated to date makes it prudent to recommend a heart-healthy diet, vigorous physical activity, maintenance of ideal body weight, and avoidance of cigarette smoking.[11]

The purpose of this chapter is to (1) assess the prevalence of different CHD risk factors as reported in cross-sectional studies of children of different ages and ethnicity; (2) examine longitudinal studies of "tracking" of CHD risk factors in children, including autopsy studies of those who were study participants earlier in their lives, and then review investigations that examine the efficacy of hygienic and pharmacologic treatment of CHD risk factors in children; (3) survey recommendations for screening children for CHD risk factors; (4) present recommendations for treatment of children found to be at high risk for CHD events later in life; and (5) outline current prevention recommendations for optimizing the cardiovascular health of all children.

Coronary Risk Factors in Youth

In the 1970s and 1980s, studies in North America documented the prevalence of CAD risk factors in children of diverse racial and ethnic backgrounds. Investigators in Bogalusa, Louisiana,[12] studied black and white children, while the National Health and Nutrition Examination Survey (NHANES) surveyed children of all major ethnicities 9 to 11 years of age nationwide.[13-15] Several other studies have focused on Latino, Native American, and Alaskan children in the United States[16,17] and indigenous First Nation children in Canada.[18] Studies in Finland have also added to the knowledge base of children's cardio-

vascular risk factors at different ages.[19] Results from these and other studies are discussed below.

Nutrition

Measurement of nutritional intake can be done by such methods as direct observation or measurement of cafeteria leftovers, but food diaries or a 24-h recall using food models are more adaptable to epidemiologic studies.[20]

More than a decade ago, Bogalusa and NHANES data indicated that children in the U.S. derive 36 to 39 percent of their calories from fat, with approximately 16 percent of calories coming from saturated fat (goals for these two indicators are 30 and 10 percent respectively). Snacks contributed approximately one-fourth of all caloric intake, with a percentage of fat similar to that of the children's regular meals.[21]

Data from the U.S. Department of Agriculture (USDA) Continuing Survey program suggest that children's diets have improved in recent years, but approximately 70 percent of children still exceed current guidelines for both total and saturated fat intake.[22] USDA investigators reported that only 1 percent of the U.S. population met recommendations for all food groups in feeding their children, but even that group exceeded fat intake guidelines.[11] Moreover, in 1995, some 72 percent of U.S. high school students ate fewer than five servings of fruits and vegetables per day.[23]

Lipids

In most of the studies reported herein, Lipid Research Clinic techniques have been used to measure total blood cholesterol (TC), HDL-C, and triglycerides. If serum triglycerides (TGs) are < 400 mg/dL, LDL-C can be calculated as LDL = TC − HDL −(TG/5).[24,25] In general, levels of TC and its subfractions are similar in boys and girls until puberty, after which HDL-C decreases significantly in boys.

Differences between children of different ethnic groups within the United States have been studied. In a multiethnic community in southern California, children of Vietnamese-American, European-American, and Latino origins had similar mean TC concentrations, ranging from 165 to 172 mg/dL.[26] Levels of TC and LDL-C in Navajo children were similar to those of children in the general U.S. population, but their HDL-C was 5 to 10 mg/dL lower and their triglyceride levels were 30 mg/dL higher.[16] In the Child and Adolescent Trial for Cardiovascular Health (CATCH), TC levels were similar among Caucasian, African-American, and Hispanic children, while HDL-C levels were higher in African-American boys and girls than children in the other two ethnic categories.[27]

Table 16–2 shows trends in TC levels among adolescents aged 12 to 17 years screened between 1966 and 1994 in three major population-based studies.[28] During this time, there has been a general decrease in mean TC levels, from 165 to 157 mg/dL, among boys and from 170 to 164 mg/dL among girls. The decline appears to have been greater among white than among black youth.

Data from NHANES Phase III (Table 16–3) show that approximately one-quarter of children still have borderline-high (170 to 199 mg/dL) TC, with another 10 percent being in the elevated (200 mg/dL or greater) category. Non-Hispanic black children have the highest cholesterol levels, with mean TC levels of 168 mg/dL in boys and 171 mg/dL in girls, compared with non-Hispanic whites, where the respective values are 162 mg/dL in boys and 166 mg/dL in girls.[28]

The multicenter Pathobiological Determinants of Atherosclerosis in Youth (PDAY) study—which evaluated coronary arteries, aortas, and blood and other specimens from over 1500 individuals 15 to 34 years old at autopsy—showed that atherosclerotic intimal surface involvement in both the aorta and right coronary arteries was positively correlated with LDL-C and very low density lipoprotein cholesterol (VLDL-C) concentrations and negatively associated with HDL-C levels.[29] Autopsy studies in Bogalusa Heart Study participants 7 to 24 years of age showed that coronary artery fatty streaks as well as aortic and coronary fibrous plaques were directly associated with levels of LDL-C measured previously.[30] Others have recently shown coronary artery calcium deposition (as documented by electron beam computed

TABLE 16–2 Trends in Mean Serum Total Cholesterol Levels Among U.S. Adolescents 12 to 17 Years of Age by Sex and Race: 1966–1970, 1971–1974, and 1988–1994

Population	NHES III* (1966–1970)			NHANES I† (1971–1974)			NHANES III‡ (1988–1994)		
	N	Mean	(SE)§	N	Mean	(SE)§	N	Mean	(SE)§
Male									
Black	471	171	(1.8)	250	165	(2.5)	389	166	(1.5)
White	3024	163	(0.7)	806	163	(1.4)	622	155	(1.6)
Total	3514	165	(0.8)	1064	164	(1.3)	1055	157	(1.3)
Female									
Black	513	172	(1.6)	259	174	(3.5)	456	168	(1.4)
White	2668	170	(0.9)	796	166	(1.4)	714	163	(1.5)
Total	3196	170	(0.8)	1062	167	(1.3)	1222	164	(1.3)
Total¶	6710	167	(0.7)	2126	165	(1.0)	2277	160	(1.1)

*National Health Examination Survey III.
†First National Health and Nutrition Examination Survey.
‡Third National Health and Nutrition Examination Survey.
§Standard error of the mean.
¶Includes other race groups in addition to white and black.
Source: Centers for Disease Control.[28]

TABLE 16–3 Serum Total Cholesterol Levels Among U.S. Children and Adolescents 4 to 19 Years of Age, by Age, Sex, and Race/Ethnicity: NHANES III, 1988–1994

Population Group	N	Mean (SE)*	Percentiles						
			5	10	25	50	75	90	95
Age[†]									
4–5 years	1707	162 (0.9)	124	132	144	161	177	194	204
6–8 years	1367	166 (1.0)	126	134	149	165	182	197	209
9–11 years	1488	171 (1.0)	131	139	151	168	187	206	222
12–15 years	1502	161 (1.2)	118	126	141	158	178	197	209
16–19 years	1435	165 (1.6)	118	124	141	158	182	207	222
12–19 years	2937	163 (1.0)	118	125	141	158	180	201	217
Total (4–19 years)	7499	165 (0.6)	121	130	145	162	181	200	216
Sex and age[†]									
Male									
4–5 years		161 (1.5)	122	132	143	159	175	191	202
6–8 years		166 (1.7)	126	134	146	164	183	202	212
9–11 years		172 (2.0)	135	140	153	170	188	208	226
12–15 years		158 (1.6)	116	124	140	157	174	192	203
16–19 years		158 (1.8)	116	122	138	155	174	199	213
12–19 years		158 (1.2)	116	123	139	156	174	195	206
Total (4–19 years)		163 (1.0)	119	127	143	161	179	198	212
Female									
4–5 years		164 (1.3)	125	133	145	162	178	196	206
6–8 years		166 (1.4)	126	135	149	165	180	196	203
9–11 years		169 (1.5)	130	137	148	166	185	204	218
12–15 years		164 (1.9)	122	129	142	159	181	201	218
16–19 years		171 (2.3)	118	128	145	163	189	217	237
12–19 years		167 (1.3)	119	128	144	161	185	209	225
Total (4–19 years)		167 (0.8)	124	132	147	163	184	202	220
Race/ethnicity and sex									
Non-Hispanic black									
Male		168 (1.0)	122	132	148	165	186	204	219
Female		171 (1.2)	122	134	149	167	189	213	226
Non-Hispanic white									
Male		162 (1.2)	118	126	143	160	178	195	207
Female		166 (1.1)	123	132	146	163	182	200	217
Mexican American									
Male		163 (1.0)	121	129	143	159	180	202	213
Female		165 (1.1)	121	128	144	161	183	201	216

*Standard error of the mean.
[†]Includes other race/ethnicity groups in addition to non-Hispanic white, non-Hispanic black, and Mexican.
Source: From Winkleby et al.,[15] with permission.

tomography, or EBCT) to be correlated with the severity of atherosclerosis in adults. In a study of 29 youths aged 11 to 23 years with familial hypercholesterolemia (mean LDL-C, 229 mg/dL), 7 had coronary calcium detected by EBCT.[31]

Blood Pressure

Measurement of blood pressure (BP) in children is subject to several potential sources of error. These include equipment differences, use of different endpoints for measuring systolic blood pressure (SBP) and diastolic blood pressure (DBP), patterns of bias by individual observers, variability among multiple determinations, and physiologic variability. The Working Group on Hypertension Control in Children and Adolescents examined several national data sets to develop normative BP tables and reported measurement standards, including preparation and positioning of the child, cuff size, and inflation and deflation rates. BP should be measured in a quiet environment after 3 to 5 min in a seated position. The BP should be recorded at least twice on each occasion, using a cuff whose width is approximately 40% of the arm circumference midway between the

olecranon and the acromion.[32] In recent years, published recommendations for notation of DBP by sphygmomanometry have varied. The First Task Force on Blood Pressure Control in Children recommended the use of phase IV Korotkoff sound (K4), and in the Bogalusa longitudinal study, Elkasabany and colleagues found that the fourth Korotkoff sound correlated better with adult BP than the fifth.[33] However, the 1996 Working Group recommended the use of phase V Korotkoff sounds for DBP measurement for children of all ages. It is recommended that BP be measured at least twice on each occasion after 3 to 5 min of rest. Readings are averaged and then compared with tables by age, gender, and height percentile. If the average SBP or DBP is at or above the 95th percentile, repeated measurements to confirm hypertension should be undertaken. With average readings below the 95th percentile but greater than or equal to the 90th percentile, the child is classified as "high normal."[32] Table 16–4 shows 95th percentile levels for blood pressure in children and adolescents by age and percentile for height.

In biracial studies of children in the U.S., African-Americans have higher blood pressure than whites. These differences persist over time, but after

TABLE 16–4 Ninety-Fifth Percentiles of Blood Pressure by Selected Ages in Girls and Boys by the 25th, 50th, and 75th Height Percentiles

Age	Girls' SBP/DBP Height Percentile			Boys' SBP/DBP Height Percentile		
	25th%	50th%	75th%	25th%	50th%	75th%
2	104/62	105/62	107/63	104/60	106/61	108/62
4	107/68	108/69	109/69	109/67	111/68	113/69
6	110/72	111/73	112/73	112/73	114/74	115/75
8	113/75	115/75	116/76	114/76	116/77	118/78
10	117/77	119/78	120/79	117/79	119/80	121/80
12	121/80	123/80	124/81	121/80	123/81	125/82
14	125/82	126/83	128/83	127/81	128/82	130/83
16	127/83	128/84	130/85	132/84	134/85	136/86

Key: SBP, systolic blood pressure; DBP, diastolic blood pressure.

Source: Adapted from the National High Blood Pressure Education Program Working Group on Hypertension Control in Children and Adolescents,[32] with permission. Blood pressures shown represent the 95th percentile levels by age, within 25th, 50th, and 75th percentile levels of height, for girls and boys.

adjustment for body size, the difference is substantially less.[34] Sociobehavioral factors are also important in hypertension development. For example, in a multisite study of young adults, black men and women who reported that they experienced racial discrimination and typically accepted this unfair treatment had significantly higher SBP and DBP than those who had not experienced discrimination or typically challenged it.[35]

In studies of children in California[36] and Chicago,[37] SBP and DBP were higher among Asian children than blacks, Latinos, and whites. In children of all ethnic groups, a strong correlation exists between obesity and blood pressure.

Obesity

Measurement of obesity is most conveniently done using body mass index (BMI), which is calculated as weight in kilograms divided by height in square meters [$kg/(m^2)$]. BMI is reasonably correlated with body fat estimates from skin-fold measurements and underwater weighing, methods more commonly used in small research studies.[38] Obesity and overweight have also been defined by percentile rank (e.g., 95th percentile) for each gender. In the U.S., the prevalence of obesity among boys and girls of all age groups has continued to increase in the past three decades, as measured in Bogalusa,[39] by the National Heart, Lung, and Blood Institute Growth and Health Study (NHLBI/GHS),[40] and by the National Health and Nutrition Examination Survey (NHANES) investigators.[41] These findings are true for each ethnic group studied, including blacks and whites in Louisiana,[39] Native Americans,[42] and Latinos.[43] Similar findings have been reported in the United Kingdom and Europe.[41] Obesity also leads to other CHD risk factors, including hypertension and dyslipidemias.[44]

Physical Inactivity

No direct measures of physical activity are suitable for large-scale studies, and indirect methods are often inconvenient or inaccurate in children. Nevertheless, the best estimates of participation by chil-

dren in aerobic activity show a dramatic downward trend in recent years.[45] In 1995, some 40 percent of high school students were not enrolled in a physical education class.[23] NHANES III data indicate that girls and boys who watch more than 4 h of television daily have greater body fat and greater BMI.[15] Obarzanek and colleagues reported similar findings after analyzing NHLBI/GHS data for physical activity and body fat in black and white girls.[40] Inactivity also adversely influences lipid levels; in one study, hours watching television were directly correlated with the likelihood the child had a total cholesterol of 200 mg/dL or greater.[46] As with other health behaviors, children are largely influenced by parents and peers in their decisions about habitual physical activity.[44]

Diabetes/Glucose Intolerance

The prevalence of non-insulin-dependent diabetes mellitus (NIDDM) among children has been rising recently, particularly in the indigenous peoples of North America (Native American children in the United States[16,17] and First Nation children in Canada). In Manitoba, for example, First Nation children are seven times more likely to have NIDDM than white children from the same region.[18] Coronary Artery Risk Development in Young Adults (CARDIA) investigators showed that physical inactivity and weight gain in children raises their fasting insulin and glucose levels.[47] Data from Bogalusa reveal persistence of elevated insulin levels—and their association with other CHD risk factors—over time.[48] Glaser has recently reviewed this subject from the genetic bases for these findings to community approaches for detection and intervention, reinforcing the efforts of primary care physicians to encourage weight reduction and physical activity as important measures to prevent the onset of diabetes in children.[49]

Smoking

Several laboratory methods exist to document cigarette smoking, including thiocyanate levels (from serum or saliva), serum cotinine, and breath analysis for carbon monoxide. For large-scale studies, however, self-report is often used.[50]

More than 1 million adolescents in the United States are daily smokers of cigarettes; two-thirds of all persons adopting the smoking habit are under age 18. These and other data are contained in periodic reports from the U.S. Surgeon General.[51] In 1995, some 35 percent of high school students had smoked cigarettes in the past month, ranging from 17 percent in Utah to 43 percent in West Virginia.[23] Even college students are smoking more now than previously.[52] In Bogalusa, Louisiana, black children who were smokers appeared to be more influenced by siblings and peers, while white children who adopted smoking were more likely to follow parents' smoking habits.[53] Nearly half of all children were given their first cigarette by family members or smoked it at home.[54] In Muscatine, Iowa, adolescent cigarette smoking was strongly correlated with friends' smoking habits.[55] A Copenhagen, Denmark, study revealed that maternal smoking doubled the likelihood that a child would become a smoker.[56]

In addition to its effect on lung function, smoking has been correlated with atherosclerosis in autopsy studies of adolescents.[57,58] In the Pathobiological Determinants of Atherosclerosis in Youth (PDAY) study, serum thiocyanate, which indicates tobacco usage, was also associated with the prevalence of raised atherosclerotic lesions, especially in the abdominal aorta.[29]

Family History

Bao and colleagues collected parental history of cardiovascular conditions from 8276 offspring. Children of parents who had experienced myocardial infarction or who were diabetic had significantly higher levels of TC, LDL-C, insulin, glucose, and body weight, as compared to those without a parental history. Children of hypertensive parents had significantly higher levels of blood pressure than their peers without such a family history. But it was concluded that because of the young age of parents, parental history information alone is not adequate to identify children needing lipid screening.[59] Whitaker and colleagues reported that among overweight chil-

dren at age 6, those with normal-weight parents have only a 24 percent chance of remaining overweight, while a child with at least one overweight parent has a 62 percent likelihood of remaining overweight.[60]

In the CARDIA study of black and white women and men aged 18 to 30 at baseline, parental risk indicators were consistently associated with increased CHD risk in their offspring. These included hypertension, glucose intolerance, obesity, and hyperlipidemia. Subjects with a parental history of myocardial infarction had higher levels of total cholesterol and blood pressure and lower levels of HDL-C.[34]

Sociodemographic Factors

Children from underserved populations, those from economically and educationally disadvantaged families, and those who live with little social support are found consistently to have higher levels of CHD risk factors. These observations have been made in North America,[61] Finland,[62] and the United Kingdom.[63]

Winkleby and colleagues analyzed data from 7686 children and young adults which were collected during the third NHANES survey. They examined risk-factor levels categorized by ethnicity (black, white, Mexican American) and by family socioeconomic status (SES) as represented by years of education of the head of household. Among study participants aged 18 to 24 whose head of household had less than 12 years of education, whites had much higher smoking rates (77 percent for men, 61 percent for women) than black and Mexican-American youth (35 percent) with similar SES levels. The rates for low-SES whites were twice as high as those for whites from higher SES groups and were nearly double the smoking rates for low-SES blacks and Mexican Americans.[15]

Cardiovascular Risk Tracking: Evidence from Longitudinal Studies

In 1973, the Bogalusa Heart Study began following cohorts of black and white children from birth through 17 years of age, noting changes in risk factors as subjects progressed through childhood and adolescence.[12] In several of the cohorts, observations have extended into young adulthood. After 15 years of surveillance, it was noted that subjects with LDL-C greater than 130 mg/dL at baseline were five times more likely to be hyperlipidemic and had double the risk of having hypertension, a low HDL-C level, and being overweight.[64]

The Cardiovascular Risk in Young Finns (CRYF) study was begun in 1980 with a cross-sectional survey of subjects 3, 6, 9, 12, 15, and 18 years of age. Subsequent examinations of these children and adolescents occurred 3 and 6 years thereafter, resulting in a total of 2236 subjects with complete follow-up data on serum lipids. The investigators found that reasonably good tracking for TC, HDL-C, and LDL-C values, particularly in boys. They noted that, when subjects were divided into quintiles, those at highest risk (high TC and LDL-C; low HDL-C) at baseline tended to become obese and to smoke cigarettes more frequently than others.[19]

The CARDIA study comprised 5115 black and white men and women aged 18 to 30 undergoing baseline examination in 1985–1986 at four centers, with follow-up at years 2, 5, 7, and 10. At the 7-year examination, approximately 80 percent of the original study cohort were evaluated. In this observational study, anthropometric, sociodemographic, health habit, blood pressure, insulin, glucose, and blood pressure measurements were made. Investigators found that, within each gender-race group, average diastolic blood pressure (DBP) was positively correlated with age, BMI, and alcohol intake; it was negatively correlated with physical activity. Blacks had higher DBP levels than whites, but the differences were attenuated greatly after accounting for obesity and the factors mentioned above.[34] They also noted that black-white differences in systolic blood pressure (SBP) were greatly reduced by taking into account experiences of racial discrimination and responses to unfair treatment recorded at the year 7 surveys.[35] In all gender-race groups, an increase in body mass during the first 7 years was associated with altered glucose and insulin metabolism.[47]

The Dietary Intervention Study in Children (DISC) was begun in 1987 to examine the efficacy and safety of long-term dietary intervention to reduce LDL-C in children with TC levels between the 80th and 98th percentiles for their age and gender. Children with higher levels were considered to be potential candidates for pharmacologic therapy. Mean age of the 362 boys was 9.7 years, while the 301 girls averaged 9.0 years. Subjects were then randomized to either usual care (notification of the children's high cholesterol levels plus educational publications) or to the intervention group, which consisted of individual and group sessions with parents and children during the subsequent 3 years, advocating a 28 percent fat diet (<8 percent of calories from saturated fat). The efficacy outcome measure was LDL-C, while measurements of height, ferritin, folate, albumin, HDL-C, triglycerides, sexual maturation, and psychosocial function were among the safety and efficacy outcomes. Levels of LDL-C decreased significantly more in the intervention group (15.4 mg/dL) than in the usual-care group (11.9 mg/dL). There were no differences in any of the safety outcome measures, indicating no adverse effects on growth or other function from the reduced-fat diet.[65] Maternal willingness to implement the study diet was significantly correlated to reduced saturated fat intake in children.[66]

In 1988, the NHLBI began its 5-year National Growth and Health Study (NGHS) of 2379 nine- and ten-year-old black and white girls at three clinical centers. Anthropometric, nutritional, blood pressure, and serum lipid measurements were done annually. At baseline, it was found that black girls were taller and heavier and had higher values of blood pressure and HDL-C. LDL-C and TC were similar in whites and blacks.[67] Body fatness correlated with both reduced energy expenditure (and increased television viewing), the percentage of saturated fat recorded on 3-day food records, and age.[40]

The Child and Adolescent Trial for Cardiovascular Health (CATCH) was a NHLBI-sponsored multicenter elementary school–based intervention study begun in 1991, which was designed to enhance heart-healthy eating, increased physical activity, and smoking abstention. Serum TC level was the primary physiologic outcome measure, while anthropometric, blood pressure, heart rate, and HDL-C measurements were also made and analyzed.[68] At each site,

24 schools were randomly assigned to one of three groups: control, school-based intervention, or school-based plus family-based intervention. Of 5106 children enrolled at baseline, 4019 were reexamined 2 1/2 years later. At that time, no significant differences were noted between the two intervention groups, so their data were pooled for analysis.[69] At the follow-up examination, children who were higher than the 85th percentile for BMI had significantly higher levels of TC, lower HDL-C values, and lower performance times on a 9-min run than less ponderous children. Being overweight and overfat at baseline was the strongest predictor of adiposity 2 1/2 years later.[70]

Nutrient intake in the intervention group showed significant improvements in all ethnic groups and in both genders. Analysis in one subsample of the CATCH population showed that total fat intake decreased from 32.7 to 30.3 percent of total calories, while saturated fat consumption dropped from 12.8 to 11.4 percent.[71] Although statistically significant differences in the children's health behaviors were noted at follow-up, both control and intervention groups had a decrease of approximately 1.0-mg/dL in serum total cholesterol. The authors speculated that the lack of significant lipid changes may have resulted from the limited intensity of the intervention (40 min per week for 12 to 15 weeks), short duration (2 1/2 years of follow-up), and suboptimal change in parental health behaviors.[69]

Recommendations for Screening

Dyslipidemias

The American Academy of Pediatrics (AAP) in their statement on cholesterol concluded that "serum cholesterol level is an imperfect predictor of future coronary vascular disease" and recommended "selective screening of children more than 2 years of age whose risk of developing coronary vascular disease can be identified by family history." They suggested that those with a parent or grandparent with coronary or peripheral artery disease before the age of 55 should have a fasting lipid profile done. Those having a par-

ent with total cholesterol level of 240 mg/dL or higher should have a nonfasting total cholesterol determination.[72] The British Hyperlipidaemia Association agrees that selective screening based on family history is appropriate but recommends a nonfasting total cholesterol test as the first step for evaluation in all children.[73]

Others have recommended one-time universal screening of children for dyslipidemia, noting that 50 percent or more of children with hypercholesterolemia would be missed using AAP screening criteria.[74–76] Of course, the yield of cases with heterozygous familial hypercholesterolemia would be low,[77] but a high prevalence of children with TC > 200 mg/dL is very likely (> 10 percent in several studies),[25,28] suggesting that behavioral intervention in families might best be started early after such identification from school-based testing [74] and intervention[71] programs. In reply, critics of such a policy have suggested that the children identified as hyperlipidemic might suffer psychologically,[78] for which there is conflicting evidence.

The National Cholesterol Education Program (NCEP) for Children and Adolescents proposed two categories of screening indicators: (1) major screening indicators, defined as a family history of early vascular disease or TC of 240 mg/dL or greater, and (2) discretionary indicators, which include smoking, diabetes, hypertension, high fat consumption, or steroid use. In their study population, Diller and colleagues found that 30 percent of children with high LDL-C levels were identified solely by the discretionary factors.[79] The NCEP recommends a scheme for risk assessment based on initial measurement of total cholesterol (Fig. 16–1) and for assessment, classification, and follow-up based on LDL-C (Fig. 16–2).[80]

High Blood Pressure

The National High Blood Pressure Education Program Working Group report provided detailed information about BP measurement methods in children but did not address the possible psychological hazards in identifying children as being hypertensive. They continue to recommend the incorporation of

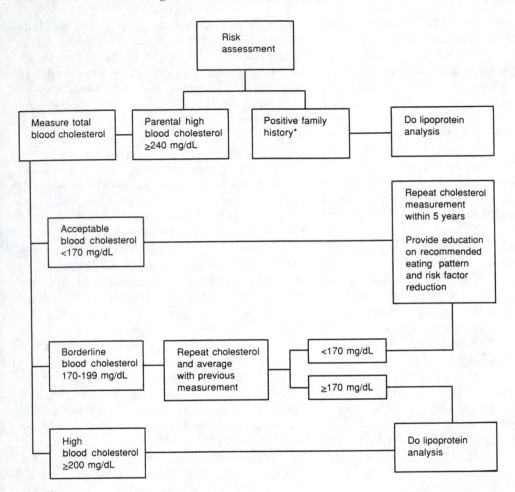

FIGURE 16–1 Risk assessment based on initial measurement of total cholesterol.
*Defined as a history of premature (before age 55) cardiovascular disease in a parent or grandparent.
(Adapted from the National Cholesterol Education Program.[80])

blood pressure measurement into the routine pediatric office examination. Values for 95th percentile values for SBP and DBP by age and percentile of height are provided in Table 16–4.[32]

Obesity

International scientific groups generally agree that calculation of BMI offers a reasonable index of adiposity in children and adolescents without a significant prevalence of stunted growth. It should be used more carefully in developing countries and in certain ethnic groups in North American populations.[81] Despite these caveats, body weight and height remain parameters that are easily and reliably assessed and should be measured at most clinical encounters. Levels of BMI above 25 kg/m^2 generally define overweight, with levels above 30 kg/m^2 indicating obesity.

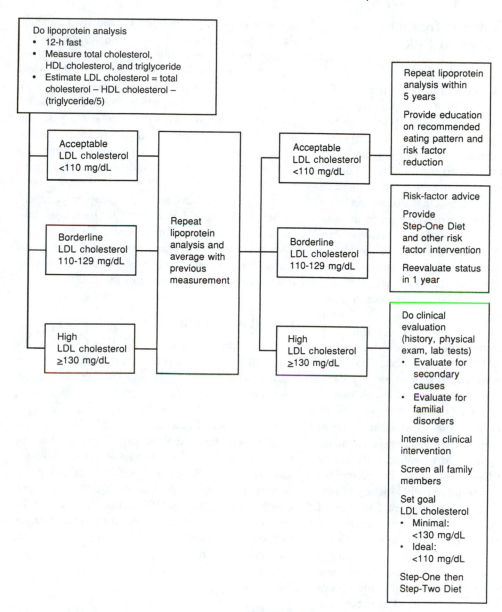

FIGURE 16–2 Classification, education, and follow-up based on low-density-lipoprotein cholesterol.
(Adapted from the National Cholesterol Education Program.[80])

Recommendations for Treatment in Children at Elevated Risk

Hyperlipidemia

The initial treatment in children above the age of 2 with elevated serum cholesterol levels is dietary management. Although a TC of 170 mg/dL or greater or an LDL-C of 130 mg/dL or greater should trigger dietary intervention (if not already implemented), the Step 1 Diet is recommended for all children above the age of 2. It consists of lowering the percentage of fat in the child's diet to less than 30 percent, with less than 10 percent of calories coming from saturated fat and less than 300 mg of cholesterol per day. The Step 2 Diet reduces saturated fat intake to less than 7 percent of caloric intake and dietary cholesterol intake to less than 300 mg/day.[72] When closely monitored, these diets have been shown not to retard growth and development. Figure 16–3 presents a schematic diagram of an initiation and follow-up schedule used for dietary intervention.[80] Aerobic exercise is important in maintaining an ideal body weight, which, in turn, contributes to lower cholesterol levels. In children above age 10 with two or more risk factors for CHD, drug therapy may be given if LDL-C remains above 160 mg/dL after at least 6 months of appropriate diet and exercise maintenance. The threshold for drug treatment in children with less than two CHD risk factors is 190 mg/dL; for those with either a positive family history of premature cardiovascular disease (before 55 years of age) or two or more risk factors (after vigorous attempts have been made to control such risk factors), the threshold is 160 mg/dL.[80] The minimum goal is an LDL-C of less than 130 mg/dL and ideally less than 110 mg/dL. Traditionally, bile-acid sequestrants such as cholestyramine and colestipol have been the first choice for treatment.[82] Nicotinic acid should be considered only in special circumstances and prescribed after referral to a lipid specialist only if cholesterol-lowering therapy by diet and bile-acid sequestrants has failed to reach therapeutic goals. Considering that nicotinic acid beneficially alters the entire lipid profile, it may be especially helpful for children and adolescents with elevated LDL-C accompanied by hypertriglyceridemia or low HDL-C.

Blood uric acid, glucose levels, and liver function should be monitored at each visit, as therapeutic dosages may be more likely to cause toxicity when used in youth or adolescents.[60] Although HMG-CoA reductase inhibitors are not generally recommended for treatment of dyslipidemia in children and adolescents, results from a recent multicenter study do suggest that they are effective in children with familial hypercholesterolemia. Compared with placebo, LDL-C levels decreased significantly (p < 0.001) by 17 percent, 24 percent, and 27 percent in those receiving dosages of 10, 20, and 40 mg/day, respectively. Although safety guidelines have not been issued for the use of these agents in children, these investigations noted that measurements of growth and sexual maturation did not differ between treatment and control groups during the course of the study.[77]

High Blood Pressure

Obese children who lose weight and successfully maintain a more ideal body weight will have substantial reductions in SBP and DBP (and improvements in lipids as well), so counseling on exercise and decreased caloric intake is essential. Cessation of smoking will likewise reduce BP. The National High Blood Pressure Education Program Working Group recommended a moderate reduction in dietary sodium through elimination of table salt and avoidance of prepared foods with high sodium content. Children whose SBP or DBP remains above the 95th percentile after implementation of hygienic methods can be treated pharmacologically. Diuretics and beta blockers have proven to be safe and useful; newer agents should be used with caution.[32]

Obesity

Investigators in children's weight-loss studies have shown that more than 80 percent of participants return to their original weight percentile. Factors favoring success include frequent contact with the intervention team, parental involvement and support in food preparation, adherence to an exercise prescription, and setting of realistic goals. For most obese children, a writing group for the American Heart Association (AHA)

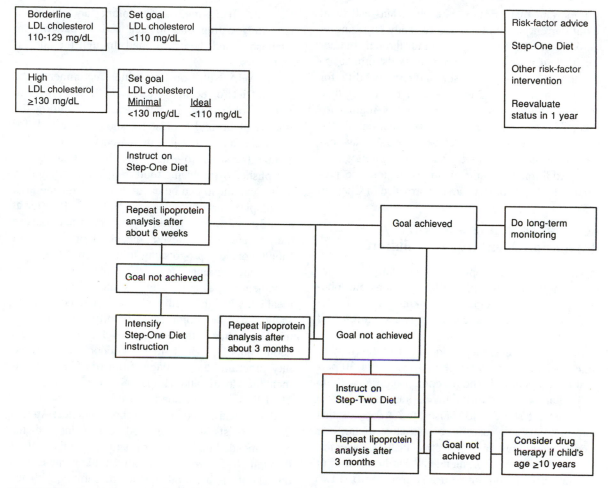

FIGURE 16–3   Follow-up schedule for dietary therapy. (Adapted from the National Cholesterol Education Program.[80])

suggests that "the primary emphasis of treatment should be prevention of weight gain above that appropriate for expected increases in height. For many children, this may mean limited or no weight gain while linear growth proceeds normally."[83] Behavioral, dietary, pharmacologic, and surgical treatments of childhood obesity have recently been reviewed.[84]

Physical Activity

As with other health behaviors, attitude and self-efficacy are important determinants of adoption of

exercise as a routine habit. An exercise "prescription" by the child's physician can complement efforts at home and school to encourage the overweight child to be aerobically active. Additional recommendations for physical activity in youth are discussed in detail in Chap. 12.

Smoking

Most adult smokers begin their habit during adolescence (or earlier).[85] Although smoking cessation programs have low success rates among adolescents, it is important that primary care physicians ask them about current smoking. Those currently engaging in smoking can be encouraged to quit through the acquisition of positive reinforcement skills, emphasizing the importance of assuming responsibility for one's own health.[86] The long-term impact of this, however, is uncertain, and prevention of regular tobacco usage is where efforts are best focused. At the community level, efforts at point-of-sale law enforcement and prohibitive pricing of cigarettes may help. Additional recommendations for tobacco prevention and control in youth are provided in Chap. 9.

Recommendations for Primary Prevention Measures in Children

Preventing the development of coronary risk factors—including dyslipidemia, hypertension, obesity, diabetes, and cigarette smoking—remains the priority of preventive cardiology in children and adolescents.

In order to prevent dyslipidemia in children more than 2 years old, an average daily intake of 30 percent of total calories should come from fat, with no more than one-third of the fat calories coming from saturated fat sources. Because the AAP holds that some parents may use more restrictive diets, their recommendations carefully state that "a lower intake of fat is not recommended." Further, "skim or low-fat milk should not be used during the first two years of life because of the high protein and electrolyte content and low calorie density of these milks."[72] Again, aerobic exercise and maintenance of an ideal body weight will help prevent dyslipidemias.

High blood pressure is best prevented by ensuring that all children are aerobically active, maintain an ideal body weight, and limit their caloric and sodium intake to recommended levels. Children with a familial history of hypertension should be monitored carefully and often to assure early detection. Smoking and alcohol should be avoided.

Nutritional strategies aimed at the prevention of obesity is a task that begins in utero; it is affected by maternal obesity, weight gain during pregnancy, and diabetes.[87] It continues during infancy and childhood as feeding, eating, and physical activity patterns are established and then continued through the adolescent years.

The AHA Nutrition Committee recommends the Step 1 Diet for normal growth and development in children older than 2 years, and that limiting the amount of fat and cholesterol should be a task for the entire family, not just the parents. After age 2, a gradual transition to a heart-healthy diet can be accomplished by replacing foods rich in fat with grains, fruits, lean meat, and other foods low in fat and high in complex carbohydrates and protein.[88] If, after at least 3 months on the Step 1 Diet, minimal goals of therapy are not achieved, the child or adolescent should consider progressing to the Step 2 Diet.[80]

At home, parents can serve as role models for engagement in physical activities and maintenance of ideal body weight. With community encouragement, schools can be prompted to modify their environment to increase the activity level of children and adolescents.[44,89] Guidelines for school and community programs are available from the U.S. Department of Health and Human Services.[90] Appendix 16–1 lists foods intended to decrease saturated fatty acid and total fat content of school lunches; Appendix 16–2 lists snack-bar foods consistent with the recommended eating pattern; and Appendixes 16–3 through 16–5 give examples of sample menus based on school or fast-food lunches to comply with the Step 1 and 2 Diets while ensuring adequate caloric intake.[80]

Major national and state efforts have targeted tobacco prevention in youth. School-based programs to help students avoid adoption of the smoking habit have been successful.[91] Although information-only programs had limited success, those based on social and behavioral approaches were more successful.

Guidelines for school health programs to prevent tobacco use and addiction are available from the U.S. Department of Health and Human Services. They recommend that all schools (1) develop and enforce a school policy on tobacco use; (2) provide instruction about the short- and long-term negative physiologic and social consequences of tobacco use, social influences on tobacco use, peer norms regarding tobacco use, and refusal skills; (3) provide tobacco-use prevention education in kindergarten through 12th grade; (4) provide program-specific training for teachers; (5) involve parents or families in support of school-based programs to prevent tobacco use; (6) support cessation efforts among students and all school staff who use tobacco; and (7) assess the tobacco-use prevention program at regular intervals.[92]

In the North Karelia Youth Project, seventh-grade students began a 2-year program aimed at preventing smoking adoption. Students learned about social pressures to begin smoking, which are exerted by peers, parents, other adults, and mass media. They were trained by demonstration and role playing to resist such pressure. Cigarette consumption, measured 15 years after the intervention, was significantly reduced.[93]

A *Report of the Surgeon General* on preventing tobacco use among young people emphasizes the community's role. It concludes that:

A crucial element of prevention is access: adolescents should not be able to purchase tobacco products in their communities. Active enforcement of age-at-sale policies by public officials and community members appears necessary to prevent minors' access to tobacco. Communities that have adopted tighter restrictions have achieved reductions in purchases made by minors. At the state and national levels, price increases have significantly reduced cigarette smoking; the young have been at least as responsive as adults to these price changes. Maintaining higher real prices of cigarettes provides a barrier to adolescent tobacco use but depends on further tax increases to offset the effects of inflation.

The results of this review thus suggest that a coordinated, multicomponent campaign involving policy changes, taxation, mass media, and behavioral education can effectively reduce the onset of tobacco use among adolescents.[51]

Conclusions

Atherosclerosis, begins in childhood, and CHD risk factors, which can be identified at an early age, are correlated with the subsequent development of coronary artery lesions and events. The prevalence of CHD risk factors varies by age and ethnicity. Longitudinal studies demonstrate "tracking" of these indicators, and autopsy studies show correlation of the risk indicators and atherosclerosis.

Guidelines have been established for screening children for CHD risk factors, for treatment of those children found to be at high risk, and for the optimization of cardiovascular health for all children. Dietary and other lifestyle approaches remain the cornerstone for the prevention and control of CHD risk factors for most children and adolescents.

Recently, a call has been made for a united effort between health care providers and parents as well as active involvement of the nation's schools to reinforce adherence to desirable lifestyle behaviors and facilitate change at a population level.[11] Although government-subsidized programs for the prevention of tobacco use have been established in virtually every state, programs that target other cardiovascular risk factors such as obesity or physical inactivity are virtually nonexistent. A comprehensive approach toward cardiovascular health promotion is needed in our schools and must be encouraged and supported both at state and national levels. Such efforts involving the entire community and family unit are essential if we are to reverse the alarming trends of increasing obesity, physical inactivity, tobacco use, and other important CHD risk factors in children and adolescents.

APPENDIX 16–1 FOODS TO PROVIDE TO DECREASE SATURATED FATTY ACID AND TOTAL FAT CONTENT OF SCHOOL LUNCHES

Milk

Low-fat milk (1 percent)

Skim milk

Meat and meat alternatives

Lean cuts of meat, such as round steak, round rump, round tip roast, tenderloin roast

Lean ground beef (85 percent extra lean) or soy protein added to regular ground beef

Chicken or turkey without skin, baked, broiled, roasted, or boiled

Fresh or frozen fish, baked, broiled, or poached

Tuna fish or salmon

Cooked dry beans and peas, such as Great Northern, kidney, lima, navy, pinto, red, black, and garbanzo beans, black-eyed peas, lentils, and split peas

Low-fat and part-skim cheeses: farmer, cottage, part-skim ricotta and mozzarella

Peanut butter

Bread or bread alternatives

Breads and bread products: bagels, breads, graham crackers, muffins, rolls, and pancakes, including whole-grain or enriched products

Noodles, rice, barley, pasta, and bulgur

Fruits and/or Vegetables

Fresh, frozen, dried, or canned fruit: apricots, cantaloupe, grapefruit, grapes, honeydew melon, peaches, plums, prunes, raisins, tangerines, and strawberries

Fresh, frozen, or canned vegetables and salads: broccoli, brussels sprouts, cabbage, carrots, cauliflower, corn, green beans, green pepper, green peas, potatoes, lettuce, okra, spinach, sweet potatoes, tomatoes, winter squash, zucchini

Fats

Mayonnaise and dressings, including reduced-calorie and modified-fat, light, or low-sodium salad dressings

Margarine or liquid vegetable oils: canola, corn, cottonseed, olive, peanut, and safflower oils

Other

Baked goods low in fat: modified cakes and cookies, including angel-food cake, fig cookies, ginger snaps, oatmeal cookies, raisin cookies

Ice milk, sherbet, low-fat puddings, and low-fat yogurt

Source: Adapted from the Child and Adolescent Trial for Cardiovascular Health (CATCH) Eat Smart School Lunch Program Guide. A Guide for Nutrition Directors, Managers, and Cooks in Elementary School Cafeterias, 1990. In: National Cholesterol Education Program.[80]

APPENDIX 16–2 SNACK BAR FOOD CONSISTENT WITH RECOMMENDED EATING PATTERN

1 percent low-fat or skim milk, low-fat cheese, low-fat or nonfat yogurt (plain or with fruit)

Fresh fruits and vegetables

Dried fruits

Fruit juices and vegetable juices; soda water with fruit juice added

Pretzels, popcorn popped in unsaturated oil, bagels, bagel chips (no fat added), baked tortilla chips

Chef's salads prepared with lean meat or water-packed tuna and low-fat cheese served with low-fat or fat-free salad dressing

Sandwiches made with sliced turkey, lean roast beef, lean ham, low-fat cold cuts, and tuna salad prepared with water-packed tuna and reduced-fat mayonnaise or salad dressing

Peanut butter* and jelly sandwiches

Hamburgers or sloppy joes made with lean, well-drained ground beef or ground turkey

Tacos made with lean, well-drained ground beef and soft corn tortillas with low-fat cheese or a small amount of regular cheese

Beef, chicken, or bean chalupa with baked (not fried) corn tortilla and low-fat cheese or a small amount of regular cheese

Pizza made with lean, well-drained ground beef and low-fat cheese or a small amount of regular cheese

Nachos with baked (not fried) corn tortilla chips and con queso made with low-fat cheese

Cookies, cupcakes, and muffins prepared with unsaturated oil or margarine

Frozen yogurt (low-fat and nonfat), ice-milk, frozen fruit bars, sherbet, fruit sorbets, low-fat pudding pops

*High in total fat; low in saturated fatty acids.

Source: Adapted from the Child and Adolescent Trial for Cardiovascular Health (CATCH) Eat Smart School Lunch Program Guide. A Guide for Nutrition Directors, Managers, and Cooks in Elementary School Cafeterias, 1990. In: National Cholesterol Education Program.[80]

APPENDIX 16–3   SAMPLE MENUS FOR CHILDREN 7 TO 10 WITH SCHOOL LUNCH

Typical	Step-One Diet	Step-Two Diet
Breakfast at Home	**Breakfast at Home**	**Breakfast at Home**
Orange juice (1/2 cup)	Orange juice (1/2 cup)	Orange juice (1/2 cup)
Oatmeal w/maple and brown sugar (1 packet)	Oatmeal w/maple and brown sugar (1 packet)	Oatmeal w/maple and brown sugar (1 packet)
Whole milk (1 cup)	1% milk (1 cup)	Margarine (2 tsp)
		Skim milk (1 cup)
School Lunch	**School Lunch**	**Bag Lunch**
Oven fried chicken w/skin	Oven fried chicken w/skin	Ham sandwich:
Mashed potatoes (1/2 cup)	Mashed potatoes (1/2 cup)	Bread (2 slices)
Green beans w/butter (1/2 cup))	Green beans w/butter (1/2 cup)	Lean ham (2 oz)
Canned pear (1/2)	Canned pear (1/2)	Mayonnaise (2 tsp)
Whole milk (1 cup)	2% milk (1 cup)	Lettuce, tomato, pickles
		Banana (1 med)
		Skim milk (1 cup)
Snack at Home	**Snack at Home**	**Snack at Home**
Ham sandwich:	Turkey sandwich:	Turkey sandwich:
Bread (2 slices)	Bread (2 slices)	Bread (2 slices)
Ham luncheon meat (1 oz)	Turkey luncheon meat (1-1/2 oz)	Turkey luncheon meat (1-1/2 oz)
Lettuce, tomato, pickle	Low-fat cheese (1 oz)	Low-fat cheese (1 oz)
Mayonnaise (1/2 tbsp)	Lettuce, tomato, pickle	Lettuce, tomato, pickle
Cola drink (1 can)	Mayonnaise (1 tsp)	Margarine (1 tsp)
	Cola drink (1 can)	Mayonnaise (1 tsp)
		Cola drink (1 can)
Dinner at Home	**Dinner at Home**	**Dinner at Home**
Tuna macaroni casserole (1 serving)	Tuna macaroni casserole* (1 serving)	Tuna macaroni casserole† (1 serving)
Carrots and peas (1/2 cup)	Carrots and peas (1/2 cup)	Carrots and peas (1/2 cup)
Roll (1 small)	Roll (1 small)	Margarine (2 tsp)
Applesauce (1/2 cup)	Margarine (1 tsp)	Applesauce (1/2 cup)
Water	Applesauce (1/2 cup)	Water
	Water	
Snack at Home	**Snack at Home**	**Snack at Home**
Chocolate brownie (2″ × 1″)	Oatmeal cookies, commercial (4 medium)	Oatmeal cookies, homemade† (4 medium)
Whole milk (1 cup)	1% milk (1 cup)	Skim milk (1 cup)
Calories: 2,008	**Calories:** 2,005	**Calories:** 1,966
Fat, % cal: 35	**Fat, % cal:** 29	**Fat, % cal:** 29
SFA, % cal: 15	**SFA, % cal:** 11	**SFA, % cal:** 7
Cholesterol, mg: 261	**Cholesterol, mg:** 188	**Cholesterol, mg:** 126

*Stick margarine used for food preparation.

†Tub margarine used for food preparation.

Source: Adapted from the National Cholesterol Education Program.[80]

APPENDIX 16–4 SAMPLE MENUS FOR GIRLS 11 TO 14 WITH FAST-FOOD LUNCH

Typical	Step-One Diet	Step-Two Diet
Breakfast at Home	**Breakfast at Home**	**Breakfast at Home**
Orange juice (1 cup)	Orange juice (1 cup)	Orange juice (1 cup)
Pre-sweetened cereal (1 cup)	Corn flakes (3/4 cup)	Corn flakes (3/4 cup)
Whole milk (1 cup)	1% milk (1 cup)	Skim milk (1 cup)
		English muffin (1/2)
		Margarine[††] (1 tsp)
Fast Food Lunch	**Fast Food Lunch**	**Sandwich Shop**
Cheeseburger	Hamburger (1/4 lb)	Tuna sandwich:
French fries (1 regular order)	French fries (1 regular order)	Bread (2 slices)
Catsup (3 packets)	Lettuce, tomato, onion, catsup	Tuna, water pack (3 oz)
Cola drink (1 small)	Animal crackers (1/2 box)	Tomato, celery, relish
	Cola drink (1 medium)	Mayonnaise (4 tsp)
		Pretzels (3/4-oz bag)
		Oatmeal cookies, homemade[††] (4)
		Cola drink (1 medium)
Snack at Home	**Snack at Home**	**Snack at Home**
Ginger snaps (2 medium)	Multigrain low-fat crackers (4)	Multigrain low-fat crackers (4)
Club soda (1 can)	Low-fat cheese (3/4 oz)	Low-fat cheese (3/4 oz)
	Club soda (1 can)	Club soda (1 can)
Dinner at Home	**Dinner at Home**	**Dinner at Home**
Fried chicken breast, breaded and fried in shortening, skin eaten	Broiled chicken, breast, no skin (3 oz)	Broiled chicken, breast, no skin (3 oz)
Boiled potato* (1)	Boiled potato[†] (1)	Boiled potato[††] (1)
Broccoli spears* (1/2 cup)	Broccoli spears[†] (4)	Broccoli spears[††] (4)
Roll (1 small)	Tomato (4 slices)	Tomato (4 slices)
Margarine[†] (1 tsp)	Bread (1 slice)	Bread (1 slice)
Iced tea (1 cup)	Strawberries (1/2 cup)	Margarine[††] (2 tsp)
	Nonfat yogurt (1 container)	Strawberries (1/2 cup)
	Water	Nonfat yogurt (1 container)
		Water
Snack at Home	**Snack at Home**	**Snack at Home**
American cheese (3/4 oz)	Cupcake, commercial (1)	Cupcake, homemade (1)
Crackers (4)	1% milk (1 cup)	Skim milk (1 cup)
Fruit drink (1/2 cup)		
Calories: 2,219	**Calories:** 2,240	**Calories:** 2,248
Fat, % cal: 35	**Fat, % cal:** 29	**Fat, % cal:** 27
SFA, % cal: 15	**SFA, % cal:** 10	**SFA, % cal:** 6
Cholesterol, mg: 264	**Cholesterol, mg:** 188	**Cholesterol, mg:** 159

*Seasoned with butter.

[†]Stick margarine used in food preparation.

[††]Tub margarine used in food preparation.

Source: Adapted from the National Cholesterol Education Program.[80]

APPENDIX 16–5   SAMPLE MENUS FOR 15 TO 19-YEAR-OLD MALES WITH FAST-FOOD LUNCH

Typical	Step-One Diet	Step-Two Diet
Breakfast at Home	**Breakfast at Home**	**Breakfast at Home**
Orange juice (1 cup)	Orange juice (1 cup)	Orange juice (1 cup)
Granola cereal (1/2 cup)	Presweetened corn flakes (3/4 cup)	Presweetened corn flakes (3/4 cup)
Whole milk (1 cup)	Margarine (1 tsp)	Margarine (2 tsp)
	Bagel (1)	Bagel (1)
	1% milk (1 cup)	Skim milk (1 cup)
Fast Food Lunch	**Sandwich Shop**	**Sandwich Shop**
Hot dog on bun w/chili (1)	Roast beef sandwich	Roast beef sandwich
Potato chips (1 oz)	Tossed salad (2 cups)	Tossed salad (2 cups)
Cola drink (12 fl oz)	Thousand island dressing	Thousand island dressing (3 tbsp)
	(2 tbsp)	Medium cola drink
	Corn chips (1-oz bag)	
	Medium cola drink	
Snack at Home	**Snack at Home**	**Snack at Home**
Chocolate candy bar (2 oz)	Ham and cheese sandwich:	Turkey and cheese sandwich:
Cola drink (12 fl oz)	Bread (2 slices)	Bread (2 slices)
	Low-fat ham (1 oz)	Turkey breast (1 oz)
	Low-fat cheese (1 oz)	Low-fat cheese (1 oz)
	Mayonnaise (2 tsp)	Lettuce, tomato, pickles
	Lettuce, tomato, pickles	Mayonnaise (2 tsp)
	Oatmeal cookies, commercial (4)	Pretzels (3/4-oz bag)
	Orange juice (1 cup)	Gingersnaps (5)
		Orange juice (1 cup)
Dinner at Home	**Dinner at Home**	**Dinner at Home**
Beef lasagna (4″ × 3″)	Chicken cacciatore (3 oz)	Chicken cacciatore (3 oz)
Tossed salad (2 cups)	Green beans (1/2 cup)*	Green beans (1/2 cup)[†]
Thousand island dressing	Rice, white (1 cup)	Rice, white (1 cup)[†]
(3 tbsp)	Margarine (1 tsp)	Margarine (1-1/2 tsp)[†]
French bread (1 slice)	Bread (1 slice)	Bread (1 slice)
Brownies (2 each 2″ × 1″)	Grapes (15)	Grapes (15)
Whole milk (1 cup)	Nonfat yogurt w/fruit flavor (1 cup)	Nonfat yogurt w/fruit flavor (1 cup)
	Water	Water
Snack at Home	**Snack at Home**	**Snack at Home**
Frozen yogurt (1 cup)	Peanut butter cookies,	Apple pie, homemade,[†]
Cola drink (12 fl oz)	homemade (6)	single crust (1/8 of 9″)
	1% milk (1 cup)	Skim milk (1 cup)

Typical		Step-One Diet		Step-Two Diet	
Calories:	2,998	**Calories:**	3,026	**Calories:**	2,993
Fat, % cal:	36	**Fat, % cal:**	30	**Fat, % cal:**	29
SFA, % cal:	15	**SFA, % cal:**	9	**SFA, % cal:**	7
Cholesterol, mg:	258	**Cholesterol, mg:**	224	**Cholesterol, mg:**	157

*Stick margarine used for food preparation.

[†]Tub margarine used for food preparation.

Source: Adapted from the National Cholesterol Education Program.[80]

References

1. Ross R: Mechanisms of disease: atherosclerosis—an inflammatory disease. *N Engl J Med* 1999; 340:115–126.
2. Enos WF, Beyer JC, Holmes R: Pathogenesis of coronary artery disease in soldiers killed in Korea. *JAMA* 1955; 148:912–914.
3. McNamara JJ, Molot MA, Stremple JF, Cutting RT: Coronary artery disease in combat casualties in Vietnam. *JAMA* 1971; 216:1185–1187.
4. Strong JP, McGill HC Jr: The natural history of coronary atherosclerosis. *Am J Pathol* 1958; 34:209–235.
5. Holman RL, McGill HC Jr, Strong JP, Geer JC: The natural history of atherosclerosis: the early aortic lesions as seen in New Orleans in the middle of the 20th century. *Am J Pathol* 1958; 34:209–235.
6. Strong JP: Coronary atherosclerosis in soldiers: a clue to the natural history of atherosclerosis in the young. *JAMA* 1986; 256:2863–2866.
7. Hirvonen J, Yla-Herttuala S, Laaksonen H, et al: Coronary intimal thickenings and lipids in Finnish children who died suddenly. *Acta Paediatr Scand* 1985; 318(suppl):221–224.
8. McGill HC Jr: Persistent problems in the pathogenesis of atherosclerosis. *Arteriosclerosis* 1984; 4:443–451.
9. Davidson DM: *Preventive Cardiology.* Baltimore, Williams & Wilkins, 1991.
10. Wattigney WA, Webber LS, Srinivisan SR, Berenson GS: The emergence of clinically abnormal levels of cardiovascular disease risk factor variables among young adults: the Bogalusa Heart Study. *Prev Med* 1995; 24:617–626.
11. VanHorn L, Greenland P: Prevention of coronary artery disease is a pediatric problem. *JAMA* 1997; 278:1779–1780.
12. Berenson GS, Srinivisan SR, Bao W, et al: Association between multiple cardiovascular risk factors and atherosclerosis in children and young adults. *N Engl J Med* 1998; 338:1650–1656.
13. Troiano RP, Flegal KM, Kuczmarski RJ, et al: Overweight prevalence and trends for children and adolescents: the National Health and Nutrition Examination Surveys, 1963 to 1991. *Arch Pediatr Adolesc Med* 1995; 149:1085–1091.
14. Andersen RE, Crespo CJ, Bartlett SJ, et al: Relationship of physical activity and television watching with body weight and level of fatness among children. Results from the Third National Health and Nutrition Examination Survey. *JAMA* 1998; 279:938–942.
15. Winkleby MA, Robinson TN, Sundquist J, Kraemer HK: Ethnic variation in cardiovascular disease risk factors among children and young adults: findings from the Third National Health and Nutrition Examination Survey, 1988–1994. *JAMA* 1999; 281:1006–1013.
16. Freedman DS, Serdula MK, Percy CA, et al: Obesity, levels of lipids and glucose, and smoking among Navajo adolescents. *J Nutr* 1997; 127(10 suppl):2120S-2127S.
17. Cook VV, Hurley JS: Prevention of type II diabetes in childhood. *Clin Pediatr* 1998; 37:123–129.
18. Dean H: NIDDM-Y in First Nation children in Canada. *Clin Pediatr* 1998; 37:89–96.
19. Porkka KVK, Viikari JSA, Akerblom HK: Tracking of serum HDL-cholesterol and other lipids in children and adolescents: the Cardiovascular Risk in Young Finns Study. *Prev Med* 1991; 20:713–724.
20. Frank GC: Environmental influences on methods used to collect dietary data from children. *Am J Clin Nutr* 1994; 59(suppl):207S-211S.
21. Frank GC, Farris RP, Cresanta JL, et al: Dietary trends of 10- and 13-year-old children in a biracial community—the Bogalusa Heart Study. *Prev Med* 1985; 14:123–139.
22. American Dietetic Association: Position of the American Dietetic Association: dietary guidance for healthy children aged 2–11 years. *J Am Diet Assoc* 1999; 99:93–101.
23. Centers for Disease Control: *Chronic Diseases and Their Risk Factors: The Nation's Leading Causes of Death.* Bethesda, MD, Centers for Disease Control, 1998.
24. Lauer RM, Clarke WR: Use of cholesterol measurements in childhood for the prediction of adult hypercholesterolemia. *JAMA* 1990; 264:3034–3038.
25. Nicklas T, Webber LS, Srinivisan SR, Berenson GS: Secular trends in dietary intake and cardiovascular risk factors in 10-year-old children: the Bogalusa Heart Study (1973–1988). *Am J Clin Nutr* 1993; 57:930–937.
26. Davidson DM, Iftner CA, Bradley BJ, et al: Family history predictors of high blood cholesterol levels in 4th grade school children. *J Am Coll Cardiol* 1989; 13:36A.
27. Webber LS, Osganian V, Luepker RV, et al: Cardiovascular risk factors among third grade children in four regions of the United States: the CATCH Study. *Am J Epidemiol* 1995; 141:428–439.
28. Third Report on Nutrition Monitoring in the United States: Volume I. U.S. Government Printing Office, Washington, D.C., 1995.
29. PDAY Research Group: Relationship of atherosclerosis in young men to serum lipoprotein cholesterol concentrations and smoking: a preliminary report from the Pathobiological Determinants of Atherosclerosis in Youth (PDAY) Research Group. *JAMA* 1990; 264:3018–3024.
30. Newman WP, Wattigney W, Berenson GS: Autopsy studies in U.S. children and adolescents: relationship of risk factors to atherosclerotic lesions. *Ann NY Acad Sci* 1991; 623:16–25.
31. Gidding SS, Bookstein LC, Chomka EV: Usefulness of electron beam computed tomography in adolescents and young adults with heterozygous familial hypercholesterolemia. *Circulation* 1998; 98:2580–2583.
32. National High Blood Pressure Education Program Working Group on Hypertension Control in Children and Adolescents: Update on the 1987 Task Force Report on high blood pressure in children and adolescents: a working

group report from the National High Blood Pressure Education Program. *Pediatrics* 1996; 98:649–658.

33. Elkasabany AM, Urbina EM, Daniels SR, Berenson GS: Prediction of adult hypertension by K4 and K5 diastolic blood pressure in children: the Bogalusa Heart Study. *J Pediatr* 1998; 132:687–692.

34. Liu K, Ruth KJ, Flack JM, et al: Blood pressure in young blacks and whites: relevance of obesity and lifestyle factors in determining differences: the CARDIA study. *Circulation* 1996; 93:60–66.

35. Krieger N, Sidney S: Racial discrimination and blood pressure: the CARDIA study of young black and white adults. *Am J Public Health* 1996; 86:1370–1378.

36. Hohn AR, Dwyer KM, Dwyer JH: Blood pressure in youth from four ethnic groups: the Pasadena Prevention Project. *J Pediatr* 1994; 125:368–373.

37. Liu K, Levinson S: Comparisons of blood pressure between Asian-American children and children from other racial groups in Chicago. *Pub Health Rep* 1996; 111(suppl 2):65–67.

38. Goran MI: Measurement issues related to studies of childhood obesity: assessment of body composition, body fat distribution, physical activity and food intake. *Pediatrics* 1998; 101:505–518.

39. Freedman DS, Srinivisan SR, Valdez RA, et al: Secular increases in relative weight and adiposity among children over two decades; the Bogalusa Heart Study. *Pediatrics* 1997; 99:420–426.

40. Obarzanek E, Schreiber GB, Crawford PB: Energy intake and physical activity in relation to indexes of body fat: the National Heart, Lung, and Blood Institute Growth and Health Study. *Am J Clin Nutr* 1994; 60:15–22.

41. Troiano RP, Flegal KM: Overweight children and adolescents: description, epidemiology and demographics. *Pediatrics* 1998; 101:497–504.

42. Salbe AD, Fontvieille AM, Harper IT, Ravussin E: Low levels of physical activity in 5-year-old children. *J Pediatr* 1997; 131:423–429.

43. Malina RM, Zavaleta AN, Little BB: Estimated overweight and obesity in Mexican-American school children. *Int J Obesity* 1986; 10:483–491.

44. Smoak CG, Burke GL, Webber LS, et al: Relation of obesity to clustering of cardiovascular disease risk factors in children and young adults: the Bogalusa Heart Study. *Am J Epidemiol* 1987; 125:364–372.

45. Kohl HW, Hobbs KE: Development of physical activity behaviors among children and adolescents. *Pediatrics* 1998; 101:549–554.

46. Wong ND, Hei TK, Qaqundah PY, et al: Television viewing and pediatric hypercholesterolemia. *Pediatrics* 1992; 90:75–79.

47. Folsom AR, Jacobs DR Jr, Wagenknecht LE, et al: Increase in fasting insulin and glucose over seven years with increasing weight and inactivity of young adults: the CARDIA study. *Am J Epidemiol* 1996; 144:235–246.

48. Bao W, Srinivisan SR, Berenson GS: Persistent elevation of plasma insulin levels is associated with increased cardiovascular risk in children and young adults: the Bogalusa Heart Study. *Circulation* 1996; 93:54–59.

49. Glaser NS: Non-insulin-dependent diabetes mellitus in childhood and adolescence. *Pediatr Clin North Am* 1997; 44:307–337.

50. Luepker RV, Pallonen UE, Murray DM, Pirie PL: Validity of telephone surveys in assessing cigarette smoking in young adults. *Am J Public Health* 1989; 79:202–204.

51. Centers for Disease Control: *Preventing Tobacco Use among Young People: A Report of the Surgeon General.* DHHS publication no. S/N 017-001-00491-0. Atlanta, GA, U.S. Department of Health and Human Services, Public Health Service, CDC, 1994.

52. Wechsler H, Rigotti NA, Gledhill-Hoyt J, Lee H: Increased levels of cigarette use among college students. *JAMA* 1998; 280:1673–1678.

53. Baugh JG, Hunter SM, Webber LS, Berenson GS: Developmental trends of first cigarette smoking experience of children: the Bogalusa Heart Study. *Am J Public Health* 1982; 72:1161–1164.

54. Greenlund KJ, Johnson CC, Webber LS, Berenson GS: Cigarette smoking attitudes and first use among third-through sixth-grade students: the Bogalusa Heart Study. *Am J Public Health* 1997; 87:1345–1348.

55. Krohn MD, Naughton MJ, Skinner MF, et al: Social disaffection, friendship patterns and adolescent cigarette use: the Muscatine Study. *J School Health* 1986; 5:146–150.

56. Osler M, Clausen J, Ibsen KI, Jensen G: Maternal smoking during childhood and increased risk of smoking in young adulthood. *Int J Epidemiol* 1995; 24:710–714.

57. McGill HC Jr, McMahan CA, Malcom GT, et al: Effects of serum lipoproteins and smoking on atherosclerosis in young men and women. *Arterioscler Thromb Vasc Biol* 1997; 17:95–106.

58. Strong JP, Malcom GT, McMahan CA, et al: Prevalence and extent of atherosclerosis in adolescents and young adults: implications for prevention from the Pathobiological Determinants of Atherosclerosis in Youth Study. *JAMA* 1999; 281:727–735.

59. Bao W, Srinivisan SR, Wattigney WA, Berenson GS: The relation of parental cardiovascular disease to risk factors in children and young adults: the Bogalusa Heart Study. *Circulation* 1995; 91:365–371.

60. Whitaker R, Wright J, Pepe M, et al: Predicting obesity in young adulthood from childhood and parental obesity. *N Engl J Med* 1997; 337:869–873.

61. Bronner YL: Nutritional status outcomes for children: ethnic, cultural and environmental contexts. *J Am Diet Assoc* 1996; 96:891–903.

62. Leino M, Porkka KV, Raitakari OT, et al: Influence of parental occupation on coronary heart disease risk factors in children: the Cardiovascular Risk in Young Finns Study. *Int J Epidemiol* 1996; 25:1189–1195.

63. Power C, Mathews S: Origins of health inequalities in a national population sample. *Lancet* 1997; 350:1584–1589.

64. Bao W, Srinivisan SR, Wattigney WA, et al: Usefulness of childhood low-density lipoprotein cholesterol level in predicting adult dyslipidemia and other cardiovascular risks: the Bogalusa Heart Study. *Arch Intern Med* 1996; 156:1315–1320.

65. DISC Collaborative Research Group: Efficacy and safety of lowering dietary intake of fat and cholesterol in children with elevated low-density lipoprotein cholesterol: the Dietary Intervention Study in Children (DISC). *JAMA* 1995; 273:1429–1435.

66. Reimers TM, Brown KM, Van Horn L, et al: Maternal acceptability of a dietary intervention designed to lower children's intake of saturated fat and cholesterol: the Dietary Intervention Study in Children (DISC). *J Am Diet Assoc* 1998; 98:31–34.

67. NHLBI Growth and Health Study Research Group: Obesity and cardiovascular disease risk factors in black and white girls: the NHLBI Growth and Health Study. *Am J Public Health* 1992; 82:1613–1620.

68. Stone EJ, Osganian SK, McKinlay SM, et al: Operational design and quality control in the CATCH multicenter trial. *Prev Med* 1996; 25:384–399.

69. Webber LS, Osganian SK, Feldman HA, et al: Cardiovascular risk factors among children after a 2 1/2 year intervention—the CATCH Study. *Prev Med* 1996; 265:432–441.

70. Dwyer JT, Stone EJ, Yang M, et al: Predictors of overweight and overfatness in a multiethnic pediatric population. *Am J Clin Nutr* 1998; 67:602–610.

71. Lytle LA, Stone EJ, Nichaman MZ, et al: Changes in nutrient intakes of elementary school children following a school-based intervention: results from the CATCH Study. *Prev Med* 1996; 25:465–477.

72. American Academy of Pediatrics Committee on Nutrition: Cholesterol in children. *Pediatrics* 1998; 101:141–147.

73. Wray R, Neil H, Rees J: Screening for hyperlipidaemia in childhood: recommendations of the British Hyperlipidaemia Association. *J R Coll Physicians Lond* 1996; 30:115–118.

74. Davidson DM, VanCamp J, Iftner CA, et al: Family history fails to detect the majority of children with high capillary blood total cholesterol. *J School Health* 1991; 61:75–80.

75. Bao W, Srinivisan SR, Wattigney WA, et al: Usefulness of childhood low-density lipoprotein cholesterol level in predicting adult dyslipidemia and other cardiovascular risks. *Arch Intern Med* 1996; 156:1315–1320.

76. Bistritzer T, Batash D, Barr J, et al: Routine childhood screening for hyperlipidemia in Israel. *Israel J Med Sci* 1996; 32:725–729.

77. Stein EA, Illingworth DR, Kwiterovich PO, et al: Efficacy and safety of lovastatin in adolescent males with heterozygous familial hypercholesterolemia. *JAMA* 1999; 281:137–144.

78. Rosenberg E, Lamping DL, Joseph L, et al: Cholesterol screening of children at high risk: behavioural and psychological effects. *Can Med Assoc J* 1997; 156:489–496.

79. Diller PM, Huster GA, Leach AD, et al: Definition and application of the discretionary screening indicators according to the National Cholesterol Education Program for Children and Adolescents. *J Pediatr* 1995; 126:345–352.

80. National Cholesterol Education Program: *Report of the Expert Panel on Blood Cholesterol Levels in Children and Adolescents.* NIH Pub 91-2732. Bethesda, MD, National Heart Lung and Blood Institute, 1991.

81. Dietz WH, Robinson TN: Use of the body mass index (BMI) as a measure of overweight in children and adolescents. *J Pediatr* 1998; 132:191–193.

82. Tonstad S, Knudtzon J, Siversten M, et al: Efficacy and safety of cholestyramine therapy in peripubertal and prepubertal children with familial hypercholesterolemia. *J Pediatr* 1996; 229:42–49.

83. Gidding SS, Leibel RL, Daniels S, et al: Understanding obesity in youth. *Circulation* 1996; 94:3383–3387.

84. Epstein LH, Myers MD, Raynor HA, Saelens BE: Treatment of pediatric obesity. *Pediatrics* 1998; 101:554–570.

85. Johnston LD, O'Malley PM, Bachman JG: *National Survey Results on Drug Use from the Monitoring the Future Study, 1975–1993.* DHHS Publication PHS 94-3809. Washington, DC, Public Health Service; 1994.

86. Franzgrote M, Ellen JM, Millsein SG, Irwin CE: Screening for adolescent smoking among primary care physicians in California. *Am J Public Health* 1997; 87:131–134.

87. Whitaker RC, Dietz WH: Role of the prenatal environment in the development of obesity. *J Pediatr* 1998; 132:768–776.

88. Fisher EA, Van Horn L, McGill HC for the Nutrition Committee: Nutrition and Children: a statement for healthcare professionals from the Nutrition Committee, American Heart Association. *Circulation* 1997; 95:2332–2333.

89. Sallis J, McKenzie T, Alcaraz J, et al: The effects of a 2 year physical education program (SPARK) on physical activity and fitness in elementary school students. *Am J Public Health* 1997; 87:1328–1334.

90. Centers for Disease Control and Prevention: Guidelines for school and community programs to promote lifelong physical activity among young people. *MMWR* 1997; 46:1–35.

91. Elder JP, Perry CL, Johnson CC, et al: Tobacco use measurement, prediction, and intervention in elementary schools in four states. *Prev Med* 1996; 25:486–494.

92. Centers for Disease Control and Prevention: Guidelines for school health programs to prevent tobacco use and addiction. *MMWR* 1994; 43:1–18.

93. Vartiainen E, Paavola M, McAlister A, Puska P: Fifteen-year follow up of smoking prevention effects in the North Karelia Youth Project. *Am J Public Health* 1998; 88:81–85.

CHAPTER 17

Seniors

Wilbert S. Aronow

Coronary heart disease (CHD) is the most common cause of death in the elderly. CHD, stroke, and peripheral arterial disease (PAD) are more common in the elderly than in younger persons. Eighty-five percent of those who die of CHD are aged 65 and older. Annually in the United States, as estimated in 1995, approximately 418,000 men and 356,000 women aged 65 years and over experience a heart attack, compared with 250,000 men and 83,000 women under the age of 65. As for strokes, more than 70 percent occur in those aged 65 and over.[1]

Among the elderly, as estimated from the Cardiovascular Health Study, the incidence per 1000 of new and recurrent heart attacks in nonblack men increases from 26.3 in those aged 65 to 74 to 53.6 in those aged 85 and older. Among nonblack women, the incidence increases from 7.8 to 24.2, respectively. In black men, these rates increase from 16.3 to 54.9, and in black women the rates range from 13.3 to 18.3, being highest in those aged 75 to 84 years. The estimated annual rate per 1000 of new and recurrent strokes among the elderly increases from 14.4 among nonblack men aged 65 to 74 to 27.9 among nonblack men aged 85 and over; among nonblack women in the same age groupings, these rates range from 6.2 to 30.6; among black men, the rates increase from 11.9 to 40.8; and among black women, the rates range from 16.1 to 22.4.[2]

All the major risk factors for CHD in younger persons remain important in the elderly, as demonstrated by the Framingham Heart Study, which compared regression coefficients for each major risk factor in those aged 65 to 94 years versus those aged 35 to 64 years (Table 17–1).[3] Although some of the coefficients, as for serum cholesterol and smoking, appear

to be attenuated in the elderly, the greater absolute risk of CHD associated with any given risk factor in the elderly more than compensates for this. The prevalence of a number risk factors—including diabetes, dyslipidemia, and hypertension—increases dramatically with age, and these conditions are quite common in the elderly. This chapter discusses the significance of these and other risk factors for CHD, stroke, and PAD in the elderly as well as strategies for risk-factor modification for the prevention of cardiovascular disease (CVD) in the elderly.

Cigarette Smoking

The Cardiovascular Health Study demonstrated in 5201 men and women of age 65 or above that more than 50 pack-years of smoking was associated with a 1.6-fold greater mortality.[2] The Systolic Hypertension in the Elderly Program pilot project showed that smoking was a predictor of first cardiovascular event and myocardial infarction (MI)/sudden death.[4] At 30-year follow-up of persons 65 years of age and above in the Framingham Heart Study, cigarette smoking was not associated with the incidence of CHD but was associated with mortality from CHD in older men and women.[5] At 12-year follow-up of men 65 to 74 years of age in the Honolulu Heart Program, the absolute excess risk of nonfatal MI and fatal CHD associated with cigarette smoking was 1.9 times higher in older men than in middle-aged men.[6]

At 5-year follow-up of 7178 persons 65 years of age and above in three communities, the relative risk for CVD mortality was 2.0 for male smokers and 1.6 for female smokers.[7] The incidence of CVD

TABLE 17–1 Effect of Risk Factors on Coronary Heart Disease Incidence: Framingham Heart Study, 30-Year Follow-Up

| | Bivariate (age-adjusted) standardized regression coefficient | | | |
| | Ages 35–64 Years | | Ages 65–94 Years | |
Risk Factor	Men	Women	Men	Women
Systolic blood pressure	0.338*	0.418*	0.401*	0.286*
Diastolic blood pressure	0.321*	0.363*	0.296*	0.082
Serum cholesterol	0.322*	0.307*	0.121	0.213*
Cigarette smoking	0.259*	0.095	−0.017	−0.034
Blood glucose	0.043	0.206*	0.166*	0.209*
Vital capacity	−0.112†	−0.331*	−0.127	−0.253*
Relative weight	0.190*	0.264*	0.177‡	0.124†

$*p < .001$
$†p < .05$
$‡p < .01$

Source: From Cupples et al.[3]

mortality in former smokers was similar to that in those who had never smoked.[6] At 40-month follow-up of 664 men, mean age 80 years, and at 48-month follow-up of 1488 women, mean age 82 years, current cigarette smoking increased the relative risk of new coronary events (nonfatal or fatal MI or sudden cardiac death) to 2.2 in men and 2.0 in women (Table 17–2).[8] At 6-year follow-up of older men and women in the Coronary Artery Surgery Study registry, the relative risk of MI or death was 1.5 for persons 65 to 69 years of age and 2.9 for persons 70 years of age and above who continued smoking as compared with quitters during the year before study enrollment.[9]

A meta-analysis of 32 studies demonstrated that cigarette smoking was a risk factor for atherothrombotic brain infarction (ABI) in men and women with a relative risk of 1.9.[10] In the Medical Research Council Trial, the incidence of stroke was 2.3 times higher in cigarette smokers than in nonsmokers.[11] Nonsmokers who received propranolol as antihypertensive therapy had a lower incidence of stroke, whereas cigarette smokers did not.[11] At 26-year follow-up in the Framingham Heart Study, cigarette smoking was associated with an increased incidence

of ABI of 1.6-fold in men and 1.9-fold in women.[12] The incidence of stroke in cigarette smokers who smoked more than 40 cigarettes daily was twice as high as in those who smoked fewer than 10 cigarettes daily. The impact of cigarette smoking did not decrease with increasing age. The risk of stroke was substantially reduced within 2 years of quitting smoking, with the incidence of stroke returning to the level of nonsmokers 5 years after cessation of smoking.[12]

At 42-month follow-up of 664 men, mean age 80 years, and at 48-month follow-up of 1488 women, mean age 82 years, current cigarette smoking was associated with an increased relative risk of new ABI of 1.5 in men and 1.9 in women (Table 17–2).[13] In a study of 1063 persons, mean age 81 years, cigarette smoking was associated with a 4.2-fold increased likelihood of significant narrowing in diameter of the extracranial, internal, or common carotid artery.[14]

Numerous studies have demonstrated that cigarette smoking is a risk factor for PAD in men and women.[15–21] In a study of 244 men and 625 women, mean age 82 years, cigarette smoking increased the

TABLE 17–2 Association of Cigarette Smoking with New Coronary Events, New Atherothrombotic Brain Infarction (ABI), and Peripheral Arterial Disease (PAD) in Elderly Men and Women

Study	No.	Mean Age, years	Follow-Up, months		Relative Risk	
			Men	Women	Men	Women
Incidence of new coronary events[8]	2152	81	40	48	2.2	2.0
Incidence of new ABI[13]	2152	81	42	48	1.5	1.9
Prevalence of PAD[21]	869	82	—	—	2.4	2.9

prevalence of PAD 2.4 times in men and 2.9 times in women (Table 17–2).[21] At 43-month follow-up of 291 persons, mean age 82 years, with PAD, cigarette smoking was an independent predictor of new coronary events with a relative risk of 1.6.[22]

Elderly men and women who smoke cigarettes should be strongly encouraged to stop smoking to reduce the development of CHD, ABI, and PAD. Smoking cessation will decrease mortality from CHD, other CVD, and all-cause mortality in elderly men and women. Approaches to smoking cessation include use of nicotine patches or nicotine gum, which are available over the counter.[23] If this therapy is unsuccessful, nicotine nasal spray or treatment with the antidepressant drug buproprion should be considered.[23,24] Concomitant behavioral therapy may also be needed.

Hypertension

Increased peripheral vascular resistance is the cause of systolic and diastolic hypertension in elderly persons. Systolic hypertension in elderly persons is diagnosed if the systolic blood pressure is 140 mmHg or higher from two or more readings on two or more visits.[25] Diastolic hypertension in elderly persons is similarly diagnosed if the diastolic blood pressure is 90 mmHg or higher.[25] In a study of 1414 persons, mean age 82 years, the prevalence of hypertension was 50 percent in elderly African Americans, 35 percent in elderly Hispanics, and 36 percent in elderly whites.[26]

Isolated systolic hypertension in elderly persons is diagnosed if the systolic blood pressure is 140 mmHg or higher with a diastolic blood pressure of less than 90 mmHg.[25] Based on an earlier systolic blood pressure threshold of 160 mmHg or higher, isolated systolic hypertension was diagnosed in 51 percent of 499 elderly persons with hypertension.[27]

Isolated systolic hypertension and diastolic hypertension are both associated with increased CVD morbidity and mortality in elderly persons.[28] Increased systolic blood pressure is a greater risk factor for CVD morbidity and mortality than is increased diastolic blood pressure.[28] The higher the systolic or diastolic blood pressure, the greater the morbidity and mortality from CHD in elderly women and men. The Cardiovascular Health Study demonstrated in 5201 elderly men and women that a brachial systolic blood pressure >169 mmHg was associated with a 2.4-fold greater 5-year mortality.[2]

At 30-year follow-up of persons 65 years of age and above in the Framingham Heart Study, systolic hypertension was related to a greater incidence of CHD in elderly men and women.[5] Diastolic hypertension correlated with the incidence of CHD in elderly men but not in elderly women.[5] At 40-month follow-up of 664 elderly men and 48-month follow-up of 1488 elderly women, systolic or diastolic hypertension was associated with a relative risk of new coronary events of 2.0 in men and 1.6 in women (Table 17–3).[8] Recent data from Framingham also suggests the importance of increased pulse pressure, a measure of large artery stiffness. Among 1924 men

TABLE 17–3 Association of Systolic or Diastolic Hypertension with New Coronary Events, New Atherothrombotic Brain Infarction (ABI), and Peripheral Arterial Disease (PAD) in Elderly Men and Women

Study	No.	Mean Age, years	Follow-Up, months		Relative Risk	
			Men	Women	Men	Women
Incidence of new coronary events[8]	2152	81	40	48	2.0	1.6
Incidence of new ABI[13]	2152	81	42	48	2.2	2.4
Prevalence of PAD[21]	869	82	—	—	1.7	1.5

and women aged 50 to 79 years, at any given level of systolic blood pressure of 120 mmHg or greater, risk of CHD over 20 years rose with lower diastolic blood pressure, suggesting that higher pulse pressure was an important component of risk.[29]

Elderly persons with hypertension should be treated with salt restriction, weight reduction if necessary, discontinuation of drugs that increase blood pressure, avoidance of alcohol and tobacco, increase in physical activity, decrease of dietary saturated fat and cholesterol, and maintenance of adequate dietary potassium, calcium, and magnesium intake.

In addition, antihypertensive drugs have been shown to reduce CVD events in elderly men and women with hypertension (Table 17–4).[30–34] The Joint National Committee on Detection, Evaluation, and Treatment of High Blood Pressure (JNC VI) recommends as initial drug treatment diuretics or beta blockers because these drugs have been found to reduce CVD morbidity and mortality in controlled clinical trials.[25] The goal of treatment in elderly persons should be the same as in younger persons to reduce the blood pressure to <140/90 mmHg, and ideally toward the optimal level of <120/80 mmHg.[25] If the systolic blood pressure is between 130 and 139 mmHg or the diastolic blood pressure is between 85 and 89 mmHg and the person has target organ damage, heart failure, renal insufficiency, and/or diabetes mellitus, drug therapy should be prescribed in addition to lifestyle modification.[25]

The choice of medication selected as monotherapy for hypertension should depend on associated

medical conditions. In uncomplicated patients, thiazide diuretics, beta blockers, or a combination of both is recommended as initial therapy in those who do not respond adequately to lifestyle modification. Diuretics are preferred in those with isolated systolic hypertension.[25] It has also been suggested that older men and women with hypertension who have had a myocardial infarction (MI) or who have angina pectoris, myocardial ischemia, or complex ventricular arrhythmias should be treated initially with a beta blocker[35] and that those who have heart failure associated with abnormal or normal left ventricular ejection fraction receive both a diuretic and an angiotensin-converting enzyme (ACE) inhibitor.[36,37] Although data on older diabetics are limited, hypertensive diabetics in general should initially be treated with an ACE inhibitor.[25]

Numerous studies have demonstrated that both systolic and diastolic hypertension increase the incidence of stroke in elderly persons.[13,15,28,30,31,33,34,38–40] The higher the systolic or diastolic blood pressure, the higher the incidence of stroke. At 30-year follow-up in the Framingham Heart Study, hypertension was the risk factor most strongly associated with stroke incidence in elderly men and women.[40] At 42-month follow-up of 664 men, mean age 80 years, and at 48-month follow-up of 1488 women, mean age 82 years, systolic or diastolic hypertension increased the relative risk of new ABI 2.2 times in men and 2.4 times in women (Table 17–2).[13]

Antihypertensive drug therapy has been demonstrated to reduce the incidence of new stroke in eld-

TABLE 17–4 Recent Trials Showing Reduction in New Coronary Events, Stroke, and Heart Failure in Elderly Persons with Hypertension Treated with Antihypertensive Drugs versus Placebo

Study	Follow-Up	Result
Swedish Trial in Old Patients With Hypertension[30] (age 70–84 years)	25 months	Drug therapy caused a 25% decrease in fatal myocardial infarctions (MIs), a 67% reduction in sudden deaths, and a 73% decrease in fatal stroke
Medical Research Council[31] (age 65–74 years)	5.8 years	Drug therapy caused a 19% borderline significant reduction in coronary events and a 25% decrease in stroke
Systolic Hypertension in the Elderly Program[32,33] (mean age 72 years)	4.5 years	Drug therapy caused a 27% decrease in nonfatal MIs plus coronary deaths, a 36% reduction in stroke, and a 49% decrease in heart failure
Systolic Hypertension in Europe[34] (mean age 70 years)	2.0 years	Drug therapy caused a 27% insignificant decrease in coronary mortality, a 30% insignificant reduction in fatal plus nonfatal MIs, and a 42% reduction in stroke

erly persons.[28,30,31,33] Elderly men and women with a systolic blood pressure equal to or greater than 140 mmHg or a diastolic blood pressure equal to or greater than 90 mmHg despite nonpharmacologic intervention should be treated with antihypertensive drug therapy to reduce the incidence of new stroke. Although there are no data showing that drug therapy for systolic blood pressures between 140 and 159 mmHg reduces the incidence of stroke or coronary events in elderly persons, those with a systolic blood pressure between 140 and 159 mmHg persisting after nonpharmacologic measures should normally be treated with antihypertensive drug therapy as in younger persons, as recommended by JNC VI.[25]

Many studies have demonstrated that hypertension is a risk factor for PAD.[15,16,18,21] In a study of 244 men and 625 women, mean age 82 years, systolic or diastolic hypertension increased the prevalence of PAD 1.7 times in men and 1.5 times in women (Table 17–2).[21]

Systolic or diastolic hypertension is also a powerful risk factor for heart failure.[41] In the Systolic Hypertension in the Elderly Program (SHEP), antihypertensive drug therapy with the step 1 drug chlorthalidone, 12.5 to 25 mg daily, and the step 2 drug atenolol, 25 to 50 mg daily, for 4.5 years was associated with a 49 percent reduction in the development of heart failure in elderly men and women (Table 17–4).[32]

Antihypertensive drug therapy may lead to orthostatic hypotension[42] or postprandial hypotension[43] in elderly persons, especially in those who are frail and institutionalized. Management of orthostatic and postprandial hypotension in elderly persons is discussed in detail elsewhere.[44] The dose of antihypertensive drug may need to be reduced or another antihypertensive drug used.

Left Ventricular Hypertrophy

Left ventricular hypertrophy (LVH) caused by hypertension or other CVD is not only a marker for CVD morbidity and mortality but also a contributor to these events in elderly men and women. Elderly men and women with electrocardiographic LVH[25,45–47] or echocardiographic LVH[25,46,48–54] have an increased risk of developing new coronary events, stroke, PAD, and heart failure. At 4-year follow-up of 406 elderly men and 735 elderly women in the Framingham study, echocardiographic LVH was 15.3 times more sensitive in predicting new coronary events in elderly men and 4.3 times more sensitive in predicting new coronary events in elderly women than was electrocardiographic LVH.[48] At 37-month follow-up of 360 men and women, mean age 82 years, with hypertension or CHD, echocardiographic LVH was 4.3 times more sensitive in predicting new coronary events and 4.0 times more sensitive in predicting new ABI than was electrocardiographic LVH.[46]

Physicians should try to prevent LVH from developing or progressing in elderly men and women with hypertension or other CVD. Framingham Heart Study data have demonstrated a reduction of CVD events in patients with regression of LVH.[55] The Cornell group has also found, in patients with uncomplicated hypertension followed for 10.2 years, that regression of LVH probably reduces the incidence of new CVD events.[56] At 10-year follow-up in the Bronx Aging Study, elderly persons in whom electrocardiographic LVH disappeared over time had a lower incidence of CVD morbidity and mortality than elderly persons with persistent LVH.[47]

A meta-analysis of 109 treatment studies found that ACE inhibitors were more effective than other antihypertensive drugs in decreasing left ventricular mass.[57] In an echocardiographic substudy of SHEP, at 3-year follow-up, the left ventricular mass index decreased by 13 percent in the active drug treatment group (a diuretic-based drug regimen) and increased by 6 percent in the placebo group.[58] Prospective studies using different types of antihypertensive drugs are necessary to determine whether regression of left ventricular mass leads to a reduction in CVD morbidity and mortality in elderly men and women.

Dyslipidemia

Numerous studies have demonstrated that a high serum total cholesterol is a risk factor for new or recurrent coronary events in elderly men and women.[5,9,59–63] Among patients 65 years of age and above with prior MI in the Framingham Heart Study, serum total cholesterol was significantly related to death from CHD and to all-cause mortality.[60] In the Established Populations for Epidemiologic Studies of the Elderly study, after 5 years of follow-up in 4066 older men and women, serum total cholesterol was a risk factor for mortality from CHD, but with apparent adverse effects of lower cholesterol levels being associated with comorbidity and frailty.[64] At 40-month follow-up of 664 elderly men and at 48-

month follow-up of 1488 elderly women, an increment of 10 mg/dL of serum total cholesterol was associated with a modest increase in the relative risk of 1.12 for new coronary events in both men and in women.[8]

A low serum high-density-lipoprotein cholesterol (HDL-C) is a risk factor for new coronary events in elderly men and women.[5,9,59,65–68] In the Framingham Heart Study,[59] in the Established Populations for Epidemiologic Studies of the Elderly,[65] and in a large cohort of convalescent home patients,[8] a low serum HDL-C was a more powerful predictor of new coronary events than was serum total cholesterol. At 40-month follow-up of 664 elderly men and at 48-month follow-up of 1488 elderly women, a decrement of 10 mg/dL of serum HDL-C increased the relative risk of new coronary events 1.70 times in men and 1.95 times in women.[8]

Hypertriglyceridemia is a risk factor for new coronary events in elderly women but not in elderly men.[9,59] At 40-month follow-up of elderly men and at 48-month follow-up of elderly women, the level of serum triglycerides was not a risk factor for new coronary events in men and was a very weak risk factor for new coronary events in women.[8]

The strongest and most consistent evidence relating cholesterol lowering to coronary event reduction in the elderly derives from recently published secondary prevention studies. At 5.4-year median follow-up of 4444 men and women (of whom 1021 were 65 to 70 years of age at study entry) with CHD and hypercholesterolemia, simvastatin compared with placebo decreased serum total cholesterol by 25 percent and serum low-density-lipoprotein cholesterol (LDL-C) by 35 percent; it increased serum HDL-C by 8 percent and decreased total mortality, coronary death, major coronary events, cerebrovascular events, new or worsening angina pectoris, and arterial bruit (Table 17–5).[69–71] In men and women 65 to 70 years of age, simvastatin decreased all-cause mortality by 34 percent, CHD mortality by 43 percent, major coronary events by 34 percent, and any atherosclerosis-related endpoint event by 44 percent.[70] Reductions in endpoint events were similar in older and younger men and women.

TABLE 17–5 Effect of Reducing Increased Serum Total and Low-Density-Lipoprotein Cholesterol by Simvastatin, Pravastatin, and Lovastatin versus Placebo in Elderly Persons

Study	Follow-Up	Result
Scandinavian Simvastatin Survival Study (4S)[69–71] (prior MI or angina)	5.4 years	Among persons aged 60 years or older, simvastatin compared with placebo, decreased total mortality by 27% and major coronary events by 29%.
Cholesterol and Recurrent Events (CARE) trial[72] (prior MI)	5.0 years	Compared with placebo, pravastatin decreased major coronary events 32% in persons 65–75 years of age at study entry, including 31% in men and 36% (n.s.) in women. Pravastatin decreased stroke 40% in this subgroup.
Long-Term Intervention with Pravastatin[73] (prior MI or unstable angina)	6.1 years	Compared with placebo, pravastatin decreased the risk of death due to CHD or nonfatal myocardial infarction by 28% in those aged 65 to 69 years and 15% (n.s.) in those aged 70–75 years.
Air Force/Texas Cardiac Atherosclerosis Prevention Study[75,76] (persons free of CHD)	5.2 years	Compared with placebo, lovastatin reduced the primary endpoint of unstable angina, fatal or nonfatal myocardial infarction, and sudden cardiac death 37%, including a 29% risk reduction in those older than 65 years.

Within the Cholesterol and Recurrent Events (CARE) trial involving pravastatin treatment for a period of 5 years in post-MI patients with cholesterol levels less than 240 mg/dL and LDL-C levels of 115 to 174 mg/dL, subset analysis of the 1283 patients aged 65 to 75 years showed a 32 percent lower risk of major coronary events and a 40 percent lower risk of stroke in the pravastatin versus the placebo group (Table 17–5).[72] Finally, the most recent supporting evidence derives from the Long-Term Intervention with Pravastatin in Ischaemic Disease (LIPID) study,[73] conducted among 9014 patients with a history of MI or unstable angina who had initial total cholesterol levels of 155 to 271 mg/dL. Although there was an overall 24 percent risk reduction in death from CHD or nonfatal MI, among the 1081 patients aged 65 to 69 years there was a significant 28 percent reduction in risk. However, those aged 70 to 75 had a nonsignificant 15 percent reduction in risk (Table 17–5).

On the basis of the above data, elderly men and women after MI who have elevated serum LDL cholesterol levels despite dietary therapy should be treated with HMG-CoA reductase inhibitor therapy. The serum LDL cholesterol level should be decreased to 100 mg/dL or less.[74]

There are also new data relating lipid reduction to coronary event reduction in elderly persons without prior CHD. At 5.2-year follow-up of 6605 men and women (21 percent 66 to 73 years of age at study entry) with serum LDL cholesterol levels between 130 to 190 mg/dL, serum HDL cholesterol levels <50 mg/dL, and no clinical evidence of CHD enrolled in the AFCAPS/TexCAPS primary prevention study, lovastatin compared with placebo caused a 37 percent decrease in the primary endpoint of unstable angina pectoris, fatal or nonfatal MI, and sudden cardiac death (Table 17–5).[75,76] Lovastatin decreased this primary endpoint by 34 percent in men, 54 percent in women, 29 percent in persons older than 65 years of age, 59 percent in smokers, 43 percent in persons with hypertension, and 43 percent in persons with diabetes mellitus. On the basis of these data, HMG-CoA reductase inhibitor therapy should be considered in addition to a prudent diet, regular exercise, and risk-factor modification in elderly persons without heart disease who have elevated serum LDL-C levels in the absence of other serious or life-limiting illness such as cancer, dementia, or malnutrition.

There are conflicting data about the association of serum lipids with stroke in men and women.[14,40,77–79] However, a meta-analysis of eight secondary prevention trials and of four primary prevention trials that used simvastatin, pravastatin, or lovastatin to decrease serum total cholesterol levels showed that HMG-CoA reductase inhibitor therapy caused a 27 percent reduction in stroke.[80] These data support the use of HMG-CoA reductase inhibitor therapy in elderly men and women with elevated serum LDL-C levels despite dietary therapy to reduce the incidence of new stroke as well as CHD events.

There are conflicting data about the association of increased serum total cholesterol[15,17–19,79,81,82] and of increased serum triglycerides[18–20,79,82] with PAD. However, a low serum HDL-C is associated with PAD.[17,19,79,82] In a study of 559 men and 1275 women, mean age 81 years, there was a 1.24 times higher probability of having PAD for a 10-mg/dL decrement of serum HDL cholesterol.[79] The Scandinavian Simvastatin Survival Study (4S) showed that compared with placebo, simvastatin reduced new intermittent claudication by 38 percent, and new carotid bruit by 48 percent.[71]

Diabetes Mellitus

Diabetes mellitus is a risk factor for new CHD events in elderly men and women.[8,83] In the Cardiovascular Health Study, an elevated fasting glucose level (>130 mg/dL) increased 5-year mortality 1.9 times.[2] At 40-month follow-up of 664 elderly men and 48-month follow-up of 1488 elderly women, diabetes mellitus increased the relative risk of new coronary events 1.9 times in men and 1.8 times in women (Table 17–6).[8]

Persons with diabetes mellitus are more often obese and have higher serum LDL-C and triglyceride levels and lower serum HDL-C levels than do nondiabetics. Diabetics also have a higher prevalence of hypertension and LVH than do nondiabetics. These risk factors contribute to the increased incidence of new CHD events in diabetics compared to nondiabetics. Increased age can further amplify these risk factor differences and contribute to greater CVD risk.

Diabetes mellitus is a risk factor for new stroke in elderly men and women.[12,40,84] Diabetes mellitus also increased the prevalence of extracranial carotid arterial disease 1.7 times among 1063 persons (mean age 81 years).[14] At 42-month follow-up of 664 elderly men and at 48-month follow-up of 1488 elderly women, diabetes mellitus increased the relative risk of new ABI 1.5 times in men and 1.5 times in women (Table 17–6).[13]

Diabetes mellitus is also a risk factor for PAD in elderly men and women.[15–18,19–21] In a study of 244 elderly men and 625 elderly women, diabetes mellitus increased the prevalence of PAD 2.4 times in men and 3.0 times in women (Table 17–6).[21]

Elderly persons with diabetes mellitus should be treated with dietary therapy, weight reduction if necessary, and appropriate drugs if necessary to control

TABLE 17–6 Association of Diabetes Mellitus with New Coronary Events, New Atherothrombotic Brain Infarction (ABI), and Peripheral Arterial Disease (PAD) in Elderly Men and Women

Study	No.	Mean Age (years)	Follow-Up, months		Relative Risk	
			Men	Women	Men	Women
Incidence of new coronary events[8]	2152	81	40	48	1.9	1.8
Incidence of new ABI[13]	2152	81	42	48	1.5	1.5
Prevalence of PAD[21]	869	82	–	–	2.4	3.0

hyperglycemia. Other risk factors such as smoking, hypertension, dyslipidemia, obesity, and physical inactivity should be controlled. These risk factors warrant special attention in the elderly, where they are often more common and/or severe.

Metabolic Syndrome

The clustering of high serum triglycerides, small LDL particles, low serum HDL-C levels, hypertension, insulin resistance (with or without glucose intolerance), and a prothrombotic state is called the metabolic syndrome (also commonly referred to as "syndrome X").[85,86] HMG-CoA reductase inhibitor therapy, alone or in combination with other lipid-altering therapy, such as niacin, should be used to reduce the atherogenic lipoproteins.[85] Hypertension should be treated in accordance with JNC-VI guidelines.[25] Nondrug therapy for insulin resistance consists of weight control and increased physical activity. Metformin and troglitazone may be useful in some persons for reducing insulin resistance. Low-dose aspirin may also be used to reduce the risk from a prothombotic state.[86]

Obesity

Obesity was an independent risk factor for new CHD events in elderly men and women in the Framingham Heart Study.[83] Disproportionate distribution of fat to the abdomen assessed by the waist-to-hip circumference ratio has also been shown to be a risk factor for cardiovascular disease, mortality from CHD, and total mortality in elderly men and women.[87,88] At 40-month follow-up of elderly men and at 48-month follow-up of elderly women, obesity was a risk factor for new CHD events in men and women by univariate analysis but not by multivariate analysis.[8]

The Framingham study found that relative weight was not a risk factor for new ABI in elderly men but was a weak risk factor for new ABI in elderly women.[40] Barrett-Connor and Khaw[84] demonstrated no association between body-mass index and new ABI in elderly men and women. At 42-month follow-up of 664 elderly men, obesity was not a risk factor for new ABI.[13] At 48-month follow-up of 1488 elderly women, obesity was a risk factor for new ABI by univariate analysis but not by multivariate analysis.[13]

The Framingham Heart Study observed that Metropolitan Life Insurance relative weight was not associated with intermittent claudication in women but was inversely associated with intermittent claudication in men.[15] In a study of 244 elderly men and 625 elderly women, obesity was insignificantly associated with PAD in men but increased the prevalence of PAD 1.8 times in women.[21]

Obese men and women with CHD, ABI, or PAD must undergo weight reduction. Weight reduction is also a first approach to controlling mild hypertension, hyperglycemia, and dyslipidemia before placing persons on long-term drug therapy. Regular aerobic exercise should be used in addition to diet to treat obesity. Clinical trials are needed to establish the efficacy of long-term drug therapy for treating obesity in the elderly.

Physical Inactivity

Physical inactivity is associated with obesity, hypertension, hyperglycemia, and dyslipidemia. At 12-year follow-up in the Honolulu Heart Program, physically active men 65 years of age or over had a relative risk of 0.43 for CHD compared with inactive men.[89] Paffenbarger et al.[90] demonstrated that persons 65 to 79 years of age with a physical activity index above 2000 kcal/week had a better survival rate than those with a physical activity index below 2000 kcal/week. Lack of moderate or vigorous exercise increased 5-year mortality in elderly men and women in the Cardiovascular Heart Study.[2] The relationship between physical inactivity and ABI is unclear.[40,91,92]

Moderate exercise programs suitable for elderly persons include walking, climbing stairs, swimming, or bicycling; however, care must be taken in prescribing any exercise program because of the high risk of injury in this age group. Group or supervised sessions, including aerobics classes, offered by senior health care plans are especially appealing. Exercise training programs are not only beneficial in preventing CHD[93] but have also been found to improve endurance and functional capacity in elderly persons after MI.[94]

Polypharmacy

Elderly persons are often taking multiple drugs, which can cause drug interactions. Only essential drugs should be prescribed to elderly persons. The initial dose of drug should be low and the increase in dose should be slow. The dose of drug should be titrated according to the elderly person's response. Appropriate use of cardiovascular drugs in elderly persons requires knowledge of age-related physiologic changes, the effects of concomitant disorders that may alter the pharmacokinetics and pharmacodynamic effects of cardiovascular drugs, and drug interactions. This subject is discussed in detail elsewhere.[95]

Summary

The significant morbidity and mortality due to CVD in the elderly warrants that this group receive special attention directed at awareness, detection, and control of important risk factors. Many of these risk factors—particularly smoking, diabetes, hypertension, dyslipidemia, obesity, and physical inactivity—continue to be important predictors of cardiovascular events in the elderly; they are largely modifiable, and in many cases reversible. Among the many older persons with preexisting cardiovascular disease, risk-factor modification is even more important, as disease will often progress rapidly otherwise. Older persons must be educated to understand that CVD is not an inevitable consequence of aging but is largely preventable, and in some cases even reversible. As large segments of populations in developed countries rapidly reach older ages, soon to be repeated in developing countries, where life spans have dramatically increased along with the incidence of cardiovascular and other chronic diseases, there is significant opportunity for prevention in the twenty-first century.

References

1. American Heart Association: *1998 Heart and Stroke Statistical Update.* Dallas, American Heart Association, 1998.
2. Fried LP, Kronmal RA, Newman AB, et al: Risk factors for 5-year mortality in older adults: The Cardiovascular Health Study. *JAMA* 1998; 279:585–592.
3. Cupples LA, D'Agostino RB: Some risk factors related to the annual incidence of cardiovascular disease and death using pooled repeated biennial measurements. In: Kannel WB, Wolf PA, Garrison RJ (eds): *Framingham Study: 30-Year Follow-Up.* National Institutes of Health Publication No. 87-2703. Springfield, VA, U.S. Department of Commerce, National Technical Information Service, 1987.
4. Siegel D, Kuller L, Lazarus NB, et al: Predictors of cardiovascular events and mortality in the Systolic Hypertension in the Elderly Program pilot project. *Am J Epidemiol* 1987; 126:385–399.
5. Kannel WB, Vokonas PS: Primary risk factors for coronary heart disease in the elderly: The Framingham study. In: Wenger NK, Furberg CD, Pitt B (eds). *Coronary Heart Disease in the Elderly.* New York, Elsevier, 1986:60–92.
6. Benfante R, Reed D, Frank J: Does cigarette smoking have an independent effect on coronary heart disease incidence in the elderly? *Am J Public Health* 1991; 81:897–899.
7. LaCroix AZ, Lang J, Scherr P, et al: Smoking and mortality among older men and women in three communities. *N Engl J Med* 1991; 324:1619–1625.
8. Aronow WS, Ahn C: Risk factors for new coronary events in a large cohort of very elderly patients with and without coronary artery disease. *Am J Cardiol* 1996; 77:864–866.
9. Hermanson B, Omenn GS, Kronmal RA, Gersh BJ: Beneficial six-year outcome of smoking cessation in older men and women with coronary artery disease: results from the CASS registry. *N Engl J Med* 1988; 319:1365–1369.
10. Shinton R, Beevers G: Meta-analysis of relation between cigarette smoking and stroke. *BMJ* 1989; 298:789–794.
11. Medical Research Council Working Party: MRC trial of treatment of mild hypertension: principal results. *BMJ Clin Res* 1985; 291:97–104.
12. Wolf PA, D'Agostino PS, Kannel WB, et al: Cigarette smoking as a risk factor for stroke: the Framingham study. *JAMA* 1988; 259:1025–1029.
13. Aronow WS, Ahn C, Gutstein H: Risk factors for new atherothrombotic brain infarction in 664 older men and 1,488 older women. *Am J Cardiol* 1996; 77:1381–1383.
14. Aronow WS, Ahn C, Schoenfeld MR: Risk factors for extracranial internal or common carotid arterial disease in elderly patients. *Am J Cardiol* 1993; 71:1479–1481.
15. Stokes J III, Kannel WB, Wolf PA, et al: The relative importance of selected risk factors for various manifestations of cardiovascular disease among men and women from 35 to 64 years old: 30 years of follow-up in the Framingham study. *Circulation* 1987; 75(suppl V):V-65–V-73.

16. Kannel WB, McGee DL: Update on some epidemiologic features of intermittent claudication: the Framingham study. *J Am Geriatr Soc* 1985; 33:13–18.

17. Pomrehn P, Duncan B, Weissfeld L, et al: The association of dyslipoproteinemia with symptoms and signs of peripheral arterial disease: the Lipid Research Clinics Program Prevalence Study. *Circulation* 1986; 73(suppl I):I-100–I-107.

18. Hughson WG, Mann JI, Garrod A: Intermittent claudication: prevalence and risk factors. *BMJ* 1978; 1:1379–1381.

19. Beach KW, Brunzell JD, Strandness DE Jr: Prevalence of severe arteriosclerosis obliterans in patients with diabetes mellitus: relation to smoking and form of therapy. *Arteriosclerosis* 1982; 2:275–280.

20. Reunanen A, Takkunen H, Aromaa A: Prevalence of intermittent claudication and its effect on mortality. *Acta Med Scand* 1982; 211:249–256.

21. Aronow WS, Sales FF, Etienne F, Lee NH: Prevalence of peripheral arterial disease and its correlation with risk factors for peripheral arterial disease in elderly patients in a long-term health care facility. *Am J Cardiol* 1988; 62:644–646.

22. Aronow WS, Ahn C, Mercando AD, Epstein S: Prognostic significance of silent ischemia in elderly patients with peripheral arterial disease with and without previous myocardial infarction. *Am J Cardiol* 1992; 69:137–139.

23. Benowitz NL: Treating tobacco addiction—nicotine or no nicotine. *N Engl J Med* 1997; 337:1230–1231.

24. Hurt RD, Sachs DPL, Glover ED, et al: A comparison of sustained-release bupropion and placebo for smoking cessation. *N Engl J Med* 1997; 337:1195–1202.

25. Joint National Committee: The Sixth Report of the Joint National Committee on the Prevention, Detection, Evaluation, and Treatment of High Blood Pressure (JNC VI). *Arch Intern Med* 1997; 157:2413–2444.

26. Aronow WS, Ahn C, Kronzon I, Koenigsberg M: Congestive heart failure, coronary events and atherothrombotic brain infarction in elderly blacks and whites with systemic hypertension and with and without echocardiographic and electrocardiographic evidence of left ventricular hypertrophy. *Am J Cardiol* 1991; 67:295–299.

27. Aronow WS, Kronzon I: Prevalence of coronary risk factors in elderly blacks and whites. *J Am Geriatr Soc* 1991; 39:567–570.

28. Applegate WB, Rutan GH: Advances in management of hypertension in older persons. *J Am Geriatr Soc* 1992; 40:1164–1174.

29. Franklin SS, Khan SA, Wong ND, Larson MG, Levy D: Is pulse pressure useful in predicting risk for coronary heart disease? The Framingham Heart Study. *Circulation* 1999; 100:354–360.

30. Dahlof B, Lindholm LH, Hansson L, et al: Morbidity and mortality in the Swedish Trial in Old Patients With Hypertension (STOP Hypertension). *Lancet* 1991; 338:1281–1285.

31. MRC Working Party: Medical Research Council Trial of treatment of hypertension in older adults: principal results. *BMJ* 1992; 304:405–412.

32. SHEP Cooperative Research Group: Prevention of stroke by antihypertensive drug treatment in older persons with isolated systolic hypertension: final results of the Systolic Hypertension in the Elderly Program (SHEP). *JAMA* 1991; 265:3255–3264.

33. Kostis JB, Davis BR, Cutler J, et al: Prevention of heart failure by antihypertensive drug treatment in older persons with isolated systolic hypertension. *JAMA* 1997; 278:212–216.

34. Staessen JA, Fagard R, Thijs L, et al: Randomised double-blind comparison of placebo and active treatment for older patients with isolated systolic hypertension. *Lancet* 1997; 350:757–764.

35. Aronow WS, Ahn C, Mercando AD, et al. Effect of propranolol versus no antiarrhythmic drug on sudden cardiac death, total cardiac death, and total death in patients ≥62 years of age with heart disease, complex ventricular arrhythmias, and left ventricular ejection fraction ≥40%. *Am J Cardiol* 1994; 74:267–270.

36. Garg R, Yusuf S, for the Collaborative Group on ACE Inhibitor Trials: Overview of randomized trials of angiotensin-converting enzyme inhibitors on mortality and morbidity in patients with heart failure. *JAMA* 1995; 273:1450–1456.

37. Aronow WS, Kronzon I: Effect of enalapril on congestive heart failure treated with diuretics in elderly patients with prior myocardial infarction and normal left ventricular ejection fraction. *Am J Cardiol* 1993; 71:602–604.

38. Garland C, Barrett-Connor E, Suarez L, Criqui MH: Isolated systolic hypertension and mortality after age 60 years. *Am J Epidemiol* 1983; 118:365–376.

39. Coope J, Warrender TS: Randomised trial of treatment of hypertension in the elderly in primary care. *BMJ* 1986; 293:1145–1151.

40. Wolf PA: Cerebrovascular disease in the elderly. In: Tresch DD, Aronow WS (eds): *Cardiovascular Disease in the Elderly Patient.* New York, Marcel Dekker, 1994:125–147.

41. Levy D, Larson MG, Vasan RS, et al: The progression from hypertension to congestive heart failure. *JAMA* 1996; 275:1557–1562.

42. Aronow WS, Lee NH, Sales FF, Etienne F: Prevalence of postural hypotension in elderly patients in a long-term health care facility. *Am J Cardiol* 1988; 62:336.

43. Aronow WS, Ahn C: Postprandial hypotension in 499 elderly persons in a long-term health care facility. *J Am Geriatr Soc* 1994; 42:930–932.

44. Aronow WS: Dizziness and syncope. In: Hazzard WR, Blass JP, Ettinger WH Jr, et al (eds): *Principles of Geriatric Medicine and Gerontology,* 4th ed. New York, McGraw-Hill, 1998.

45. Kannel WB, Dannenberg AL, Levy D: Population implications of electrocardiographic left ventricular hypertrophy. *Am J Cardiol* 1987; 60:851–931.

46. Aronow WS, Koenigsberg M, Schwartz KS: Usefulness of echocardiographic and electrocardiographic left ventricular hypertrophy in predicting new cardiac events and atherothrombotic brain infarction in elderly patients with systemic hypertension or coronary artery disease. *Am J Noninvas Cardiol* 1989; 3:367–370.

47. Kahn S, Frishman WH, Weissman S, et al: Left ventricular hypertrophy on electrocardiogram: prognostic implications from a 10 year cohort study of older subjects: a report from the Bronx Longitudinal Aging Study. *J Am Geriatr Soc* 1996; 44:524–529.

48. Levy D, Garrison RJ, Savage DD, et al: Left ventricular mass and incidence of coronary heart disease in an elderly cohort: the Framingham Heart Study. *Ann Intern Med* 1989; 110:101–107.

49. Aronow WS, Koenigsberg M, Schwartz KS: Usefulness of echocardiographic left ventricular hypertrophy in predicting new coronary events and atherothrombotic brain infarction in patients over 62 years of age. *Am J Cardiol* 1988; 61:1130–1132.

50. Aronow WS, Epstein S, Koenigsberg M, Schwartz KS: Usefulness of echocardiographic left ventricular hypertrophy, ventricular tachycardia, and complex ventricular arrhythmias in predicting ventricular fibrillation or sudden cardiac death in elderly patients. *Am J Cardiol* 1988; 62:1124–1125.

51. Aronow WS, Gutstein H, Hsieh FY: Risk factors for thromboembolic stroke in elderly patients with chronic atrial fibrillation. *Am J Cardiol* 1989; 63:366–367.

52. Aronow WS, Ahn C, Kronzon I, Gutstein H: Association of plasma renin activity and echocardiographic left ventricular hypertrophy with frequency of new coronary events and new atherothrombotic brain infarction in older persons with systemic hypertension. *Am J Cardiol* 1997; 79:1543–1545.

53. Bikkina M, Levy D, Evans JC, et al: Left ventricular mass and risk of stroke in an elderly cohort: the Framingham Heart Study. *JAMA* 1994; 272:33–36.

54. Aronow WS, Ahn C, Kronzon I, et al: Association of extracranial carotid arterial disease, prior atherothrombotic brain infarction, systemic hypertension, and left ventricular hypertrophy with the incidence of new atherothrombotic brain infarction at 45-month follow-up in 1,482 older patients. *Am J Cardiol* 1997; 79:991–993.

55. Kannel WB, D'Agostino RB, Levy D, et al: Prognostic significance of regression of left ventricular hypertrophy (abstr). *Circulation* 1988; 78(suppl II):II-89.

56. Koren MJ, Savage DD, Casale PN, et al: Changes in left ventricular mass predict risk in essential hypertension (abstr). *Circulation* 1990; 82(suppl III):III-29.

57. Dahlof B, Pennert K, Hansson L: Reversal of left ventricular hypertrophy in hypertensive patients: a meta-analysis of 109 treatment studies. *Am J Hypertens* 1992; 5:95–110.

58. Ofili EO, Cohen JD, St. Vrain JA, et al: Effect of treatment of isolated systolic hypertension on left ventricular mass. *JAMA* 1998; 279:778–780.

59. Castelli WP, Wilson PWF, Levy D, Anderson K: Cardiovascular disease in the elderly. *Am J Cardiol* 1989; 63:12H–19H.

60. Wong ND, Wilson PWF, Kannel WB: Serum cholesterol as a prognostic factor after myocardial infarction: the Framingham study. *Ann Intern Med* 1991; 115:687–693.

61. Benfante R, Reed D: Is elevated serum cholesterol level a factor for coronary heart disease in the elderly? *JAMA* 1990; 263:393–396.

62. Barrett-Connor E, Suarez L, Khaw K-T, et al: Ischemic heart disease risk factors after age 50. *J Chronic Dis* 1984; 37:903–908.

63. Rubin SM, Sidney S, Black DM, et al: High blood cholesterol in elderly men and the excess risk for coronary heart disease. *Ann Intern Med* 1990; 113:916–920.

64. Corti MC, Guralnik JM, Salive ME, et al: Clarifying the direct relation between total cholesterol levels and death from coronary heart disease in older persons. *Ann Intern Med* 1997; 126:753–760.

65. Corti MC, Guralnik JM, Salive ME, et al: HDL cholesterol predicts coronary heart disease mortality in older persons. *JAMA* 1995; 274:539–544.

66. Zimetbaum P, Frishman WH, Ooi WL, et al: Plasma lipids and lipoproteins and the incidence of cardiovascular disease in the very elderly: the Bronx Aging Study. *Arterioscler Thromb* 1992; 12:416–423.

67. Aronow WS, Ahn C: Correlation of serum lipids with the presence or absence of coronary artery disease in 1,793 men and women aged ≥62 years. *Am J Cardiol* 1994; 73:702–703.

68. Lavie CJ, Milani RV: National Cholesterol Education Program's recommendations, and implications of "missing" high-density lipoprotein cholesterol in cardiac rehabilitation programs. *Am J Cardiol* 1991; 68:1087.

69. Scandinavian Simvastatin Survival Study Group: Randomised trial of cholesterol lowering in 4444 patients with coronary heart disease: the Scandinavian Simvastatin Survival Study (4S). *Lancet* 1994; 344:1383–1389.

70. Miettinen TA, Pyorala K, Olsson AG, et al: Cholesterol-lowering therapy in women and elderly patients with myocardial infarction or angina pectoris: findings from the Scandinavian Simvastatin Survival Study (4S). *Circulation* 1997; 96:4211–4218.

71. Pedersen TR, Kjekshus J, Pyorala K, et al: Effect of simvastatin on ischemic signs and symptoms in the Scandinavian Simvastatin Survival Study (4S). *Am J Cardiol* 1998; 81:333–336.

72. Lewis SJ, Moye LA, Sacks FM, et al. Effect of pravastatin on cardiovascular events in older patients with myocardial infarction and cholesterol levels in the average range: results of the Cholesterol and Recurrent Events (CARE) Trial. *Ann Intern Med* 1998; 129:681–689.

73. The Long-Term Intervention with Pravastatin in Ischaemic Disease (LIPID) Study Group: Prevention of cardiovascular events and death with pravastatin in patients with coronary heart disease and a broad range of initial cholesterol levels. *N Engl J Med* 1998; 339:1349–1357.

74. Grundy SM, Balady GJ, Criqui MH, et al: When to start cholesterol-lowering therapy in patients with coronary heart disease: a statement for health care professionals from the American Heart Association Task Force on Risk Reduction. *Circulation* 1997; 95:1683–1685.

75. Gotto AM: Presentation of the Air Force/Texas Cardiac Atherosclerotic Prevention Study at the Annual Scientific Meeting of the American Heart Association, Dallas, November 1997.

76. Downs JR, Clearfield M, Weis S, et al: Primary prevention of acute coronary events with lovastatin in men and women with average cholesterol levels: results of AFCAPS/TexCAPS. *JAMA* 1998; 279:1615–1622.

77. Iso H, Jacobs DR Jr, Wentworth D, et al: Serum cholesterol levels and six-year mortality from stroke in 350,977 men screened for the Multiple Risk Factor Intervention Trial. *N Engl J Med* 1989; 320:904–910.

78. Bihari-Varga M, Szekely J, Gruber E: Plasma high-density lipoproteins in coronary, cerebral and peripheral vascular disease: the influence of various risk factors. *Atherosclerosis* 1981; 40:337–345.

79. Aronow WS, Ahn C: Correlation of serum lipids with the presence or absence of atherothrombotic brain infarction and peripheral arterial disease in 1,834 men and women aged ≥62 years. *Am J Cardiol* 1994; 73:995–997.

80. Crouse JR III, Byington RP, Hoen HM, Furberg CD: Reductase inhibitor monotherapy and stroke prevention. *Arch Intern Med* 1997; 157:1305–1310.

81. Criqui MH, Browner D, Fronek A, et al: Peripheral arterial disease in large vessels is epidemiologically distinct from small vessel disease: an analysis of risk factors. *Am J Epidemiol* 1989; 129:1110–1119.

82. Fowkes FGR, Housley E, Riemersma RA, et al: Smoking, lipids, glucose intolerance, and blood pressure as risk factors for peripheral atherosclerosis compared with ischemic heart disease in the Edinburgh Artery Study. *Am J Epidemiol* 1992; 135:331–340.

83. Vokonas PS, Kannel WB: Epidemiology of coronary heart disease in the elderly. In: Tresch DD, Aronow WS (eds): *Cardiovascular Disease in the Elderly Patient.* New York, Marcel Dekker, 1994:91–123.

84. Barrett-Connor E, Khaw K-T: Diabetes mellitus: an independent risk factor for stroke. *Am J Epidemiol* 1988; 128:116–123.

85. Grundy SM: Small LDL, atherogenic dyslipidemia, and the metabolic syndrome. *Circulation* 1997; 95:1–4.

86. Grundy SM: Hypertriglyceridemia, atherogenic dyslipidemia, and the metabolic syndrome. *Am J Cardiol* 1998; 81(4A):18B–25B.

87. Kannel WB, Cupples LA, Ramaswami R, et al: Regional obesity and risk of cardiovascular disease. *J Clin Epidemiol* 1991; 44:183–190.

88. Folsom AR, Kaye SA, Sellers TA, et al: Body fat distribution and 5-year risk of death in older women. *JAMA* 1993; 269:483–487.

89. Donahue RP, Abbott RD, Reed DM, Yano K: Physical activity and coronary heart disease in middle-aged and elderly men: the Honolulu Heart Program. *Am J Public Health* 1988; 78:683–685.

90. Paffenbarger RS Jr, Hyde RT, Wing AL, et al: Physical activity, all-cause mortality, and longevity of college alumni. *N Engl J Med* 1986; 314:605–613.

91. Paffenbarger RS Jr, Wing AL: Characteristics in youth predisposing to fatal stroke in later years. *Lancet* 1967; 1:753–754.

92. Paffenbarger RS Jr: Factors predisposing to fatal stroke in longshoremen. *Prev Med* 1972; 1:522–527.

93. Wenger NK: Physical inactivity as a risk factor for coronary heart disease in the elderly. *Cardiol Elderly* 1994; 2:375–379.

94. Williams MA, Maresh CM, Aronow WS, et al: The value of early out-patient cardiac exercise programmes for the elderly in comparison with other selected age groups. *Eur Heart J* 1984; 5(suppl E):113–115.

95. Aronow WS: Cardiovascular drug therapy in the elderly. In: Frishman WH, Sonnenblick EH (eds): *Cardiovascular Pharmacotherapeutics.* New York, McGraw-Hill, 1997:1267–1281.

CHAPTER 18

African Americans

Keith C. Norris
Charles K. Francis

Despite overall declines in age-adjusted cardiovascular disease (CVD) morbidity and mortality during the past three decades in African Americans, the rates of illness and death from coronary heart disease (CHD), stroke, heart failure, and other CVDs have not improved to the same extent as they have in whites.[1–3]

Of the major factors contributing to racial disparities in health over the last decade, differing rates of improvement in lifestyle and control of risk factors for CVD may be among the most important. For many Americans, national and regional programs in risk-factor education and public health measures have led to improved control of lipids and blood pressure and decreased CVD risk. African Americans have not experienced a comparable improvement in lifestyle and control of risk factors. Modifiable risk factors—such as hypertension, hypercholesterolemia, smoking, diabetes, obesity, and sedentary lifestyle—remain more prevalent and severe among African Americans and other minority populations. Differences in the frequency of risk-factor clustering as well as adverse socioeconomic status, lower educational attainment, insufficient numbers of minority health care providers, reduced access to health care, and the effects of suspected racism may be translated into disparities in CVD prevalence, clinical management, and outcomes in African-American populations.

This chapter discusses the epidemiology of CVD in African Americans and examines CVD prevention efforts in this group. It also explores—from the perspective of the individual patient, the health care provider, the community, and the population at large—how these findings may be translated into new strategies for reduction of racial disparities in CVD prevalence and outcomes.

Epidemiology of Cardiovascular Diseases in African Americans

CVD affects nearly 13 million Americans and is the leading cause of death in the United States.[4] Nearly a million deaths were attributed to CVD in 1996 and approximately 58 million persons in the United States have one or more types of CVD.[4] In 1996, death rates from CVD (per 100,000 population) were 46.5 percent higher in black males than white males (315.9 versus 215.6, respectively) and 67.0 percent higher in black females than white females (209.3 versus 125.3, respectively) (Fig. 18–1).[4] Although the age-adjusted mortality rate for CVD has fallen by 19 percent over the last 10 years, the absolute rate fell only 2 percent owing to the increasing age of the U.S. population.[4]

Coronary Artery Disease

The estimated prevalence of CHD among American adults is 7.2 percent for the general population. For non-Hispanic whites, the estimated rate was 7.5 percent; for non-Hispanic blacks, 6.9 percent; and for Mexican Americans, 5.6 percent—with similar trends noted for the estimated prevalence of angina pectoris across ethnic/racial groups.[4] Despite a 7 percent lesser prevalence of CHD, the 1996 death rates (per 100,000 population) were 4.3 percent higher in

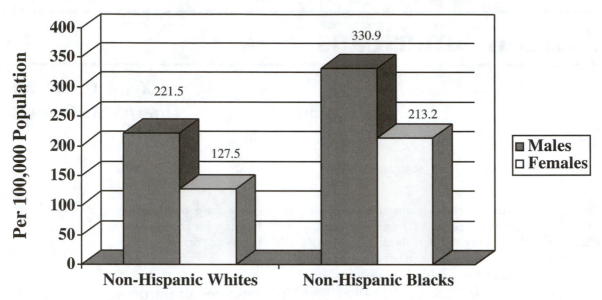

FIGURE 18–1 1996 Cardiovascular disease mortality rates. (From the American Heart Association,[4] with permission.)

black males than white males (125.4 versus 120.2, respectively) and 35.8 percent higher in black females than white females (80.0 versus 58.9, respectively).[4] In the Cardiovascular Health Study of older Americans, the rate (per 100,000 population) of new and recurrent heart attacks per year in men ages 65 to 74 was 16.3 for black men versus 26.3 for white men; in ages 75 to 84, the rate was 54.9 and 39.7, respectively; and in men older than 85 years, the rate was 40.8 and 53.6, respectively.[4] Other national data shows age- and gender-adjusted risks for coronary deaths among African American men 25 to 44 years old and women 25 to 54 years old to be twice that of whites. Moreover, socioeconomic status explained half or more of all excess risks for African Americans.[5]

Angina pectoris is also common in African Americans, but there are significant racial and gender differences. Data from the third National Health and Nutrition Examination Survey (NHANES III) indicate that angina pectoris is more prevalent in non-Hispanic black women, 5.2 per 100,000 population, compared with 4.1 in non-Hispanic white women and 4.6 in Mexican-American women. However, the prevalence of angina pectoris is lowest in black men, 2.6 per 100,000 population, compared with 3.4 in both non-Hispanic white men and Mexican-American men.[6]

Congestive Heart Failure

Congestive heart failure (CHF) is now responsible for at least 200,000 deaths per year at an annual cost of nearly $20 billion.[4] The 1996 mortality rates (per 100,000) for CHF were about 33 percent higher for African Americans than for whites: 6.7 for white males and 8.8 for black males; 5.3 for white females and 7.2 for black females.[4] Excess hospitalizations among African Americans for CHF were reported to be largely explained by the higher prevalence CVD

risk factors, predominantly hypertension and diabetes, although in younger women these risk factors
did not completely explain the excess risk.[7] For
African Americans below the age of 65, CHF mortality was reported to be approximately 2.5 times that
of whites.[8]

Race-specific variations in heart failure death rates
may be related to the higher prevalence, greater
severity, and poorer control rates of hypertension
among African Americans.[1] Long-term hypertension
trials suggest that blood pressure reduction would be
the most effective measure for slowing the progression of heart failure.[9] Other explanations for the
racial variation in CHF mortality include neurohormonal differences, delayed treatment owing to reduced access to care, influences of other risk factors
on the atherosclerotic processes, and the socioeconomic and cultural environment.[1]

In a report from the Studies on Left Ventricular
Dysfunction (SOLVD), the frequency of hypertension as an etiology of heart failure was ninefold
higher in African Americans than in whites. Excep-
tionally high rates of hypertensive heart diseases
were noted among African Americans, and hospital
admission rates for African Americans were also
twice those of whites.[10] CHF mortality among racial
groups in SOLVD after 1-year follow-up was similar, suggesting that access to care and appropriate intervention can improve CHF outcomes for African
Americans.[11] From 34-month follow-up in SOLVD,
Dries et al. found an approximately 30 percent
greater mortality rate among black versus white subjects after adjusting for age and coexisting medical
conditions.[12]

Stroke

Stroke is the third leading cause of death for African
Americans, behind heart disease and cancer. Stroke
prevalence, morbidity, and mortality are increased in
African Americans, perhaps owing to differences in
pathogenesis, stroke management, and risk-factor
control. The estimated prevalence of stroke for
African-American men is 1.8 times and women 2.5
times that of their white counterparts. The mortality
rates (per 100,000) for stroke in 1996 were 26.3 for

white males and 50.9 for black males; they were 22.9
for white females and 39.2 for black females—93.5
and 71.2 percent higher for black males and black
females, respectively.[4] In addition, young African
Americans have a two- to threefold greater risk of
ischemic stroke and are 2.5 times more likely to die
of stroke than are whites.[4] Stroke mortality also
varies with geographic distribution, with a dramatically higher incidence and mortality rate reported
from the southeastern United States.[13–15]

In the population-based Atherosclerosis Risk in
Communities (ARIC) study, hypertension was more
frequent in African Americans than whites and was
associated with subclinical cerebrovascular atherosclerosis, as determined by ultrasound-measured
carotid artery intima-media thickness.[16] Among several other CVD risk factors, hypertension contributes
substantially to the high rate of stroke in the African-
American community. Indeed, most hypertension
trials have shown an even greater reduction in stroke
events in comparison to coronary events.[17,18] Like
European Americans, African Americans with a positive family history of stroke have a higher risk of
stroke than those without such a history, consistent
with the expression of genetic susceptibility and/or
a shared environment in the etiology of stroke.[19]

Renal Disease

For African Americans, CVD and renal disease are
inextricably linked. Hypertension is a determining
factor in the pathogenesis, prevalence, and outcomes
of both cardiovascular and renal disease in African
Americans. End-stage renal disease (ESRD) is perhaps the most vivid example of racial differences
in health outcomes in the United States. African-
American men between the age of 24 and 44 are
nearly 20 times more likely to suffer from hypertension-related ESRD than are white men.[20,21] This
increased incidence may not be accounted for by a
higher prevalence of hypertension[22] or socioeconomic factors alone,[23] suggesting a genetic predisposition to hypertension-related ESRD among
African Americans. ESRD is four times more common among African Americans than among their
white counterparts, with a rate of 818 per million in

African Americans and 194 per million in whites.[21] Diabetes and hypertension are responsible for over 70 percent of patients beginning ESRD treatment.[21] Increased prevalence of both hypertension and diabetes in African Americans contributes to the excess ESRD in this population.

Peripheral Vascular Disease

Peripheral vascular disease (PVD) remains a major cause of disability among African Americans. The high prevalence of both diabetes and smoking greatly increase the risk for PVD complications for African Americans, although an independent racial predisposition to lower-leg vascular differences has been suggested.[24] Variations in treatment also affect the debility PVD imposes on the African-American community. A review of over 7000 cases of angioplasty, bypass surgery, or amputation for lower-extremity PVD revealed that, compared with white counterparts, African Americans were 2.5 times as likely to have an amputation performed than to undergo angioplasty or bypass surgery. Whether this reflects differences in the extent of vascular disease or biases in clinician practices is unclear.[25] Regardless, the impact on both the individual and the African-American community is substantial.

Cardiovascular Disease Risk Factors in African Americans

The relationship between risk factors and CVD appears applicable to both African-American and white populations.[26-29] The traditional risk factors include hypertension, hyperlipidemia (especially hypercholesterolemia), smoking, diabetes, sedentary lifestyle, and obesity. These risk factors have been shown to be important, not only in early life but also with advancing age.[30] Although total CVD risk is acknowledged to be multifactorial, the relative influence of individual risk factors and whether their impact differs between racial and ethnic groups remain topics of debate.

Familial aggregation of risk has been demonstrated in both African-American and white siblings of persons with premature CHD.[31] Several studies suggest that risk-factor clustering in African Americans occurs at 1.5 times the rate in whites, further contributing to the high mortality rate of CHD,[32,33] although rates can vary depending upon the risk factors examined. Some of these risk factors exert their effects in an exponential fashion.[34,35]

In addition to physiologic risk factors, socioeconomic status has been shown to greatly influence CVD mortality, even after controlling for other well-recognized CVD risk factors.[26,36] For African Americans and the overall population, understanding the interaction of culture and environment with specific risk factors is critical to the identification and treatment of high-risk individuals and for the development and implementation of effective population-based strategies for CVD risk reduction.

Hypertension

Hypertension is an important risk factor for CVD—including heart attack, stroke, congestive heart failure, peripheral vascular disease, and renal failure.[17,37-39] African Americans suffer disproportionately from hypertension and its sequelae, likely due to a combination of socioeconomic and genetic factors.[1,26] Essential hypertension was the most common diagnosis made by physicians in 1993,[40] thus generating a frequent opportunity for health care providers to initiate dialogue regarding coexisting CVD risk factors for a large group of at risk individuals. Although blood pressure control for the nation has improved since the first NHANES, it is still unacceptably low.[41,42] NHANES III reported the prevalence of hypertension among all age groups to be nearly 50 percent higher among African Americans than among whites (Fig. 18–2) and an overall rate of blood pressure control less than 30 percent as has been reported nationally (Fig. 18–3).[41]

Several studies have reported a two- to threefold greater prevalence of severe hypertension (defined as 180/110 mmHg or greater) among African Americans, as compared to whites, further contributing to the higher rate of hypertension-related complications.[38,41,43] The 1996 age-adjusted mortality rate from high blood pressure was more than three times greater for African Americans than for whites.[4,44]

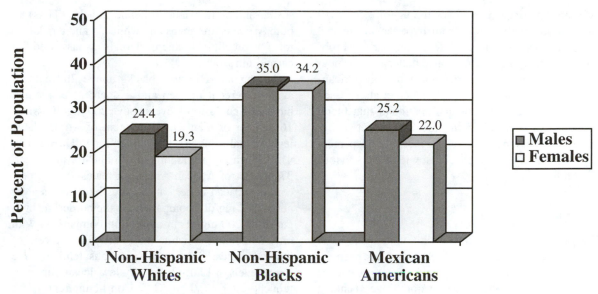

FIGURE 18–2 Estimated prevalence of high blood pressure by sex and race. (From the Centers for Disease Control/National Center for Health Statistics.[44])

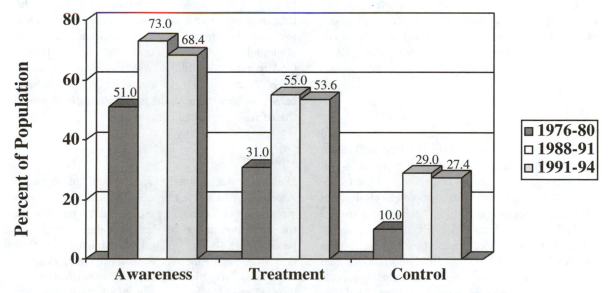

FIGURE 18–3 High blood pressure awareness, treatment and control rates (systolic blood pressure of 140 mmHg or greater and/or a diastolic blood pressure of 90 mmHg or greater or reporting the use of antihypertensive medication). (From the Centers for Disease Control/National Center for Health Statistics.[6])

African-American men under the age of 45 are 10 times more likely to die from hypertension-related complications than their white counterparts.[45] Probably even more important is the challenge of achieving standard blood pressure control in many African-American communities.[46,47] Kotchen et al. assessed over 500 African Americans and found that blood pressure was controlled in only 26 percent of hypertensive persons, despite the fact that 64 percent reported having seen a physician within the previous 3 months.[47]

Smoking

The risk of CVD associated with smoking is independent of age and gender.[48] Smoking has been associated with a more than fourfold greater prevalence of severe, uncontrolled hypertension (stage 3) among inner-city African Americans.[49] By contrast, smoking cessation is associated with a nearly 50 percent reduction in CVD.[51,52] Although the prevalence of smoking among African Americans is greater than[52] or similar to[53] that among whites, African Americans smoke fewer cigarettes.[52,53] African-American males and individuals with less than a high school education are consistently reported as more frequent smokers.[53] Similarly, those with less than a high school education and ethnic minorities are among those least likely to quit smoking.[54–57]

Dyslipidemia

The benefits of cholesterol-lowering for primary and secondary prevention of CHD have been well established.[58–60] Accurate assessment of a patient's risk for CHD must include not only levels of total cholesterol but also low-density-lipoprotein cholesterol (LDL-C), high-density-lipoprotein cholesterol (HDL-C), and triglycerides.[61] Evaluation of serum triglycerides is especially important in patients with diabetes.[62] Recently, certain lipid subfractions that may be independently linked with cardiovascular outcomes have received much attention. ARIC investigators reported mean lipoprotein(a) levels were more than twice as high for African Americans than for whites and were an independent risk factor for

stroke and/or transient ischemic attacks (TIAs) in both African Americans and whites,[63] and a risk factor for preclinical atherosclerosis as assessed by carotid ultrasound.[64]

Among non-Hispanic blacks above 20 years of age, 46 percent of men and 47 percent of women have total cholesterol levels above 200 mg/dL, while 16 percent of men and 20 percent of women have levels equal to or greater than 240 mg/dL (Fig. 18–4).[4,6] Furthermore, among youth age 19 and under, 37 percent of African-American males and 46 percent of African-American females have levels at or above 170 mg/dL (comparable to the borderline high cutoff of 200 mg/dL in adults), in comparison with only 27 percent of white males and 31.5 percent of white females.[4,6] African Americans tend to have lower levels of LDL-C and very low density lipoprotein cholesterol (VLDL-C).[65] Conflicting reports exist as to lower,[65] similar,[52,66] or higher[6,52,67,68] levels of HDL-C in African Americans. Despite the demonstrated efficacy of cholesterol lowering as an effective risk-reduction strategy for CVD, the medical community has not done an adequate job of ensuring that the millions of patients who could benefit from lipid-lowering therapy actually receive the treatment they require.[69,70] Awareness of hypercholesterolemia remains low in the African-American community.[46] Moreover, despite the fact that HMG-CoA reductase inhibitors have been shown to effectively decrease LDL-C levels in African Americans,[71–73] this therapy remains underutilized within the African-American community.[46,70]

Diabetes

Diabetes affects nearly 7.3 percent of African-American men and 9.1 percent of African-American women, a rate nearly 50 percent greater than that in the white population but less than that among Hispanics (Fig. 18–5).[74] The 1996 adjusted mortality rate for African Americans was more than twice that for whites.[4] This is only partially explained by socioeconomic factors.[75] The particularly high prevalence among African-American women is due in large part to the high prevalence of obesity and the subsequent development of insulin resistance among

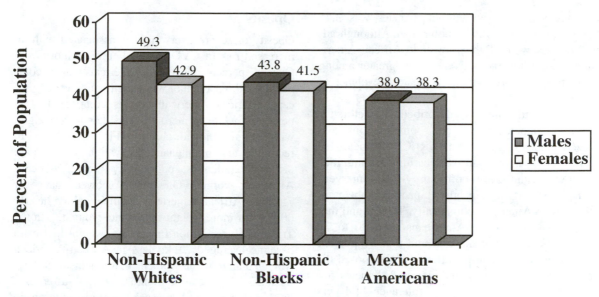

FIGURE 18–4 Estimated percentage of Americans age 20 and older with LDL-C of 130 mg/dL or greater by race and sex. (From the Centers for Disease Control/National Center for Health Statistics.[6])

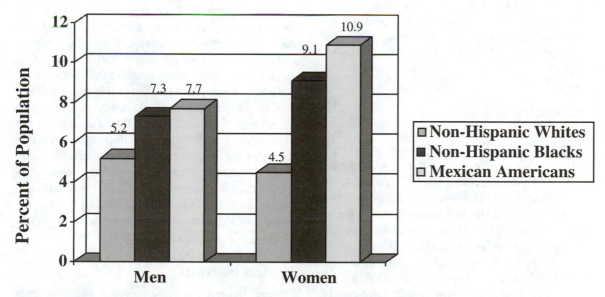

FIGURE 18–5 Estimated prevalence of physician-diagnosed diabetes in adults age 20 and above by sex and race. (From Harris et al.,[74] with permission.)

them, which has been described as an independent risk factor for CVD.[76,77] Thus, significant CVD risk-factor clustering occurs intrinsically in patients with type II diabetes. Folsom et al. reported that, among 13,446 middle-aged men and women free of CHD at baseline, the relative risk of CHD for people with diabetes versus those without diabetes was 3.45 among women and 2.52 among men. Although adjusted rates were slightly lower in African Americans, overall adverse outcomes were greater among African Americans owing to a greater prevalence of diabetes.[78]

Herman and colleagues described risk factors for diabetes, diabetes prevalence, complications, and care practices from project DIRECT (Diabetes Intervention Reaching and Educating Communities Together), a multilevel community-based intervention project highlighting the impact of diabetes in the African-American community. They found that 52 percent of African Americans aged 20 to 74 years reported being inactive and that 51 percent were overweight. The prevalence of diagnosed diabetes was 5.2 percent, undiagnosed diabetes 5.7 percent, and impaired glucose tolerance 11.4 percent. Also, African Americans with diabetes were significantly more likely than nonblacks with diabetes to have uncontrolled hypertension, to smoke cigarettes, and to lack health insurance or a private health care provider.[79] These multiple risk factors in diabetic patients further contribute to the disproportionately high CVD rates in African Americans.[28,34]

Hyperinsulinemia

Hyperinsulinemia, is associated with an increased risk for the subsequent development of multiple CVD risk factors—including diabetes, hypertension, hyperlipidemia, and CHD.[80–83] In the ARIC study, high serum insulin levels as well as increased body mass index (BMI) and waist-hip ratio were independently predictive of the development of diabetes, hypertension, and/or dyslipidemia in patients who had none of these metabolic abnormalities at baseline.[27,84] Whereas hyperinsulinemia and other characteristic features of syndrome X have consistently been noted in white populations, a different spectrum appears to occur in African-American patients with hyperinsulinemia in whom associations with hypertension,[85] high triglycerides, and lower HDL-C,[86] and increased CHD[86] have been questioned.[85–87]

Obesity

Obesity or severe overweight is associated with an increased risk of CVD in racial/ethnic minorities.[89] Over 57 percent of African-American males (compared to 59.6 percent of white men), and over 66 percent of African-American females (compared to 45.5 percent of white women) are considered overweight, with similar trends for children (Fig. 18–6).[4] Weight reduction and maintenance of weight loss remain difficult challenges, particularly among African-American women. One study showed that over 7 years, African-American women gained nearly 60 percent more weight than white women.[90] In the Trials of Hypertension Prevention, weight loss from baseline averaged 2.2 kg less in African-American women than in white women at 18 months of follow-up and 2.7 kg less at 36 months.[91] Racial differences in obesity and blood pressure are already present in 9- to 11-year-old children.[92,93] Obesity was directly associated with atherogenic plasma lipids, systolic blood pressure, serum glucose and insulin, and prevalence of diabetes mellitus; it was independently associated with CVD in young and middle-aged African Americans and whites in the Coronary Artery Risk Development in Young Adults (CARDIA) and ARIC studies.[28] Among more than 11,000 subjects in NHANES it was noted that the likelihood of diabetes was 75 percent greater for African Americans than for whites at low (<22 kg/m^2) BMI but equivalent at high (≥32 kg/m^2) BMI.[94] Effective intervention strategies are difficult to implement and, particularly in African-American women, one must consider issues such as the cultural tolerance for overweight and obesity as well as the importance of family and social networks in the dissemination of health information.[95,96]

Physical Inactivity

Physical inactivity is more prevalent among women than men, among African Americans and Hispanics than whites, among older than younger adults, and among the less affluent than the more affluent.[4] Regular physical activity has been associated with reduced CVD risk factors and improved outcomes.[97–102] In addition, cardiac rehabilitation re-

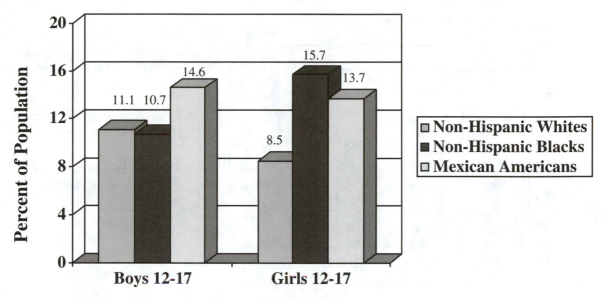

FIGURE 18–6 Estimated prevalence of overweight in children and adolescents by sex, age, and race. (From the Centers for Disease Control and Prevention[6]; age-specific 95th percentile cutoff points from revised CDC/NCHS growth charts and the American Heart Association,[4] with permission.)

duces post–myocardial infarction mortality rates and improves functional capacity in patients with CHF.[103] Recent studies show that among African Americans age 18 and older, 42.7 percent of women and 33.1 percent of men report no leisure-time physical activity (Fig. 18–7).[4] As with diet, poor patterns of exercise among the younger African-American community can contribute to greater risk for CVD with advancing age. Efforts to increase awareness and promote physical activities among children and young adults can help develop lifestyles associated with a low risk for CVD. For older persons, physical activity can also improve CVD risk factors and outcomes.[104,105] A 12-week course of moderate-intensity aerobic exercise and a T'ai Chi program of light activity were both effective in reducing systolic blood pressure (8.4 and 7.0 mmHg, respectively) and diastolic blood pressure (3.2 and 2.4 mmHg, respectively) among 62 sedentary older adults (45 percent black, 79 percent women, aged ≥60 years) with stage 1 hypertension receiving nonpharmacologic treatment.[106] Similarly, a weight-loss and exercise program for older African Americans with non-insulin-dependent diabetes improved both glycemic and blood pressure control.[107]

Moderate-intensity exercise has been reported to reduce blood pressure in hypertensive African Americans while having only a modest effect on serum lipid levels.[108] Regular exercise reduced blood pressure and left ventricular hypertrophy in African-American men aged 35 to 76 with severe hypertension.[108] The need for improved awareness of the benefit of regular physical activity and innovative ways to implement it remains a major challenge for many African-American communities. Many African Americans live in socioeconomically depressed neighborhoods where walking in the streets or parks is dangerous. Organized group activities can both help allay some of the fears and motivate people to action. Given the marked benefits of physical activity for improving multiple CVD risk factors, exercise is an extremely cost-effective approach to reducing CVD risk in the African-American community.

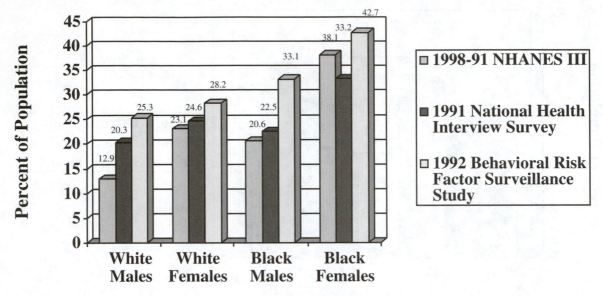

FIGURE 18–7 Estimated percentage of Americans age 18 and above who report no leisure-time physical activity by race and sex. (*Physical Activity and Health: A Report of the Surgeon General.* Washington, DC, United States Department of Health and Human Services, 1996.)

Diet

Nutrition plays a significant role in many of the CVD-associated risk factors. Several studies support a relationship between blood pressure and dietary cations.[109–114] In most studies, African Americans have been noted to have a greater sodium intake,[115] higher sodium/potassium intake,[116] lower potassium,[117,118] lower magnesium,[117] and/or lower calcium intake.[117,118] This may be related to a combination of socioeconomic factors and dietary customs within the African-American community associated with a high intake of salt and fat.[118] Several traditional African-American food preparations are related partly to a continuation of cooking practices developed during slavery, when African-American slaves were often given only old leftovers to eat and thus used generous amounts of seasonings, salts, and gravies to make the food palatable. Sodium restriction,[119–121] potassium supplementation,[111,122] and, to a lesser extent, calcium supplementation[114] have been associated with an improvement of hypertension in both black and white populations. Appel and colleagues from the multicenter Dietary Approaches to Stop Hypertension (DASH) study reported that a diet rich in fruits and vegetables with a low saturated and total fat content was particularly effective in reducing blood pressure, independent of weight loss, in nearly 500 healthy men and women (60 percent African American) with a baseline systolic blood pressure less than 160 mmHg and diastolic blood pressure 80 to 95 mmHg.[123]

Most studies support the presence of a dietary influence on CVD and hypertension among ethnic/racial minorities. A cross-sectional analysis of data from the NHANES II (1976–1980) and the Hispanic Health and Nutrition Examination Survey (1982–1984) suggested that dietary cation intake did not alter the magnitude of the ethnic differences in prevalence of hypertension.[116] However, the available data overall support the promotion of dietary modification as well as continued research into dietary constituents as important factors to improve CVD risk factors and outcomes.[124,125] Although the challenge of altering hundreds of years of traditional dietary customs is daunting, subtle modifications can produce significant reductions in the sodium and fat content of many traditional African-American meals, and these measures can often be implemented at both the individual and community levels.

Gender

Postmenopausal women receiving hormone replacement therapy (HRT) have a substantially lower risk for CVD mortality than those not receiving HRT.[126–128] However, concerns of complications such as uterine and breast cancer have led to cautions regarding the use of HRT,[129–131] although more recent reports suggest that the risk of HRT-associated cancers may no longer exist with the newer therapies.[128] Multiple cardiovascular benefits of HRT in postmenopausal women have been reported.[132–136] There are no reports of any significant racial differences in these mechanisms. One report suggests that only 13 percent of women are receiving HRT on a consistent basis[137] and HRT use may be even lower among minorities.[138]

Like women in general, African-American women are often less likely to receive the full benefit of available cardiovascular treatments; this compound problem further worsens the CVD risk profile of African-American women. Postmenopausal African-American women with heart disease were less likely to use lipid-lowering medication, unlikely to meet the LDL cholesterol treatment goal,[70] and more likely to have excessive CVD risk factors.[139] The compounding of low HRT use and other CVD risk-reduction therapies and reduced cardiovascular treatments among older African-American women further contributes to the even greater disparity in CVD outcomes noted between African-American and white women as compared with African-American and white men.[4]

Homocysteine

An elevation in plasma homocysteine levels has recently been described as an independent risk factor for coronary and peripheral vascular diseases.[140] Homocysteine may cause direct injury to the endothelial cell, stimulate smooth muscle cell growth, and increase thrombogenicity.[141] Limited data exists as to homocysteine levels in African Americans. A group of healthy premenopausal African-American women were reported to have increased plasma total homocysteine levels as compared with white women of a similar relatively advantaged socioeconomic status.[139] By contrast, polymorphism of the gene encoding for 5,10-methylene tetrahydrofolate reductase, which gives rise to a thermolabile form of the enzyme and is associated with increased levels of homocysteine, was less common in African Americans than in whites.[142] Further studies examining the role of homocysteine levels in CVD outcomes for African Americans are warranted.

Psychosocial Factors and Stress

Stress may be associated with a variety of neurohormonal changes that contribute to CVD,[143] and stress-reduction therapies may improve the associated risks.[144,145] Worsening psychosocial stresses arising from indigent lives and disenfranchisement from our health care system are additional putative contributors to increased CVD in African Americans. Several investigators have suggested that the increased incidence of hypertension in African Americans was due largely to internalized demands arising from socioeconomic stresses.[146–148] This phenomenon is frequently termed "active coping" or "John Henryism." The Charleston Heart Study revealed an increased incidence of hypertension associated with darker skin color in African Americans.[147] However, this association was abolished when adjusted for social class. Klag and associates reported an increased incidence of hypertension associated with darker skin color only in subjects in the lower levels of socioeconomic status, further supporting the influence of environmental factors on blood pressure in African Americans.[149] Both Waitzman and Smith[146] and Dressler[150,151] reported similar findings. Given that the excess of hypertension and other CVD risk factors may be mediated in part by behavioral factors operating through biological mechanisms, interventional studies are warranted to assess their efficacy in African-American communities.[152]

Risk Assessment and Treatment

Effective risk-reduction strategies can markedly reduce the incidence of both primary and secondary cardiovascular events. The American Heart Association (AHA) recommends that all primary care providers offer their patients counseling to promote physical activity, a healthy diet, and smoking cessation as part of the preventive health examination.[153] Despite the strong body of evidence documenting their efficacy, risk-reduction therapies continue to be underutilized or ineffectively implemented.[154] This is particularly evident within the African-American community, where comprehensive changes in health care delivery systems are needed to ensure that risk-reduction strategies become a routine part of care for patients with CVD.[155]

A thorough assessment by the clinician should include the evaluation of blood pressure, family history of CHD, smoking, weight/height, age, level of physical activity, diet, and measurement of lipids.[61] The opportunity of screening first-degree relatives should be undertaken with a view to primary prevention.[156] General recommendations for CVD prevention include smoking cessation, reduction of dietary fat intake to less than 30 percent of total energy, achieving optimal weight, and regular aerobic exercise. Addressing specific risk factors such as hypertension, diabetes, or hypercholesterolemia remains an important aspect of overall CVD prevention and treatment and may often warrant pharmacologic therapy, especially if multiple risk factors are present. The high prevalence of multiple risk factors within the African-American community magnifies the need for early risk-factor assessment and family screening as well as addressing these issues in a positive, proactive manner for both the family and the community.

Evaluation and Treatment of Hypertension in African Americans

Hypertension has been reported to be one of the most important modifiable risk factors for coronary disease.[157] Extensive investigations have delineated the effectiveness of both nonpharmacologic and pharmacologic therapies. African Americans have disproportionate burden of hypertension and offer a unique challenge to our standard approach to the treatment of hypertension owing to variations in its pathogenesis and the response to treatment in this population. A greater understanding of the pathophysiology of hypertension in African Americans enhances the appreciation of strategies for risk-factor reduction as well as the rationale for pharmacologic interventions.

Pathophysiology of Hypertension in African Americans

Idiopathic or essential hypertension is the most common form of hypertension and is a multifactorial disorder related to environmental, genetic (polygenic), and structural/anatomic factors. Several pathophysiologic changes that contribute to the development of hypertension appear to be related to race/ethnicity. African Americans have an increased prevalence of salt sensitivity.[158-161] Wilson and Grim have hypothesized a genetic component based on the African slave trade, where many slaves perished during the middle passage due to diarrheal diseases and dehydration; only those who were the most avid sodium retainers survived.[162] Several additional pathophysiologic changes may be present among African Americans that could lead to a salt-sensitive state. Su et al.[163] reported an amiloride-sensitive sodium channel variant in African Americans. Such alterations can result in constitutive activation of the channel and enhanced renal sodium reabsorption, consistent with a salt-sensitive state. An impaired rise in atrial natriuretic peptide (ANP) in response to sodium loading in African Americans could lead to a salt-sensitive hypertensive state.[164,165] Likewise, deficient or impaired renal nitric oxide production may lead to an increase in sodium and water retention and elevate blood pressure.[166,167] Other reported genetic associations for hypertension in African Americans include alterations in the beta$_2$-adrenergic receptor[168-170] and the alpha$_2$-adrenergic receptor.[171]

Treatment of Hypertension in African Americans

As outlined by the *Sixth Report of the Joint National Committee on Prevention, Detection, Evaluation, and Treatment of High Blood Pressure* (JNC VI), if lifestyle modifications are unable to control blood pressure, pharmacologic intervention with either diuretics or beta blockers is recommended as first line therapy.[17] Specific CVD risk factors or coexisting disease may modify the choice to an angiotensin-converting enzyme (ACE) inhibitor (i.e., CHF, diabetes), an alpha blocker (i.e., prostatic enlargement, hypercholesterolemia), or other agents. Despite studies reporting lower blood pressure response rates among African Americans to several antihypertensive agents—in contrast to diuretics and calcium channel blockers[172–176]—ethnicity should not be the primary criterion for selecting a given type of antihypertensive therapy. The overriding issues should include assessment of coexisting risk factors and cultural/socioeconomic factors.[177] Restriction of beta blockers[178] and/or possibly ACE inhibitors in African Americans with specific CVD risk factors or previous myocardial infarction could contribute to their increased mortality from CVD diseases. The most definitive treatment data are likely to come from the final report of the National Institutes of Health–sponsored Antihypertensive and Lipid Lowering Therapy to Prevent Heart Attack Trial (ALL-HAT), which has enrolled approximately 40,000 patients aged 55 years and older with multiple cardiac risk factors.[179] This report is particularly important, since many of the previously completed trials excluded the complex patients who are frequently encountered in clinical practice.

Evaluation and Treatment of Diabetes in African Americans

The strong association between diabetes and adverse cardiovascular events is well established. The high prevalence of diabetes (diagnosed and undiagnosed) and impaired glucose tolerance among African Americans makes their evaluation and treatment critical for reducing CVD in this population. Although current recommendations for diabetes screening are to begin at age 45 years, a recent evaluation of the cost-effectiveness of diabetes screening for persons above 25 years of age noted that screening was more cost-effective among younger persons and African Americans.[180] There has recently been a lowering in the fasting glucose threshold as a diagnostic criterion for diabetes from the previous value of 140 mg/dL to the new value of 126 mg/dL.[181] However, this lower value has recently been challenged, as Davidson and colleagues reported 60 percent of patients diagnosed with diabetes using the new criteria had normal HbA1c levels, noting that this could lead to the mislabeling of patients, with potential negative insurance, employment, social and psychological consequences.[182] Such mislabeling could be even more detrimental in socioeconomically fragile minority patients. Thus, patients with mildly elevated fasting blood glucose values should have their HbA1c levels measured and be given the diagnosis of diabetes only if the HbA1c level is more than 1 percent above the upper limit of normal.[182] If the HbA1c level is less than 1 percent above the upper limit of normal, close observation with appropriate diet and exercise counseling remain important components of treatment, as these patients are still at high risk.

Evaluation and Treatment of Dyslipidemia in African Americans

Because of mixed reports regarding lipid abnormalities among African Americans,[6,52,65–68] it is plausible that some health care providers may not focus on this issue as a significant risk factor in comparison to other risk factors, such as hypertension and diabetes. Treatment for hyperlipidemia in African Americans should be no different than that for the general population. There should be an equally high sensitivity for screening high-risk individuals and for providing treatment when appropriate.[183] According to current guidelines, the goal of therapy in patients with clinical atherosclerotic disease, including CHD, is to decrease LDL-C to 100 mg/dL or lower.[184] Delaying the use of drug therapy in most young adult men (<35 years) and premenopausal women with

LDL-C levels in the range of 160 to 220 mg/dL who are otherwise at low risk for CHD in the near future is prudent as long as close follow-up is maintained. If needed, pharmacologic therapy should be initiated, as it has been shown to effectively improve serum lipids in African Americans.[71–73] Likewise, high-risk elderly patients who are otherwise in good health are candidates for cholesterol-lowering therapy regardless of race or gender, as recommended by the National Cholesterol Education Program.[184]

Evaluation and Treatment of Smoking in African Americans

A careful evaluation of tobacco use should include the number of cigarettes smoked, the brand, the manner of inhalation, and number of puffs per cigarette. This allows a detailed assessment and initiates an in-depth dialogue between clinician and patient. It is an important and hopefully more effective approach, since a brief physician-based smoking cessation message was not an effective strategy for use with African-American smokers in a large urban public general hospital.[185] In addition to physician counseling, treatment with a nicotine patch[186] and referral to a smoking-cessation program may be of benefit for African Americans.[187,188] Unfortunately, the effectiveness of many smoking-cessation programs has not been consistently demonstrated.[189,190] Another approach is to integrate several of the family members if they are willing and motivated to be supportive of smoking cessation. Despite the suboptimal results of many smoking-cessation interventions, a particular approach may work well for a given patient; thus multiple attempts and strategies to achieve smoking cessation should be pursued.

Evaluation of Cardiovascular Disease

Presenting symptoms of ischemic-type chest pain and their correlation to myocardial infarction differ between races. In a study of 3401 African-American and 6600 white patients with symptoms suggestive of acute cardiac ischemia presenting to the emergency room, a diagnosis of acute myocardial infarction was confirmed in only 6 percent of African-American men and 4 percent of African-American women—in contrast to 12 percent of white men, and 8 percent of white women, respectively.[191] The lower prevalence of confirmed myocardial infarction among African Americans with chest pain may be related to a lesser prevalence of ischemic heart disease and a greater prevalence of left ventricular hypertrophy.[192,193] In addition, the high prevalence of abnormal electrocardiographic findings among African Americans[194] contributes to the concern of acute myocardial infarction in the setting of acute chest pain.

It appears that left ventricular hypertrophy in hypertension carries greater physiologic morbidity for African Americans than for whites. Ethnic differences in coronary arteriolar autoregulation and vasoreactivity may help explain the higher case fatality from coronary heart disease but lesser amounts of atherosclerotic CAD.[195] Among 91 African Americans and 81 whites referred for cardiac catheterization because of suspected myocardial ischemia but who were found to have no significant coronary stenosis, African Americans were typified by a marked reduction coronary flow reserve and an increased frequency of abnormal thallium tests.[195] However, abnormalities in cardiac vasoreactivity in patients referred for chest pain in normal coronary arteries was related to the presence of left ventricular hypertrophy (LVH, more common among African Americans), but not ethnicity.[196] Thus, diminished coronary reserve and altered microvascular relaxation associated with LVH may be an important key to the high rate of CVD among African Americans.

Access to Health Care and Impact on Treatment

Barriers in health care access and delivery further contribute to adverse CVD outcomes for African Americans. Several large studies have demonstrated marked variations in the utilization of cardiovascular procedures for African Americans as opposed to whites. If all populations are to reap the benefits of new therapeutic advances, it is critical that the treatment of CVD include not only the continuous development of effective treatments but equal access to and delivery of quality care. Pavlik and colleagues found that Hispanics and African Americans were significantly more likely to be in poor blood pressure control than whites after adjustment for multiple variables, suggesting the increased need for education of primary care providers in more aggressive blood pressure control, especially in minorities.[197]

Among nearly 4000 coronary bypass surgery patients with similar medical insurance coverage, survival was worse for African Americans than whites at 1 year (84 versus 92 percent, respectively) and at 5 years (64 versus 82 percent, respectively).[198] Women and African Americans hospitalized with myocardial infarctions at both teaching and non-teaching hospitals were less likely to have coronary angiography, coronary artery bypass graft surgery, and thrombolytic therapy. African Americans were also less likely to have coronary angioplasty.[199] A recent report noted that among 720 primary care physicians who viewed recorded interviews with actors portraying patients with cardiac symptoms, women and African Americans were only 60 percent as likely to be referred for cardiac catheterization, despite the same clinical picture.[200] Several other reports have noted disparities in health care related to racial background and/or insurance status.[201–205] The lack of a primary care physician was significantly associated with poor adherence to drug treatment for hypertension,[206] emphasizing the role of the physician-patient relationship and access to health care as critical variables influencing CVD outcomes in minorities.

By contrast, Pettinger and colleagues[207] provided free antihypertensive medication and follow-up medical care for 36 months to 79 patients (mostly African American and indigent) with severe hypertension and renal insufficiency. Compliance was 95 percent, and all patients had either stabilization or improvement in their renal function. When free medications were provided for patients receiving stepped care in the Hypertension Detection and Follow-up Program (HDFP) in comparison to usual care, 5-year mortality rates among African Americans were 23 percent less.[208] And in the MRFIT trial, the special-intervention group achieved better compliance and blood pressure control than the usual-care group for both African Americans and whites.[52] In the Thrombolysis in Myocardial Infarction II Trial, African Americans and Hispanics had mortality rates, after adjustment for baseline variables, that were similar to those of whites, suggesting no independent effect of race on outcome.[209]

Scott and colleagues reported on 5-year follow-up data for percutaneous transluminal coronary angioplasty in over 2000 patients [1939 (90.8 percent) white and 76 (3.6 percent) African American]. There were no significant differences between groups in mortality, myocardial infarction, coronary artery bypass grafting, or repeat coronary angioplasty, although very few African Americans were evaluated.[210] An analysis of almost 5000 patients found that white patients were three times as likely to undergo cardiovascular procedures as were African Americans prior to the development of ESRD. However, they had nearly identical rates after developing ESRD, at which time Medicare covered all patients.[211] Leape and coworkers analyzed whether cardiovascular procedures were utilized when needed rather than comparing crude use rates between ethnic/gender/socioeconomic groups. They reported that women, ethnic minorities, and the uninsured did receive needed interventions, although overall rates were less at hospitals that did not provide on-site revascularization.[212] However, the issues of appropriate preventive and early care were not addressed.

These data suggest that although CVD outcomes in general practice for racial/ethnic minorities, women, and the uninsured remain worse, the apparent deleterious effects of race and poverty on adverse cardiovascular related outcomes can often be abolished or attenuated in more controlled settings with ready access to high-quality medical care and medications. Despite the multiple reports of disparate health outcomes independent of insurance status,[213,214] there is optimism that managed care may deliver less biased care in some settings,[215–218] although not all agree.[219,220]

Interracial Variations

In addition to the classically described CVD risk factors, additional assessments may be helpful in the risk stratification of African Americans. Genetic, geographic, socioeconomic, and educational variations within the African-American community play an important role both in CVD risk assessment and the effective implementation of strategies for risk-factor reduction.[221–223] One study showed no difference in the incidence of hypertension among middle-class African Americans and whites with similar levels of baseline blood pressure and BMI followed for 7 years.[224] This suggests that higher socioeconomic status and educational attainment for African Americans is associated with hypertension incidence rates lower than rates reported for disadvantaged African Americans. In assessing mortality rates in residents of New York City, Southern-born African Americans had substantially higher and Caribbean-born African Americans substantially lower CVD mortality rates than those born in the Northeast. African Americans born in the South, 25 to 44 years of age, had a rate of death from coronary heart disease that was 30 percent higher than among those born in the Northeast and four times that of those born in the Caribbean of the same sex and age.[223]

Community Prevention Programs

The paucity of clinical trials demonstrating the feasibility and effectiveness of interventions in African Americans has, in part, impeded reduction of CVD rates in African Americans. Generalizations should not be made that effective or ineffective interventions in white communities are similarly effective or ineffective in African-American communities. Risk-factor management should be emphasized with culturally sensitive strategies[225] for the implementation of community-based programs. Six years of experience in a large community-based CVD prevention program in a predominantly minority urban setting suggested that such programs can be effective; however, they are unlikely to be sustained effectively without external resources.[226] A community-oriented

primary care approach for the detection, treatment, and control of hypertension was effective in every race-sex stratum of hypertensive patients utilizing the neighborhood health center; a particularly good response was noted for men and for African Americans.[227] The use of schools is also effective in many instances. One semester of aerobic exercise reduced systolic blood pressure more than the standard physical education in high-risk, predominantly African-American adolescent girls with blood pressure above the 67th percentile, thus reinforcing physical education in school as a feasible and effective health-promotion strategy for high-risk adolescent girls.[228]

Communitywide intervention efforts and messages improved knowledge of cardiovascular risk factors in a biracial South Carolina community with a generally low level of education. However, greater changes in most of these behaviors and knowledge were observed among white adults, further emphasizing the need for different strategies to reach African Americans.[229] A comprehensive work-site health promotion program among 4000 city of Birmingham employees significantly reduced systolic blood pressure in African-American participants. This study suggests that educational intervention tailored to the specific health perceptions and working conditions of a low-literacy population is feasible and is an effective way to improve hypertension control.[230] Another novel approach includes alliance formation, such as the Baltimore Alliance for the Prevention and Control of Hypertension and Diabetes, which was established to promote care to the underserved community of West Baltimore, Maryland, and to improve outcomes of hypertension and diabetes. This alliance of university, community health programs, church-based programs, managed care, and pharmaceutical company partners and a health policy and services research group is under evaluation; such a unique combination should better address cultural relevance and hopefully lead to improved outcomes.[231]

The church has been a particularly effective partner in the African-American community for implementing health care strategies. Church programs have been developed for smoking cessation,[232] and a church-based high blood pressure program for

African-American women led to improved blood pressure control in over 70 percent of participants and sustained weight loss in over 65 percent.[233] The use of registered nurses as church health educators led to a significant increase in knowledge scores and improved blood pressure levels from pre- to posttesting.[234] Some persons in the congregation can be trained to take the blood pressures of members of the congregation regularly, record weights, and assist with weight-control and food-preparation techniques and/or serve as smoking-cessation counselors. Another project developed a picture book about hypertension for children that was disseminated through Sunday school classes.[235]

Thus, community-based programs at various locations where people congregate—such as churches, barbershops, beauty salons, firehouses, housing projects, and work sites—can play a valuable role in improving the cardiovascular health of African Americans.[236] Health care professionals can be a potent force for the development of these programs by defining the scope and function of lay volunteers and promoting these programs in a variety of other ways. Intraracial diversity is an important factor to be considered in the development of community blood pressure control programs for African Americans, accounting for age, gender, educational background, socioeconomic status, health behaviors, and access to health care.[221,237]

Public Health Strategies

A widened disparity across educational groups in knowledge of cardiovascular risk factors was documented over the period of 1980–1990 among 2455 women and men from three population-based cross-sectional surveys in two northern California cities. These findings raise legitimate concerns that reformation of policies and strategies related to cardiovascular risk-reduction education are greatly needed.[238] Much of the health care disparity between ethnic minorities and whites in America has been attributed to socioeconomic factors. Although racial differences may necessitate changes in therapeutic intervention for relevant subgroups, it appears that race-specific differences account for less than 50 percent of the health outcomes among African Americans.[36]

One example of public health intervention involves smoking, where policy interventions to control tobacco use are among the most cost-effective approaches to prevent CVD. Restrictions on tobacco advertising and promotion, policies limiting youth access to tobacco, comprehensive school health programs, excise taxes, and other economic incentives have been very effective.[239] Similarly, efforts to control hypertension should encompass primary prevention, early detection, and adequate awareness and treatment of high blood pressure.[240–242]

These observations emphasize the need for population approaches to promote physical activity and prevention of CVD and other chronic illnesses, including federal, state, and local legislation and regulation, as well as policy development and implementation, and environmental support.[243]

Summary

Both primary and secondary prevention programs targeted at African-American populations need to include education at the level of the health care provider, the individual, the immediate family, and the community. The use of primary prevention education programs using established groups such as schools, social clubs, and churches to promote risk-factor awareness should be considered. Often churches can provide a place for education with regard to appropriate diet, weight control, exercise, high blood pressure control, smoking cessation, and alcohol abstinence in a culturally sensitive manner that can seldom be duplicated in most structured, government-developed programs. When feasible, simultaneous efforts to provide cholesterol, weight, blood pressure, smoking, alcohol, and other risk factor screening, counseling, and/or referral services should be made available. Physicians, nurses, and other health care professionals should be encouraged to lead or participate in many of these efforts and can often be an invaluable resource for many medically related questions and concerns within the community.

Secondary prevention measures can also be addressed through community programs, since most of these community-based risk-reduction strategies will mirror those of primary prevention. Improving patients' knowledge of proven interventions to reduce post–myocardial infarction mortality rates can stimulate them to enter into a more detailed dialogue with their primary care providers and hopefully improve their health. Since there is no evidence to support a different secondary prevention goal for African Americans in contrast to whites, it is important that health care providers and health management systems make specific secondary prevention therapies and needed cardiovascular interventions widely available.

Hopefully, by using innovative individual/family and community-based approaches for primary and secondary CVD prevention, we will soon see significant improvements in the health of the African-American community.

References

1. Francis CK: Research in coronary heart disease in blacks: issues and challenges. *J Health Care Poor Underserved* 1997; 8:250–269.
2. Karter AJ, Gazzaniga JM, Cohen RD, et al: Ischemic heart disease and stroke mortality in African-American, Hispanic, and non-Hispanic white men and women, 1985 to 1991. *West J Med* 1998; 169:139–145.
3. Cardiovascular Health Branch, Division of Chronic Disease Control and Community Intervention, National Center for Chronic Disease Prevention and Health Promotion, CDC: Trends in ischemic heart disease mortality—United States, 1980–1988. *MMWR* 1992; 41:548–556.
4. American Heart Association: *1999 Heart and Stroke Statistical Update.* Dallas, American Heart Association, 1998.
5. Escobedo LG, Giles WH, Anda RF: Socioeconomic status, race, and death from coronary heart disease. *Am J Prev Med* 1997; 13:123–130.
6. Centers for Disease Control/National Center for Health Statistics: *National Health and Nutrition Examination Survey III (NHANES III) 1988–94.* Bethesda, MD, CDC/NCHS, 1995.
7. Alexander M, Grumbach K, Selby J, et al: Hospitalization for congestive heart failure: explaining racial differences. *JAMA* 1995; 274:1037–1042.
8. Gillum RF: Epidemiology of heart failure in the United States. *Am Heart J* 1993; 126:1042–1047.
9. Moser M, Hebert PR: Prevention, left ventricular hypertrophy and congestive heart failure in hypertension treatment trials. *J Am Coll Cardiol* 1996; 27:1214–1218.
10. The SOLVD Investigators: Effect of enalapril on survival in patients with reduced ejection fractions and congestive heart failure. *N Engl J Med* 1991; 335:293–302.
11. Bourassa MG, Gurne O, Bangdiwala SI, et al: Natural history and patterns of current practice in heart failure: the Studies of Left Ventricular Dysfunction (SOLVD) investigators. *J Am Coll Cardiol* 1993; 22(suppl A):14A–19A.
12. Dries DL, Exner DV, Gersh BJ, et al: Racial differences in the outcome of left ventricular dysfunction. *N Engl J Med* 1999; 340:609–616.
13. Miller JP, Perry HM Jr, Rossiter JE, et al: Regional differences in mortality during 15-year follow-up of 11,936 hypertensive veterans. *Hypertension* 1994; 23:431–438.
14. Gillum RF, Ingram DI: The relation between residence in the southeast region of the United States and stroke incidence and death: the NHANES I epidemiologic follow-up study. *Am J Epidemiol* 1996; 144:665–667.
15. Perry HM, Roccella EJ: Conference report on stroke mortality in the southeastern United States. *Hypertension* 1998; 31:1206–1215.
16. Arnett DK, Tyroler HA, Burke G, et al: Hypertension and subclinical carotid artery atherosclerosis in blacks and whites: the Atherosclerosis Risk in Communities Study. ARIC investigators. *Arch Intern Med* 1996; 156:1983–1989.
17. The Sixth Report of the Joint National Committee on Prevention, Detection, Evaluation, and Treatment of high blood pressure. *Arch Intern Med* 1997; 157:2413–2446.
18. Mulrow CD, Cornell JA, Herrera CR: Hypertension in the elderly: implications and generalization of randomized trials. *JAMA* 1994; 272:1932–1938.
19. Liao D, Myers R, Hunt S, et al: Familial history of stroke and stroke risk: the Family Heart Study. *Stroke* 1997; 28:1908–1912.
20. Jones CA, Agodoa L: Kidney disease and hypertension in blacks: scope of the problem. *Am J Kidney Dis* 1993; 21(4 suppl):6–9.
21. U.S. Renal Data System (USRDS): *1998 Annual Data Report.* Bethesda, MD, National Institutes of Health, National Institute of Diabetes and Digestive and Kidney Diseases, April 1998.
22. McClellan W, Tuttle E, Issa A: Racial differences in the incidence of end-stage renal disease (ESRD) are not entirely explained by differences in the prevalence of hypertension. *Am J Kidney Dis* 1988; 12:285–290.
23. Klag MJ, Stamler J, Brancati FL, et al: End-stage renal disease in African-American and white men: 16-year MRFIT findings. *JAMA* 1997; 277:1293–1298.
24. Bond V Jr, Thompson GD, Franks BD, et al: Racial differences in minimum lower leg vascular resistance in normotensive young adults with positive and negative

parental histories of hypertension. *J Cardiovasc Risk* 1996; 3:423–426.

25. Tunis SR, Bass EB, Klag MJ, Steinberg EP: Variation in utilization of procedures for treatment of peripheral arterial disease: a look at patient characteristics. *Arch Intern Med* 1993; 153:991–998.

26. Otten MW Jr, Teutsch SM, Williamson DF, Marks JS: The effect of known risk factors on the excess mortality of black adults in the United States. *JAMA* 1990; 263:845–850.

27. Schmidt MI, Duncan BB, Watson RL, et al: A metabolic syndrome in whites and African-Americans: the Atherosclerosis Risk in Communities baseline study. *Diabetes Care* 1996; 19:414–418.

28. Folsom AR, Burke GL, Byers CL, et al: Implications of obesity for cardiovascular disease in blacks: the CARDIA and ARIC studies. *Am J Clin Nutr* 1991; 53(6 suppl):1604S–1611S.

29. Vaccaro O, Stamler J, Neaton JD: Sixteen-year coronary mortality in black and white men with diabetes screened for the Multiple Risk Factor Intervention Trial (MRFIT). *Int J Epidemiol* 1998; 27:636–641.

30. Howard G, Manolio TA, Burke GL, et al: Does the association of risk factors and atherosclerosis change with age? An analysis of the combined ARIC and CHS cohorts. The Atherosclerosis Risk in Communities (ARIC) and Cardiovascular Health Study (CHS) investigators. *Stroke* 1997; 28:1693–1701.

31. Becker DM, Yook RM, Moy TF, et al: Markedly high prevalence of coronary risk factors in apparently healthy African-American and white siblings of persons with premature coronary heart disease. *Am J Cardiol* 1998; 82:1046–1051.

32. Genest JJ, McNamara JR, Salem DN, Schaefer EJ: Prevalence of risk factors in men with premature coronary artery disease. *Am J Cardiol* 1991; 67:1185–1189.

33. Rowland ML, Fulwood R: Coronary heart disease risk factor trends in blacks between the first and second National Health and Nutrition Examination Surveys, United States, 1971–1980. *Am Heart J* 1984; 108(3 Pt 2):771–779.

34. Suarez L, Barrett-Connor E: Interaction between cigarette smoking and diabetes mellitus in the prediction of death attributed to cardiovascular disease. *Am J Epidemiol* 1984; 120:670–675.

35. Hopkins PN, Williams RR, Hunt SC: Magnified risks from cigarette smoking for coronary prone families in Utah. *West J Med* 1984; 141:196–202.

36. Davey Smith G, Neaton JD, Wentworth D, et al: Mortality differences between black and white men in the USA: contribution of income and other risk factors among men screened for the MRFIT. MRFIT research group. Multiple Risk Factor Intervention Trial. *Lancet* 1998; 351:934–939.

37. Hennekens CH: Lessons from hypertension trials. *Am J Med* 1998; 104:50S–53S.

38. Klag MJ, Whelton PK, Randall BL, et al: Blood pressure and end-stage renal disease in men. *N Engl J Med* 1996; 334:13–18.

39. Deubner DC, Tyroler HA, Cassel JC, et al: Attributable risk, population attributable risk and population attributable fraction of death associated with hypertension in a biracial population. *Circulation* 1975; 52:901–908.

40. Nelson C, Woodwell D: National ambulatory medical care survey: 1993 summary. *Vital Health Stat* [13] 1998; 136:iii–vi, 1–99.

41. Burt VL, Whelton P, Roccella EJ, et al: Prevalence of hypertension in the U.S. adult population: results from the third National Health and Nutrition Examination Survey, 1988–1991. *Hypertension* 1995; 25:305–313.

42. Coca A: Actual blood pressure control: are we doing things right? *J Hypertens Suppl* 1998; 16:S45–S51.

43. The Joint National Committee on Detection, Evaluation, and Treatment of High Blood Pressure: The fifth report of the Joint National Committee on Detection, Evaluation and Treatment of High Blood Pressure (JNC V). *Arch Intern Med* 1993; 153:154–183.

44. Centers for Disease Control/National Center for Health Statistics: *Health United States 1998*. Bethesda, MD: CDC/NCHS, 1998.

45. Magnus MH. Cardiovascular health among African-Americans: a review of the health status, risk reduction, and intervention strategies. *Am J Health Promotion* 1991; 5:282–290.

46. Nieto FJ, Alonso J, Chambless LE, et al: Population awareness and control of hypertension and hypercholesterolemia: the Atherosclerosis Risk in Communities study. *Arch Intern Med* 1995; 155:677–684.

47. Kotchen JM, Shakoor-Abdullah B, Walker WE, et al: Hypertension control and access to medical care in the inner city. *Am J Public Health* 1998; 88:1696–1699.

48. U.S. Department of Health and Human Services: *The Health Consequences of Smoking: Cardiovascular Disease: A Report of the Surgeon General*. DHHS publication No. (PHS) 84-50204. Washington, DC: Office on Smoking and Health, U.S. Government Printing Office, 1983.

49. McNagny SE, Ahluwalia JS, Clark WS, Resnicow KA: Cigarette smoking and severe uncontrolled hypertension in inner-city African Americans. *Am J Med* 1997; 103:121–127.

50. Hermanson B, Omenn GS, Kronmal RA, Gersh BJ: Beneficial six-year outcome of smoking cessation in older men and women with coronary artery disease: results from the CASS registry. *N Engl J Med* 1988; 319:1365–1369.

51. Rosenberg L, Kaufman DW, Helmrich SP, Shapiro S: The risk of myocardial infarction after quitting smoking in men under 55 years of age. *N Engl J Med* 1985; 313:1511–1514.

52. Connett JE, Stamler J: Responses of black and white males to the special intervention program of the

Multiple Risk Factor Intervention Trial. *Am Heart J* 1984; 108(3 pt 2):839–848.

53. Centers for Disease Control/National Center for Health Statistics: *National Health Interview Survey, 1995.* Bethesda, MD: CDC/NCHS, 1995.

54. Royce JM, Corbett K, Sorensen G, Ockene J: Gender, social pressure, and smoking cessations: the Community Intervention Trial for Smoking Cessation (COMMIT) at baseline. *Soc Sci Med* 1997; 44:359–370.

55. Feigelman W, Lee J: Probing the paradoxical pattern of cigarette smoking among African Americans: low teenage consumption and high adult use. *J Drug Educ* 1995; 25:307–320.

56. Rogers RG, Nam CB, Hummer RA: Demographic and socioeconomic links to cigarette smoking. *Soc Biol* 1995; 42:1–21.

57. Royce JM, Hymowitz N, Corbett K, et al: Smoking cessation factors among African Americans and whites: COMMIT Research Group. *Am J Public Health* 1993; 83:220–226.

58. Gotto AM Jr: Assessing the benefits of lipid-lowering therapy. *Am J Cardiol* 1998; 82:2M–4M.

59. White CW: Benefit of aggressive lipid-lowering therapy: insights from the post coronary artery bypass graft study and other trials. *Am J Med* 1998; 105:63S–68S.

60. Jones PH: Future of lipid-lowering trials: what else do we need to know? *Am J Cardiol* 1998; 82:32M–38M.

61. Shepherd J. Profiling risk and new therapeutic interventions: looking ahead. *Am J Med* 1998; 104:19S–22S.

62. Kreisberg RA. Diabetic dyslipidemia. *Am J Cardiol* 1998; 82:67U–73U.

63. Schreiner PJ, Chambless LE, Brown SA, et al: Lipoprotein(a) as a correlate of stroke and transient ischemic attack prevalence in a biracial cohort: the ARIC study. Atherosclerosis Risk in Communities. *Ann Epidemiol* 1994; 4:351–359.

64. Schreiner PJ, Morrisett JD, Sharrett AR, et al: Lipoprotein[a] as a risk factor for preclinical atherosclerosis. *Arterioscler Thromb* 1993; 13:826–833.

65. Wilson PW, Savage DD, Castelli WP, et al: HDL-cholesterol in a sample of black adults: the Framingham minority. *Metabolism* 1983; 32:328–332.

66. Sprafka JM, Burke GL, Folsom AR, Hahn LP: Hypercholesterolemia prevalence, awareness, and treatment in blacks and whites: the Minnesota Heart Survey. *Prev Med* 1989; 18:423–432.

67. Linn S, Fulwood R, Rifkind B, et al: High density lipoprotein cholesterol levels among U.S. adults by selected demographic and socioeconomic variables: the Second National Health and Nutrition Examination Survey 1976–1980. *Am J Epidemiol* 1989; 129:281–294.

68. Gidding SS, Liu K, Bild DE, et al: Prevalence and identification of abnormal lipoprotein levels in a biracial population aged 23–35 years (the CARDIA Study). The

Coronary Artery Risk Development in Young Adults study. *Am J Cardiol* 1996; 78:304–348.

69. Gotto AM Jr: Risk factor modification: rationale for management of dyslipidemia. *Am J Med* 1998; 104:6S–8S.

70. Schrott HG, Bittner V, Vittinghoff E, et al: Adherence to National Cholesterol Education Program Treatment goals in postmenopausal women with heart disease: the Heart and Estrogen/Progestin Replacement Study (HERS). The HERS research group. *JAMA* 1997; 277:1281–1286.

71. Jacobson TA, Chin MM, Curry CL, et al: Efficacy and safety of pravastatin in African Americans with primary hypercholesterolemia. *Arch Intern Med* 1995; 155:1900–1906.

72. Prisant LM, Downton M, Watkins LO, et al: Efficacy and tolerability of lovastatin in 459 African-Americans with hypercholesterolemia. *Am J Cardiol* 1996; 78:420–424.

73. Fong RL, Ward HJ: The efficacy of lovastatin in lowering cholesterol in African Americans with primary hypercholesterolemia. *Am J Med* 1997; 102:387–391.

74. Harris MI, Flegal KM, Cowie CC, et al: Prevalence of diabetes, impaired fasting glucose, and impaired glucose tolerance in U.S. adults: the Third National Health and Nutrition Examination Survey, 1988–1994. *Diabetes Care* 1998; 21:518–524.

75. Brancati FL, Whelton PK, Kuller LH, Klag MJ: Diabetes mellitus, race, and socioeconomic status: a population-based study. *Ann Epidemiol* 1996; 6:67–73.

76. Reaven GM: Pathophysiology of insulin resistance in human disease. *Physiol Rev* 1995; 75:473–486.

77. Reaven GM: Role of insulin resistance in human disease (syndrome X): an expanded definition. *Annu Rev Med* 1993; 44:121–131.

78. Folsom AR, Szklo M, Stevens J, et al: A prospective study of coronary heart disease in relation to fasting insulin, glucose, and diabetes: the Atherosclerosis Risk in Communities (ARIC) study. *Diabetes Care* 1997; 20:935–942.

79. Herman WH, Thompson TJ, Visscher W, et al: Diabetes mellitus and its complications in an African-American community: project DIRECT. *J Natl Med Assoc* 1998; 90:147–156.

80. Maheux P, Jeppesen J, Sheu WH, et al: Additive effects of obesity, hypertension, and type 2 diabetes on insulin resistance. *Hypertension* 1994; 24:695–698.

81. Reaven GM, Laws A: Insulin resistance, compensatory hyperinsulinaemia, and coronary heart disease. *Diabetologia* 1994; 37:948–952.

82. Weir MR, Hanes DS: Hypertension in African Americans: a paradigm of metabolic disarray. *Semin Nephrol* 1996; 16:102–109.

83. Nabulsi AA, Folsom AR, Heiss G, et al: Fasting hyperinsulinemia and cardiovascular disease risk factors in nondiabetic adults: stronger associations in lean versus obese subjects. Atherosclerosis Risk in Communities study investigators. *Metabolism* 1995; 44:914–922.

84. Liese AD, Mayer-Davis EJ, Tyroler HA, et al: Development of the multiple metabolic syndrome in the ARIC cohort: joint contribution of insulin, BMI, and WHR: atherosclerosis risk in communities. *Ann Epidemiol* 1997; 7:407–416.

85. Osei K, Schuster DP: Effects of race and ethnicity on insulin sensitivity, blood pressure, and heart rate in three ethnic populations: comparative studies in African-Americans, African immigrants (Ghanaians), and white Americans using ambulatory blood pressure monitoring. *Am J Hypertens* 1996; 9(12 pt 1):1157–1164.

86. Cappuccio FP: Ethnicity and cardiovascular risk: variations in people of African ancestry and South Asian origin. *J Hum Hypertens* 1997; 11:571–576.

87. Haffner SM: Progress in population analyses of the insulin resistance syndrome. *Ann NY Acad Sci* 1997; 827:1–12.

88. Osei K, Schuster DP: Ethnic differences in secretion, sensitivity, and hepatic extraction of insulin in black and white Americans. *Diabet Med* 1994; 11:755–762.

89. Sowers JR: Obesity and cardiovascular disease. *Clin Chem* 1998; 44(8 pt 2):1821–1825.

90. Lewis CE, Smith DE, Wallace DD, et al: Seven-year trends in body weight and associations with lifestyle and behavioral characteristics in black and white young adults: the CARDIA study. *Am J Public Health* 1997; 87:635–642.

91. Kumanyika SK, Obarzanek E, Stevens VJ, et al: Weight-loss experience of black and white participants in NHLBI-sponsored clinical trials. *Am J Clin Nutr* 1991; 53(6 suppl):1631S–1638S.

92. Obesity and cardiovascular disease risk factors in black and white girls: the NHLBI Growth and Health Study. *Am J Public Health* 1992; 82:1613–1620.

93. Figueroa-Colon R, Franklin FA, Lee JY, et al: Prevalence of obesity with increased blood pressure in elementary school-aged children. *South Med J* 1997; 90:806–813.

94. Resnick HE, Valsania P, Halter JB, Lin X: Differential effects of BMI on diabetes risk among black and white Americans. *Diabetes Care* 1998; 21:1828–1835.

95. Melnyk MG, Weinstein E: Preventing obesity in black women by targeting adolescents: a literature review. *J Am Diet Assoc* 1994; 94:536–540.

96. Morris RI: Bridging cultural boundaries: the African American and transcultural caring. *Adv Pract Nurs Q* 1996; 2:31–38.

97. Rodriguez BL, Curb JD, Burchfiel CM, et al: Physical activity and 23-year incidence of coronary heart disease morbidity and mortality among middle-aged men: the Honolulu Heart Program. *Circulation* 1994; 89:2540–2544.

98. Lee IM, Paffenbarger RS Jr, Hennekens CH: Physical activity, physical fitness and longevity. *Aging* 1997; 9:2–11.

99. Burnham JM: Exercise is medicine: health benefits of regular physical activity. *J La State Med Soc* 1998; 150:319–323.

100. Rose G: Physical activity and coronary heart disease. *Proc R Soc Med* 1969; 62:1183–1188.

101. Ekelund LG, Haskell WL, Johnson JL, et al: Physical fitness as a predictor of cardiovascular mortality in asymptomatic North American men. *N Engl J Med* 1988; 318:1379–1384.

102. Blair SN, Kohl HW III, Paffenbarger RS Jr, et al: Physical fitness and all-cause mortality: a prospective study of healthy men and women. *JAMA* 1989; 262:2395–2401.

103. Shaw LW: Effects of a prescribed supervised exercise program on mortality and cardiovascular morbidity in patients after myocardial infarction: the National Exercise and Heart Disease Project. *Am J Cardiol* 1981; 48:39–46.

104. LaCroix AZ, Leveille SG, Hecht JA, et al: Does walking decrease the risk of cardiovascular disease hospitalizations and death in older adults? *J Am Geriatr Soc* 1996; 44:113–120.

105. Villeneuve PJ, Morrison HI, Craig CL, Schaubel DE: Physical activity, physical fitness, and risk of dying. *Epidemiology* 1998; 9:626–631.

106. Young DR, Appel LJ, Jee S, Miller ER III: The effects of aerobic exercise and T'ai Chi on blood pressure in older people: results of a randomized trial. *J Am Geriatr Soc* 1999; 47:277–284.

107. Agurs-Collins TD, Kumanyika SK, Ten Have TR, Adams-Campbell LL: A randomized controlled trial of weight reduction and exercise for diabetes management in older African-American subjects (see comments). *Diabetes Care* 1997; 20:1503–1511.

108. Kokkinos PF, Narayan P, Colleran J, et al: Effects of moderate intensity exercise on serum lipids in African-American men with severe systemic hypertension. *Am J Cardiol* 1998; 81:732–735.

109. Cutler JA, Follmann D, Allender PS: Randomized trials of sodium reduction: an overview. *Am J Clin Nutr* 1997; 65(2 suppl):643S–651S.

110. Stamler J: The INTERSALT Study: background, methods, findings, and implications. *Am J Clin Nutr* 1997; 65(2 suppl):626S–642S.

111. Whelton PK, He J, Cutler JA, et al: Effects of oral potassium on blood pressure: meta-analysis of randomized controlled clinical trials. *JAMA* 1997; 277:1624–1632.

112. Freudenheim JL, Russell M, Trevisan M, Doemland M: Calcium intake and blood pressure in blacks and whites. *Ethn Dis* 1991; 1:114–122.

113. McCarron DA, Metz JA, Hatton DC. Mineral intake and blood pressure in African Americans. *Am J Clin Nutr* 1998; 68:517–518.

114. Allender PS, Cutler JA, Follmann D, et al: Dietary calcium and blood pressure: a meta-analysis of randomized clinical trials. *Ann Intern Med* 1996; 124:825–831.

115. Gerber AM, James SA, Ammerman AS, et al: Socioeconomic status and electrolyte intake in black adults: the Pitt County study. *Am J Public Health* 1991; 81:1608–1612.

116. Bauer UE, Mayne ST: Do ethnic differences in dietary cation intake explain ethnic differences in hypertension prevalence? Results from a cross-sectional analysis. *Ann Epidemiol* 1997; 7:479–485.

117. Ford ES: Race, education, and dietary cations: findings from the Third National Health and Nutrition Examination Survey. *Ethn Dis* 1998; 8:10–20.

118. Shimakawa T, Sorlie P, Carpenter MA, et al: Dietary intake patterns and sociodemographic factors in the atherosclerosis risk in communities study: ARIC study investigators. *Prev Med* 1994; 23:769–780.

119. He J, Whelton PK: Role of sodium reduction in the treatment and prevention of hypertension. *Curr Opin Cardiol* 1997; 12:202–207.

120. Whelton PK, Appel LJ, Espeland MA, et al: Sodium reduction and weight loss in the treatment of hypertension in older persons: a randomized controlled trial of nonpharmacologic interventions in the elderly (TONE): TONE collaborative research group. *JAMA* 1998; 279:839–846.

121. Whelton PK, Kumanyika SK, Cook NR, et al: Efficacy of nonpharmacologic interventions in adults with high-normal blood pressure: results from phase 1 of the Trials of Hypertension Prevention: Trials of Hypertension Prevention collaborative research group. *Am J Clin Nutr* 1997; 65(2 suppl):652S–660S.

122. Brancati FL, Appel LJ, Seidler AJ, Whelton PK: Effect of potassium supplementation on blood pressure in African Americans on a low-potassium diet: a randomized, double-blind, placebo-controlled trial. *Arch Intern Med* 1996; 156:61–67.

123. Appel LJ, Moore TJ, Obarzanek E, et al: A clinical trial of the effects of dietary patterns on blood pressure. *N Engl J Med* 1997; 336:1117–1124.

124. Adrogue HJ, Wesson DE: Role of dietary factors in the hypertension of African Americans. *Semin Nephrol* 1996; 16:94–101.

125. Gates G, McDonald M: Comparison of dietary risk factors for cardiovascular disease in African-American and white women. *J Am Diet Assoc* 1997; 97:1394–1400.

126. Stampfer MJ, Willett WC, Colditz GA, et al: A prospective study of postmenopausal estrogen therapy and coronary heart disease. *N Engl J Med* 1985; 313:1044–1049.

127. Grodstein F, Stampfer MJ, Colditz GA, et al: Postmenopausal hormone therapy and mortality. *N Engl J Med* 1997; 336:1769–1775.

128. Barrett-Connor E, Wenger NK, Grady D, et al: Hormone and nonhormone therapy for the maintenance of postmenopausal health: the need for randomized controlled trials of estrogen and raloxifene. *J Womens Health* 1998; 7:839–847.

129. Barrett-Connor E, Grady D: Hormone replacement therapy, heart disease, and other considerations. *Annu Rev Public Health* 1998; 19:55–72.

130. Colditz GA: Relationship between estrogen levels, use of hormone replacement therapy, and breast cancer. *J Natl Cancer Inst* 1998; 90:814–823.

131. Colditz GA, Stampfer MJ, Willett WC, et al: Type of postmenopausal hormone use and risk of breast cancer: 12-year follow-up from the Nurses' Health Study. *Cancer Causes Control* 1992; 3:433–439.

132. Brown SA, Hutchinson R, Morrisett J, et al: Plasma lipid, lipoprotein cholesterol, and apoprotein distributions in selected US communities: the Atherosclerosis Risk in Communities (ARIC) study. *Arterioscler Thromb* 1993; 13:1139–1158.

133. Stevenson JC: Various actions of oestrogens on the vascular system. *Maturitas* 1998; 20;30:5–9.

134. Nasr A, Breckwoldt M: Estrogen replacement therapy and cardiovascular protection: lipid mechanisms are the tip of an iceberg. *Gynecol Endocrinol* 1998; 12:43–59.

135. Vogel RA: Coronary risk factors, endothelial function, and atherosclerosis: a review. *Clin Cardiol* 1997; 20:426–432.

136. Shahar E, Folsom AR, Salomaa VV, et al: Relation of hormone-replacement therapy to measures of plasma fibrinolytic activity: Atherosclerosis Risk in Communities (ARIC) study investigators. *Circulation* 1996; 93:1970–1975.

137. Johannes CB, Crawford SL, Posner JG, McKinlay SM: Longitudinal patterns and correlates of hormone replacement therapy use in middle-aged women. *Am J Epidemiol* 1994; 140:439–452.

138. Egeland GM, Matthews KA, Kuller LH, Kelsey SF: Characteristics of noncontraceptive hormone users. *Prev Med* 1988; 17:403–411.

139. Gerhard GT, Sexton G, Malinow MR, et al: Premenopausal African American women have more risk factors for coronary heart disease than white women. *Am J Cardiol* 1998; 82:1040–1045.

140. Refsum H, Ueland PM, Nygard O, Vollset SE: Homocysteine and cardiovascular disease. *Annu Rev Med* 1998; 49:31–62.

141. van der Molen EF, Hiipakka MJ, van Lith-Zanders H, et al: Homocysteine metabolism in endothelial cells of a patient homozygous for cystathionine beta-synthase (CS) deficiency. *Thromb Haemost* 1997; 78:827–833.

142. McAndrew PE, Brandt JT, Pearl DK, Prior TW: The incidence of the gene for thermolabile methylene tetrahydrofolate reductase in African Americans. *Thromb Res* 1996; 83:195–198.

143. Kubzansky LD, Kawachi I, Weiss ST, Sparrow D: Anxiety and coronary heart disease: a synthesis of epidemiological, psychological, and experimental evidence. *Ann Behav Med* 1998; 20:47–58.

144. Schneider RH, Nidich SI, Salerno JW, et al: Lower lipid peroxide levels in practitioners of the Transcendental Meditation program. *Psychosom Med* 1998; 60:38–41.

145. Alexander CN, Schneider RH, Staggers F, et al: Trial of stress reduction for hypertension in older African Americans: II. Sex and risk subgroup analysis. *Hypertension* 1996; 28:228–237.

146. Waitzman NJ, Smith KR: The effect of occupational class transitions on hypertension: racial disparities among working-age men. *Am J Public Health* 1994; 84:945–950.

147. Keil JE, Tyroler HA, Sandifer SH, Boyle E Jr: Hypertension: effects of social class and racial admixture. *Am J Public Health* 1977; 64:634–639.

148. Krieger N, Sidney S. Racial discrimination and blood pressure: the CARDIA Study of young black and white adults. *Am J Public Health* 1996; 86:1370–1378.

149. Klag MJ, Whelton PK, Coresh J, et al: The association of skin color with blood pressure in U.S. blacks with low socioeconomic status. *JAMA* 1991; 265:599–602.

150. Dressler WW: Social identity and arterial blood pressure in the African-American community. *Ethn Dis* 1996; 6:176–189.

151. Dressler WW: Hypertension in the African American community: social, cultural, and psychological factors. *Semin Nephrol* 1996; 16:71–82.

152. Barnes V, Schneider R, Alexander C, Staggers F: Stress, stress reduction, and hypertension in African Americans: an updated review. *J Natl Med Assoc* 1997; 89:464–476.

153. Grundy SM, Balady GJ, Criqui MH, et al: *Guide to Primary Prevention of Cardiovascular Diseases 1997.* A Statement for Healthcare Professionals from the task force on risk reduction. *Circulation* 1997; 95:2329–2331.

154. Missed opportunities in preventive counseling for cardiovascular disease. *MMWR* 1998; 47:91–95.

155. Smith SC Jr: Risk reduction therapies for patients with coronary artery disease: a call for increased implementation. *Am J Med* 1998; 104(2A):23S–26S.

156. Wood D: European and American recommendations for coronary heart disease prevention. *Eur Heart J* 1998; 19(suppl A):A12–A19.

157. He J, Whelton P: Epidemiology and prevention of hypertension. *Med Clin North Am* 1997; 81:1077–1097.

158. Dustan HP, Valdes G, Bravo EL, Tarazi RC: Excessive Na+ retention as a characteristic of salt-sensitive hypertension. *Am J Med Sci* 1986; 29:67–74.

159. Campese, VM, Romoff MS, Levitan D, et al: Abnormal relationship between Na+ intake and sympathetic nervous system activity in salt-sensitive patients with essential hypertension. *Kidney Int* 1982; 21:371–378.

160. Weinberger MH, Miller JZ, Luft FC, Grim CE, Fineberg NS: Definitions and characteristics of Na+ sensitivity and blood pressure resistance. *Hypertension* 1986; 8:II-127–II-134.

161. Grim CE, Miller JZ, Luft FC, et al: Genetic influences on renin, aldosterone, and the renal excretion of sodium and potassium following volume expansion and contraction in normal man. *Hypertension* 1979; 1:583–590.

162. Wilson TW, Grim CE: Biohistory of slavery and blood pressure differences in blacks today: a hypothesis. *Hypertension* 1991; 17(suppl I):I-122–I-128.

163. Su YR, Rutkowski MP, Klanke CA, et al: A novel variant of the beta-subunit of the amiloride-sensitive sodium channel in African Americans. *J Am Soc Nephrol* 1996; 7:2543–2549.

164. Campese VM, Tawadrous M, Bigazzi R, et al: Salt intake and plasma atrial natriuretic peptide and nitric oxide in hypertension. *Hypertension* 1996; 28:335–340.

165. Rutledge DR, Sun Y, Ross EA: Polymorphism within the atrial natriuretic peptide gene in essential hypertension. *J Hypertens* 1995; 13:953–955.

166. Thorup C, Persson AEG: Nitric oxide and renal blood pressure regulation. *Curr Opin Nephrol Hypertens* 1998; 7:197–202.

167. Campese VM, Amar M, Anjali C, et al: Effect of L-arginine on systemic and renal haemodynamics in salt-sensitive patients with essential hypertension. *J Hum Hypertens* 1997; 11:527–532.

168. Svetkey LP, Chen YT, McKeown SP, et al: Preliminary evidence of linkage of salt sensitivity in black Americans at the beta$_2$-adrenergic receptor locus. *Hypertension* 1997; 29:918–922.

169. Kotanko P, Binder A, Tasker J, et al: Essential hypertension in African Caribbeans associates with a variant of the beta$_2$-adrenoceptor. *Hypertension* 1997; 30:773–776.

170. Watkins LL, Dimsdale JE, Ziegler MG: Reduced beta$_2$-receptor mediated vasodilation in African Americans. *Life Sci* 1995; 57:1411–1416.

171. Lockette W, Ghosh S, Farrow S, et al: Alpha$_2$-adrenergic receptor gene polymorphism and hypertension in blacks. *Am J Hypertens* 1995; 8:390–394.

172. Veterans Administration Cooperative Study Group on Antihypertensive Agents: Comparison of propanolol and hydrochlorothiazide for the initial treatment of hypertension: I. Results of short-term titration with emphasis on racial differences in response. *JAMA* 1982; 248:1996–2003.

173. Wassertheil-Smoller S, Oberman A, Blaufox MD, et al: The Trial of Antihypertensive Interventions and Management (TAIM) Study: final results with regards to blood pressure, cardiovascular risk, and quality of life. *Am J Hypertens* 1992; 5:37–44.

174. Saunders E, Weir MR, Kong BW, et al: A comparison of the efficacy and safety of a beta blocker, a calcium channel blocker, and a converting enzyme inhibitor in hypertensive blacks. *Arch Intern Med* 1990; 150:1707–1713.

175. Applegate WB, Phillips HL, Schnaper H, et al: A randomized controlled trial of the effects of three antihypertensive agents on blood pressure control and quality of life in older women. *Arch Intern Med* 1991; 151:1817–1823.

176. Materson BJ, Reda DJ, Cushman WC, et al: Single drug

therapy for hypertension in men: a comparison of six antihypertensive agents with placebo. *N Engl J Med* 1993; 328:914–921.

177. Jamerson K, DeQuattro V: The impact of ethnicity on response to antihypertensive therapy. *Am J Med* 1996; 101:22S–32S.

178. Gottlieb SS, McCarter RJ, Vogel RA: Effect of beta-blockade on mortality among high-risk and low-risk patients after myocardial infarction (see comments). *N Engl J Med* 1998; 339:489–497.

179. Davis BR, Cutler JA, Gordon DJ, et al: Rationale and design for the Antihypertensive and Lipid Lowering Treatment to Prevent Heart Attack Trial (ALLHAT): ALLHAT research group. *Am J Hypertens* 1996; 9(4 pt 1):342–360.

180. CDC Diabetes Cost-Effectiveness Study Group, Centers for Disease Control and Prevention: The cost-effectiveness of screening for type 2 diabetes. *JAMA* 1998; 280:1757–1763.

181. Report of the Expert Committee on the Diagnosis and Classification of Diabetes Mellitus. *Diabetes Care* 1997; 20:1183–1197.

182. Davidson MB, Schriger DL, Peters AL, Lorber B: Relationship between fasting plasma glucose and glycosylated hemoglobin: potential for false-positive diagnoses of type 2 diabetes using new diagnostic criteria. *JAMA* 1999; 281:1203–1210.

183. Rifai N, Neufeld E, Ahlstrom P, et al: Failure of current guidelines for cholesterol screening in urban African-American adolescents. *Pediatrics* 1996; 98(3 pt 1):383–388.

184. National Cholesterol Education Program: Second report of the expert panel on Detection, Evaluation, and Treatment of High Blood Cholesterol in Adults (Adult Treatment Panel II). *Circulation* 1994; 89:1333–1445.

185. Allen B Jr, Pederson LL, Leonard EH: Effectiveness of physicians-in-training counseling for smoking cessation in African Americans. *J Natl Med Assoc* 1998; 90:597–604.

186. Ahluwalia JS, McNagny SE, Clark WS: Smoking cessation among inner-city African Americans using the nicotine transdermal patch (see comments). *J Gen Intern Med* 1998; 13:1–8.

187. Orleans CT, Boyd NR, Bingler R, et al: A self-help intervention for African American smokers: tailoring cancer information service counseling for a special population. *Prev Med* 1998; 27(5 pt 2):S61–S70.

188. Fisher EB, Auslander WF, Munro JF, et al: Neighbors for a smoke free north side: evaluation of a community organization approach to promoting smoking cessation among African Americans. *Am J Public Health* 1998; 88:1658–1663.

189. Resnicow K, Vaughan R, Futterman R, et al: A self-help smoking cessation program for inner-city African Americans: results from the Harlem Health Connection Project. *Health Educ Behav* 1997; 24:201–217.

190. Resnicow K, Royce J, Vaughan R, et al: Analysis of a multicomponent smoking cessation project: what worked and why. *Prev Med* 1997; 26:373–381.

191. Maynard C, Beshansky JR, Griffith JL, Selker HP: Causes of chest pain and symptoms suggestive of acute cardiac ischemia in African-American patients presenting to the emergency department: a multicenter study. *J Natl Med Assoc* 1997; 89:665–671.

192. Gardin JM, Wagenknecht LE, Anton-Culver H, et al: Relationship of cardiovascular risk factors to echocardiographic left ventricular mass in healthy young black and white adult men and women: the CARDIA study—Coronary Artery Risk Development in Young Adults. *Circulation* 1995; 92:380–387.

193. Arnett DK, Rautaharju P, Crow R, et al: Black-white differences in electrocardiographic left ventricular mass and its association with blood pressure (the ARIC study)—Atherosclerosis Risk in Communities. *Am J Cardiol* 1994; 74:247–252.

194. Vitelli LL, Crow RS, Shahar E, et al: Electrocardiographic findings in a healthy biracial population: Atherosclerosis Risk in Communities (ARIC) study investigators. *Am J Cardiol* 1998; 81:453–459.

195. Houghton JL, Prisant LM, Carr AA, et al: Racial differences in myocardial ischemia and coronary flow reserve in hypertension. *J Am Coll Cardiol* 1994; 23:1123–1129.

196. Houghton JL, Smith VE, Strogatz DS, et al: Effect of African-American race and hypertensive left ventricular hypertrophy on coronary vascular reactivity and endothelial function. *Hypertension* 1997; 29:706–714.

197. Pavlik VN, Hyman DJ, Vallbona C: Hypertension control in multi-ethnic primary care clinics. *J Hum Hypertens* 1996; 10(suppl 3):S19–S23.

198. Gray RJ, Nessim S, Khan SS, et al: Adverse 5-year outcome after coronary artery bypass surgery in blacks. *Arch Intern Med* 1996; 156:769–773.

199. Weitzman S, Cooper L, Chambless L, Rosamond W, Clegg L, Marcucci G, Romm F, White A. Gender, racial, and geographic differences in the performance of cardiac diagnostic and therapeutic procedures for hospitalized acute myocardial infarction in four states. *Am J Cardiol* 1997; 79:722–726.

200. Schulman KA, Berlin JA, Harless W, et al: The effect of race and sex on physician's recommendations for cardiac catheterization. *N Engl J Med* 1999; 340:618–626.

201. Centers for Disease Control/National Center for Health Statistics: *Third National Health and Nutrition Examination Survey, 1988–1991 (Phase 1)*. Bethesda, MD: CDC/NCHS/National Heart, Lung, and Blood Institute Chartbook of U.S. National Data on Socioeconomic Status and Cardiovascular Health and Disease, June 1995.

(Working group: Stamler J, Chair, Hazuda HP, Haywood LJ, House JS, Kaplan GA, Tyroler HA.)

202. Gittelsohn KG, Halpern J, Sanchez RI: Income, race and surgery in Maryland. *Am J Public Health* 1991; 81:1435–1441.

203. Wennecker MB, Epstein AM: Racial inequities in the use of procedures for patients with ischemic heart disease in Massachusetts. *JAMA* 1989; 261:253–257.

204. McBean AM, Warren JL, Babish JD: Continuing differences in the rates of percutaneous transluminal coronary angioplasty and coronary artery bypass graft surgery between elderly black and white Medicare beneficiaries. *Am Heart J* 1994; 127:287–295.

205. Agency for Health Policy and Research: *Gender, Race/Ethnicity and Treatment of Adults in Hospital by Diagnosis.* AHCPR Publication #96-0011. Washington, DC, U.S. Department of Health and Human Services, December 1995.

206. Shea S, Misra D, Ehrlich MH, et al: Correlates of nonadherence to hypertension treatment in an inner-city minority population. *Am J Public Health* 1992; 82:1607–1612.

207. Pettinger WA, Lee HC, Reisch J, Mitchell HC: Long-term improvement in renal function after short-term strict blood pressure control in hypertensive nephrosclerosis. *Hypertension* 1989; 13:766–772.

208. Hypertension Detection and Follow-up Program Cooperative Group: Educational level and 5-year all-cause mortality in the Hypertension Detection and Follow-up program. *Hypertension* 1987; 9:641–646.

209. Taylor HA, Chaitman BR, Rogers WJ, et al: Race and prognosis after myocardial infarction: results of the thrombolysis in myocardial infarction (TIMI) phase II trial. *Circulation* 1993; 88(4 pt 1):1484–1494.

210. Scott NA, Kelsey SF, Detre K, et al: Percutaneous transluminal coronary angioplasty in African-American patients (the National Heart, Lung, and Blood Institute 1985–1986 Percutaneous Transluminal Coronary Angioplasty Registry). *Am J Cardiol* 1994; 73:1141–1146.

211. Daumit GL, Hermann JA, Coresh J, Powe NR: Use of cardiovascular procedure among black persons and white persons: a 7-year nationwide study in patients with renal disease. *Ann Intern Med* 1999; 130:173–182.

212. Leape LL, Hilbourne LH, Bell R, et al: Underuse of cardiac procedures: do women, ethnic minorities, and the uninsured fail to receive needed revascularization? *Ann Intern Med* 1999; 130:183–192.

213. Carlisle DM, Leake BD, Shapiro MF: Racial and ethnic disparities in the use of cardiovascular procedures: associations with type of health insurance. *Am J Public Health* 1997; 87:263–267.

214. Carlisle DM, Leake BD, Shapiro MF: Racial and ethnic differences in the use of invasive cardiac procedures among cardiac patients in Los Angeles County, 1986 through 1988. *Am J Public Health* 1995; 85:352–356.

215. Taylor AJ, Meyer GS, Morse RW, Pearson CE: Can characteristics of a health care system mitigate ethnic bias in access to cardiovascular procedures? Experience from the Military Health Services System. *J Am Coll Cardiol* 1997; 30:901–907.

216. Clancy CM, Franks P: Utilization of specialty and primary care: the impact of HMO insurance and patient-related factors. *J Fam Pract* 1997; 45:500–508.

217. Selby JV, Zhang D: Risk factors for lower extremity amputation in persons with diabetes. *Diabetes Care* 1995; 18:509–516.

218. Preston JA: Management of geriatric hypertension in health maintenance organizations. *J Am Geriatr Soc* 1991; 39:683–690.

219. Saag KG, Doebbeling BN, Rohrer JE, et al: Variation in tertiary prevention and health service utilization among the elderly: the role of urban-rural residence and supplemental insurance. *Med Care* 1998; 36:965–976.

220. Ware JE Jr, Bayliss MS, Rogers WH, et al: Differences in 4-year health outcomes for elderly and poor, chronically ill patients treated in HMO and fee-for-service systems: results from the Medical Outcomes Study. *JAMA* 1996; 276:1039–1047.

221. Dressler WW, Bindon JR, Neggers YH: Culture, socioeconomic status, and coronary heart disease risk factors in an African American Community. *J Behav Med* 1998; 21:527–544.

222. Hahn RA, Heath GW, Chang MH: Cardiovascular disease risk factors and preventive practices among adults—United States, 1994: a behavioral risk factor atlas. Behavioral Risk Factor Surveillance System state coordinators. *MMWR* 1998; 47:35–69.

223. Fang J, Madhavan S, Alderman MH: The association between birthplace and mortality from cardiovascular causes among black and white residents of New York City. *N Engl J Med* 1996; 335:1545–1551.

224. He J, Klag MJ, Appel LJ, et al: Seven-year incidence of hypertension in a cohort of middle-aged African Americans and whites. *Hypertension* 1998; 31:1130–1135.

225. Pearson TA, Jenkins GM, Thomas J: Prevention of coronary heart disease in black adults. *Cardiovasc Clin* 1991; 21:263–276.

226. Shea S, Basch CE, Wechsler H, Lantigua R: The Washington Heights-Inwood Healthy Heart Program: a 6-year report from a disadvantaged urban setting. *Am J Public Health* 1996; 86:166–171.

227. O'Connor PJ, Wagner EH, Strogatz DS: Hypertension control in a rural community: an assessment of community-oriented primary care. *J Fam Pract* 1990; 30:420–424.

228. Ewart CK, Young DR, Hagberg JM: Effects of school-based aerobic exercise on blood pressure in adolescent girls at risk for hypertension. *Am J Public Health* 1998; 88:949–951.

229. Smith NL, Croft JB, Heath GW, Cokkinides V: Changes in cardiovascular disease knowledge and behavior in a low-education population of African-American and white adults. *Ethn Dis* 1996; 6:244–254.

230. Fouad MN, Kiefe CI, Bartolucci AA, et al: A hypertension control program tailored to unskilled and minority workers. *Ethn Dis* 1997; 7:191–199.

231. Gerber JC, Stewart DL: Prevention and control of hypertension and diabetes in an underserved population through community outreach and disease management: a plan of action. *J Assoc Acad Minor Phys* 1998; 9:48–52.

232. Stillman FA, Bone LR, Rand C, et al: Heart, body, and soul: a church-based smoking-cessation program for Urban African Americans. *Prev Med* 1993; 22:335–349.

233. Kumanyika SK, Charleston JB: Lose weight and win: a church-based weight loss program for blood pressure control among black women. *Patient Educ Couns* 1992; 19:19–32.

234. Smith ED, Merritt SL, Patel MK: Church-based education: an outreach program for African Americans with hypertension. *Ethn Health* 1997; 2:243–253.

235. Jackson AL: Operation Sunday school—educating caring hearts to be healthy hearts. *Public Health Rep* 1990; 105:85–88.

236. Kong BW: Community-based hypertension control programs that work. *J Health Care Poor Underserved* 1997; 8:409–415.

237. Shakoor-Abdullah B, Kotchen JM, Walker WE, et al: Incorporating socio-economic and risk factor diversity into the development of an African-American community blood pressure control program. *Ethn Dis* 1997; 7:175–183.

238. Davis SK, Winkleby MA, Farquhar JW: Increasing disparity in knowledge of cardiovascular disease risk factors and risk-reduction strategies by socioeconomic status: implications for policymakers. *Am J Prev Med* 1995; 11:318–323.

239. Brownson RC, Koffman DM, Novotny TE, et al: Environmental and policy interventions to control tobacco use and prevent cardiovascular disease. *Health Educ Q* 1995; 22:478–498.

240. Speers MA, Schmid TL: Policy and environmental interventions for the prevention and control of cardiovascular diseases. *Health Educ Q* 1995; 22:476–477.

241. Lackland DT. An international working party on assessing hypertension control in populations: a proposal. *J Hum Hypertens* 1996; 10(suppl 1):S29–S31.

242. Gyarfas I: Lessons from worldwide experience with hypertension control. *J Hum Hypertens* 1996; 10(suppl 1):S21–S25.

243. King AC, Jeffery RW, Fridinger F, et al: Environmental and policy approaches to cardiovascular disease prevention through physical activity: issues and opportunities. *Health Educ Q* 1995; 22:499–511.

CHAPTER 19

Hispanic Americans

Stanley L. Bassin

Approximately 40 million persons of Hispanic origin constitute the largest minority group in the United States. This diverse group includes Cubans, Mexicans, Spaniards, other Latinos, and an estimated more than 4 million living here without legal documents.[1] With approximately 600,000 new immigrants a year and an estimated half of them entering the country illegally, Hispanics will comprise 50 million residents within the next 6 years.[2] In the next decade, Mexican Americans are projected to be the majority population in the United States, with 7 of 10 persons currently under the age of 35, while less than half of non-Hispanics are in the same age group. On the other hand, three times as many non-Hispanics are over the age of 65 in comparison with their Hispanic counterparts.

Although overall mortality rates and those from cardiovascular disease (CVD) are lower in Hispanics than in whites, certain risk factors—particularly diabetes, obesity, and physical inactivity—are among the highest in the Hispanic population and continue to be on the increase.[3,4] This chapter examines cultural and epidemiologic issues related to CVD in Hispanics as well as strategies for the prevention of CVD in this population.

Demographic and Cultural Issues

Approximately 6 of 10 Hispanics are of Mexican heritage, reside predominantly in the Southwest and several major metropolitan areas throughout the United States, and make up the largest minority population.[5] Another 16 percent of Hispanics in the United States are Cubans residing in the Northeast, Florida, and New York and Puerto Ricans living in the Northeast

and Puerto Rico. Of the remaining Hispanics, many originate from Central America and live primarily in Arizona and California.[2]

There are marked differences in culture, history, and lifestyle among Hispanics. Spanish is the common language, but more than one-third do not speak it well or are illiterate in their native tongue. Despite a shared language, broad diversity exists among Hispanics, with a core ancestry that can be traced to numerous Spanish-speaking countries and distinct national histories, traditions, and lifestyles. Mexican Americans and Central Americans have a complicated background despite a common history of Spanish origin.[5,6] Some diseases that seem to be prevalent among indigenous North Americans also seem to be present among Mexican Americans but are not as pronounced among other Hispanics. Thus, the generalization of specific health findings to other Hispanic groups should be minimized. Some of the surveys suggest that Hispanics are over-represented among uninsured and medically underserved populations. They are the second lowest (just ahead of African Americans) of major ethnic groups in earnings, and their health status reflects this level of poverty.

Epidemiology and Risk Factors

Overview

Heart disease and stroke are among the leading causes of death among Hispanics, as they are for whites. However, the death rate (per 100,000 population) appears to be actually lower for Hispanics (52.6) than for whites (75.7).[7] Diseases of the heart and stroke still remain the leading causes of death, both in

Hispanic males (26.9 percent of all deaths) and in Hispanic females (33.3 percent of all deaths).[4] While significant research on CVD prevention has been conducted among middle-class whites, only recently have sufficient data become available on Hispanics. Most studies have involved relatively small samples, have failed to recognize Hispanics' diverse cultural groups, have been cross-sectional in nature, or have involved limited follow-up. Some tracking studies began with young adults but were limited to narrow geographical areas. The Hispanic Health and Nutrition Examination Survey (HHANES) was the first national study to assess the health and nutritional status of the Latino population, including mainland Puerto Ricans.[8] This report disclosed that a greater percentage of Hispanics smoked cigarettes and were obese, diabetic, and/or hypertensive. Their rates of heart conditions were lower than those of whites but comparable to those of African Americans.[9]

Much of the burden of CVD among Hispanics may result from obesity, hypertension, inadequate physical activity and fitness, high cholesterol, and tobacco use.[10] Some studies have shown evidence of a greater prevalence of obesity or elevated cholesterol or triglycerides among Hispanic populations than among whites.[10,11] Moreover, Mexican Americans are three to five times as likely to have non-insulin-dependent diabetes than whites.[12] A 7- to 8-year follow-up of the San Antonio Heart Study was used to estimate CVD mortality and its association with baseline risk factors. Overall the traditional risk factors accounted for 55 percent of CVD mortality in Mexican Americans but only 46 percent in whites.[13]

Although in many cases risk factors among Hispanics were shown to be worse than those among whites, mortality rates were lower—opposite of what would have been expected from a generally poorer and undereducated population. These surprising statistics underlie the Hispanic epidemiologic paradox.[11] When examined in relation to migration and socioeconomic status, those with the lowest socioeconomic status had a threefold greater risk of death than those with the highest status. Foreign-born Mexican Americans had the lowest mortality rate, while those born in the United States and whites had equivalent rates when socioeconomic status was accounted for. This suggests that the Hispanic paradox of traditionally lower mortality rates may have to be questioned in the light of more acculturation data.[13]

During the 1990s, while CVD mortality rates have fallen in the general U.S. population, mortality data reported in the five southwestern states find that Mexican Americans and whites have similar rates but Mexican-American men have slightly lower rates than white men. Mortality following myocardial infarction (MI) is greater among Mexican Americans than among whites.[3]

The Corpus Christi (Texas) study[14] found Mexican Americans to have received fewer cardiovascular medications than whites, and women fewer than men. They also reported in a 25-month follow-up after hospitalization for MI, age-adjusted all-cause mortality rates among those who survived the initial 28 days to be similar among Mexican-American women and non-Hispanic white women (17.8 and 18.1 percent, respectively), but 70 percent higher among Mexican-American men than among non-Hispanic white men (17.4 and 10.2 percent, respectively).[15] For both men and women, greater hospitalization rates for MI were observed among Hispanics than among whites. The effect of diabetes on the severity of acute MI and post-MI survival rates was also studied. Despite a similar infarction size, diabetic subjects had a higher incidence of heart failure and poorer prognosis than did nondiabetics. The higher incidence of diabetes among Mexican Americans may contribute to lower survival rates in those with CVD.[13,16]

The Hispanic paradox seems in need of revision because today it seems to apply only to Mexican-American men. Many Hispanics underutilize preventive health services and employ emergency treatment only once an illness has become life-threatening.[6] Unfortunately the next decade may find the Hispanic population in poorer health, needing improved preventive and medical services that meet both their medical and linguistic needs. Only with this can we effect a reduction in their CVD risk.

Hypertension

An estimated 50 million Americans have high blood pressure. Among Mexican Americans, data from the National Health and Nutrition Examination Survey

(NHANES) III collected in 1988 to 1994[4] showed the prevalence of hypertension to be 25.2 percent in men and 22.0 percent in women, slightly higher than that of white men (24.4 percent) but similar to that of white women (19.3 percent). Lower prevalences were reported in Cuban Americans and in Puerto Ricans. The 1980s HHANES data demonstrated lower or similar hypertension rates in Mexican Americans compared to whites. Other investigators also discovered that many Mexican Americans were identified as undiagnosed hypertensives, with blood pressure prevention and control programs underutilized.[17,18] Data from NHANES III and other studies have shown, in Mexican Americans as in whites, progressive increases in systolic and diastolic blood pressure as people age. Among Mexican Americans aged 60 years and over, more than 50 percent of men and nearly two-thirds of women have hypertension. Overall (all ages, 20 to 74 years), during 1988 to 1991, 20 percent of Hispanic men and 15 percent of Hispanic women had hypertension, which meant little change since NHANES II in 1976 to 1980. This is in contrast to substantial reductions in hypertension prevalence among both whites and African Americans during the same time period (Table 19–1).[19–23] In California, data on Hispanics show high blood pressure prevalence at 22 percent in men and 25 percent in women, which is nearly equivalent to that of whites but substantially lower than that of blacks (Fig. 19–1).[24] Among youth, between 5 and 8 percent of the Hispanic youngsters had blood pressure readings above the 90th percentile, the national standards used to define high normal blood pressure in children and adolescents.[21,25]

The association between blood pressure and weight has been established across most gender and racial groups. Among Hispanics, the relative risk of developing hypertension among the obese is five to six times that among lean individuals. The prevalence of overweight among hypertensive men ranges from 39 to 60 percent and among women from 44 to 74 percent. Also, only 9 percent of these hypertensives had been treated. Percent of body fat is the most sensitive anthropometric measurement in predicting blood pressure.[25]

The National Institute of Aging examined over 9700 middle-aged adults in its health and retirement cross-sectional survey. It found higher rates of hypertension and diabetes but lower rates of heart disease—regardless of income, education, and accumulated wealth—among Mexican Americans as compared to whites. Ethnic-specific data can be misleading unless sociodemographic information is taken into account. Although awareness of hypertension is very good, the rate of control in Hispanics is only about 25 percent, similar to that in whites.[25]

The Stanford Five-City Study examined the sociodemographic influences on blood pressure in Mexican Americans and whites matched for age, gender, education, and residential neighborhood. Mean levels of systolic and diastolic blood pressure were essentially identical, even though Mexican Americans had higher levels of obesity.[26]

Lipids

Blood lipids and lipoproteins are associated with several metabolic disorders. The best available evidence suggests that behaviors associated with increased CVD are acquired early in life and may accelerate the development of CVD.[27] High blood cholesterol is one of the most influential factors and can account for a substantial role in heart disease. Among Mexican Americans aged 20 years and over, 47 percent of men and 43 percent of women have total cholesterol levels over 200 mg/dL, which is similar to those of African-American men and women (46 percent) but lower than those of white men (52 percent) and white women (51 percent). In addition, 18 percent of Mexican Americans have total cholesterol levels of 240 mg/dL or higher.[4] Mean total cholesterol levels are similar among Mexican Americans and whites in most age groups except for a tendency toward higher mean levels in Mexican Americans aged 20 to 29 and 70 to 79 (Figs. 19–2 and 19–3). Further, whereas among Mexican Americans, 39 percent of men and 38 percent of women have low-density-lipoprotein cholesterol (LDL-C) levels of 130 mg/dL or higher, only 15 percent of men and 6 percent of women have levels of high-density-lipoprotein cholesterol (HDL-C) levels of less than 35 mg/dL (Table 19–2).[4,23]

Studies of cholesterol screening have shown, regardless of geographic area, that participants are

TABLE 19-1 Percentage of Adults 20 Years of Age and Older Who Have Hypertension by Age, Sex, and Race/Ethnicity, 1960–1962, 1971–1974, 1976–1980, 1988–1991

Sex, Age, Race, and Hispanic Origin	NHES I (1960–1962)			NHANES I (1971–1974)			NHANES II (1976–1980)			NHANES III (1988–1991)		
	Sample Size	%	SE	Sample Size	%	SE	Sample Size	%	SE	Sample Size	%	SE
20–74 years, age-adjusted												
Both sexes	6023	36.8	1.25	12,827	38.4	0.84	11,665	39.0	1.27	6726	23.3	0.72
Male*	2855	39.7	1.88	4962	42.6	1.13	5566	44.0	1.68	3473	26.3	1.06
Female†	3168	33.9	1.13	7865	34.3	0.90	6099	34.1	1.03	3253	20.4	0.70
White male	2466	39.0	1.93	4114	41.9	1.18	4853	43.6	1.78	2441	25.0	1.15
White female†	2708	31.9	1.15	6353	32.4	0.90	5281	32.4	1.09	2243	19.1	0.73
Black male	329	48.3	3.34	2211	51.1	2.93	600	48.9	2.30	949	37.6	1.29
Black female†	409	51.2	2.16	784	49.9	2.01	708	47.8	1.74	934	30.7	1.08
White, non-Hispanic male	...	...	...	...	...	...	4620	44.0	1.83	1400	25.2	1.19
White, non-Hispanic female†	...	...	...	...	...	...	5022	32.1	1.08	1310	19.0	0.74
Black, non-Hispanic male	...	...	...	...	...	...	590	48.9	2.50	939	37.4	1.30
Black, non-Hispanic female†	...	...	...	...	...	...	700	47.9	1.74	918	30.8	1.12
Mexican-American male‡	...	...	...	...	...	...	1460	25.2	1.34	1011	27.1	1.37
Mexican-American female†‡	...	...	...	...	...	...	1798	21.8	0.88	910	20.5	0.98
20–74 years, crude												
Both sexes*	6023	39.1	1.30	12,827	39.7	0.84	11,665	39.7	1.09	6726	23.5	0.78
Male*	2855	41.7	1.91	4962	43.3	1.37	5566	44.0	1.60	3473	25.7	1.12
Female*†	3168	36.7	1.77	7865	36.5	1.06	6099	35.6	1.48	3253	21.3	1.08
White male	2466	41.0	1.87	4114	42.8	1.47	4853	43.8	1.73	2441	25.0	1.18
White female†	2708	35.1	1.73	6353	34.9	1.14	5281	34.2	1.59	2243	20.4	1.15
Black male	329	50.5	3.78	784	52.1	3.18	600	47.4	2.54	949	34.3	1.77
Black female†	409	52.0	3.39	1427	50.2	2.36	708	46.1	2.34	934	28.7	1.70
White, non-Hispanic male	...	...	...	...	...	...	4620	44.3	1.83	1400	25.8	1.29
White, non-Hispanic female†	...	...	...	...	...	...	5022	34.4	1.68	1310	20.7	1.23
Black, non-Hispanic male	...	...	...	...	...	...	590	47.5	2.54	939	34.2	1.80
Black, non-Hispanic female†	...	...	...	...	...	...	700	46.1	2.32	918	29.0	1.74
Mexican-American male‡	...	...	...	...	...	...	1460	18.8	1.08	1011	19.6	1.89
Mexican-American female†‡	...	...	...	...	...	...	1798	16.7	0.93	910	14.9	1.78

... Category not applicable.
* Includes data for race-ethnic groups not shown separately.
† Excludes pregnant women.
‡ Data for Mexican Americans are for 1982–1984.

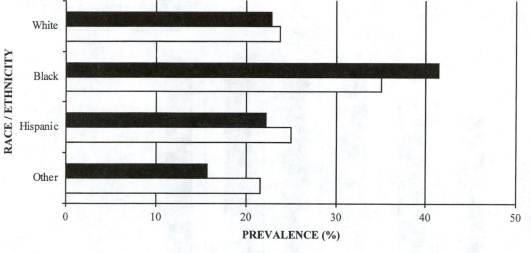
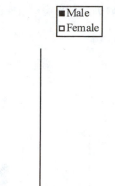

FIGURE 19–1 Prevalence of high blood pressure among California adults by race and gender, 1996. Data age-adjusted to 1990 California population.
(From Gazzaniga et al[24] with permission.)

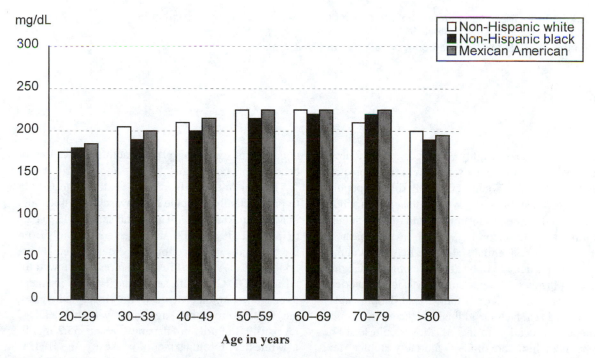

FIGURE 19–2 Mean serum total cholesterol level for males 20 years of age and older by age and race/ethnicity, 1988–1991.
(From the *Third Report on Nutrition Monitoring in the United States.*[23])

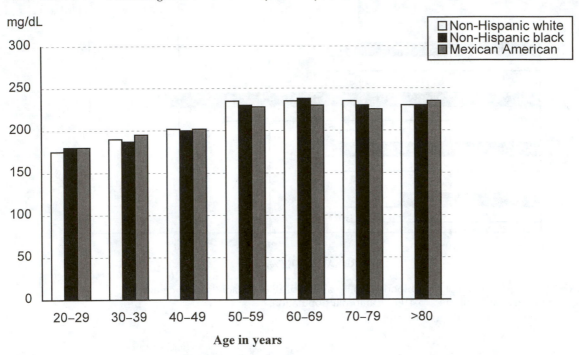

mg/dL

☐ Non-Hispanic white
■ Non-Hispanic black
▨ Mexican American

Age in years

FIGURE 19–3 Mean serum total cholesterol level for females 20 years of age and older by age and race/ethnicity, 1988–1991.
(From the *Third Report on Nutrition Monitoring in the United States.*[23])

often white, female, highly educated, and have never smoked.[28] Reaching other segments of the population has been difficult. Young, ethnically diverse populations below age 45, who have less than a high school education, lack health insurance, and may be subject to official data recording, which may appear to threaten their residential status, are frequently unmotivated to participate in health screenings. Thus, data on lipid levels is meager among Mexican-American youngsters and adults. On the basis of the previously mentioned risk factors, adding socioeconomic conditions and education to the equation would lead one to predict a high rate of CVD mortality among Mexican Americans. Although studies frequently claim a lower CVD mortality in Hispanics than in whites, this needs to be reconsidered in the light of probable

under- or misreporting of risk factors and causes of death in this population.[11,29–31]

The San Antonio Heart Study is the largest study to prospectively examine cardiovascular risk factors in Mexican Americans. The initial sample, 1220 participants (1979 to 1982), was selected randomly from three socially and economically distinct neighborhoods of San Antonio, Texas. The results showed total and LDL-C in both sexes and HDL-C in males to be similar among Mexican Americans and whites, but white women had significantly higher HDL-C levels (49.9 mg/dL in Hispanics versus 55.2 mg/dL in whites). After adjustment for obesity, the HDL-C gap between ethnic groups was diminished. Mexican Americans of both sexes had higher triglyceride levels than their white counterparts. Since adiposity

TABLE 19–2 Percentage of People 20 Years of Age and Older with Low Levels of Serum High-Density-Lipoprotein Cholesterol (<35 mg/dL), by Sex, Age, and Race/Ethnicity, 1988–1991

Sex and Age	Total Population*			Non-Hispanic White			Non-Hispanic Black			Mexican American		
	Sample Size	%	SE	Sample Size	%	SE	Sample Size	%	SE	Sample Size	%	SE
Male												
20–29 years	793	10.3	1.35	202	11.6	2.30	230	5.4	1.51	329	13.4	2.18
30–39 years	699	14.1	1.65	263	14.6	2.21	194	10.2	2.19	218	11.3	2.50
40–49 years	600	20.8	2.07	238	23.2	2.79	162	11.4	2.52	174	25.4	3.84
50–59 years	472	19.8	2.29	258	21.3	2.59	100	10.1[†]	[†]	94	12.2[†]	[†]
60–69 years	558	20.0	2.12	251	21.2	2.63	129	12.0	2.89	168	20.1	3.60
70–79 years	458	19.1	2.30	300	19.4	2.32	84	13.0	3.71	69	14.7[†]	[†]
80 years and over	340	15.4	2.45	291	16.4	2.21	19	—	—	25	23.1[†]	[†]
Total	**3920**	**16.3**	**1.13**	**1803**	**17.8**	**1.32**	**918**	**9.2**	**1.16**	**1077**	**15.2**	**1.67**
Female												
20–29 years	783	4.5	1.10	224	4.8[†]	[†]	232	1.5[†]	[†]	303	4.7	1.27
30–39 years	740	7.8	1.46	260	8.6	1.95	216	4.1[†]	[†]	239	3.5[†]	[†]
40–49 years	582	3.4[†]	[†]	221	3.3[†]	[†]	153	5.2[†]	[†]	176	9.1	2.26
50–59 years	434	6.6	1.77	214	7.5	2.02	115	2.7[†]	[†]	93	7.3[†]	[†]
60–69 years	549	5.4	1.44	245	5.8	1.69	135	3.5[†]	[†]	157	6.2[†]	[†]
70–79 years	412	6.2	1.77	261	6.8	1.75	90	3.4[†]	[†]	50	5.3[†]	[l]
80 years and over	356	7.2	2.04	292	7.6	1.75	38	3.8[†]	[†]	22	7.6[†]	[†]
Total	**3856**	**5.7**	**0.72**	**1717**	**6.2**	**0.86**	**979**	**3.3**	**0.69**	**1040**	**5.5**	**1.08**

* Includes data for race-ethnic groups not shown separately.

† Indicates a statistic that is potentially unreliable because of small sample size or large coefficient of variation.

— Observed percent is 0.0.

Source: From the Third Report on Nutrition Monitoring in the United States.[23]

is greater among Mexican Americans, it is not surprising to see higher triglycerides and central body fat patterning more often among them.[32]

Hixon and colleagues[33] examined the relative contributions of the environment and genetics to lipids and other risk factors. Up to three generations of 42 families were studied from the San Antonio Heart Study. For the lipid and lipoprotein phenotypes, age, gender, and environmental covariates accounted for less than 15 percent of the total phenotypic variation, whereas genetic factors accounted for double to triple the percentage of the phenotypic variation.[16] Valdez and coworkers looked at the two groups of

San Antonio study subjects and comparable Mexico City residents to further discriminate between genetic and environmental (e.g., lifestyle) influences on blood measurements. While they found fasting and 2-h insulin levels to have a genetic component, fasting and 2-h glucose were consistently higher in Mexican Americans than in the other two groups. A clear environmental effect was suggested, with Mexican Americans and whites having higher levels of triglycerides and lower HDL-C levels, but higher amounts of total and LDL-C, regardless of gender than those living in Mexico City. The authors suggested that the average Mexico City diet, which is higher in carbohydrates (65 percent to 49 percent), may have accounted for the lipid differences. They also suggested a genetic effect of obesity on insulin levels, whereas lipid levels seem to be determined more by lifestyle.[34]

Findings from NHANES III showed mean cholesterol levels to peak at 219 mg/dL for Mexican-American men and 229 mg/dL for Mexican-American women in the seventh decade of life. Compared with whites and African Americans, these numbers were similar for men but lower for women (Figs. 19–2 and 19–3).[23] Others find even lower cholesterol levels for Mexican-American women.[35] The substantial levels of obesity in this population do not appear to be associated with the higher expected levels of serum cholesterol. Culturally appropriate services should be provided to manage lipid problems in this population.

Obesity in Hispanic Adults

Nearly 55 percent of American adults are considered overweight or obese, an increase from 43 percent in 1960.[23,36] More than one-third of Americans are considered overweight, using a standard of body-mass index (BMI) greater than 25 to 30 kg/m^2, and one-sixth are overweight using the definition of greater than 30 kg/m^2 to define obesity.[7] The prevalence of obesity is greater among Mexican Americans, exceeding that among whites and matching that among African Americans.[37,38] Among Mexican Americans between the ages of 20 and 74, some 67 percent of men and 68 percent of women are overweight or obese (using a definition of BMI of 25 kg/m^2 or greater), with 23 percent of men and 34 percent of women being defined as obese (BMI of 30 kg/m^2 or greater).[4] This contrasts with 59.6 percent of white men and 45.5 percent of white women who are overweight or obese (20.0 and 24.4 percent, respectively, are obese). Among African Americans, 57.5 percent of males and 66.5 percent of females are overweight (21.3 and 37.3 percent, respectively, are obese).[4] Using a definition of BMI of 27.8 kg/m^2 or higher in men and 27.3 kg/m^2 or higher in women after age 40, more than half of Mexican-American men and women are overweight (Table 19–3).[23] In California, the prevalence of over-

weight among Hispanics aged 18 and over is 35 percent in men and 43 percent in women.[24]

Other studies conducted within the last two decades have also seen that Mexican Americans are more overweight and have higher levels of obesity than whites.[10,39] Hispanic adults, when evaluated by U.S. national standards, are found to be overweight with a less favorable, centralized distribution of body fat, increasing the risks for diabetes and other cardiovascular risk factors.[10,37] The San Antonio Heart Study found that Mexican Americans were overweight and had greater adiposity than non-Hispanic white Texans.[40] It was reported that overweight in Mexican Americans began at an earlier age, and their ranking regarding levels of obesity in comparison with other ethnic groups did not change with advancing age. Some studies have shown that Mexican Americans reach their prevalence peak in obesity prior to age 40, while other ethnic groups peak at later periods in life.[41] Both white and Hispanic men show a steady increase in overweight prevalence; however, by the fifth decade of life, 57 percent of Hispanic men but only 38 percent of white men are overweight (Table 19–3).[23] Among Hispanic women, however, there seems to be an even greater divergence in the prevalence of overweight, especially among young women.

Surveys on diet and physical activity have shown that Hispanics have adverse dietary intake, low physical activity levels, and a lower level of concern about obesity than whites in the same community.[40,42] These findings coincide with other investigations that regard obesity as a problem of energy imbalance, with more calories consumed than expended. In addition, genetic composition may also play a major role in how individuals express their metabolism in an environment that focuses on consumption of calorie-dense foods. The decrease in physical activity level across all youth makes the population ripe for obesity.[36,43] This portends an even greater level of adult obesity within the next two decades.

Obesity and Body Fat Distribution

Because of their generally shorter stature, the greater prevalences of obesity in Mexican Americans is due

TABLE 19–3 Percentage of People 20 Years of Age and Older Who Are Overweight (High BMI) by Sex, Age, and Race/Ethnicity, 1988–1991

Sex and Age	Total Population*			Non-Hispanic White			Non-Hispanic Black			Mexican American		
	Sample Size	%	SE	Sample Size	%	SE	Sample Size	%	SE	Sample Size	%	SE
Male												
Total	4209	31.4	0.93	1896	32.3	1.40	1045	30.9	1.86	1136	35.5	1.85
20–29 years	858	20.2	1.85	218	19.2	2.78	251	30.0	2.94	353	24.1	2.28
30–39 years	759	27.4	2.19	277	28.3	2.83	223	26.1	2.99	233	29.4	2.98
40–49 years	643	37.0	2.57	247	38.1	3.22	186	34.4	3.55	185	56.9	3.64
50–59 years	493	42.1	3.01	262	42.5	3.19	110	38.0	4.71	98	51.6	5.05
60–69 years	588	42.2	2.75	262	43.6	3.20	150	31.6	3.86	167	54.0	3.86
70–79 years	495	35.9	2.91	318	36.0	2.81	99	34.6	4.87	72	41.0	5.80
80 years and over	373	18.0	2.69	312	18.4	2.29	26	16.1[†]	[†]	28	24.1[†]	
Female[‡]												
Total	4050	35.2	0.98	1818	32.8	1.43	1067	48.6	1.99	1039	46.7	2.02
20–29 years	755	20.1	1.83	224	17.7	2.55	230	31.0	3.53	277	34.4	2.85
30–39 years	770	34.1	2.14	274	31.2	2.80	236	47.7	3.76	234	48.2	3.27
40–49 years	623	37.6	2.43	233	32.5	3.07	169	59.8	4.37	188	57.1	3.61
50–59 years	465	51.8	2.90	228	50.9	3.31	128	59.3	5.03	98	56.8	5.00
60–69 years	595	42.5	2.54	260	40.3	3.04	159	63.3	4.42	162	52.3	3.92
70–79 years	446	37.2	2.87	277	35.4	2.87	103	49.0	5.70	53	49.7	6.87
80 years and over	396	26.2	2.77	322	25.2	2.42	42	36.5	8.60	27	30.60[†]	[†]

* Includes data for race-ethnic groups not shown separately.

[†] Indicates a statistic that is potentially unreliable because of small sample size or large coefficient of variation.

[‡] Excludes pregnant women.

Note: BMI is an index used to relate weight to stature. For men, overweight is defined as a BMI greater than or equal to 27.8 kg/m²; for women, it is defined as a BMI greater than or equal to 27.3 kg/m².

Source: From the *Third Report on Nutrition Monitoring in the United States*.[23]

in part to excess weight for stature.[12,44] Mexican Americans have greater upper body adiposity than whites, but the ethnic difference in central adiposity index is greater than what would be expected based on the difference in waist/hip ratio.[45,46] The failure of lifestyle measures to change either of the two fat deposit sites suggests that genetic factors may be the regulating agent in determining body fat distribution. One might also find that excess fat tissue represents an increase in weight, with at least some of the additional weight accounted for by excess adiposity. This has been suggested by skinfold thicknesses recorded by many investigators at central and peripheral sites as measures of subcutaneous adipose tissue.[39,46–49] Haffner et al. also suggest that the distributions of centrality index (subscapular/triceps) and waist/hip ratio may be used as distinct independent predictors of metabolic diseases for this population.[46] Body fat distribution is an additional component of obesity risk; in particular, upper body fat has been associated with increased risk for diabetes.[50] Each of the indices of fat patterning measures separate aspects of intermediate metabolism—e.g., lipids, lipoproteins, and triglycerides. Thus, every effort should be made to assess regional areas of body fat dispersal. If only one measure is possible, the waist/hip ratio appears to be most practical, with the best sensitivity for assessing central body fat patterning. A panel from National Academy of Sciences suggests the waist/hip ratio is a very useful measure for determining increased risk for CVD, with a ratio of 0.8 or greater representing an appropriate standard for beginning intervention.[51]

Obesity in Hispanic Youth

Obesity has been an especially significant health problem, especially in lower-income Mexican-American youth.[12] There is a growing body of literature suggesting that obesity acquired during childhood is maintained throughout the adult years. Gortmaker et al.[52] have reported that the level of obesity among U.S. adolescents was relatively steady until the mid1970s, but showed an increasingly upward trend until 1994. It is estimated that about 25 percent of U.S. adolescents are currently obese.[53] When HHANES I data standards for youth height and weight are compared to data collected a decade later, a substantial weight gain was seen among the younger age groups without a proportional increase in stature.[39,53] The weight increases are progressively higher across all percentiles, with the widest gap seen at the 90th percentile. The excessive weight for stature seems to be related to excessive fat tissue and not to lean muscle mass.[54] With a positive energy balance, body mass increases to accommodate the increases in energy stores. Hill and Peters suggest that the gain in body mass restores the energy balance at the next level.[43] The growing increase in youth body fatness above the 50th percentile has been associated with adverse changes in lipid and carbohydrate metabolism, leading to adult centralized obesity and increased risk of adult-onset diabetes.[47,55] The average age of diagnosis of noninsulin-dependent diabetes mellitus (NIDDM) in Mexican Americans is several years below that in whites, which may be a reflection of a longer period of excessive overweight.[56]

Recently, NHANES III found that young Hispanic males and females (primarily Mexican Americans) were the groups most likely to be overweight as compared with whites and other ethnic groups and that obesity patterns in Hispanics showed higher waist/hip ratios. Bassin et al. found, in a sample of nearly 1300 (aged 8 to 13 years) children in Los Angeles County during a 6-year period, that over 55 percent were obese, based on skinfold measurement and body mass index classification.[54,57,58] These findings coincide with findings in adult Hispanics in the American Southwest.[2,9,36]

Sociocultural Factors for Obesity

The development of obesity seems to begin at an even earlier age among Mexican Americans than among non-Hispanic whites because of sociocultural and socioeconomic factors linked to diet and physical inactivity.[44,59] Numerous reports have documented the level of obesity from cross-sectional studies, but there have been limited data on secular changes. Popkin and Udry reexamined thousands of ethnically diverse adolescents for body composition, stratified by socioeconomic status, and focused on generations living in the United States, yielding three different generational waves. The data categorized by generation and location of birth revealed a 24 percent increase in weight between first and second generation but hardly any change with second- and third-generation youth. The major differences in obesity prevalence were seen among Hispanic teenagers born in another country as opposed to those born in the United States. The acculturation process appears to be a very powerful force in the development of obesity.[60]

Although the health hazards of obesity are easily discussed on a biological level, the contributions of socioeconomic status and assimilation into the society are rarely examined or expressed. Findings from the San Antonio Heart Study suggest that while there are connections between obesity and lifestyle factors, there are also gender- and age-specific differences. Among men of higher socioeconomic status, there was a greater prevalence of obesity and centralized fat patterning. However, women of higher socioeconomic status demonstrated lower levels of obesity and more favorable body fat distribution.

Within the same social class, Mexican Americans were shorter and slightly heavier than non-Hispanic whites.[7,40] A weak and inconsistent relationship was found between socioeconomic status and being overweight in teenage girls and boys, whereas a stronger relationship appears to be present for whites.[7]

Diabetes

Over the last 65 years, diabetes has ranked among the 10 leading causes of morbidity and mortality in the United States. The San Antonio Heart Study has made significant efforts to examine diabetes in the Mexican-American population. Cross-sectional surveys of adults have shown a substantial increase, as compared with whites, in the prevalence of non-insulin-dependent diabetes mellitus (NIDDM).[10,46,49,61] From NHANES III, the prevalence of diabetes among Mexican Americans aged 20 and above is 8 percent for men and 11 percent for women. These rates are significantly higher than those among whites. Moreover, up to an additional 5 percent of Mexican-American men and 4 percent of Mexican-American women may have undiagnosed diabetes, based on the American Diabetes Association cutoff defining diabetes as

a fasting blood glucose of 126 mg/dL or greater.[4] In California, which has the nation's largest Mexican-American population, the prevalence of diabetes among Hispanics in 1996 was 13 percent—three times higher than that among whites (Fig. 19–4).[24]

The underreported prevalence of NIDDM may be of even greater concern among Mexican Americans. Diehl and Stern report undiagnosed diabetes in Texas, Colorado, New Mexico, and California to significantly impact the reported prevalence of diabetes for both men and women. They also point out that the NIDDM prevalence rates are related to socioeconomic status, with those in the lowest socioeconomic classes having the highest prevalence of NIDDM.[10] More complex analyses, which controlled for both social class and obesity, found Mexican Americans of both sexes to have a higher prevalence of NIDDM than whites.[62] One of the most interesting investigations of Mexican Americans by the San Antonio Heart Study involved the use of skin color as an index of Native-American heritage for predicting NIDDM. Very high rates of diabetes have been reported among Native Americans who inhabit the Southwest. The rates of the disease related closely to the degree of blending between the two

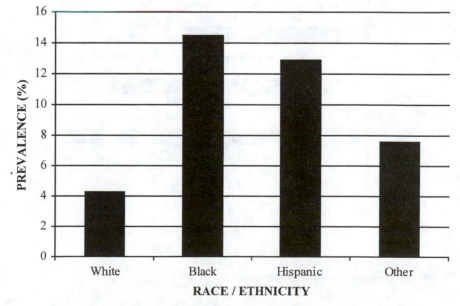

FIGURE 19–4

Prevalence of diabetes among California adults by race, 1996.

Data age-adjusted to 1990 California population.

(From Gazzaniga et al.,[24] with permission.)

ethnic groups. The authors concluded that NIDDM was highest in the segment of the Mexican-American population whose origins could be traced most closely to those of Native-American ancestry.[63]

It is now likely that a greater proportion of the Mexican-American as compared to the white population is prediabetic. The increasing level of childhood obesity puts the Mexican-American population at even greater risk of NIDDM. The San Antonio Heart Study investigators found that approximately 50 percent of the sample were previously undiagnosed diabetics and were less likely to seek medical care because they had no insurance. What makes the situation even more dangerous is that underutilization of screening for diabetes seems to be related to folk medicine and religious beliefs. In addition to traditional medicine, patients may employ folk healers who use herbs and other potions as well as prayers to treat the disease. Some of the less educated and strongly religious patients believe that it is

a higher being or fate that determines whether they will have diabetes.[64]

Cigarette Smoking

The adverse effects of smoking have been widely advertised, but the message has not penetrated the Mexican-American community to the extent that it has in the white community. National prevalence rates of smoking among Mexican Americans are 22 percent for men and 15 percent for women, but among youth in grades 9 to 12, they are markedly higher—36 percent of boys and 32 percent of girls smoke.[4] California smoking prevalence data in adults reveal that Mexican-American women have the lowest prevalence rate, but Mexican-American men smoke only 3 percent (19 percent) less than whites (Fig. 19–5).[24] The report suggests that the low smoking rate among Mexican Americans continues; however, men are 40 percent more likely to smoke than women.

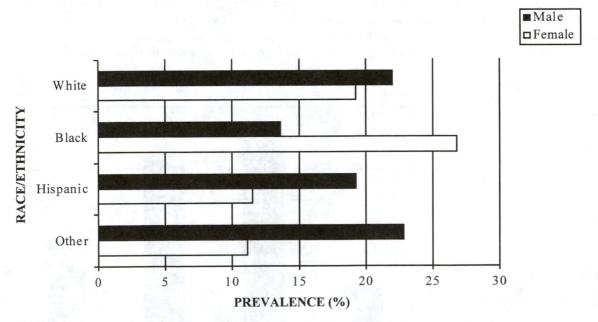

FIGURE 19–5 Prevalence of cigarette smoking among California adults by race and gender, 1996.
Data age-adjusted to 1990 california population.
(From Gazzaniga et al.,[24] with permission.)

Less information is available about Hispanics than about whites and African Americans regarding short- and long-term trends in smoking. National and statewide efforts have been launched to prevent youth from smoking experimentation.[65] School-based programs, which target all children, assume that preventing the youth from smoking will dampen the interest in smoking during adulthood. The HHANES found the prevalence of smoking to decline substantially with higher levels of education— i.e., those who had completed high school or had more education had a lower prevalence of smoking. There was seen only a small decline among the population who had never attended high school. The reduction in smoking was greater among women than in men. On the other hand, youngsters were most inclined to experiment with tobacco use, with the same frequency as other groups. Smoking had greater acceptance and social support with fewer years of formal education. The social and economic experiences of living in a low-income community, with a materialistic and socially conscious culture, may have lowered the resistance to smoking.[66,67] The lower level of education along with increased social pressure exposes a vulnerability to tobacco advertising and smoking. Morris et al. found Mexican-American youngsters starting to smoke at younger ages than was previously reported.[68] The smoking increase among Mexican-American young people should be viewed with alarm because of its adult health consequences. Substantial efforts should be made to further reduce the prevalence of smoking in all ethnic groups, especially among those with less than a high school education. Without individually tailored intervention strategies for youth, there will likely be an increase in adult tobacco use.

Physical Activity

The inverse relation of physical activity to cardiovascular disease has only been scientifically established over recent decades, despite being well-known since Plato's time.[69] Only 24 percent of Americans are physically active on a regular basis (20+ min per day three or more times per week). Among Hispanics, 62 percent of both men and women report a sedentary lifestyle.[3] An even higher proportion of Hispanics in California report little or no physical activity in the past month (70 percent of men and 66 percent of women).[24]

In addition, among Mexican Americans, 35 percent of women who were of acceptable weight exercised three or more times per week compared to only 27 percent of those who were overweight (Table 19–4A); among men, 48 percent of those who were underweight compared to only 41 percent of those who were overweight exercised three or more times per week (Table 19–4B).[23] Participation in physical activity among Mexican-American women is substantially lower than among white women (32 versus 52 percent, respectively). Furthermore, in California, 70 percent of Hispanic men and 66 percent of Hispanic women were physically inactive (reporting little or no leisure-time physical activity in the past month), substantially higher than in whites (50.2 percent for men and 50.6 percent for women).[24]

Since Mexican Americans have among the lowest socioeconomic status and the highest educational dropout rates,[70] significant efforts are needed to increase their rates of physical activity participation.[71,72] Many physical activity surveys were originally designed for men and do not take into account energy expenditure in home or on-the-job activities. Ransdell and Wells reported that findings in Mexican-American women supported the view that females who are over age 40 and less than college educated seldom exercise. Interestingly, marital status was a strong predictor for engaging in any exercise, and social support was a primary ingredient to encourage physical activity among women.[73] In youth, physical activity is encouraged and becomes prevalent when viewed as a social behavior that is learned and developed. But there has traditionally been a lack of interest in identifying social and cultural determinants, as well as developing appropriate measuring instruments, which has hampered participation in physical activity.[74] While there are significant data from the Youth National Fitness Test, ethnically diverse populations have not been extensively studied, resulting in reliance on general U.S. population reports.

TABLE 19–4A Percentage of Women* 20 Years of Age and Older Who Exercised Three or More Times per Week during Leisure Time by Age, Race-Ethnicity, and Body Weight Status, 1988–1991

Sex, Age, and Body Weight Status	Total Population[†]			Non-Hispanic White			Non-Hispanic Black			Mexican American		
	Sample Size	%	SE	Sample Size	%	SE	Sample Size	%	SE	Sample Size	%	SE
Total												
Underweight	179	48.0	6.77	101	49.9	8.27	45	37.6	6.82	22	54.5*	*
Acceptable weight	2119	54.0	2.25	1052	56.3	2.40	480	42.5	2.99	519	35.1	1.87
Overweight	1656	41.9	2.69	581	44.8	3.33	528	38.7	2.97	502	26.7	3.59
Total	**3954**	**49.3**	**1.90**	**1734**	**52.1**	**2.16**	**1053**	**40.4**	**2.35**	**1043**	**31.5**	**2.11**
20–39 years old												
Underweight	88	53.6	7.97	40	54.4	9.88	28	46.7*	*	15	59.2*	*
Acceptable weight	895	56.1	2.87	327	58.9	3.04	252	46.6	3.44	285	36.7	2.36
Overweight	542	43.7	4.06	127	45.6	5.23	186	50.6	4.49	215	26.3	4.38
Total	**1525**	**52.4**	**2.35**	**494**	**55.2**	**2.54**	**466**	**48.1**	**2.37**	**515**	**33.0**	**2.67**
40–59 years old												
Underweight	30	37.7[‡]	[‡]	20	44.5[‡]	[‡]	6	. . .[§]	. . .[§]	1	. . .[§]	. . .[§]
Acceptable weight	496	53.3	4.00	247	55.2	4.72	106	45.3	7.42	121	33.9	5.03
Overweight	558	42.9	3.31	187	47.5	4.44	184	32.9	4.46	167	28.1	4.50
Total	**1084**	**48.0**	**2.52**	**454**	**51.6**	**3.22**	**296**	**37.4**	**4.00**	**289**	**30.4**	**2.62**
60 years and over												
Underweight	61	44.4	7.35	41	44.4	7.03	11	. . .	. . .	6	. . .	. . .
Acceptable weight	728	50.9	2.71	478	53.2	2.64	122	25.6	4.47	113	29.3	6.17
Overweight	556	38.4	3.59	267	40.9	4.19	158	27.1	4.78	120	24.3	3.82
Total	**1345**	**45.7**	**2.69**	**786**	**48.2**	**2.85**	**291**	**25.9**	**3.95**	**239**	**27.1**	**3.49**

* Excludes pregnant women.

[†] Includes data for race-ethnic groups not shown separately.

[‡] Indicates a statistic that is potentially unreliable because of small sample size or large coefficient of variation.

[§] Does not meet minimum sample size requirements.

Note: Based on self-reported leisure-time physical activity. BMI is an index used to relate weight to stature. Underweight is defined as a BMI less than or equal to the 15th percentile, acceptable weight as a BMI between the 16th and 84th percentiles, and overweight as a BMI equal to or greater than the 85th percentile, based on BMI for 20- to 29-year-old females.

Source: VIMS, Third National Health and Nutrition Examination Survey, 1988–91.

Despite the importance of physical activity in reducing weight, improving the cardiovascular system, and insulin resistance, Mexican Americans are more likely to be sedentary. There is a need to understand the factors that encourage Mexican Americans to participate in physical activity because of its important health consequences.

Conclusions

During the past half-century, there has been major progress in understanding risk factors for CVD; however, many epidemiologic and clinical investigations have been limited to whites. Only in the past two decades have efforts targeted the Hispanic popula-

TABLE 19–4B   Percentage of Men 20 Years of Age and Older Who Exercised Three or More Times per Week during Leisure Time by Age, Race-Ethnicity, and Body Weight Status, 1988–1991

Sex, Age, and Body Weight Status	Total Population*			Non-Hispanic White			Non-Hispanic Black			Mexican American		
	Sample Size	%	SE	Sample Size	%	SE	Sample Size	%	SE	Sample Size	%	SE
Total												
Underweight	341	52.2	4.27	132	50.7	5.47	120	63.2	5.76	74	48.2	6.67
Acceptable weight	2400	62.8	2.24	1093	64.4	2.44	593	61.8	2.29	625	46.6	2.61
Overweight	1381	55.1	2.19	593	56.1	2.68	328	58.7	3.09	431	41.1	2.38
Total	**4122**	**59.5**	**1.79**	**1818**	**60.7**	**2.06**	**1041**	**61.0**	**2.28**	**1130**	**44.7**	**1.59**
20–39 years old												
Underweight	177	50.0	5.38	55	47.5	6.56	59	73.6	7.67	55	51.6	7.18
Acceptable weight	1025	64.1	3.23	317	65.0	3.95	283	72.0	3.14	381	48.6	2.39
Overweight	418	59.9	2.99	123	59.2	3.77	132	72.2	4.68	153	44.2	5.95
Total	**1620**	**61.5**	**2.38**	**495**	**61.6**	**2.91**	**474**	**72.2**	**3.05**	**589**	**47.7**	**1.43**
40–59 years old												
Underweight	48	66.8	6.92	16	64.2[†]	[†]	25	73.8[†]	[†]	4	...[‡]	...[‡]
Acceptable weight	606	62.0	2.81	287	64.5	3.31	163	54.6	3.79	124	39.1	5.07
Overweight	480	51.1	2.63	203	53.8	3.24	108	48.2	5.61	155	38.3	8.16
Total	**1134**	**57.9**	**2.09**	**506**	**60.1**	**2.58**	**296**	**53.2**	**2.69**	**283**	**38.2**	**4.59**
60 years and over												
Underweight	116	49.0	6.40	61	53.0	7.41	36	22.6	5.58	15	35.6*	*
Acceptable weight	769	60.4	2.44	489	63.0	2.53	147	38.4	4.83	120	46.0	5.23
Overweight	483	54.0	4.55	267	55.6	5.01	88	45.2	5.97	123	37.3	2.93
Total	**1368**	**57.2**	**2.65**	**817**	**59.5**	**2.84**	**271**	**38.5**	**3.07**	**258**	**41.4**	**2.66**

* Includes data for race-ethnic groups not shown separately.

[†] Indicates a statistic that is potentially unreliable because of small sample size or large coefficient of variation.

[‡] Does not meet minimum sample size requirements.

Note: Based on self-reported leisure-time physical activity. BMI is an index used to relate weight to stature. Underweight is defined as a BMI less than or equal to the 15th percentile, acceptable weight as a BMI between the 16th and 84th percentiles, and overweight as a BMI equal to or greater than the 85th percentile, based on BMIs for 20- to 29-year-old males.

Source: From the *Third Report on Nutrition Monitoring in the United States.*[23]

tion and has progress been made. The paucity of research on CVD in Mexican Americans is probably related to the small number of scientists in represented geographic areas and, until recently, the lack of national funding priorities. Using available data, physicians and health promotion personnel should be taught to consider ancestry and culture when imple-

menting CVD prevention efforts in Hispanics. A small reduction in levels of risk factors such as obesity and diabetes would likely reduce morbidity and mortality from future CVD and related conditions, including diabetes, in these population groups.

Recent reports have found that Hispanics' advantage in terms of traditionally lower CVD rates is disappearing with growing assimilation. Further information about Hispanics' major risk factors for heart disease and stroke relative to country of birth, generation in United States, degree of acculturation, traditional diet, and other lifestyle factors is needed. Only with this can effective preventive health strategies be developed.

References

1. Kingston RS, Smith JP: Socioeconomic status and racial and ethnic differences in functional status associated with chronic diseases. *Am J Public Health* 1997; 87:805–810.
2. U.S. Bureau of the Census: *Hispanic Americans Today: Current Population Reports.* Series P-23, No. 183. Washington, DC, U.S. Government Printing Office, 1993.
3. Sorlie PD, Backlund MS, Johnson NJ, Rogot E: Mortality by Hispanic status in the United States. *JAMA* 1993; 270:2464–2468.
4. American Heart Association: *Hispanics and Cardiovascular Disease.* Biostatistical Fact Sheets, 1999. Dallas, American Heart Association, 1999.
5. Ramirez AG: Hypertension in Hispanic Americans: overview of the population. *Public Health Rep* 1996; III(2):25–29.
6. *Progress Report for Hispanic Americans.* Washington, DC, U.S. Department of Health and Human Services, 1993.
7. National Center for Health Statistics: *Health, United States, 1993.* Hyattsville, MD, Public Health Service, 1994.
8. Public Health Service: Plan and Operation of the Hispanic Health and Nutrition Examination Survey 1982–84. *Vital Health Statistics [1] 1985*: DHHS publication PHS 85-1321. Hyattsville, MD, Public Health Service, 1985.
9. Bernard MA, Lampley-Dallas V, Smith L: Common health problems among minority elders. *J Am Diet Assoc* 1997; 97:771–776.
10. Diehl AC, Stern MP: Special health problems of Mexican Americans: obesity, gall bladder disease, diabetes mellitus and cardiovascular disease. *Adv Intern Med* 1989; 34:73–96.
11. Markides KS, Coreil J: The health of Hispanics in the southwestern United States: an epidemiological paradox. *Public Health Rep* 1986; 101:253–265.
12. Hazuda HP, Haffner SM, Stern MP, et al: Effects of acculturation and socioeconomic status on obesity and diabetes in Mexican-Americans. *Am J Epidemiol* 1988; 128:1289–1301.
13. Wei M, Valdez RA, Mitchel BD, et al: Migration status, socioeconomic status and mortality rates in Mexican

Americans and non-Hispanic whites: the San Antonio Heart Study. *Ann Epidemiol* 1996; 6:307–313.
14. Goff DC, Nichaman MZ, Chau W, et al: Greater incidence of hospitalized myocardial infarction among Mexican Americans than non-Hispanic whites: the Corpus Christi Heart Project, 1988–1992. *Circulation* 1997; 95:1433–1440.
15. Goff DC Jr, Ramsey DJ, Wear MC: Mortality after hospitalization for myocardial infarction among Mexican Americans and non-Hispanic whites: the Corpus Christi Heart Project. *Ethn Dis* 1993; 3:55–63.
16. Wei M, Mitchell BD, Haffner SM Stern MP: Effects of cigarette smoking, diabetes, high cholesterol and hypertension on all-cause mortality and cardiovascular disease mortality in Mexican Americans: the San Antonio Heart Study. *Am J Epidemiol* 1996; 141:1058–1065.
17. Maldonado MM: Hypertension in Hispanics, Asians and Pacific-Islanders and Native Americans. *Circulation* 1991; 83:1467–1469.
18. Haffner SM, Stern MP: Decreased prevalence of hypertension in Mexican Americans. *Hypertension* 1990; 16:225–232.
19. Crespo CJ, Loria CM, Burt VL: Hypertension and other cardiovascular risk factors among Mexican Americans, Cuban Americans and Puerto Ricans from the Hispanic Health and Nutrition Examination Survey. *Public Health Rep* 1996; 111(suppl 2):7–10.
20. Pappas G, Gergen PJ, Carol M: Hypertension prevalence and the status of awareness, treatment, and control in the Hispanic Health and Nutrition Examination Survey (HHANES) 1982–84. *Am J Public Health* 1990; 80:1431–1436.
21. National Institutes of Health, National Heart, Lung, Blood Institute: The Fifth Report of the Joint National Committee on Detection, Evaluation and Treatment of High Blood Pressure. National High Blood Pressure Education Program Publication (NIH) 93-1088. Bethesda MD, National Heart, Lung, Blood Institute, 1992.
22. Sorel JE, Ragland DR, Syme SL: Blood pressure in Mexican Americans, whites, blacks: The Second National Health and Nutrition Examination Survey and the Hispanic Health and Nutrition Examination Survey. *Am J Epidemiol* 1991; 134:370–378.
23. Third Report on Nutrition Monitoring in The United States: vol II. Washington, DC, U.S. Government Printing Office, 1995
24. Gazzaniga JM, Kao C, Cowling DW, et al: *Cardiovascular Disease Risk Factors among California Adults, 1984–1996.* CORE Program, University of California. Sacramento, CA, San Francisco and California Department of Health Services, 1998.
25. Havas S, Sherwin R: Putting it all together: Summary of the NHLBI Workshop on hypertension in Hispanic American, Native American, and Asian/Pacific Islander population. *Public Health Rep* 1996; 111 2(suppl):77–79.

26. Fortman SP: Effect of long-term community health education on blood pressure and hypertension control: the Stanford Five-City Project. *Am J Epidemiol* 1990; 132:629–646.

27. Berenson GS, Wattigney MS, Tracy RE: Atherosclerosis of the aorta and coronary arteries and cardiovascular risk factors in persons aged 6 to 30 studied at necropsy (the Bogalusa Heart Study). *Am J Cardiol* 1992; 70:851–858.

28. Muscat JE, Axelrad C, Ray K, et al: Cholesterol screening in a community health promotion program: epidemiological results from a biracial community. *Public Health Rep* 1994; 109:93–98.

29. Mitchell BD, Stern MP, Haffner SM, et al: Risk factors for cardiovascular mortality in Mexican Americans. *Int J Obesity* 1990; 14:623–629.

30. Schoen R, Nelson VE: Mortality due to all causes among Spanish-surnamed Californians 1969–1971. *Soc Sci Q* 1981; 62:259–272.

31. Poe GS, Powell-Griner E, McLaughlin JK: Comparability of death certificates and 1986 mortality followback survey. In: *Vital Health Statistics 1993*. DHHS Pub no. (PHS) 94-1392. Hyattsville, MD, Public Health Service, 1993.

32. Haffner SM, Stern MP, Hazuda HP, et al: The role of behavioral variables and fat patterning in explaining ethnic differences in serum lipids and lipoproteins. *Am J Epidemiol* 1986; 123:830–839.

33. Hixon JE, Henkel RD, Sharp RM, Comuzzie AG: Genetic and environmental contributions to cardiovascular risk factors in Mexican Americans: the San Antonio Family Heart Study. *Circulation* 1996 94:2159–2170.

34. Valdez R, Gonzalez-Villalpando C, Mitchell BD, et al: Differential impact of obesity in related populations. *Obesity Res* 1995; 3:223–232.

35. Winklely MA, Kramer HC, Ahn DK, Vanady AN: Ethnic and socioeconomic differences in cardiovascular disease risk factors: findings for women from the Third National Health and Nutrition Examination Survey, 1988–1994. *JAMA* 1998; 280:356–362.

36. U.S. Department of Health and Human Services: Update: prevalence of overweight among children, adolescents, and adults—United States, 1988–94. *MMWR* 1997; 46:199–202.

37. Pawson IG, Martorel R, Mendoza FE: Prevalence of overweight and obesity in U.S. Hispanic population. *Am J Nutr* 1995; 53:15,225–15,228.

38. Jeffrey RW: Population perspectives on the prevention and treatment of obesity in minority populations. *Am J Clin Nutr* 1991; 53:1621–1624.

39. Roche AE, Guo S, Bumgartner RN, et al: Reference data for weight, stature, and weight/stature in Mexican Americans from the Hispanic Health and Nutrition Examination Survey (HHANES) 1982–1984. *Am J Clin Nutr* 1990; 51(suppl):917–245.

40. Stern MP, Pugh JA, Gaskell SP, Hazuda HP: Knowledge, attitudes, and behavior related to obesity and dieting in Mexican American and Anglos: the San Antonio Heart Study. *Am J Epidemiol* 1992; 115:917–927.

41. Centers for Disease Control: Prevalence of overweight for Hispanics-United States, 1982–1984. *JAMA* 1990; 263:631–632.

42. Rand CSW, Kuldau JM: The epidemiology of obesity and self-defined weight problems in the general population: gender, race, age, and social class. *Int J Eating Dis* 1990; 9:329–343.

43. Hill JO, Peters JC: Environmental contributions to obesity epidemic. *Science* 1998; 28:1371–1374.

44. Malina RM, Little BB, Stern MP, et al: Ethnic and social class differences in selected anthropometric characteristics of Mexican-American and Anglo adults: the San Antonio Heart Study. *Hum Biol* 1983; 55:867–883.

45. Haffner SM, Stern MP, Hazuda HP, et al: Do upper-body and central adiposity measure different aspects of regional body-fat distribution? Relationship to non-insulin-dependent diabetes mellitus, lipids, and lipoproteins. *Diabetes* 1987; 36:43–51.

46. Haffner SM, Stern MP, Hazuda HP, et al: Upper body and centralized obesity in Mexican Americans and Non-Hispanic whites: relationship to body mass index and demographic variables. *Int J Obesity* 1986; 10:493–502.

47. Mueller WH, Joos SK, Havis CL, et al: The Diabetes Alert Study: growth, fatness, fat patterning, adolescence through adulthood in Mexican Americans. *Am J Phys Anthropol* 1984; 64:389–99.

48. Stern SP, Haffner SM: Do anthropometric differences between Mexican Americans and non-Hispanic whites explain ethnic differences in metabolic variables? *Acta Med Scand Suppl* 1989; 723:37–44.

49. Joos SK, Mueller WH, Hanis CL, Schull WS: Diabetes Alert Study: weight history, and body adiposity in diabetic and non-diabetic Mexican American adults. *Ann Hum Biol* 1984; 11:161–171.

50. Kumanyika SK: Special issues regarding obesity in minority populations. *Ann Intern Med* 1993; 119(7 pt 2):650–654.

51. U.S. Department of Health and Human Services: *Physical Activity and Health: A Report of the Surgeon General*. Atlanta, GA, U.S. Department of Health and Human Services, Centers for Disease Control and Prevention, National Center for Chronic Disease Prevention and Health Promotion, 1996.

52. Gortmaker SL, Dietz WH, Wehler CA: Increasing obesity in the United States. *Am J Dis Child* 1987; 141:535–554.

53. Troiano RP, Flegal KM, Kuczmarski RJ, et al: Overweight prevalence and trends for children and adolescents. *Arch Pediat Adolesc Med* 1995; 149:1085–1091.

54. Bassin SL, Gustin W, Morris GS, et al: Hispanic youth obesity: body fat and cardiovascular risk factors (abstr). *Circulation* 1995; 92:1481.

55. Stern MP, Haffner SM, Hazuda HP, et al. Hyperinsulinemia in a population at high risk for non-insulin-dependent diabetes mellitus. *N Engl J Med* 1986; 315:220–224.

56. Raymond CA: Diabetes in Mexican Americans: pressing problem in a growing population. *JAMA* 1988; 259:1772.

57. Wong ND, Bassin SL, Dietrick R: Relationship of blood lipids to anthropometric measures and family medical history in an ethnically diverse school-aged population. *Ethn Dis* 1991; 1:351–363.

58. Bassin SL, Khan SA, Gustin W, et al: Measures of obesity and their relation to cardiovascular risk factors in Hispanic youth. Submitted.

59. Troiano RP, Flegal KM: Overweight children and adolescents: description, epidemiology and demographics. *Pediatrics* 1998; 101(suppl):497–504.

60. Popkin BM, Udry JR: Adolescent obesity increases significantly in second and third generation U.S. immigrants: the National Longitudinal Study of Adolescent Health. *J Nutr* 1998; 128:701–706.

61. Stern MP, Haffner SM: Body fat distribution and hyperinsulinemia as risk factors for diabetes and cardiovascular disease. *Arteriosclerosis* 1986; 6:123–130.

62. Stern MP, Haffner SM: Type II diabetes and its complications in Mexican Americans. *Diabetes Metab Rev* 1990; 6:29–40.

63. Knowler WC, Pettitt DJ, Saad MF, et al: Obesity in the Pima Indians: Its magnitude and relationship with diabetes. *Am J Clin Nutr* 1991; 53(suppl):1543S–1551S.

64. Zaldivar A, Smolowitz J: Perceptions of the importance of religion and folk medicine by non-Mexican American Hispanic adults with diabetes. *Diabetes Educ* 1994; 20:363–366.

65. Escobedo LG, Anda RF, Smith PF, et al: Sociodemographic characteristics of cigarette smoking initiation in the United States: implications for smoking prevention policy. *JAMA* 1990; 264:1550–1556.

66. Escobedo LG, Remington PL: Birth cohort analysis of smoking prevalence among Hispanics in the United States. *JAMA* 1989; 261:66–69.

67. Escobedo LG, Peddicord JP: Smoking prevalence in U.S. birth cohorts: the influence of gender and education. *Am J Public Health* 1996; 86:231–236.

68. Morris GS, Vo AN, Bassin S, et al: Prevalence and sociobehavioral correlates of tobacco use among Hispanic children: the tobacco resistance activity program. *J Sch Health* 1993; 63:391–396.

69. Paffenbarger RS, Hyde RT, Wing AL, Jung IM, et al: The association of changes in PA level and other lifestyle characteristics with mortality among men. *N Engl J Med* 1993; 328:538–545.

70. Farrell SW, Kampert JB, Kohl HW III, et al: Influences of cardiorespiratory fitness levels and other predictors of cardiovascular disease mortality in men. *Med Sci Sports Exerc* 1998; 3:899–905.

71. Pate RR, Pratt ME, Blair SN, et al: Physical activity and public health: a recommendation from the Centers for Disease Control and Prevention and the American College Of Sports Medicine. *JAMA* 1995; 273:402–407.

72. Sallis JF, Patterson TL, Buono MJ, et al: Aggregation of physical activity habits in Mexican American and Anglo families. *J Behav Med* 1988; 11:13–41.

73. Ransdell LB, Wells CL: Physical activity in urban white, African-American, and Mexican-American women. *Med Sci Sports Exerc* 1998; 3:1608–1615.

74. Moller JH, Taubert KA, Allen HD, et al: Cardiovascular health and disease in children: current status—AHA Medical/Scientific Statement Special Report. *Circulation* 1994; 89:923–930.

CHAPTER 20

Prevention of Coronary Heart Disease in Asian Populations

Prakash C. Deedwania
Rajeev Gupta

The Asian countries have traditionally had a low prevalence of coronary heart disease (CHD). However, with modernization of Asia, there has been an alarming increase in its incidence.[1] This region is undergoing unprecedented economic growth, rapid technological changes, urbanization, and major changes in lifestyle. The very high CHD death rates in Singapore, which are similar to those of the United States and Australia, provide a warning that Asia should expect a surge in CHD similar to that observed in the United States and other developed countries in the 1950s and 1960s.[2] Most recent estimates suggest about 36 percent of all deaths in Asian/Pacific Islanders living in the United States are due to cardiovascular diseases, as compared with about 41 percent of the entire population. The age-adjusted annual CHD mortality rate per 1000 declined from 4.7 to 2.9 between 1966 and 1984. Stroke incidence rates per 1000 also declined markedly (from 5.1 to 2.4).[3,4] Some reports, however, suggest the age-adjusted prevalence of CHD among Asian immigrants to the United States to be higher than that among their Caucasian counterparts.[5]

Studies reviewed below from different Asian populations living both within and beyond the United States show that the level of cardiovascular risk in Asians is becoming increasingly similar to that of Caucasian populations. Table 20–1 shows estimated cardiovascular risk factor prevalences as most recently estimated for the Asian/Pacific Islander population in the United States.[4] Consideration must be given to applying the lessons in prevention learned

TABLE 20–1 Estimated Cardiovascular Risk Factor Prevalences (%) in Asian/Pacific Islanders, United States

Risk Factor	Men	Women
High blood pressure	9.7%	8.4%
Smoking	29.4%	4.3%
High blood cholesterol	27.4%	25.8%
Physical inactivity	56.6%	64.7%
Overweight	10.8%	10.1%
	(65.5% in Native Hawaiians)	(62.6% in Native Hawaiians)
Diabetes	3.4%	2.4%

Source: Data from the American Heart Association,[4] with permission.

over the past half-century in other populations to prevent the emerging epidemic of CHD in Asian countries and populations.

Coronary Risk Factors and Disease in Asian Populations

Japanese

At the beginning of the Seven Countries Study in 1958, Japanese cohorts had the lowest saturated fat intake, the lowest levels of serum cholesterol, and one of the lowest incidences of CHD. In the Japanese rural areas of Tanushimaru, among men 40 to 64 years of age, mortality rates from myocardial infarction have remained stable at 0.3 to 0.5 per 1000 per year from 1958 to 1992.[6] Overall in Japan, the crude death rates from CHD increased up to 1972 but remained stable thereafter. Although the age-adjusted death rate from CHD is decreasing, there is an alarming increase in other heart disease death rates. This may be related to mortality from hypertensive heart disease.[7] From one study in the Tokyo area, 49.8 percent of sudden deaths examined at autopsy have been attributed to CHD.[8]

The situation among emigrant Japanese is entirely different. Initial studies in Honolulu showed that the cholesterol levels in subjects living there were significantly greater than in Japanese cohorts but lower than those in the United States.[9] The incidence of CHD was also lower than in Caucasians.[10] Cholesterol levels in Japanese subjects living in the United States were almost equal to those in Caucasians, and the incidence of CHD was similar,[9,10] suggesting that acculturation may play a significant role in determining CHD risk.

The Ni-Hon-San Study of the Japanese living in Japan, Hawaii, and the mainland United States provides a classic example of the influence of Western lifestyle and dietary changes on CHD incidence in a low-incidence population. The average annual mortality rates from CHD in Japanese men 55 to 59 years of age in the late 1960s were 1.4 per 1000 in Japan, 1.7 per 1000 in Honolulu, and 4.8 per 1000 in San Francisco.[10] Mean levels or prevalences of selected coronary risk factors within each of these three population groups are shown in Table 20–2. There is a trend toward an increase in the prevalence of obesity as well as in high lipid levels among those living in Japan, Honolulu, and San Francisco (in order of increasing levels). Although the values of biochemical variables are significantly greater in the Japanese living in the United States (Hawaii and California),[9] levels of blood pressure and the prevalence of hypertension are not significantly different.[11] Obesity and biochemical risk factors may partly explain the greater CHD mortality among the Japanese in the United States.

The Honolulu Heart Study is the largest and longest-running epidemiologic study of heart disease

TABLE 20–2 Coronary Risk Factor Means (±SD) and Prevalences in Japanese Men—Ni-Hon-San Study

	Age Group	Japan	Honolulu	San Francisco
Total cholesterol	45–49	179.8 ± 2.2	219.4 ± .09	223.4 ± 1.3
	50–54	182.5 ± 1.7	219.4 ± 0.7	228.2 ± 1.7
	55–59	181.5 ± 1.7	218.7 ± 1.0	226.8 ± 2.2
Triglycerides	45–49	142.0 ± 37.2	—	192.0 ± 12.7
	50–54	136.0 ± 19.3	182.0 ± 6.7	182.0 ± 12.6
	55–59	124.0 ± 9.2	180.0 ± 7.5	170.0 ± 14.7
Systolic blood pressure	45–49	126.0 ± 22.8	131.0 ± 21.8	123.0 ± 18.0
	50–54	130.0 ± 23.4	134.0 ± 24.6	132.0 ± 17.4
	55–59	136.0 ± 25.2	135.0 ± 24.4	139.0 ± 21.8
Diastolic blood pressure	45–49	81.0 ± 13.7	80.0 ± 13.0	79.0 ± 12.8
	50–54	82.0 ± 13.6	86.0 ± 13.7	84.0 ± 10.0
	55–59	85.0 ± 14.0	82.0 ± 13.0	88.0 ± 13.8
Obesity (%) (>120% ideal body weight)	45–49	17.8	63.2	38.1
	50–54	23.9	52.6	54.5
	55–59	24.7	50.4	57.6

Source: Adapted from Worth et al.,[10] with permission.

in Asian Americans. It has provided repeated assessments of a wide range of cardiovascular risk factors and has followed the morbidity and mortality status of 8006 men of Japanese ancestry born between 1900 and 1919 who have been followed since 1965 with a series of laboratory and medical examinations as well as assessments of dietary habits and physical activity. This study has documented many of the same risk factors for CHD found in Caucasian populations, including a strong, recently reported relation of total cholesterol to CHD and total mortality.[12] Hypertension is also quite common in this population, being prevalent in over half of the men aged 60 to 75 and in 67 percent of those aged 75 to 81.[13]

Chinese

CHD has long been known to clinicians to be relatively uncommon in China. However, recent data from a nationwide survey of pathologic material and studies of hospitalized cardiac patients have provided evidence suggesting that the incidence of CHD has increased in the last two decades.[14] A corresponding rise in mean serum cholesterol level has also been noted, although the level attained is still significantly lower than that in the United States and other western European countries. The changes observed in general disease patterns in China since the late 1950s show a decline in mortality from infectious diseases and an increase in average life expectancy at birth. Mortality rates from CHD and stroke have reportedly increased substantially, and the major cardiovascular diseases are now the leading cause of death.[15]

Although, in their broad generic grouping, cardiovascular diseases are the leading cause of death in both China and the United States, there are important differences in the pattern of specific cardiovascular diseases between the two countries. Mortality from CHD represents more than 50 percent of deaths caused by all types of cardiovascular diseases in the United States but only 20 percent for urban China and 10 percent for rural China. Correspondingly, mortality from CHD accounts for about two-thirds of all heart disease deaths among Americans but only 50 percent for urban Chinese and 25 per-

cent for rural Chinese. CHD death rates per 100,000 people are much higher for the United States than for China. Stroke deaths outnumber coronary deaths in China, whereas the reverse prevails in the United States. Complex biomedical and socioeconomic factors are responsible for these differences.[15]

Data on cardiovascular risk factors in Chinese who have emigrated to the United States are lacking. However, important differences in coronary risk factors in urban as compared with rural Chinese have been noted. The People's Republic of China—United States Cardiovascular and Cardiopulmonary Epidemiology Research Group data[15] in four Chinese samples 35 to 54 years of age show that levels of mean systolic and diastolic blood pressure, lipids (cholesterol, triglycerides), and body-mass index were considerably lower in rural as compared with urban subjects. The prevalence of hypertension and hypercholesterolemia was also lower among rural Chinese. The highest prevalence of these risk factors was found in urban Beijing, followed by semiurban and rural Beijing, urban Guangzhou, and rural Guangzhou (Table 20–3). The possibility exists that dietary and other lifestyle practices, which differ between northern and southern provinces and between urban and rural communities, may play a role in these risk factor differences. In fact, a more recent analysis showed that the Key's score for dietary fat was significantly related to levels of total cholesterol.[16]

Mean values as well as the prevalences of hyperlipidemia and hypertension are lower in Chinese than in middle-aged populations in Western industrialized countries. In contrast to the United States, where hypertension is more common among rural Americans, it is more prevalent in urban subjects in China. This rural-urban differential suggests the role of dietary and socioeconomic factors in its genesis. In the United Kingdom, Chinese men and women, as compared with Caucasians, had lower total and LDL cholesterol levels, body-mass index, and smoking prevalence, although the Chinese women had higher blood pressure levels.[17] In the United States, however, Asian-born Chinese living in New York City's Chinatown had higher total cholesterol levels than did either urban or rural Chinese living in Shanghai, China. Those living in the United States also had

TABLE 20–3   Urban-Rural Differences in Coronary Risk Factors in China—34 to 54 Years

	Beijing		Guangzhou	
	Urban	**Rural**	**Urban**	**Rural**
Men				
Body-mass index (kg/m^2)	23.5 ± 3.0	22.3 ± 3.0	20.6 ± 2.4	19.8 ± 2.0
Systolic blood pressure, mmHg	123.1 ± 17.6	127.0 ± 20.0	113.3 ± 13.9	114.6 ± 14.3
Diastolic blood pressure, mmHg	82.3 ± 11.9	80.9 ± 11.9	75.4 ± 9.5	73.0 ± 9.5
Hypertension: Blood pressure ≥140/90 (%)	47.1	39.0	14.2	10.0
Total cholesterol (mg/dL)	184.8 ± 37.8	171.3 ± 38.1	181.6 ± 31.8	158.7 ± 30.9
Triglycerides (mg/dL)	110.1 ± 73.5	116.3 ± 38.1	104.7 ± 85.9	80.9 ± 78.5
High cholesterol ≥200 mg/dL (%)	29.2	21.8	26.3	9.1
Smoking (%)	71.4	77.7	72.7	76.7
Women				
Body-mass index (kg/m^2)	24.3 ± 3.7	22.7 ± 3.3	21.8 ± 3.0	19.6 ± 2.1
Systolic blood pressure, mmHg	123.1 ± 21.6	121.7 ± 19.2	115.7 ± 17.6	109.8 ± 13.7
Diastolic blood pressure, mmHg	79.0 ± 11.7	75.9 ± 11.3	75.6 ± 10.5	69.8 ± 8.8
Hypertension: Blood pressure ≥140/90 (%)	41.0	27.3	18.2	5.5
Total cholesterol (mg/dL)	187.6 ± 42.4	168.1 ± 40.8	187.5 ± 33.2	154.9 ± 28.7
Triglycerides (mg/dL)	118.4 ± 83.1	108.9 ± 64.9	100.1 ± 89.4	75.7 ± 44.2
High cholesterol ≥200 mg/dL (%)	33.0	18.9	32.1	6.5
Smoking (%)	23.2	30.9	3.2	7.5

Source: From the People's Republic of China—United States Cardiovascular and Cardiopulmonary Epidemiology Research Group,[15] with permission.

prevalences of cholesterol levels classified as borderline-high (35 percent) and high (23 percent) according to the National Cholesterol Education Program; these Chinese were similar to a comparable group of screened Caucasians (32 percent borderline-high and 36 percent high).[18]

South Asians

The prevalence of CHD is increasing rapidly in South Asian countries. Cardiovascular diseases, especially CHD, are major contributors to mortality and morbidity in India.[19,20] Conservative estimates suggest that in 1990, cardiovascular diseases caused 2.39 million deaths and the nation incurred a loss of 28.59 million disability-adjusted life years.[19] Demographic shifts in the population age profile combined with lifestyle-related increases in the levels of cardiovascular risk factors are accelerating the CHD epidemic in India.[21] A doubling of deaths due to CHD between 1985 and 2015 has been projected. In men, the projected death rates per 100,000 population are 145 in 1985, 253 in 2000, and 295 in 2015; in women, these rates are projected to be 126, 204 and 239, respectively. Cardiovascular diseases, mainly CHD, are likely to account for at least 33.5 percent of total deaths by the year 2015 and would replace infectious diseases as the number-one killer of Indians. CHD prevalence has shown a significant increase in India since the 1950s. The increase is significantly greater in urban subjects than in rural, as in other parts of

Asia.[20] CHD prevalence increased in urban populations from 1.05 percent (Delhi) in 1960 to 9.67 percent (Delhi) and 7.90 percent (Jaipur) in 1995. In rural areas, it increased from 2.03 percent (Haryana) in 1974 to 3.70 percent (Rajasthan) in 1994. This increase has been associated with a steep increase in major coronary risk factors in the Indian population. The prevalence of hypertension has shown a significant increase in both urban and rural subjects.[22] In urban populations, earlier studies of Dotto (1949), Dubey (1954), and Sathe (1959) showed a hypertension prevalence of 1.2, 4.2, and 3.0 percent in populations of Calcutta, Kanpur, and Bombay, respectively. Recent studies using the same guidelines [World Health Organization (WHO) 1959] from Ludhiana (1985) and Jaipur (1995) show that the prevalence has increased to 14.1 and 11.0 percent, respectively. Age-adjusted analysis also shows a steep increase in mean systolic blood pressure (BP) in Indians. In men aged 40 to 49 years, mean systolic BP has increased from 112 to 128 mmHg. Similarly, in New Delhi, mean population cholesterol levels have increased from 162 mg/dL in 1982 to 190 mg/dL in 1992.[23]

Among civil servants in Kathmandu, Nepal, a prevalence of CHD of 4.7 percent has been reported, with tobacco use noted to be the major risk factor. A prevalence of hypertension ranging from 5 to 6 percent in rural areas to 8 to 10 percent in urban areas in the Kathmandu region has also been reported. As these data were based on WHO criteria from 1978 defining hypertension as 160/95 mmHg or above, the prevalence would be substantially greater by today's standards. Comparing urban versus rural areas, obesity was noted to be twice as common (24 versus 12 percent) and a sedentary lifestyle three times as common (35 versus 11 percent).[24]

A considerable excess of CHD among expatriate South Asian communities has been reported from several countries.[25] From 1979 to 1983, age-standardized CHD mortality was 40 percent higher in men and women of South Asian extraction than in the general population of England and Wales, irrespective of social class or religious group.[26] The falling CHD mortality rates experienced by most of the Western world over the past two decades contrast

sharply with rising CHD mortality in westernized South Asian communities.[25,27] Among UK-based South Asians, CHD mortality increased by 6 percent in men and 13 percent in women in the decade from 1970 to 1980. Excess mortality from CHD in South Asians is especially striking in young men.[28]

To determine the coronary risk factors that may be important in Indians, epidemiologic studies in urban and rural populations in Rajasthan were performed. In cross-sectional surveys in randomly selected urban[29] and rural[30] areas of Rajasthan in Western India, 3397 men (1415 urban, 1982 rural) and 1963 women (797 urban, 1166 rural) 20 years of age and above were studied. Blood samples were obtained from a random 10 percent. CHD prevalence diagnosed by history and electrocardiographic (ECG) changes was greater in the urban than in the rural areas (men, 6.0 versus 3.4 percent; women, 10.5 versus 3.7 percent; $p < .01$). The prevalence of ECG changes alone was also greater in urban areas (men, 3.5 versus 2.8 percent; women, 8.4 versus 3.3 percent; $p < .05$). In the urban areas as compared with the rural, risk factors significantly ($p < .01$) more prevalent included hypertension (men, 30 versus 24 percent; women, 34 versus 17 percent), diabetes history (men, 1.1 versus 0.1 percent; women, 1.0 versus 0.1 percent), obesity (both sexes, 11 versus 6 percent), truncal obesity (men, 26 versus 4 percent; women, 17 versus 5 percent), physical inactivity in men (86 versus 82 percent), and smoking in women (19 versus 5 percent). However, in rural men, smoking was more prevalent (51 versus 39 percent) (Table 20–4).[31]

Gupta compared CHD and risk-factor prevalences in urban and rural populations of Haryana.[32] CHD prevalence in urban subjects was twice that in rural subjects. The Haryana studies showed a greater prevalence of hypertension, obesity, and sedentary lifestyle in urban subjects; furthermore, factors such as diabetes, truncal obesity, and higher cholesterol levels were also more prevalent in urban subjects. A higher prevalence of sedentary lifestyle, truncal obesity, and diabetes is suggestive of an insulin-resistant state in urban subjects. The Indian Council of Medical Research Task Force

TABLE 20–4 Urban-Rural Difference in Coronary Risk Factor Prevalence in India, percent

	Urban	Rural	χ^2 (p value)
Men	**(n = 1415)**	**(n = 1982)**	
Smoking and tobacco use	548 (38.7)	1006 (50.8)	47.65 (<.001)
Leisure-time activity	202 (14.3)	363 (18.3)	9.43 (.002)
Diabetes history	15 (1.1)	4 (0.2)	9.44 (.002)
Hypertension: blood pressure 140/90 mmHg	417 (29.5)	470 (23.7)	13.88 (<.001)
Hypertension: blood pressure 160/95 mmHg	146 (10.3)	150 (7.6)	7.51 (.006)
Obesity (BMI) 27 kg/m^2	161 (11.4)	104 (5.2)	42.30 (<.001)
Truncal obesity >0.95	64/252 (25.4)	17/399 (4.3)	61.41 (<.001)
Cholesterol ≥200 mg/dL	52/199 (26.1)	45/202 (22.3)	0.62 (.433)
HDL cholesterol <35 mg/dL	47/199 (23.5)	49/202 (24.2)	0.01 (.97)
Women	**(n = 797)**	**(n = 1166)**	
Smoking and tobacco use	149 (18.7)	54 (4.6)	99.48 (<.001)
Leisure-time activity	64 (8.0)	88 (7.5)	0.09 (.76)
Diabetes history	8 (1.0)	2 (0.1)	4.93 (.026)
Hypertension: blood pressure ≥140/90 mmHg	267 (33.5)	197 (16.9)	71.40 (<.001)
Hypertension: blood pressure ≥160/95 mmHg	97 (12.2)	72 (6.2)	20.87 (<.001)
Obesity (BMI) 27 kg/m^2	87 (10.9)	74 (6.4)	12.53 (<.001)
Truncal obesity >0.95	33/193 (17.1)	5/104 (4.8)	8.08 (.001)
Cholesterol ≥200 mg/dL	NA	22/98 (22.5)	NA
HDL cholesterol <35 mg/dL	NA	40/98 (40.8)	NA

Key: BMI, body-mass index; HDL, high-density lipoprotein; NA, not available.
Source: Adapted from Gupta,[31] with permission.

Project on coronary risk-factor prevalence in urban and rural subjects in Delhi also reported a greater prevalence of coronary risk factors (smoking, obesity, truncal obesity, hypertension, diabetes, and hypercholesterolemia) in urban subjects.[33] South Asian Indians have also been noted to be more prone than Malays or Chinese to central obesity, with insulin resistance and glucose intolerance as well as higher lipoprotein(a) values, which may relate to their higher propensity to develop "syndrome X."[34] Thus, the risk factors that occur more in urban Japanese, Chinese, and South Asians and are associated with a greater prevalence of CHD also need to be controlled in Indians for prevention of CHD (Table 20–5).

TABLE 20–5 Coronary Risk Factors with Greater Frequency in Urban Asians Compared with Rural Asians

Sedentary lifestyle

Hypertension

Body-mass index, obesity waist:hip ratio, truncal obesity

Total and low-density-lipoprotein cholesterol, hypercholesterolemia

Triglyceride levels

Fasting insulin levels, insulin resistance

Source: Adapted from Hughes,[34] with permission.

Multiethnic Studies of Asians Living in the United States

A large study of more than 1700 Asian Americans living in California showed these individuals to be less knowlegeable about hypertension and less likely to be under treatment or in control than hypertensive persons of other races. The study also noted Filipinos to have the highest prevalence of hypertension (60 percent of men and 65 percent of women aged 50 or older) as compared with other Asian groups.[35]

More recently, a large cross-sectional study of 13,081 Asians living in the United States showed a higher body-mass index and smoking prevalence among U.S.-born men and a higher prevalence of hypertension in Chinese U.S.-born men but no difference in cholesterol levels among those born versus not born in the United States.[36] This study also showed body-mass index and smoking prevalence to be lowest in Chinese men and women, total cholesterol levels highest in Japanese men and women, and hypertension prevalence highest in Filipino men and women.

A study among Southeast Asian refugee children has noted systolic blood pressures among Hmong boys and diastolic blood pressures among Hmong boys and girls and of Cambodian girls to be greater than those of African Americans and Caucasians of the same sexes.[37] Recent data also suggest high smoking prevalence rates in certain Asian-American immigrant populations, including 72 percent in Laotian, 71 percent in Cambodian, and 42 percent in Native Hawaiians.[38]

Why Is Coronary Heart Disease Increasing in Asians?

The epidemiologic evolution or transition has been characterized by six stages described by indices of acculturation, urbanization, affluence, saturated-fat intake, salt intake, and smoking.[39] The prevalence of atherosclerotic diseases, CHD, and hypertension initially increases with a rise in these factors, then stabilizes, and finally decreases.

In Indians, the social and economic indices of epidemiologic transition explain the increasing CHD prevalence.[21,23] There has been a marked increase in urbanization in India. In 1901, only 11 percent of the population was living in urban areas (towns with population of >20,000). This proportion increased to 20.2 percent in 1971 and 26.1 percent in 1991. The increase in urbanization in most Asian countries is greater than that in most of the developed countries of Europe, North America, and elsewhere. There is a strong correlation between urbanization and increase in CHD prevalence ($r=.76$) in urban communities.

Affluence is measured by evaluating per capita net domestic product, growth of production, and human development index.[40,41] The per capita net domestic product in India has approximately doubled in the past 30 years. The average annual growth rate in gross domestic product (GDP) was 3.4 percent in 1970 to 1980 and increased to 5.4 percent in 1980 to 1991. This increase of 2 percent in GDP is greater than that in many developed countries, most of which showed a decline in this variable.

The World Health Organization[42] has reported that the dietary changes taking place as Indian populations move up the socioeconomic scale include: (1) increased intake of legumes, vegetables, milk, and— in the case of nonvegetarians—foods of animal origin; (2) substitution of coarse grain by polished grains, resulting in a decreased fiber intake; (3) increased intake of edible fat with increasing consumption of saturated hydrogenated fat in the middle class and Indian ghee in more prosperous segments; (4) increased intake of calories and sweets; and (5) increased overall energy intake in relation to expenditure, resulting in obesity.

Per capita consumption of major fats and oils has increased in the last 30 years.[43] In 1958 it was 5.62 kg/year, which showed an increasing (but not insignificant) trend from 5.79 in 1961 to 5.23 in 1966, 5.85 in 1971, 5.21 in 1976, 6.48 in 1981, and 6.97 in 1986. This consumption is much lower than in European Economic Community (EEC) countries (38.98), the United States (39.72), Canada (34.83), and Japan (19.84). However, the diet of 17 percent of the rural poor does not include any edible oil; about 5 percent of the population consumes nearly 40 percent of the available fat.[44] National Nutrition Monitoring Bureau data on the average intake of fat in different socioeconomic groups show that with an increase in income, consumption of fats and oils increases.[44] In 1981, the daily fat intake (grams per day) was 46 in high-income groups, 35 in middle-income groups, 22 in low-income groups, and 13 in urban slum dwellers. We reported that the intake of saturated fats (percent of energy/day) was 14.0 in high-income groups, 11.6 in middle-income groups, and 6.6 in low-income groups.[23] The intake of polyunsaturated fats was similar in all the income groups, but low-income groups consumed more monounsaturated fats. The consumption of fats and oils (grams per day) among rural subjects has remained constant from 1976 (10.8) to 1982 (9.8).[44]

Per capita consumption of total fats did not show a significant increase ($r = .64$, $p = .168$), but intake of hydrogenated fats increased significantly from 1956 to 1986 ($r = .99$, $p = .016$).[43] In urban subjects, serum cholesterol levels increased from 157 ± 29 mg/dL (Delhi) in 1982 to 199 ± 39 mg/dL (Delhi) and 176 ± 43 mg/dL (Jaipur) in 1996.[23]

Per capita tobacco consumption per adult person per year in kilograms was 0.7 in 1974 to 1976 and 0.8 in 1990. It is projected to increase to 0.9 in the year 2000.[45] This is in contrast to countries with established market economies, where there is decline in cardiovascular disease mortality and the tobacco consumption is projected to decrease from 2.9 in 1974–1976 and 2.2 in 1990 to 1.8 in the year 2000. Per capita consumption of salt increased from 10.5 g/day in 1970 to 16.8 g/day in 1994.[40]

Thus, we hypothesize that the increasing prevalence of CHD in Indians and other Asians can be explained by lifestyle and dietary changes due to epidemiologic transition. Rapid shift from a rural subsistence economy to an urban, market-oriented industrial economy is associated with new health problems, as presently seen in India. The above data show that the prevalence of CHD has increased rapidly in India. During this period there has been an increase in urbanization, gross domestic product, and human development index. These factors have led to more affluent lifestyles, involving an increased dietary intake of calories and saturated fat and leading to increased levels of serum cholesterol. Improvements in transportation tend to increase the preva-

lence of sedentary lifestyles, contributing further to obesity, hypertension, detrimental serum lipid profiles, and insulin resistance.

Strategies for Prevention

The decline in CHD mortality in Western countries has been mainly due to a decrease in coronary risk factors, achieved by aggressive public education programs regarding their control. This is known as primary prevention or avoidance of disease. Patients with established heart disease should also use similar measures to decrease the risk of a second heart attack. Primary prevention is based on control of atherosclerosis risk factors. Of major and modifiable coronary risk factors, smoking, sedentary lifestyle, generalized and truncal obesity, hypertension, hypercholesterolemia, and insulin resistance are already widespread among urban Asians (Tables 20–2 to 20–5).

Do we need more scientific studies before prevention efforts are initiated or can we learn from the studies performed so far? Migrant studies within the native country of origin (e.g., China) and transnational migration studies have clearly shown that CHD is a significant problem among Asians. Coronary risk factors such as hypertension, smoking, lack of physical activity, obesity and truncal obesity, and improper diet are fairly widespread. These populations are not very different from Caucasians and other ethnic groups where CHD is endemic, although some of the risk factors may be different.[46] Onset of CHD in younger subjects is a cause for concern. Also, genetic factors that are modified by environment could be important.

Williams[28] has summarized the coronary risk factors of South Asians living in the United Kingdom that are associated with a greater CHD incidence in this ethnic group (Table 20–6). Although some of the major coronary risk factors—such as hypertension, smoking, and hypercholesterolemia—are similar in indigenous populations and emigrant Asians, certain unconventional risk factors (e.g., obesity and diabetes) emerge. Prevention should be directed toward these risk factors also.

TABLE 20–6 Coronary Risk Factors in United Kingdom–based Asians versus the Indigenous United Kingdom Population

Risk factors similar (between groups):

Hypertension

Smoking

Body-mass index

Total cholesterol

Apolipoprotein B

Risk factors greater in Asians than in Caucasians

Sedentary lifestyle

Truncal obesity

Hyperinsulinemia and insulin resistance

Decreased beta-cell function

Diabetes mellitus (NIDDM)

Lipoprotein(a) levels

Triglyceride levels

Low-HDL cholesterol

Increased plasminogen activator inhibitor

Decreased tissue plasminogen activator

Key: NIDDM, non-insulin-dependent diabetes mellitus; HDL, high-density-lipoprotein cholesterol.

Source: Adapted from Williams,[28] with permission.

Sedentary lifestyle is an important cause of many of these and the focus of preventive efforts should clearly be in this direction.

Preventive medicine in Asia is as old as history. The ancient Indian science of Ayurveda deals with the influence of lifestyle modifications to promote health and avoid sickness. Long before Hippocrates, Aristotle, and Galen, a couplet from the Bhagavad Gita, emphasized the importance of balanced food, exercise and other lifestyle variables in disease prevention: "One who observes control over his diet, takes regular exercise, has time to relax, does the right toil in discharge of his duties, observes proper hours of sleep and awakening and is balanced in his actions and reactions, emotions and reason, duties and rewards, conquers disease."[47] This is a summary of current lifestyle changes recommended to prevent CHD. In the modern context, it is important that ap-

propriate strategies are developed and effectively implemented.

A wide range of cardiovascular benefits of acupuncture has also been reported, including some therapeutic effects on hypertension,[48–49] angina pectoris,[50–51] and acute myocardial infarction.[52] A recent review of acupuncture's beneficial effects on the cardiovascular system has been published.[53]

The efficacy of traditional medicines, including herbal product mixtures, based on the belief that several individual ingredients may have synergistic effects (e.g., antioxidant, hypocholesterolemic, or other antiatherosclerotic effects), also needs further investigation. The hypotensive effect of herbal therapies is being investigated[54] and has been documented to be efficacious in controlling at least milder forms of hypertension.[55] A Tibetan herbal complex, widely marketed in Europe, has been shown to increase pain-free walking distance in those with intermittent claudication.[56] Larger-scale clinical trials are needed to document the effectiveness of these therapies used alone or in combination with established Western pharmacologic therapy to control cardiovascular risk factors and prevent cardiovascular disease.

Population Strategy

We have identified many traditional coronary risk factors as important among Asians. Most of these can be changed by adopting healthier lifestyles, since preventing heart disease calls for establishing these lifestyles as norms for the entire population. Several important lifestyle-related changes applicable especially to urban and emigrant populations can be suggested:[57]

1. Control of hypertension can be achieved by reducing the intake of salt, alcohol, and calories as well as by exercise, stress management, and greater intake of calcium, potassium, magnesium, and fiber.
2. Control of hypercholesterolemia and decrease in mean LDL-cholesterol levels can be achieved by reducing the intake of saturated fats, meat, and dairy products and increasing the intake of polyunsaturated fats and fiber.

3. Low HDL-cholesterol levels can be influenced by greater intake of monounsaturated fats, fruits and green vegetables, and exercise.
4. Truncal obesity can be reduced by regular exercise.
5. Peripheral insulin resistance can also be improved by regular physical activity.
6. Smoking control requires a variety of measures, including but not limited to government restrictions on smoking in the workplace and in public, bans on advertising and sponsorship by tobacco companies, enhanced community education programs, and physician-supervised counseling on smoking cessation.

Behavioral and environmental changes relevant to these risk factors include changes in eating patterns, drinking, smoking, physical activity, and other psychosocial factors.

Eating Patterns

The production and consumption of the following foods should be preferred, emphasized, and supported: foods of plant origin; cereal grains, vegetables, beans, and fruits; fish, poultry, and low-fat meat; low-fat milk and dairy products; and liquid vegetable oils and soft margarines. The production and consumption of the following should be decreased: high-fat meats, meat products, and lard; high-fat dairy products such as whole milk, cheeses, cream, and butter; whole eggs; salt and salty products; sugar and sweet products; and commercial bakery products with a high content of fat and empty calories.

The importance of maintaining cultural beliefs in eating and other lifestyle habits needs to be considered. A study of middle-school Chinese schoolchildren showed that those living in China as opposed to the United States showed less consumption of meat, dairy products, fat, sweets, and fast foods and greater consumption of vegetables and fruits.[58] Additionally, a study of elderly Chinese immigrants aged 60 to 96 showed that they displayed similar characteristics as those found among urban Chinese. Specifically, they were physically active, seldom obese, and consumed a diet low in fat, high in car-

bohydrates, and had lower lipids as compared to elderly whites.[59]

The marketing of low-fat food products should be targeted more aggressively to Asian media, and educational materials and dietary assessment tools need to be produced that are culturally sensitive to the diversity of Asian population groups.

Smoking

The smoking habit became epidemic with the growth of the cigarette manufacturing industry. It is thus a recent, widespread, and essentially unnatural behavior. In the whole population, smoking, especially of cigarettes, should be reduced in amount and frequency with the final aim of eliminating the habit completely. Until that time, children, adolescents, pregnant women, and women on oral contraceptives need special protection. Low-tar, low-nicotine cigarettes offer no alternative solution to the abandonment of smoking as far as the heart is concerned.

The consumption of smokeless tobacco is another important problem in Asian groups. In both Chinese and South Asians, tobacco is consumed in many other forms—e.g., bidi (tobacco rolled in the *Diospyrus melanoxylon* leaf), Indian pipe tobacco (chillum, hookah), chewing tobacco in many forms. Bidi is the most common form of tobacco smoked in India. Its smokers may face similar risks of hypertension and CHD as cigarette smokers,[60] despite the fact that the tobacco content is less than one-fourth that of regular cigarettes. This may be because of smoking habits (bidi smoke must be inhaled more frequently than cigarette smoke in order to keep the leaf burning) and the fact that bidi may contain unidentified toxic substances.[61] Habits of smoking and the use of smokeless tobacco must be curtailed among Asians. Social and economic taboos are needed to accomplish this goal.

Finally, the problem of environmental tobacco exposure cannot be underestimated. One of the most convincing studies of the harmful effect of passive smoking was conducted in China among nonsmoking women with CHD and matched controls. The investigators showed greater odds of CHD among women with husbands who smoked or were exposed to tobacco smoke in the workplace. A nearly twofold greater odds of CHD among women who were exposed to tobacco at work persisted after adjustment for other risk factors, and a linear trend with the amount of tobacco exposure was observed.[62]

Physical Activity

Coincident with the switch from hunger and deficient nutrition to overeating in the first two-thirds of this century, the mean level of habitual physical activity has also decreased substantially among Asians. This has resulted in increased body-mass index and obesity. The problem is greater among Asians who have recently undergone this metamorphosis both socially and physically. Obesity contributes to CHD through its effects on blood pressure, cholesterol levels, diabetes mellitus, and insulin resistance. The urbanization of Asian countries has also substantially contributed to decreased levels of physical activity, particularly in the larger cities.

Regular physical activity should again become a normal part of everyday adult life, and—as in media and other forms of advertising targeted to Caucasian populations—needs to be integrated more successfully into the Asian culture. The natural inclination of children and young people to engage in vigorous physical activity should be encouraged, supported, and maintained through the formative years. Enjoyable forms of exercise should be available to everyone.

Psychosocial Factors

The importance of psychological and social factors in contributing to the risk of CHD is obvious. These factors are especially important in migrant populations, whether the migration is from villages to cities in Asia or to developed countries of the West. Indirect estimates of this stress can be gauged by poor living conditions, low levels of education, increasing adult and juvenile crime, smoking and alcohol habits, and breakdown of the family unit among these groups. Not only is the behavior of the individual important, but that of the community as a whole is to be understood in this context. The need for equalizing access to health and social services is important in this regard.

A reassessment of the social value system should be promoted. Social norms that put more value on health, human relations, culture, and preservation of nature should be encouraged. Such changes may result in less tension, aggressive drive, competitiveness, and frustration, all of which promote personality patterns that are believed to enhance CHD risk.

Summary

Coronary heart disease among Asians can be prevented by controlling the intake of tobacco, salt, saturated fats, alcohol, and calories; by increasing both work-related and leisure-time physical activity; by increasing consumption of heart-healthy foods such as fruits and vegetables, high-fiber cereals, oils containing balanced amounts of polyunsaturated and monounsaturated fats (e.g., canola oil, soybean oil), and spices and cereals with a high flavonoid content. Stress-management techniques, especially yoga, may be important. Reverting to traditional Asian social lifestyles (joint families, small families, good education) is also important.

Prevention efforts should begin in childhood, when health-risk behaviors begin. Parents, teachers, and peer groups are important in imparting health education to children. In Indian adolescent children, there is a high prevalence of high dietary fat intake, obesity, hypertension, and hypercholesterolemia.[63]

High-Risk Approach

The *Oxford Textbook of Medicine* mentions East Asian race as an atherosclerosis risk factor,[64] consistent with the observation of high CHD mortality among this group. Thus, all Asians, especially South Asians, should be targets for primary prevention strategies. The effectiveness of intervention in these high-risk populations depends directly on practicing physicians and other health care workers. In order to integrate prevention and treatment at the primary health care level, greater emphasis on prevention is needed in the daily practice of medicine. This requires an active interest on the part of physicians, a willingness on the part of patients to accept and act on preventive advice, and the acceptance by governments and health insurance organizations for the cost of preventive services, like that of curative care, should be fully reimbursed.[65] Physicians and other health care providers serving Asian/Pacific Islander populations need to be educated as to the specific cultural barriers and opportunities that would encourage cardiovascular disease prevention practices to be implemented.

The American Heart Association recently published guidelines for secondary prevention of CHD.[66] These are based on compelling scientific evidence in patients with CHD demonstrating that risk-factor interventions extend overall survival, improve quality of life, decrease the need for interventional procedures such as angioplasty and coronary bypass grafting, and reduce the incidence of subsequent myocardial infarction. The interventions are smoking cessation, lipid management, physical activity, weight management, estrogen replacement in postmenopausal women, and blood pressure control. In addition, nutritional guidelines need to be formulated. The WHO has formulated certain population nutrition goals that are useful in the prevention of CHD.[42]

Conclusions

The need to contain the epidemic of cardiovascular disease and minimize its toll on Asians is obvious and urgent. National strategies to meet this objective must be developed and effectively implemented. Regional and global initiatives by international agencies concerned with health care are also required. A large number of social issues that are determinants of health behavior in Asians must be considered before embarking on such a policy (Table 20–7).

Asians are minority groups in most of the developed countries. The high incidence of CHD in emigrants as compared with native populations underlines the importance of population prevention strategies. These strategies should be directed toward prevention of acquisition or augmentation of coronary risk factors in these communities (primordial prevention) combined with programs to reverse and reduce the risk-factor elevations observed in the ur-

TABLE 20–7 Determinants of Health Behavior among Asians

Educational status, illiteracy

Family structure, breakdown of traditional family system

Peer influence, improper guidance

Caste system and social hierarchy

Lack of media awareness

Lack of motivation to change

ban and migrant communities (primary prevention).

However, as always, the demand for prevention should come from within the population. Increasing levels of affluence and acculturation lead to a greater recognition that measures to prevent chronic diseases are useful and cost-effective. Ultimately, it is expected that with proper control of the behavioral and lifestyle risk factors for CHD, Asians can advance to higher stages of the epidemiologic transition[39] where, while maintaining a modern lifestyle, a return to their ancestral low rates of cardiovascular disease will be possible. The roles of literacy and better health education in promoting favorable lifestyles are important, and urgent population and individual measures are needed to control the emerging CHD epidemic among the Asians living in Asia or elsewhere.

References

1. Janus ED, Postiglione A, Singh RB, et al, for the Council of Arteriosclerosis of the International Society and Federation of Cardiology: The modernization of Asia: implications for coronary heart disease. *Circulation* 1996; 94:2671–2673.
2. Reddy KS, Yusuf S: Emerging epidemic of cardiovascular disease in developing countries. *Circulation* 1998; 97:596–601.
3. Enas EA, Garg A, Davidson MA, et al: Coronary heart disease and its risk factors in first-generation immigrant Asian Indians to the United States of America. *Indian Heart J* 1996; 48:343–353.
4. American Heart Association. *Asian/Pacific-Islander and Cardiovascular Diseases Biostatistical Fact Sheet.* Dallas, AHA, 1999.

5. Centers for Disease Control and Prevention: *Chronic Diseases and Their Risk Factors: The Nation's Leading Cause of Death.* Washington, DC, U.S. Department of Health and Human Services, 1998.

6. Koga Y, Hashimoto R, Adachi H, et al: Recent trends in cardiovascular disease and risk factors in the Seven Countries Study: Japan. In: Toshima H, Koga Y, Blackburn H (eds): *Lessons for Science from the Seven Countries Study.* Tokyo, Springer-Verlag, 1994:63–74.

7. Baba S, Ozawa H, Sakai Y, et al: Heart disease deaths in a Japanese urban area evaluated by clinical and police records. *Circulation* 1994; 89:109–115.

8. Ueshima H, Tatara K, Asakura S: Declining mortality from ischemic heart disease and changes in coronary risk factors in Japan, 1956–1980. *Am J Epidemiol* 1987; 125:62–72.

9. Nichaman MZ, Hamilton HB, Kagan A, et al: Epidemiologic studies of coronary heart disease and stroke in Japanese men living in Japan, Hawaii and California: distribution of biochemical risk factors. *Am J Epidemiol* 1975; 102:491–501.

10. Worth RM, Kato H, Rhoads GG, et al: Epidemiologic studies of coronary heart disease and stroke in Japanese men living in Japan, Hawaii and California: mortality. *Am J Epidemiol* 1975; 102:481–490.

11. Winkelstein W, Kagan A, Kato H, et al: Epidemiologic studies of coronary heart disease and stroke in Japanese men living in Japan, Hawaii and California: blood pressure distributions. *Am J Epidemiol* 1975; 102:502–513.

12. Iribarren C, Reed DM, Burchfiel CM, Dwyer JH: Serum total cholesterol and mortality: confounding factors and risk modification in Japanese-American men. *JAMA* 1995; 273:1926–1932.

13. Curb JD, Aluli NE, Huang BJ, et al: Hypertension in elderly Japanese-Americans and adult native Hawaiians. *Public Health Rep* 1996; 111(suppl 2):53–55.

14. Tao S, Huang Z, Wu W, et al: Coronary heart disease and its risk factors in the People's Republic of China. *Int J Epidemiol* 1989; 18(suppl 1):S159-S163.

15. People's Republic of China—United States Cardiovascular and Cardiopulmonary Epidemiology Research Group: An epidemiological study of cardiovascular and cardiopulmonary disease risk factors in four populations in the People's Republic of China—baseline report from the PRC-USA Collaborative Study. *Circulation* 1992; 85:1083–1096.

16. Zhou B, Rao X, Dennis BH, et al: The relationship between dietary factors and serum lipids in Chinese urban and rural populations of Beijing and Guangzhou: PRC–USA Cardiovascular and Cardiopulmonary Research Group. *Int J of Epidemiol* 1995; 24:528–534.

17. Harland JO, Unwin N, Bohpal RS, et al: Low levels of cardiovascular risk factors and coronary heart disease in a UK Chinese population. *J Epidemiol Commun Health* 1997; 51:636–642.

18. Pinnelas D, De La Torre R, Pugh J, et al: Total serum cholesterol levels in Asians living in New York City: results of a self-referred cholesterol screening. *NY State J Med* 1992; 92:245–249.

19. Reddy KS: Cardiovascular diseases in India. *WHO Stat Q* 1993; 46:101–107.

20. Gupta R, Gupta VP. Meta-analysis of coronary heart disease prevalence in India. *Indian Heart J* 1996; 48:241–245.

21. Gupta R, Singhal S: Coronary heart disease in India. Letter. *Circulation* 1997; 96:3785.

22. Gupta R, Al-Odat NA, Gupta VP: Hypertension epidemiology in India: meta-analysis of fifty year prevalence rates and blood pressure trends. *J Hum Hypertens* 1996; 10:465–472.

23. Gupta R, Singhal S: Epidemiological evolution, fat intake, cholesterol levels and increasing coronary heart disease in India. *JAMA-India* 1997; 21:50–54.

24. Pandey MR: Hypertension in Nepal. *Bib Cardiol* 1997; 42:68–76.

25. McKeigue PM, Miller GJ, Marmot MG: Coronary heart disease in South Asians overseas: a review. *J Clin Epidemiol* 1989; 42:597–609.

26. Balarajan R, Adelstein AM, Bulusu L, et al: Patterns of mortality among migrants to England and Wales from the Indian subcontinent. *BMJ* 1984; 289:1185–1187.

27. Marmot MG: Coronary heart disease: rise and fall of a modern epidemic. In: Marmot MG, Elliot P (eds.): *Coronary Heart Disease Epidemiology: From Aetiology to Public Health.* Oxford, UK, Oxford University Press, 1992:3–19.

28. Williams B: Westernized Asians and cardiovascular disease: nature or nurture? *Lancet* 1995; 345:401–402.

29. Gupta R, Prakash H, Majumdar S, et al: Prevalence of coronary heart disease and coronary risk factors in an urban population of Rajasthan. *Indian Heart J* 1995; 47:331–338.

30. Gupta R, Prakash H, Gupta VP, et al: Prevalence and determinants of coronary heart disease in a rural population of India. *J Clin Epidemiol* 1997; 50:203–209.

31. Gupta R, Gupta VP. Urban-rural differences in coronary risk factors do not fully explain greater urban coronary heart disease prevalence. *J Assoc Physicians India* 1997; 45:683–686.

32. Gupta SP, Malhotra KC: Urban-rural trends in epidemiology of coronary heart disease. *J Assoc Physicians India* 1975; 23:885–892.

33. Reddy KS, Shah P, Shrivastava U, et al: Coronary heart disease risk factors in an industrial population of north India (abstr). *Can J Cardiol* 1997; 13(suppl B):26B.

34. Hughes K, Aw TC, Kuperan P, Choo M. Central obesity, insulin resistance, syndrome X, lipoprotein(a), and cardiovascular risk in Indians, Malays, and Chinese in Singapore. *J Epidemiol Commun Health* 1997; 51:394–399.

35. Stavig FR et al: Hypertension and related health issues among Asians and Pacific Islanders in California. *Public Health Rep* 1988; 103:28–37.

36. Klatsky AL, Tekawa IS, Armstrong MA: Cardiovascular risk factors among Asian Americans. *Public Health Rep* 1996; 111(suppl 2):62–64.

37. Munger RG, Gowez-Marin O, Prineas RJ, et al: Elevated blood pressure among Southeast Asian refugee children in Minnesota. *Am J Epidemiol* 1991; 133:1257–1265.

38. U.S. Department of Health and Human Services: *Preventing Tobacco Use among Young People: A Report of the Surgeon General.* Atlanta, GA, U.S. Department of Health and Human Services, Public Health Services, 1994.

39. Gillum RF: The epidemiology of cardiovascular disease in black Americans. *New Engl J Med* 1996; 335:1597–1599.

40. Government of India: *Economic Survey 1994–95.* New Delhi, Ministry of Finance (Economic Division), 1995.

41. Technical notes. In: *Human Development Report 1993. United Nations Development Report.* New York, Oxford University Press, 1993:100–114.

42. World Health Organization, WHO Study Group: *Diet, Nutrition, and the Prevention of Chronic Diseases.* Technical Report Series 797. Geneva, World Health Organization, 1990:49–50.

43. Gulati VP, Phansalkar SJ: *Oilseeds and Edible Oil Economy of India.* New Delhi, Vikas Publishing House, 1994: 230–231.

44. Gopalan C: Trends in food consumption patterns: impact of developmental transition. In: Biswas MR, Gabr M (eds): *Nutrition in the Nineties: Policy Issues.* Delhi, Oxford University Press, 1994:34–54.

45. World Bank: Population and health data. In: *World Development Report 1993: Investing in Health.* New York: Oxford University Press, 1993:195–324.

46. Rose G: Causes of the trends and variations in coronary heart disease mortality in different countries. *Int J Epidemiol* 1989; 18(suppl 1):S174-S179.

47. Gupta KD: Prevention: the key to progress. *South Asian J Prev Cardiol* 1997; 1:57–58.

48. Tam KC, Yiu HH: The effect of acupuncture on essential hypertension. *Am J Chinese Med* 1975; 3:369–375.

49. Chiu YJ, Chi A, Reid IA: Cardiovascular and endocrine effects of acupuncture in hypertensive patients. *Clin Exper Hypertens* 1997; 19:1047–1063.

50. Richter A, Herlitz J, Hjalmarson A: Effect of acupuncture in patients with angina pectoris. *Eur Heart J* 1991; 12:175–178.

51. Ballegaard S, Meyer CN, Trojaborg W: Acupuncture in angina pectoris: does acupuncture have a specific effect? *J Intern Med* 1991; 229:357–362.

52. Bao YX, Lu HH, Yu GR, et al: The immediate effect on acute myocardial infarction treated by puncturing Neiguan. *Chin Acupunct Moxib* 1981; 1:2–5.

53. Longhurst JC. Acupuncture's beneficial effects on the cardiovascular system. *Prev Cardiol* 1998; 4:21–33.

54. Wang XS: Progress of Chinese herbal medicines on hypotensive effect. *Cung-Kuo Chung His I Chieh Ho Tsa Chih* 1994; 14:123–126.

55. Wong ND, Ming S, Zhou HY, Black HR: A comparison of Chinese and Western medical approaches for the treatment of mild hypertension. *Yale J Biol Med* 1991; 64:79–87.

56. Drabaek H, Mehlsen J, Petersen JP, et al: Padma-28, a herbal preparation, increases walking distance in patients with intermittent claudication. *Ugeskr Laeger* 1994; 156:6207–6209.

57. Gupta R, Gupta VP: Lessons for prevention from a coronary heart disease epidemiology study in Western India. *Curr Sci* 1998; 43:253–258.

58. Sun WY, Chen WW: A preliminary study of potential dietary risk factor for coronary heart disease among Chinese American adolescents. *J School Health* 1994; 64:368–371.

59. Choi ES, McGundy RD, Dallal GE, et al: The prevalence of cardiovascular risk factors among elderly Chinese Americans. *Arch Intern Med* 1990; 150:413–418.

60. Gupta R, Sharma SC, Gupta VP, Gupta KD: Smoking and alcohol intake in a rural Indian population and correlation with hypertension and coronary heart disease prevalence. *J Assoc Physicians India* 1995; 43:253–258.

61. Pakhale SS, Jayant KM, Bhide SV: Chemical analysis of smoke of Indian cigarettes, bidis, and other indigenous forms of smoking, levels of steam, volatile phenol, hydrogen cytanide, and bendo(a)pyrene. *Ind J Chest Dis Allied Sci* 1990; 32:75–81.

62. He Y, Lam TH, Li LS, et al: Passive smoking at work as a risk factor for coronary heart disease in Chinese women who have never smoked. *BMJ* 1994; 308:380–384.

63. Gupta R, Goyle A, Kashyap S, et al: Prevalence of atherosclerosis risk factors in adolescent school children. *Indian Heart J* 1998; 50:511–515.

64. Scott J: The pathogenesis of atherosclerosis. In: Weatherall DJ, Ledingham JGG, Warrel DA (eds): *Oxford Textbook of Medicine,* 3rd ed. Oxford, UK, Oxford University Press, 1996:2289–2294.

65. Thompson B, Pertschuk M: Community intervention and advocacy. In: Ockene IS, Ockene JK (eds): *Prevention of Coronary Heart Disease.* Boston. Little Brown, 1992:493–515.

66. Smith SC, Blair SN, Criqui MH, et al, for the Secondary Prevention Panel: Preventing heart attack and deaths in patients with coronary disease. AHA medical/scientific statement. *Circulation* 1995; 92:2–4.

CHAPTER 21

Native Americans

David R. Baines

Background

The term *Native American* refers to American Indians and Alaska Natives. Alaska has three distinct racial aboriginal groups: the American Indians (Athabascan, Tlingit, Tsimpsian, and Haida tribes), Eskimos, and Aleuts. Native Hawaiians, although technically Native Americans, are considered under the Asian/Pacific Island group. They do, however, have similar health problems, and much of what is said about American Indians and Alaska Natives can be applied to Native Hawaiians. Although Native Americans are the first Americans, they are the smallest and most diverse minority group. There are over 2 million American Indians and Alaska Natives, representing 0.8 percent of the U.S. population (Fig. 21–1).[1] They reside in every state and come from over 550 federally recognized tribes.[2] Nearly 50 percent of the population is in the West, with 29 percent in the South, 17 percent in the Midwest, and 6 percent in the Northeast.[3] Some 38 percent live on Reservation Trust lands, in tribal areas, or in Alaska Native Village areas, and nearly two-thirds live in urban areas.[4]

Health Status, Heart Disease, and Stroke

Diseases of the heart and stroke represent the leading cause of death in American Indians and Alaska Natives, accounting for 26 percent of all deaths in 1995, followed by accidents, cancer, chronic liver disease, and suicides (Fig. 21–2).[5] There is wide variation in mortality rates from heart disease in different areas of the country, corresponding to differ-

ent rates between the tribes (Fig. 21–3).[6] Although Albuquerque, Tucson, and California rates are much lower than the U.S. All-races rate of 144.3 per 100,000, those living in Bemidji and Aberdeen have rates that are appreciably higher. A similar pattern is seen for cerebrovascular disease, with Aberdeen and Billings having the highest rates (Fig. 21–4).[6] Although cardiovascular disease ranks as the leading cause of death for many Native American communities, data comparing the Native American population to all races in the United States show particularly higher death rates among Native Americans for tuberculosis, chronic liver disease and cirrhosis, accidents, and diabetes mellitus (Fig. 21–5).

Mortality surveillance in the Strong Heart Study, a large epidemiologic study among three American Indian populations—including over 4500 participants aged 45 to 74 from 12 tribes located in Arizona, Oklahoma, and South/North Dakota—showed overall 5-year cardiovascular disease (CVD) mortality rates to be similar between the communities (96 per 1000, 107 per 1000, and 114 per 1000, respectively).[7] These rates, while close to those of the U.S. African-American population and the overall U.S. population average in Arizona and Oklahoma, were more than two times higher than those in South/North Dakota. Among American Indians, CVD was the leading cause of death in Oklahoma and South/North Dakota, but diabetes led among Arizona women.[7]

An extensive review of the medical literature reveals that coronary heart disease (CHD) was uncommon for many decades earlier in the twentieth century.[8–27] These studies were primarily done in the Southwest. More recently, studies have shown that

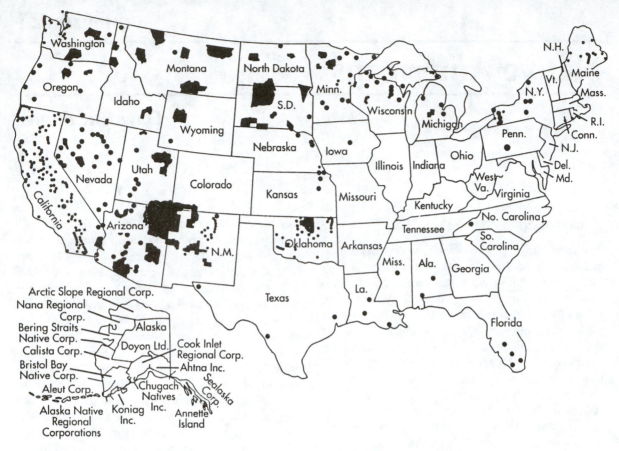

FIGURE 21–1   Federally recognized Indian reservations and Alaska native regional corporations, 1985. (*Source*: Indian Health Services.)

FIGURE 21–2
Mortality rates for leading causes, Indians and Alaska Natives, calendar years 1991–1993. The two leading causes of death for American Indians and Alaska Natives (1991–1993) and the U.S. All-races and White populations (1992) were diseases of the heart and malignant neoplasms. This is a change for the Indian population; accidents had been the second leading cause of death.

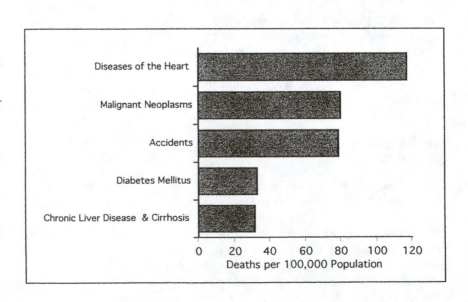

FIGURE 21–3 Age-adjusted diseases of the heart mortality rates, calendar years 1991–1993. In 1991–1993, the age-adjusted diseases of the heart mortality rate for the IHS service area population was 132.4. When the 3 IHS areas with apparent problems in underreporting of Indian race on death certificates are excluded, the rate is 143.3. This is essentially the same as the U.S. All-races rate in 1992, i.e., 144.3. The Albuquerque, Tucson, and Navajo Area rates are well below the U.S. rate. (*Source:* Indian Health Services.[6])

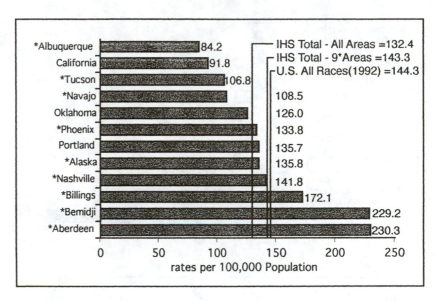

FIGURE 21–4 Age-adjusted cerebrovascular diseases mortality rates, calendar years 1991–1993. In 1991–1993, the age-adjusted cerebrovascular diseases mortality rate for the IHS service area population was 25.3. When the 3 IHS areas with apparent problems in underreporting of Indian race on death certificates are excluded, the rate is 29.0. This is 11 percent higher than the U.S. All-races rate of 26.2 for 1992. The Billings Area rate of 44.7 was 2.3 times the Navajo Area rate of 19.8. (*Source:* Indian Health Services.[6])

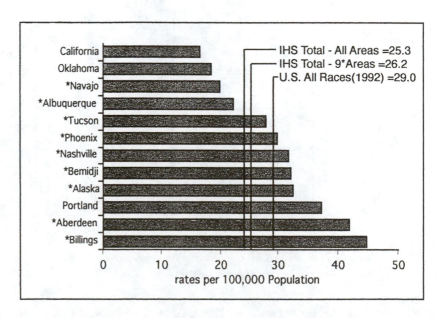

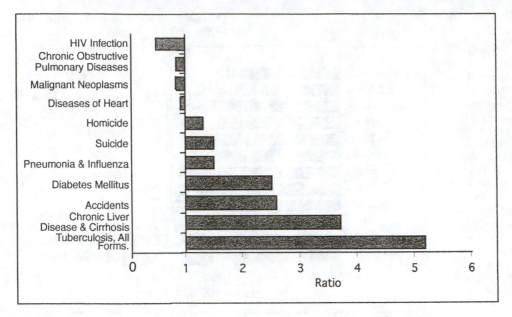

FIGURE 21–5 Selected age-adjusted death rates, ratio of Indians (1991–1993) to U.S. All races (1992). The American Indian and Alaska Native age-adjusted mortality rates for 1991–1993 were above those of the U.S. All races (1992) for tuberculosis, chronic liver disease and cirrhosis, accidents, diabetes mellitus, pneumonia and influenza, suicide, and homicide. Indian rates were below those of the U.S. All races for HIV infection, chronic obstructive pulmonary diseases, malignant neoplasms, and diseases of the heart. (*Source:* Indian Health Services.[6])

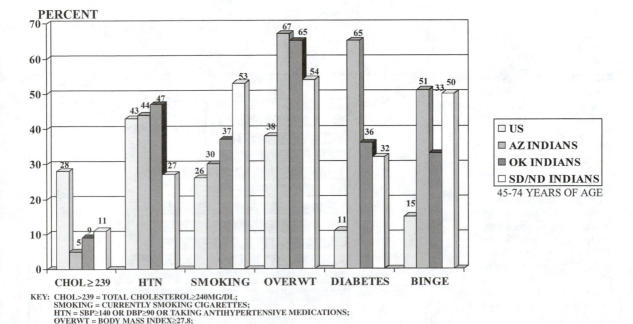

KEY: CHOL>239 = TOTAL CHOLESTEROL≥240MG/DL;
      SMOKING = CURRENTLY SMOKING CIGARETTES;
      HTN = SBP≥140 OR DBP≥90 OR TAKING ANTIHYPERTENSIVE MEDICATIONS;
      OVERWT = BODY MASS INDEX≥27.8;
      BINGE = 5 OR MORE DRINKS ON OCCASION IN LAST YEAR.

FIGURE 21–6 Cardiovascular disease risk factors, U.S. All races or white and American Indian Men Strong Heart Study, 1989–1991. (*Source:* Welty TK,[38,52] with permisssion.)

Key: HTN, hypertension; Overwt, overweight; Binge, binge drinking.

PERCENT

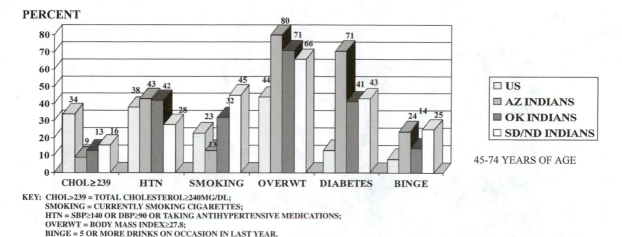

KEY: CHOL>239 = TOTAL CHOLESTEROL≥240MG/DL;
SMOKING = CURRENTLY SMOKING CIGARETTES;
HTN = SBP≥140 OR DBP≥90 OR TAKING ANTIHYPERTENSIVE MEDICATIONS;
OVERWT = BODY MASS INDEX≥27.8;
BINGE = 5 OR MORE DRINKS ON OCCASION IN LAST YEAR.

FIGURE 21–7 Cardiovascular disease risk factors, U.S. All races or white and American Indian Women Strong Heart Study, 1989–1991. (*Source:* Welty TK,[38,52] with permission.)

Key: HTN, hypertension; Overwt, overweight; Binge, binge drinking.

certain tribes had CHD rates that were similar to or exceeded those of the general U.S. population.[28–30] Currently, CHD is the number one cause of mortality in the American Indian and Alaska Native populations.[5,7] There are many potential reasons for this: (1) Westernization of the diet; (2) more sedentary lifestyles; (3) increasing obesity; (4) increasing diabetes rates; (5) recreational, rather than ceremonial, tobacco use; (6) poor social and economic status of the population; (7) lack of consistent and adequate access to care; and (8) cultural factors. There was also a corresponding decrease in infectious diseases, which were the primary cause of mortality in the mid-1900s.[31]

Until recently there were no large multicenter studies on American Indians. The majority of studies were retrospective and involved tribes in the Southwest. In 1989, the National Heart, Lung, and Blood Institute funded the Strong Heart Study, which involved 13 tribes in four states.[32] Multiple reports have been published on this study, involving risk factors, disease prevalence, and mortality[32–52] (Figs. 21–6 and 21–7).[38,52] These data show risk factors such as cigarette smoking, overweight, diabetes, and binge drinking to be substantially more common among Native American groups as compared to the general U.S. population both in men and women. However, this pattern does not seem to hold for elevated cholesterol levels and hypertension, which appear to be of similar or lower prevalence among most Native American groups studied. Prior to this study, American Indians and Alaska Natives represented such small numbers in research studies that they were included in other categories.

Cardiovascular Risk Factors

Hypertension

In 1963, Clifford et al. noted lower prevalences of hypertension among White Mountain Apaches as compared to U.S. rates and predicted that as civilization slowly changed this population's lives, eating habits, and living conditions, the disease patterns would change.[23] He predicted that the lower rates of hypertension and CHD would not continue but would approach or exceed the rates for all races in the United States. Other authors agreed or noted rates similar to or higher than rates for other groups.[47,53–57] Hypertension accounts for 42 percent of all Indian Health Service ambulatory visits, exceeded only by upper respiratory infections, otitis media, and diabetes.[58] Important is its strong linkage with diabetes and the synergistic increase in morbidity when hypertension and diabetes occur together. The Strong Heart Study found, in Oklahoma and Arizona, that the rates of hypertension were similar to U.S. rates despite higher rates of obesity and diabetes. Rates for North and South Dakota

PERCENT

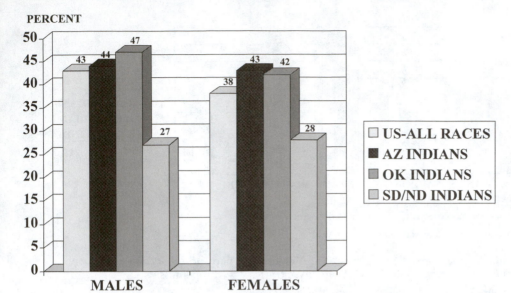

FIGURE 21–8 Hypertension* Prevalence NHANES III/Strong Heart Studies, U.S., 1988–1991; American Indian, 1989–1991. (*Source:* Welty TK,[38] with permission.) *SBP≥140 or DBP≥90 or taking BP medications.

Key: AZ, Arizona; OK, Oklahoma; SD/ND, South Dakota/North Dakota.

were less (Fig. 21–8).[38] Among 4549 American Indians aged 45 to 74 from 13 communities in the Strong Heart Study, the prevalence of hypertension (as defined by a systolic blood pressure of ≥ 140 mmHg or a diastolic blood pressure of ≥ 90 mmHg, or taking antihypertensive medication) ranged from 28 to 47 percent across tribal areas. Overall, the prevalence was 39.0 percent among Native American men and 37.7 percent among Native American women.[38] Although more than 70 percent were aware of the diagnosis, only slightly more than 50 percent were receiving treatment and only 30 percent had their hypertension controlled by medication. Blood pressure was significantly related to glucose intolerance, age, obesity, and alcohol consumption but not to plasma insulin.[57]

Lipids

There is wide variation in studies that looked at lipids among American Indians and Alaska Natives. Some studies have shown lower levels of total and low-density-lipoprotein cholesterol (LDL-C) compared to U.S. whites,[12,31,40,59,60] while others showed comparable[61] or higher levels.[62] These studies indicate that

each population must be looked at individually. In the Strong Heart Study, mean total cholesterol levels ranged from 177 to 199 mg/dL in men and 181 to 202 mg/dL in women, and LDL-C levels ranged from 102 to 122 mg/dL in men and 105 to 120 mg/dL in women, depending on the community studied. Those living in North and South Dakota as compared to Arizona and Oklahoma Indians generally had higher levels, but levels for all groups were generally lower than those for all U.S. races[38] (Fig. 21–9).[38,52] Overall, about 26 percent of Native American men and 29 percent of women are estimated to have high blood cholesterol.[5] In one Arizona Indian tribe, however, prevalence of hypercholesterolemia tended to be lower (19 percent of men and 14 percent of women).[60] Approximately 20 percent of Native American men and women have elevated triglycerides (≥200 mg/dL) (slightly higher than for U.S. women of all races, but slightly lower for men). Some 24 to 28 percent of men and 9 to 14 percent of women have low high-density-lipoprotein cholesterol (HDL-C) levels, a higher prevalence than that seen among all U.S. races combined (19 percent for men and 6 percent for women) (Fig. 21–10).[38,52]

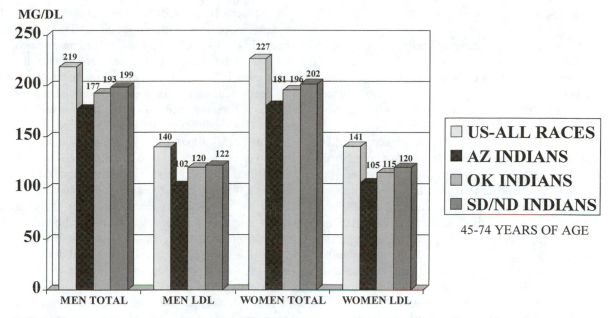

FIGURE 21–9   Mean total and LDL cholesterol concentrations NHANES III/Strong Heart Studies, U.S., 1988–1991; American Indian, 1989–1991. (*Source:* Welty TK,[38,52] with permission.)

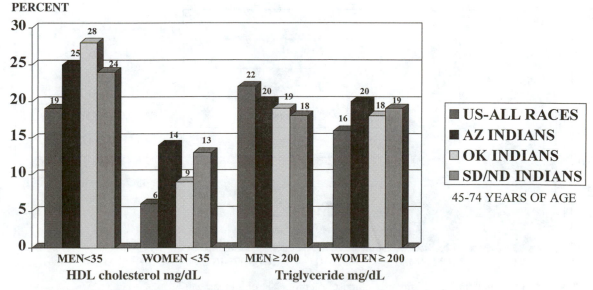

FIGURE 21–10   Abnormal lipids NHANES II/Strong Heart Studies, U.S., 1976–1980; American Indian, 1989–1991. (*Source:* Welty TK,[38,52] with permission.)

Diabetes

Diabetes has been extensively studied in southwestern Indian tribes, where the rate far exceeds that of the general population. However, prevalence rates are highly variable, depending on the tribe. Some living in Arizona have among the highest prevalence rates of diabetes (65 percent of men and 71 percent of women), while the prevalence is nearly half that among those living in Oklahoma or North and South Dakota;[38] however, rates of impaired glucose tolerance appear to be similar among all three populations (Fig. 21–11).[38] Among the Inuit tribes of the Northwest Territories, there are only 4 cases per 1000 population.[63] Among the Pascua Yaqui Indian tribe in Arizona, diabetes was the second most common risk factor (superseded only by obesity), present in 35 percent of men and 39 percent of women.[64] The Pima have the highest rate of diabetes of any population in the world,[65] with a reported 500 cases per 1000 population. Diabetes has been noted to be an increasing problem in other groups as well.[66–69]

The Strong Heart Study showed that diabetes was strongly associated with prevalent CHD in each group (Fig. 21–12).[52] These investigations showed diabetes to be the most important risk factor for CVD, especially among women.[37] Among the Navajos, nearly half of all diagnosed myocardial infarctions have been reported to occur in persons with diabetes; one study showed the age-adjusted rate of CHD to be 5.2 times that of persons without diabetes. For cerebrovascular disease, the relative risk was 10.2, and for peripheral vascular disease, the relative risk was 6.8.[66] Diabetes mortality rates among Native Americans more than four times those of whites have also been reported.[63] This health burden comes from diabetic complications. For instance, kidney disease resulting in end-stage renal disease is nearly six times more common among Native Americans than among whites; among the Pima Indians, the rate of kidney failure is more than 20 times that of the general U.S. population. But the southwestern tribes had lower rates of CHD despite their higher rates of diabetes. The Strong investigators felt that smoking rates and lower cholesterol levels made up

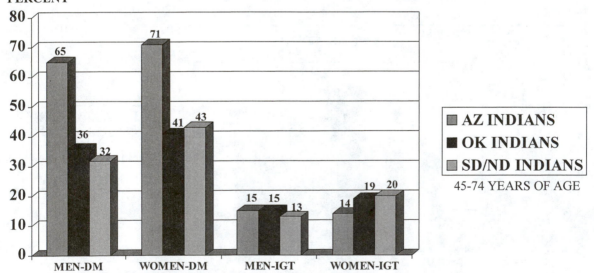

FIGURE 21–11 Diabetes* and impaired glucose tolerance† Strong Heart Study. (*Source:* Welty TK,[38] with permission.)
*On diabetes medications or post 75 gm glucose load ≥200mg/dL.
†Post 75 gm glucose load 140–199 mg/dL.

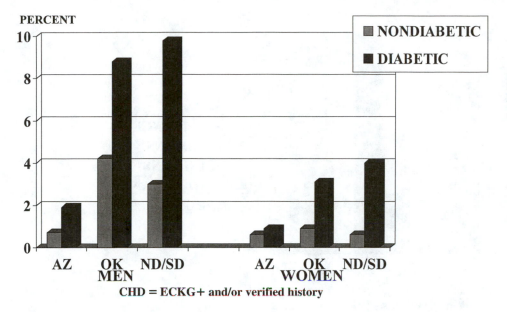

PERCENT

CHD = ECKG+ and/or verified history

FIGURE 21–12 Relation of diabetes with prevalence of CHD in the Strong Heart Study. (*Source:* Welty TK,[52] with permission.)

for some of this difference.[50] Within this population, diabetes appears to be positively associated with age, level of obesity, degree of Indian ancestry, and parental diabetes status.

There is evidence for the efficacy of community programs aimed at diabetes control. The Zuni Diabetes Project is a community-based exercise and weight-control program designed to encourage weight loss and improve glycemic control in people with diabetes. It was initiated by the Indian Health Service and is now managed by the Zuni Wellness Center. Regular aerobic exercise classes are held, as are clinics to monitor weight, serum glucose, and blood pressure. Some 92 percent of patients have completed the 10-week program, and most people keep weight off after a 50-week follow-up period. Patients also showed significant drops in blood glucose levels and decreases in diabetes medications as compared to nonparticipants.[70]

Obesity and Physical Inactivity

Obesity and physical inactivity are common problems[38,53,71–73] in the Native American population and have been associated with an increased risk of

cardiovascular disease.[53,80] Whereas the overall (all races) U.S. prevalence of overweight [based on a body-mass index (BMI) $\geq$ 27.8 kg/m^2 for males and $\geq$ 27.3 kg/m^2 for females] was 38 percent in men and 44 percent in women, prevalence rates among the American Indian tribes studied in the Strong Heart Study ranged from 54 to 67 percent in men and 66 to 80 percent in women studied over the same period. The prevalence of obesity tended to be highest among southwestern tribes as compared to North and South Dakota tribes (Fig. 21–13).[38] Both weight and BMI are also higher among these three American Indian populations as compared to all U.S. races (Fig. 21–14).[38] Another recent cross-sectional investigation showed obesity to be the most common risk factor among the Pascua Yaqui Indian tribe in Tucson, Arizona, where the prevalence was 69 percent among women and 40 percent among men.[64] Some of the risk is associated with increased diabetes in some populations, as well as increased blood pressure.

The change to a sedentary lifestyle has contributed greatly to this problem. This has replaced the traditionally active lifestyle, where hunting, fishing, and gathering were the rule. American Indians in the

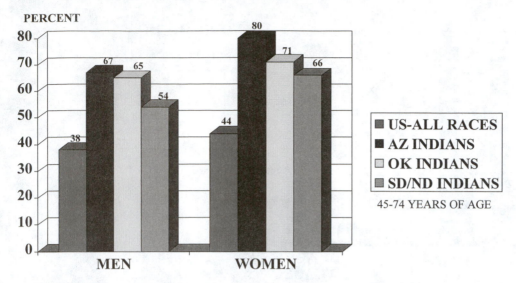

FIGURE 21–13 Overweight* prevalence NHANES III/Strong Heart Studies, U.S., 1988–1991; American Indian, 1989–1991. (*Source:* Welty TK,[38] with permission.) *Males BMI≥27.8; Females BMI≥27.3.

Strong Heart Study report watching an average of 3 h of television daily, and 38 percent of men and 48 percent of women report no activity during the preceding week (17 percent of men and 20 percent of women report no activity in the preceding year).[38]

Recently, a larger and larger proportion of Native Americans are living off reservations. Therefore, the available data reporting consistently higher rates of obesity among Native Americans as compared to whites has been questioned. Recent data among Na-

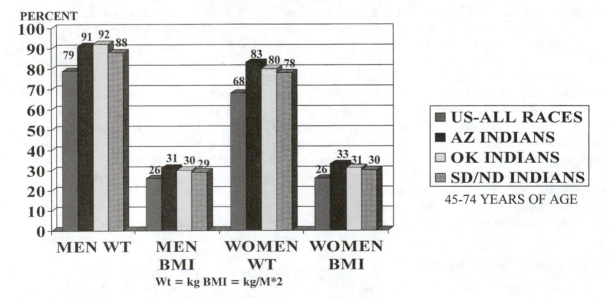

FIGURE 21–14 Mean weight and body mass index NHANES II/Strong Heart Studies, U.S., 1976–1980; American Indian, 1989–1991. (*Source:* Welty TK,[38] with permission.)

tive American girls in public schools do not show consistent age-specific differences as compared to other ethnic groups.[73]

Tobacco

Tobacco is a sacred substance that the tribes consider to have been given to them for ceremonial use. Men smoke tobacco and the dried leaves, roots, and bark of other plants on ceremonial and social occasions. In some tribes, the smoking of tobacco increases the efficacy of a request and makes an obligation or agreement more binding. Recreational use of tobacco occurred after contact with Europeans.[74] National smoking prevalence rates among Native Americans in 1987–1991 were reported to be 33 percent among men and 27 percent among women (compared to 26 percent for white men and 23 percent for white women), but rates as high as 53 percent among men and 45 percent among women have been noted in North and South Dakota tribes.[38] As reported by the Strong Heart Study, there is great variation in smoking prevalence by tribe (Fig. 21–15).[38] Reportedly

lower rates are seen among those living in certain southwestern tribes (24 percent among women and 43 percent among men).[52,64] Overall among Native Americans, studies have shown variable rates of recreational tobacco use, with low rates in the Southwest, high rates in the northern plains, and overall rates generally higher than for the general population.[75–81]

Although Native American men smoke more than their female counterparts, data from the Adolescent Indian Health Survey comprising 13,454 students in grades 7 to 12 suggest that the opposite is true of younger persons. Among them, in every grade after the seventh, females were more likely to be daily cigarette smokers (9 percent in junior high school to 18 percent in high school) than were males of the same age (8 to 15 percent, respectively).

The use of cigars, pipes, and smokeless tobacco tends to be relatively uncommon, however,[5] although it represents a fraction of regular cigarette smoking prevalence. By one report among Eastern Band Cherokee women, prevalence rates for current smokeless tobacco use and smoking were 8 and 39

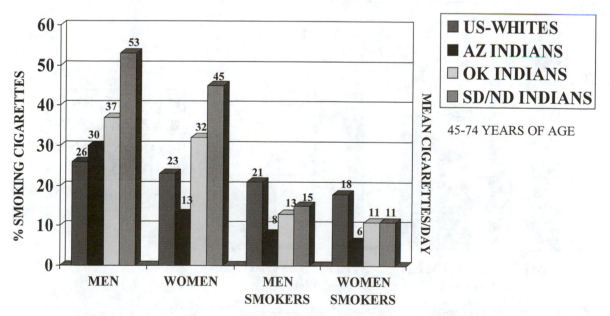

FIGURE 21–15 Cigarette smoking CDC/Strong Heart Studies, U.S., 1987–1991; American Indian, 1989–1991. (*Source:* Welty TK,[38] with permission.)

percent, respectively. Lower education status and having consulted an Indian healer tended to predict the use of smokeless tobacco, whereas young age, alcohol use, no yearly physical examination, separated or divorced marital status, and lack of friends or church participation predicted cigarette smoking.[82] The number of cigarettes consumed per day tended to be fewer in all areas as compared to that among non-Indians. Smoking is felt to be a major factor in the higher rate of CVD among the Sioux.[50] A number of studies[83-85] have shown that a wide variety of interventions can be beneficial in lowering recreational tobacco use in this population.

Alcohol

Among Native Americans compared to whites, the prevalence of alcohol use has been reported to be lower; among users, however, binge drinking is much higher among Native Americans.[50] Binge drinking has been associated with high blood pressure[57] and sudden death.[86] This problem causes many adverse

effects, and CVD is just one small part of the plague affecting this population. Among participants in the Strong Heart Study, the prevalence of current alcohol use ranged from 49 to 60 percent among men and 28 to 38 percent among women, depending on the tribe. Among drinkers, binge drinking was highly variable, but as many as 44 percent of men and 18 percent of women engaged in this practice (Fig. 21-16).[38,52]

Nutritional Practices

Over the last 30 years, traditional foods such as corn, buffalo, and venison have been replaced by processed and commercially prepared foods. Data from the Strong Heart Study show mean total fat intake as a percentage of total calories to be consistently above the recommended level of 30 percent and fiber intake below the recommended daily 20 to 30 g.[87] But significant variation also exists among communities; the Pima Indians had the highest consumption fat and cholesterol, but also the highest fiber intake among the three communities studied.[88]

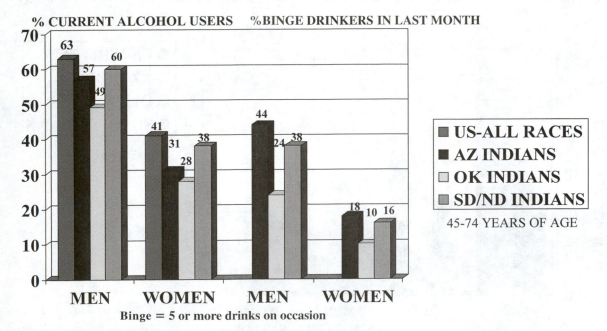

FIGURE 21-16 Alcohol use CDC-BRFS/Strong Heart Studies, U.S., 1987-1991; American Indian, 1989-1991. (*Source:* Welty TK,[38,52] with permission.)

Although sodium intake among the Pima Indians is close to the recommended levels, Pima Indians consume too much of their fat as saturated fat and have average levels of cholesterol intake above the recommended level of less than 300 mg/day.[89]

Estrogen Replacement Therapy

Data from the Strong Heart Study suggest that the use of hormone replacement therapy (HRT) among postmenopausal women aged 45 to 74 is low. Current HRT use varied from 5 percent in Arizona to 21 percent in Oklahoma. As compared to nonusers, users had significantly lower levels of LDL-C (-6.4 mg/dL) and fibrinogen (-26.2 mg/dL) and a lower waist/hip ratio (-0.02) as well as higher levels of HDL-C (5 mg/dL).[90] Greater efforts of educating the Native American community about the potential cardiovascular benefits of HRT in postmenopausal women are needed.

Socioeconomic Status

In 1990, the median Native American family income was $19,897, compared to $31,435 for whites: 31.6 percent lived below the poverty level, compared to 9.8 percent for whites, and unemployment was three times higher for Native Americans than for whites.[5] Only 65.3 percent graduated from high school, compared to 77.9 percent of whites, and only 8.9 percent get bachelor's degrees, compared to 21.5 percent of whites.[5]

The Native American population is young, with a median age of 24.2 years, compared to 34.4 years for whites. This is due to a high birth rate (26.6 per 1000 population, compared to 15.0 per 1000 population of whites[5]) and the fact that only 3.7 percent of deaths occur before age 45, compared to 12 percent for all races in the United States.[91] The Strong Heart Study has linked lower socioeconomic status to higher rates of CVD.[41] The limited funding available from the Indian Health Service may also be a factor. Access to care continues to be a major problem for much of this population.

Preventive Strategies

In order to make an impact on reducing CVD incidence in the Native American population, it is essential that we enhance efforts to improve the screening and identification of those at highest risk and target resources toward risk reduction. Local hospitals and clinics should be provided with the resources to conduct community-based screening efforts to, in particular, identify the large numbers of Native Americans untreated or inadequately treated for hypertension, diabetes, and/or dyslipidemia. Primary care clinics focusing on risk-factor reduction should be empowered to treat those with elevated cardiovascular risk factors. Physicians should be made aware of standards for the identification, classification, and management of these conditions, as discussed in depth in earlier chapters of this text.

Since guidelines specific for the management of cardiovascular risk factors among individual Native American groups do not exist, the adoption of guidelines published for the population as a whole will be a prudent strategy until further data become available on the effectiveness of proven and recommended strategies in these populations. As much as possible, culturally appropriate strategies (see below) should be used to complement proven medical approaches.

Broad recommendations regarding promotion of cardiovascular health among Native Americans, titled *Building Healthy Hearts for American Indians and Alaska Natives: A Background Report* have been recently published by the National Institutes of Health.[75] This report has recommended that, based on the available epidemiologic data, the following CVD risk factors and target audiences be identified as possible targets for intervention:

1. Cigarette smoking in tribes living in the Midwestern United States and Alaska
2. Cigarette smoking among youth living on reservations
3. Diabetes in all tribes, especially those living in the southwestern and midwestern United States
4. High blood pressure in tribes with a high prevalence of diabetes

5. Obesity and physical inactivity in all tribes with an emphasis on family intervention and childhood obesity prevention programs
6. Comprehensive health-promotion approaches incorporating heart-healthy lifestyle changes

This report also recommends that to build and maintain interest in the interventions targeted, that community members should participate actively in all aspects of the program. Traditional healers, community health representatives, nutrition aides, students in health fields at American Indian colleges, and others should be recruited as volunteers or staff. Also, school boards, health boards, and community health programs can be channels for incorporating family activities and community events such as powwows into the program. Finally, professional training opportunities for health care providers of native professional associations and other professional health groups should be encouraged to incorporate both Western and traditional medicine, as in annual national conferences.

Although there are no published data on the comparative effectiveness of different risk-reducing therapies among Native Americans as compared to other ethnic groups, the personal experience of the author with several tribes suggests response to antihypertensive and lipid-lowering therapy among Native Americans to be most similar to that among white populations—Native Americans do not appear to be salt-sensitive and have a good response to the major classes of antihypertensive therapy. Further documentation of these reports is needed through carefully controlled trials.

Increased community awareness regarding healthy lifestyles is an essential component of primary prevention. In an effort to prevent and combat diabetes, advisory groups and coalitions have formed in some tribes in order to increase community awareness and strengthen the infrastructure necessary to promote healthy lifestyles.[92] Comprehensive obesity prevention programs are also promising.[93] The utilization of group or communitywide strategies may be more effective than an individual approach in this population. Stressing the benefits of therapy for the entire family (e.g., diet healthy for all) rather than just for the individual will likely be more successful.

Ongoing Community-Based Health Programs

A few community-based prevention programs have demonstrated success in the Native American community. PATHWAYS is a multisite school-based obesity prevention program sponsored by the National Heart, Lung, and Blood Institute designed to reduce the prevalence of obesity among school-aged children by promoting healthful eating and physical activity. It is conducted in cooperation with seven Indian reservations in Arizona, New Mexico, and South Dakota and involves a classroom curriculum for children in grades 3, 4, and 5.[75] The Southwestern Cardiovascular Curriculum is a multifactorial, culturally oriented curriculum created for American Indian students in rural northwestern New Mexico that is intended to increase knowledge about health and healthy behavior by teaching students about healthier lifestyles and ways to achieve them.[75]

Cultural Issues

Culture can be a major barrier to adequate care. Sir William Osler stated, "It is more important to know what sort of patient has a disease, than what sort of disease a patient has."[91] Provider background can have a significant impact on health care delivery.[94] Beliefs on health, disease, and healing are often very different from the traditional Western or European concept. Some understanding of Native American culture can help improve the outcome of the physician-patient encounter. Health in Native American culture is not the absence of disease but rather harmony with oneself (mind, body, and spirit), harmony with others, and harmony with one's surroundings or environment. When harmony is lost, illness is enabled to enter.

Spirituality or religion is inseparable from health. Traditional Indian healers use spiritual means to diagnose and heal. They are viewed as healing from the inside of the body because they treat the cause of the illness or whatever led to the loss of harmony. Western medicine is viewed as healing from the outside of the body—treating the symptoms (e.g., headache, dyspepsia, etc.). Both methods are viewed as compatible and are not considered competitive. They have the same goal—a healthy patient! Traditional healers do not feel it is their place to prolong life but simply to try to make it better.

Cultural norms are different too. The Native American handshake is gentle, to show respect. It is not a test of strength or a show of domination. Eye contact means a lack of trust. The person looking into your eyes during an encounter is looking to see if you are telling the truth. There is no clock fixation, and some languages have no future tense. There are many more differences, but these are a few important ones.

Some guidelines for those working with patients from another culture are as follows:

1. Remember you are the foreigner. Adapt to their ways. Do not expect them to adapt to your ways (cultural imposition).
2. Respect them. Do not be condescending or paternalistic or ethnocentric.
3. Be patient. Do not show haste.
4. Do not use professional jargon. Speak to your listeners at a level they can understand. Ask them if you explained yourself clearly enough. Indians consider it impolite to ask questions, so they probably will not, as this would imply that you had done a bad job, and that would be disrespectful.
5. Go to social events and learn by watching. Do not ask a lot of questions, as this would show that you were not paying attention.
6. Develop relationships with staff from the culture with which you are working. They can help you learn a lot about their ways.
7. Respect the culture's traditional beliefs and customs.

There are also some lessons regarding elders that should be considered:

1. Respect others' ways. You do not need to understand them in order to respect their ways.

2. There is a spiritual side to healing. With all the high-tech wizardry at our disposal, it is often easy to forget this.
3. The healer is not the source of the healing but simply a conduit, for the healing powers of the creator can get to the patient. It is not to our credit that we are smart and can help others. These are gifts, and they need to be looked upon as gifts if they are to be there for us.

Some qualities observed to be successful in Native American communities are the following:

1. Native Americans truly respect us and our ways.
2. They are interested in our ways.
3. They really care about our people.
4. They are patient and try to learn our ways so they can better adapt to our culture.

Health Care

The Indian Health Service (IHS), an agency of the Public Health Service, provides health care for about 60 percent of this population.[5] The remainder are covered by Medicare, Medicaid, or third-party insurance or are uninsured. The IHS is predominantly on reservations and a few urban settings that have large Native American populations.[43] Some tribes have taken over the administration of the health care under Public Law 93-638 but still get varying degrees of support from the IHS.

The IHS is made up of 12 regional administrative units or area offices. Combining tribal and IHS-operated facilities, there are 144 service units, 49 hospitals, and 484 ambulatory centers.[6] The IHS does not operate in all eligible locations owing to financial and personnel limitations. There is a misconception that all American Indians and Alaska Natives can get free care or that the IHS provides universal coverage for the Native American community. In reality, the IHS predominantly provides primary care services and contracts for services it cannot provide. The IHS has limited funding and resources; often, eligible patients cannot get services because of lack of contract care funds. In 1996, the per capita funding for health care in the United States was $3046 and the IHS average was $1200, according to the Indian Health Service Office of Planning.[95]

Conclusion

CVD is the leading cause of death among American Indians and Alaska Natives. A study of trends and risk factors suggests that this will continue, as this population has adopted Western lifestyles. Culturally appropriate and sensitive intervention programs[96–99] can be effective. With improvements in funding of the IHS, it is hoped that there will be increased opportunities for CVD prevention and treatment, which will, one hopes, reverse the trend of increasing CVD in this population.

References

1. *Cancer Facts and Figures 1997.* Atlanta, GA, American Cancer Society, 1997.
2. *Healthy People 2000.* National Health Promotion and Disease Prevention Objectives. DHHS Pub. No. (PHS) 91-50212. Washington, DC, U.S. Department of Health and Human Services, U.S. Government Printing Office, 1991.
3. *Documentation of the Cancer Research Needs of American Indians and Alaska Natives.* Native American Monograph No. 1. NIH Pub. No. 93-3603. Washington, DC, National Cancer Institute, 1993.
4. *Chronic Disease in Minority Populations: African Americans, American Indians and Alaska Natives, Asian and Pacific Islanders, Hispanic Americans 1994.* Atlanta, GA, Centers for Disease Control and Prevention, 1994.
5. American Heart Association: *American Indian/Alaska Natives and Cardiovascular Diseases: Biostatistical Fact Sheet.* Dallas, AHA, 1995.
6. *Regional Differences in Indian Health 1996.* Rockville, MD, Division of Program Statistics. Office of Planning, Evaluation and Legislation, Indian Health Services, U.S. Department of Health and Human Services, 1996.
7. Lee ET, Cowan LD, Welty TK, et al: All-cause mortality and cardiovascular disease mortality in three American Indian populations, aged 45–74 years, 1984–1988: the Strong Heart Study. *Am J Epidemiol* 1998; 147:995–1008.
8. Salsbury CG: Disease incidence among the Navajos. *Southwest Med* 1937; 21:230.
9. Kraus BS: *The Disease Picture in Indian Health in Arizona.* Tucson, AZ, University of Arizona Press, 1954, pp 75–109.
10. *Heart Disease Among Indians in the U.S., 1955.* Washington, DC, U.S. Department of Health, Education, and Welfare, Public Health Service, Division of Indian Health, U.S. Government Printing Office, 1957.
11. Silbert J: Absence of coronary thrombosis in Navajo Indians. *Calif Med* 1955; 82:114.
12. Page IH, Lewis LA, Gilbert J: Plasma, lipids, and proteins and their relationship to coronary disease among Navajo Indians. *Circulation* 1956; 13:675.
13. Smith RL: Recorded and expected mortality among the Navajo with special reference to cancer. *J Natl Cancer Inst* 1956; 17:77.
14. Adair J: Patterns of health and disease among the Navajos. *Ann Am Acad Pol Soc Sci* 1957; 311:80.
15. Smith RL: Cardiovascular, renal, and diabetes deaths among the Navajos. *Public Health Rep* 1957; 72:33.
16. Leo TF: Cardiovascular Survey in a Population of Arizona Indians. *Circulation* 1958; 18:748.
17. Hesse FG: Evidence of cholecystitis and other diseases among Pima Indians of southern Arizona. *JAMA* 1959; 170:1789.
18. Streeper RB: An electrocardiographic and autopsy study of coronary heart disease in the Navajo. *Dis Chest* 1960; 38:305.
19. Deuschle K: Interdisciplinary approach to public health on the Navajo Indian reservation: medical and anthropological aspects. *Ann NY Acad Sci* 1960; 84:887.
20. Clifford NJ, Kelly JJ, Leo TF, Eder HA: Coronary heart disease and hypertension in the White Mountain Apache Tribe. *Circulation* 1963; 28:926.
21. Fulmer HS: Coronary heart disease among the Navajo Indians. *Ann Intern Med* 1963; 59:740.
22. Hesse FG: Incidence of disease in the Navajo Indian: a necropsy study of coronary and aortic atherosclerosis, cholelithiasis, and neoplastic disease. *Arch Pathol (Chicago)* 1964; 77:553.
23. Kravetz RE: Disease distribution in southwestern American Indians: analysis of 211 autopsies. *Arizona Med* 1964; 21:628.
24. Sievers ML: Myocardial infarction among southwestern American Indians. *Ann Intern Med* 1967; 67:800–807.
25. Ingelfinger JA., Bonnett PH, Liebow IM, Miller M: Coronary heart disease in the Pima Indians: electrocardiographic findings and postmortem evidence of myocardial infarction in a population with high prevalence of diabetes mellitus. *Diabetes* 1976; 25:561–565.
26. Becker TM, Wiggins C, Key CR, Samet JM: Ischemic heart disease mortality in Hispanics, American Indians and non-Hispanic whites in New Mexico, 1958–1982. *Circulation* 1988; 78:302–309.
27. Middaugh JP: Cardiovascular deaths among Alaska Natives, 1980–1986. *Am J Public Health* 1990; 80:282–285.
28. Pinkerton RE, Badke FR: Coronary heart disease: an epidemiologic study of Crow and Northern Cheyenne Indians. *Rocky Mountain Med J* 1974; 71:577–583.

29. Sievers ML: Diseases of North American Indians, in Rothchild HR (ed): *Bio-cultural Aspects of Disease.* New York. Academic Press, 1981.

30. Hrabovsky SL, Welty TK, Coulehan JL: Acute myocardial infarction and sudden death in Sioux Indians. *West Med J* 1989; 150:420–422.

31. Gillum RF, Billum BS, Smith N: Cardiovascular risk factors among urban American Indians: blood pressure, serum lipids, smoking, diabetes, health knowledge, and behavior. *Am Heart J* 1984; 107:765–776.

32. Lee ET, Welty TK, Fabsitz R, et al: The Strong Heart Study. A study of cardiovascular disease in American Indians: design and methods. *Am J Epidemiol* 1990; 132:1141–1155.

33. Howard BV: Associations of lipoproteins with obesity in American Indians: the Strong Heart Study, in Oomura Y, Tarui S, Shimazu T (eds): *Progress in Obesity Research, 1990.* John Libbey, 1990, pp 291–294.

34. Howard BV, Welty TK, Fabsitz RR, et al: Risk factors for coronary heart disease in diabetic and non-diabetic Native Americans: the Strong Heart Study. *J Diabetes Care* 1992; 41(suppl 2):4–11.

35. Lowe LP, Travel D, Wallace RB, Welty TK: Type II diabetes and cognitive function: a population-based study of Native Americans. *J Diabetes Care* 1994; 17:891–896.

36. Lee ET, Howard BV, Savage PJ, et al: Diabetes and impaired glucose tolerance in three American Indian populations aged 45–74 years: the Strong Heart Study. *Diabetes Care* 1995; 18:599–610.

37. Howard BV, Lee ET, Cowan LD, et al: Coronary heart disease prevalence and its relation to risk factors in American Indians: the Strong Heart Study. *Am J Epidemiol* 1995; 142:254–268.

38. Welty TK, Lee ET, Yeh J, et al: Cardiovascular disease risk factors among American Indians: the Strong Heart Study. *Am J Epidemiol* 1995; 42:269–287.

39. Robbins DC, Knowler WC, Lee ET, et al: Regional differences in albuminuria among American Indians: an epidemic of renal disease. *Kidney Int* 1996; 49:557–563.

40. Robbins DC, Welty TK, Wang WY, et al: Plasma, lipids, and lipoprotein concentrations among American Indians: comparison with the U.S. population. *Curr Opin Lipidol* 1996; 7:188–195.

41. Lee ET, Go OT: Socioeconomic status and cardiovascular health and disease in American Indians: the Strong Heart Study, in *Proceedings of the National Institutes of Health Conference on Socioeconomic Status and Cardiovascular Disease and Health, November 1995.* Bethesda, MD, NIH, 1996.

42. Cowan LD, Go OT, Howard BV, et al: Parity, postmenopausal estrogen use and cardiovascular disease risk factors in American Indian women: the Strong Heart Study. *J Women Health* 1997; 6:441–449.

43. Zephier EM, Ballew C, Mokdad A, et al: Intake of nutrients related to cardiovascular disease risk among three groups of American Indians: the Strong Heart Study. *Prev Med* 1997; 26:508–515.

44. Devereux RB, Roman MJ, de Simone G, et al: Relations of left ventricular mass to demographic and hemodynamic variables in American Indians: the Strong Heart Study. *Circulation* 1997; 96:1416–1423.

45. Devereux RB, Roman MJ, Paranicas M, et al: Relations of Doppler stroke volume and its components to left ventricular stroke volume in normotensive and hypertensive American Indians: the Strong Heart Study. *Am J Hypertens* 1997; 10:619–628.

46. Oopik AJ, Dorogy M, Devereux RB, et al: Major electrocardiographic abnormalities among American Indians aged 45–74 years: the Strong Heart Study. *Am J Cardiol* 1996; 78:1400–1405.

47. Howard BV, Lee ET, Yeh JL, et al: Hypertension in adult American Indians: the Strong Heart Study. *Hypertension* 1996; 28:256–264.

48. Gray RS, Robbins DC, Wang W, et al: Relation of LDL size to the insulin resistance syndrome and coronary heart disease in American Indians: the Strong Heart Study. *Arterioscler Thromb Vasc Biol* 1997; 17:2713–2720.

49. Kataoka S, Robbins DC, Cowan LD, et al: Apolipoprotein E polymorphism in American Indians and its relation to plasma lipoproteins and diabetes: the Strong Heart Study. *Arterioscler Thromb Vasc Biol* 1996; 16:918–925.

50. Howard BV, Lee ET, Fabsitz RR, et al: Diabetes and coronary heart disease in American Indians: the Strong Heart Study. *Diabetes* 1996; 45(suppl 3):S6–S13.

51. Welty TK, Coulehan JL: Cardiovascular disease among American Indians and Alaska Natives. *Diabetes Care* 1993; 16:277–283.

52. Welty TK: Principal investigator: Strong Heart Study. Personal communication, 1998.

53. Strotz CR, Shorr GI: Hypertension in the Papago Indians. *Circulation* 1973; 48:1299–1303.

54. Sievers ML: Historical overview of hypertension among American Indians and Alaska Natives. *Arizona Med* 1977; 34:607–610.

55. Destefano F, Coulehan JL, Wiant MK: Blood pressure survey on the Navajo Indian reservation. *Am J Epidemiol* 1979; 190:335–345.

56. Gillum RF, Prineas RJ, Palta M, Horibe H: Blood pressure of urban Native American school children. *J Hypertens* 1980; 2:744–749.

57. Howard BV: Blood pressure in 13 American Indian communities: the Strong Heart Study. *Public Health Rep* 1996; 111(suppl 2):47–48.

58. National Heart, Lung and Blood Institute: *Hypertension in Hispanic Americans, American Indians and Alaskan Natives, and Asian and Pacific Islanders.* Bethesda, MD, National Institutes of Health, 1996.

59. Savage PJ, Hamman RF, Bartha G, et al: Serum cholesterol in American (Pima) Indian children and adolescents. *J Pediatr* 1976; 58:274–282.

60. Campos-Gutealt D, Ellis J, Aickin M, et al: Prevalence of cardiovascular disease risk factors in a southwestern Native American tribe. *Public Health Rep* 1995; 110:742–748.

61. Mendlein JM, Freedman DS, Peter DG, et al: Risk factors for coronary heart disease among Navajo Indians: findings from the Navajo Health and Nutrition Survey. *J Nutr* 1997; 127:2099S–2105S.

62. Sugarman JR, Gilbert TJ, Perry CA, Peter DG: Serum cholesterol concentrations among Navajo Indians. *Public Health Rep* 1992; 107:92–99.

63. National Institute of Diabetes and Digestive and Kidney Diseases: *Diabetes in America,* 2d ed. NIH Pub. No. 95-1468. Bethesda, MD, National Institutes of Health, 1995.

64. Campos-Outcalt D, Ellis J, Aickin M, et al: Prevalence of cardiovascular disease risk factors in a southwestern Native American tribe. *Public Health Rep* 1995; 110:742–748.

65. Howard BV, Knowler WC, Davis MP, et al: Diabetes and atherosclerosis in the Pima Indians. *M Sinai J Med* 1982; 49:169–175.

66. Hoy W, Light A, Megill D: Cardiovascular disease in Navajo Indians with type 2 diabetes. *Public Health Rep* 1995; 110:87–94.

67. Delisle HF, Rivard M, Ekoe JM: Prevalence estimates of diabetes and of other cardiovascular risk factors in the two largest Algonquin communities of Quebec. *J Diabetes Care* 1995; 18:1255–1259.

68. Gilliland FD, Owen C, Gilliland SS, Carter JS: Temporal trends in diabetes mortality among American Indians and Hispanics in New Mexico: birth cohort and period effects. *Am J Epidemiol* 1997; 145:422–431.

69. Casper M, Rith-Najarian S, Croft J, et al: Blood pressure, diabetes, and body mass index among Chippewa and Menominee Indians: the Inter Tribal Heart Project preliminary data. *Public Health Rep* 1996; 3:37–39.

70. Heath GW, Wilson RH, Smith J, Leonard BE: Community-based exercise and weight control: diabetes risk reduction and glycemic control in Zuni Indians. *Am J Clin Nutr* 1991; 53:1642S–1646S.

71. Gruber E, Anderson MM, Ponton L, DiClemente R: Overweight and obesity in Native-American adolescents: comparing nonreservation youths with African-American and Caucasian peers. *Am J Prev Med* 1995; 11:306–310.

72. Fitzgerald SJ, Kriska AM, Pereira MA, de Courten MP: Associations among physical activity, television watching, and obesity in adult Pima Indians. *Med Sci Sports Exerc* 1997; 29:910–915.

73. Freedman DS, Serdula MK, Percy CA, et al: Obesity, levels of lipids and glucose, and smoking among Navajo adolescents. *J Nutr* 1997; 127:2120S–2127S.

74. Gillum RF, Gillum BS, Smith N: Cardiovascular risk factors among urban American Indians: blood pressure, serum lipids, smoking, diabetes, health knowledge and behavior. *Am Heart J* 1984; 107:765–776.

75. National Institutes of Health: *Building Healthy Hearts for American Indians and Alaska Natives: A Background Report.* National Institute of Health, Bethesda, MD, February 1999.

76. Spangler JG, Dignan MB, Michielutte R: Correlates of tobacco use among Native American women in western North Carolina. *Am J Public Health* 1997; 87:108–111.

77. Kaplan SD, Lanier AP, Merritt RK, Siegel PZ: Prevalence of tobacco use among Alaska Natives: a review. *Prev Med* 1997; 26:460–465.

78. Nelson DE, Moon RW, Holtzman D, et al: Patterns of health risk behavior for chronic disease: a comparison between adolescent and adult American Indians living on or near reservations in Montana. *Soc Adolesc Med* 1997; 21:25–32.

79. Kimball EH, Goldberg HI, Oberle MW: The prevalence of selected risk factors for chronic disease among American Indians in Washington State. *Public Health Rep* 1996; 111:264–271.

80. Spangler JG, Dignan MG, Michielutte R: Correlates of tobacco use among Native American women in western North Carolina. *Am J Public Health* 1997; 87:108–111.

81. Davis SM, Lambert LC, Cunningham-Sabo L, Skipper BJ: Tobacco use: baseline results from Pathways to Health: a school-based project for southwestern American Indian youth. *Prev Med* 1995; 24:454–460.

82. Glasgow RE, Lichtenstein E, Wilder D, et al: The Tribal Tobacco Policy Project: working with Northwest Indian Tribes on smoking policies. *Prev Med* 1995; 24:434–440.

83. Lando HA, Johnson KM, Graham-Tomasi RP, et al: Urban Indians' smoking patterns and interest in quitting. *Public Health Rep* 1992; 107:340–344.

84. Lichtenstein E, Glasgow RE, Lopez K, et al: Promoting tobacco control policies in Northwest Indian Tribes. *Am J Public Health* 1995; 85:991–994.

85. Johnson K, Lando HA, Schmid LS, Solberg LI: The Gains Project: Outcome of smoking cessation strategies in four urban Native American clinics. *J Addict Behav* 1997; 22:207–218.

86. May PA: Alcohol abuse and alcoholism among American Indians: an overview, in Watts TD, Wright R (eds): *Alcoholism in Minority Populations.* Springfield, IL, Charles C Thomas, 1989, pp 95–119.

87. Federation of American Societies for Experimental Biology: *Third Report on Nutrition Monitoring in the United States*: Vol 1. Prepared for the Interagency Board for Nutrition Monitoring and Related Research. Washington DC, U.S. Government Printing Office, 1995.

88. National Cholesterol Education Program: Second Report of the Expert Panel on Detection, Evaluation, and Treatment of High Blood Cholesterol in Adults. Washington,

DC, National Heart Lung, and Blood Institute, National Institutes of Health, 1993.

89. Smith CJ, Nelson RG, Hardy SA, et al: Survey of the diet of Pima Indians using quantitative food frequency assessment and 24-hour recall. *J Am Diet Assoc* 1996; 96:778–783.

90. Cowan LD, Go OT, Howard BV, et al: Parity, post-menopausal estrogen use, and cardiovascular disease risk factors in American Indian women: the Strong Heart Study. *J Womens Health* 1997; 6:441–449.

91. Day TW: Cross cultural medicine at home. *Minn Med* 1992; 75:15–17.

92. Hood VL, Kelly B, Martinez C, et al: A Native American community initiative to prevent diabetes. *Ethn Health* 1997; 2:277–285.

93. Broussard BA, Sugarman JR, Bachman-Carter K, et al: Toward comprehensive obesity prevention programs in Native American communities. *Obesity Res* 1995; 3(suppl 2):289s–297s.

94. Moy E, Bartman BA: Physician race and care of minority and medically indigent patients. *JAMA* 1995; 273:1515–1520.

95. Opening Statement before the Indian Affairs Committee of the U.S. Senate 5/15/97. Michael Trujillo, M.D., MPH, Assistant Surgeon General. Director, Indian Health Service, Department of Health and Human Services. Budget Oversight Hearing FY 1998 Budget Request.

96. Cheadle A, Pearson D, Wagner E, et al: A community based approach to preventing alcohol use among adolescents on an American Indian reservation. *Public Health Rep* 1995; 110:439–447.

97. Wilson R, Smith J, Martin AM, Helgerson S: A low cost competitive approach to weight reduction in a Native American community. *Int J Obesity* 1989; 13:731–738.

98. Stegmayer P, Levrien FC, Smith M, et al: Designing a diabetes nutrition education program for a Native American community. *Diabetes Educ* 1984; 14:64–66.

99. Harris MB, Davis SM, Ford VL, Tso H: The checkerboard cardiovascular curriculum: a culturally oriented program. *J Schol Health* 1988; 58:104–107.

Part **V**

Comprehensive Approaches to Prevention

CHAPTER 22

Primary Prevention

Thomas A. Pearson

General Approaches to Primary Prevention

A variety of approaches might be considered to reduce the populationwide burden of heart disease, stroke, and peripheral vascular disease. While *secondary prevention* refers to the prevention of death or recurrence of disease in those who are already symptomatic, *primary prevention* pertains to the prevention of the onset of disease in persons without prior symptoms of cardiovascular disease (CVD). Another approach would be so-called *primordial prevention,* in which the factors causative of the disease, the so-called risk factors (see below), would be prevented, thereby reducing the likelihood of development of the disease itself. The distinction between primary and secondary prevention has lessened owing to a large overlap resulting from increasingly sensitive technologies. These technologies can identify pathophysiologic states, early lesions, or silent disease in persons who have never been symptomatic. Therefore, primary prevention can be redefined as the prevention of the atherosclerotic disease process itself, with secondary prevention being treatment of the atherosclerotic disease process.[1]

Key to the primary prevention of CVD is the notion of risk factors. A correlation of clinical, epidemiologic, and experimental studies has established the role of traits as agents etiologically related to atherosclerotic CVD. In considering these factors as part of an effort to prevent CVD, it may be useful to subclassify these factors as nonmodifiable, behavioral, and physiologic (Fig. 22–1).[2] *Nonmodifiable* factors—such as age, sex, race, and family history of CVD—might be used to identify high-risk groups benefiting from special programs. *Behavioral* risk factors—such as a sedentary lifestyle, unhealthful diet, heavy alcohol consumption, and cigarette smoking—might be approached on either a population-wide or individual basis. These behaviors and all nonmodifiable factors may, in turn, be related to the physiologic risk factors (hypertension, obesity, lipid disorders, diabetes) that are generally measured clinically and managed pharmacologically. The distinction between behavioral and physiologic risk factors takes on added importance in primary prevention: behavioral risk factors can be approached on a populationwide basis and physiologic risk factors are often targets of the high-risk approach (see below).

In general, there are two approaches to primary prevention: *the population approach* and the *high-risk approach.*[3] Consider the distribution of risk or a risk factor in the population. In Fig. 22–2,[4] the distribution of serum cholesterol levels in the U.S. population identifies an entire population at higher risk than populations who have a lower burden of coronary disease, such as the Japanese. At the same time, there is a variation in the level of serum cholesterol (the same applies to other risk factors). Most people are found in the middle of the bell-shaped distribution of values, but a "tail" exists of persons with higher values. One public health intervention would be the so-called high-risk approach, in which individuals with high values are identified and intensively treated. This results in the reduction of those persons' risk to that of the middle of the curve (Fig. 22–2A). This is, in essence, what a clinician does when a patient's high cholesterol or blood pressure is assessed and drugs are prescribed to reduce the levels into the "normal" range.

Nonmodifiable risk factors

Physiological risk factors

Endpoints

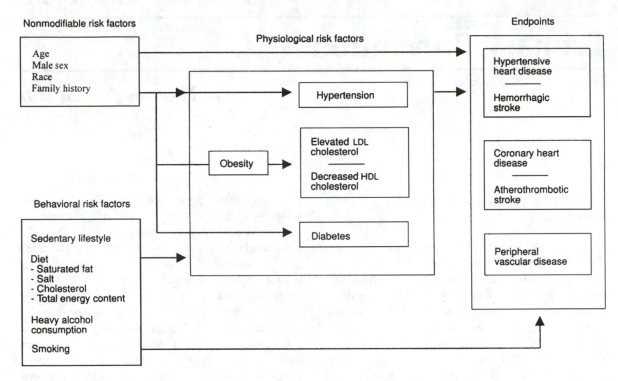

FIGURE 22–1 Relationships between cardiovascular risk factors and cardiovascular diseases.

The problem with sole reliance on the high-risk approach is that most cases of CVD do not occur in high-risk subjects. While the rate of CVD is higher for these individuals, high-risk subjects account for a small percentage of those who suffer with CVD. Most cases of CVD occur among those falling within the "average" risk group. True reduction in the population burden of CVD may result only from shifting the entire population level of risk factors (Fig. 22–2*B*).

The two approaches need not be exclusive. In reality, combinations of high-risk and population approaches are usually employed in practice (Fig. 22–2*C*). The purpose of this chapter is to discuss these practical strategies as applied to populations and individuals.

The Population Approach to Primary Prevention

The Conceptual Framework for the Population Approach

The rationale for the population approach to CVD prevention is derived not only from the observation that most cases of CVD have average or slightly above average risks. Rather, CVD might be considered a disease of Occidental culture, with markedly higher rates of CVD associated with populations who adopt the Western lifestyle of a high-fat, high-cholesterol diet, tobacco use, and lack of physical activity. Epidemiologic evidence for this cultural basis of CVD is extensive and derived from multiple sources, including comparisons of risk factors and

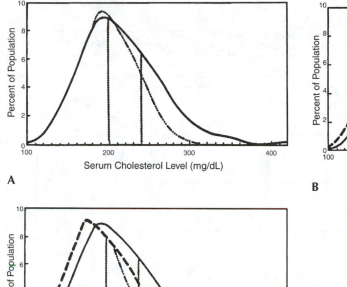

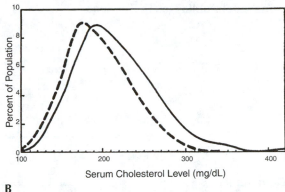

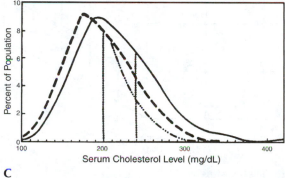

FIGURE 22–2 *A.* Cholesterol distribution in U.S. population aged 20 to 74 years from the *National Health and Nutrition Examination Survey II* (1976–1980) and potential changes in the distribution. Expected shift in population distribution of serum cholesterol values with application of high-risk approach (Adult Treatment Panel Guidelines of National Cholesterol Education Program). Dashed line shows effect of recommendations. *B.* Expected shift in population distribution of serum cholesterol values with application of public health approach (Population Panel of the National Cholesterol Education Program). Dashed line shows effect of recommendations. *C.* Anticipated combined effects of high-risk (dotted-dashed line) and public health approaches (dashed line) of the National Cholesterol Education Program. (From Carleton et al.,[4] with permission.)

CVD rates between populations, trends in CVD rates, studies of migrants to high-risk societies, and results of public health trials.[5] The basic tenet of the population approach is: If the basis of CVD is social and economic, the solution to the CVD epidemic must be social and economic.[3]

In considering populationwide resources to control CVD, the major targets are often those populationwide behaviors that can be causative of the physiologic risk factors [e.g., a high-fat diet, which contributes to elevated low-density-lipoprotein (LDL) cholesterol] as well as directly causative of CVD (e.g., cigarette smoking). A conceptual framework can then be developed as to how these risk factors and risk behaviors might be approached on a population basis (Fig. 22–3). This requires the application of essential public health services such as surveillance, education, organizational partnerships, assurance of personal health services, and legislation/policy[6] in a variety of community settings

Essential Public Health Services

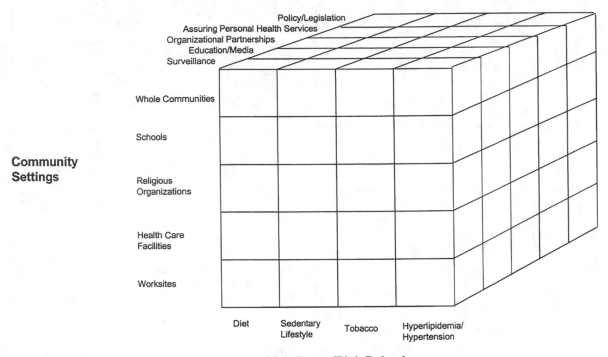

Risk Factor/Risk Behavior

FIGURE 22–3 A conceptual framework for public health practice in cardiovascular disease prevention.

including work sites, health care facilities, religious organizations, schools, and whole communities.[7] The result is a grid in which specific behaviors might be addressed through specific means in specific community settings, which, in aggregate, constitute an entire population (Fig. 22–3).

Strategies for Communitywide Prevention of Cardiovascular Disease

Overview In considering populationwide behaviors that affect CVD risk, it is worthwhile to consider the complex array of influences on that behavior. Consider the factors in the food chain that influence eating patterns (Fig. 22–4). This includes the science base, the food manufacturers, distributors and retailers, restaurants and other food service organizations, economic considerations, cultural factors, and taste.

In attempting to alter these factors, it is likely that a number of strategies might need to be employed. Major approaches include (1) surveillance of CVD and its risk factors, (2) public education and mass media, (3) community organizations and partnerships, and (4) policies, regulations, and legislation.

Surveillance and populationwide data A number of strategies are available for influencing populationwide CVD prevention, including surveillance of the burden of CVD in the population.[8] In most countries in western Europe, North America, and Australia/New Zealand, CVD has been recognized as the leading cause of death for half a century. Only recently, however, has attention focused on CVD as the major cause of disability and death in developing countries.[9] Data on mortality for CVD can be misleading, as case-fatality rates from myocardial in-

Food Science Base	Food Manufacture	Food Distribution	Food Purchasing	Food Preparation	Food Consumption	Food – Consumption Outcomes
Nutritional Biochemical Preservation Genetics	Agriculture Synthesis Processing Additives Modifiers Hybridizers Mass Prep.	Wholesale Retail Prod.-Specific Route-Specific	Cost Culture Advertising Knowledge Health	In-House Restaurants Institutional	Socialization Education Nutr. Value Health Culture Taste Cost Mood	Pleasure Health Deficiencies Surpluses

OTHER MAJOR INFLUENCES ON THE FOOD CHAIN

Advertising
Agribusiness
Conglomerates
Culinary Education
Food Science Education
General Education
Government Agencies
Grocery Chains

Health Professionals
Media
Nutrition Education
Profitability
Special Interest Groups
Subsidies
Taxation

FIGURE 22–4 Major elements in the food chain that determine eating patterns in a population. (From Carleton and Lasater,[8] with permission.)

farction, angina, and stroke decline. Morbidity data are much more difficult to obtain and often show little change in incidence and possibly an increase in prevalence, along with increased health care costs. Risk-factor prevalence data are available at the state level in the United States from sources like the Behavioral Risk Factor Survey. These data suggest that certain risk factors such as obesity and probably hypertension are, in fact, increasing. Such data may be useful in creating the political and social will to target populationwide behaviors at all levels.[10,11]

Public health education/media Community interventions have frequently used a variety of different channels of communication to increase awareness of CVD to modify public behaviors. Several community interventions to control CVD have used mass media and print media extensively. A useful consideration in selecting media for intervention is the audience and the message to be conveyed. Flora et al.[12] have proposed a framework in which the me-

dia might be selected (Fig. 22–5). Selection of a medium might focus on reaching a large number of people minimally or targeting a select group of the population more intensely. The message might serve to alert the audience or get them to contemplate the issue. The major types of mass media can thus be classified. Other types of media can be tailored to the local community, such as posters, church bulletins, etc.

Community organizations and partnerships A cornerstone of the Victoria Declaration on Heart Health[10] was the recognition that a large number of sectors of the community would have to become actively involved if the mass epidemic of CVD were to be controlled. These sectors would include (1) health, media, education, and social science professionals; (2) the scientific research community; (3) governmental agencies concerned with health, education, trade, commerce, and agriculture; (4) the private sector, including health, food, and transportation

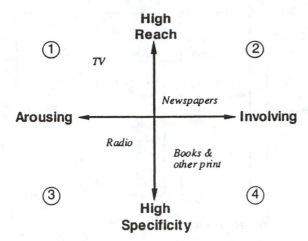

FIGURE 22–5 Dimensions of mass media in communication of health messages to a population. (From Flora et al.,[12] with permission.)

industries; (5) international organizations and agencies concerned with health and economic development; (6) community health coalitions and voluntary health organizations such as heart associations and foundations; (7) employers and employee organizations, such as unions. Coalition building would be essential to tackle a problem of this magnitude.

Policy and legislation Another approach to modification of populationwide behaviors could be the development of policies which affect the environments in which people live and the regulations by which they live.[7] In the United States, government policies involving tobacco have continued to evolve, including taxation, restriction of smoking in various buildings and work sites, control of sales of tobacco to children, elimination of advertising, etc. These policies are by no means limited to governments, with numerous private companies instituting their own regulations on clean air, increased health care and life insurance premiums for smokers, and even hiring criteria favoring nonsmokers. Similarly, policies related to physical activity might relate to requirements for physical education curricula in the schools, reimbursement for physical activity counseling by health care professionals, and development of facilities (gymnasia, walking/bicycling paths,

etc.), that would encourage safe physical activity. Finally, nutrition policy can be effective in changing eating behaviors through price supports and taxation, dietary guidelines, food assistance programs, school meals, etc.[13] The health care professional may also need to serve as an advocate to advance these policy goals.[11]

Evidence for Effectiveness in Various Settings

Interventions in whole communities Over the past 30 years, a number of studies to reduce the entire population's risk of CVD have been carried out in Europe, Africa, North America, and Australia.[14] These often include programs in specific community settings, such as work sites, schools, religious organizations, etc. Although the trials have differed considerably in their approach, a common theme was to change behavior not only in the individual but also in the family, society, and culture targeted for intervention. These communitywide interventions typically used multiple media, provided multiple health education messages, and had multiple target groups.[15,16]

Two early projects provided preliminary evidence for the efficacy of this approach. The Stanford Three Community Study (1972–1975) used two approaches, one with a mass media campaign (radio, television, print media) and intensive instruction of high-risk residents and the other using the media campaign alone, compared with no intervention in a comparison community.[17] The intervention communities demonstrated a 23 percent reduction in coronary heart disease (CHD) risk score compared with the comparison community.[18] The North Karelia Project (1972 to the present) consisted of a comprehensive, populationwide intervention in the Finnish province of North Karelia, which at the time had one of the highest CVD mortality rates in the world.[19] A similar province was used as a comparison group. The intervention consisted of a public education campaign using radio, newspapers and other printed material, group education, and environmental interventions. Striking reductions in smoking, fat consumed in the diet, blood pressure, and blood cholesterol were observed, and between 1972 and 1978,

FIGURE 22–6 Mortality from coronary heart disease in men 35 to 64 years of age in North Karelia versus the rest of Finland, 1968–1992. (From Puska et al.,[19] with permission.)

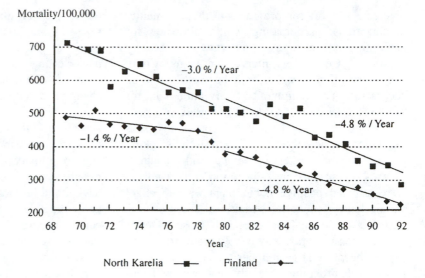

CVD mortality in North Karelia decreased faster than that in the comparison province and Finland as a whole (Fig. 22–6). These two projects provided the basis for a large number of additional programs to investigate the process of community interventions for CVD prevention in more detail.[14]

Three large U.S. trials were initiated to further explore community intervention in theory and in practice:[14] the Stanford Five-City Project (1980–1986),[20] the Minnesota Heart Health Program (1981–1988),[21] and the Pawtucket Heart Health Program (1984–1991).[22] Among the three projects, 13 communities with over 900,000 people were studied, using a nonrandomized assignment of some communities to intervention and others as comparison communities. A large number of materials were developed and field-tested (Table 22–1). The Stanford Five-City Project demonstrated reductions in smoking, cholesterol, blood pressure, and CHD risk, though the biggest changes occurred early in the comparison.[20] Evaluation of the Minnesota Heart Health Program suggested that physical activity increased and smoking decreased in women.[21] The Pawtucket Heart Health Program also showed a reduction in CHD risk.[22] All programs demonstrated success in organizing and in implementing various aspects of their intervention strategies.

These three large U.S. projects generally had less effect and less sustenance than hypothesized, for reasons that are not entirely clear.[7,14,23] There does seem to be consensus that community-based interventions—with multiple messages, multiple target groups, and using multiple media—can change the knowledge, attitudes, and behavior of individuals

TABLE 22–1 Materials Developed for Use in the Minnesota Heart Health Program, the Stanford Five-City Project, and the Pawtucket Heart Health Program

Mass media

Other print (kits, brochures, direct mail)

Events and contests

Screenings

Group and direct education

School programs

Worksite interventions

Physician and medical setting programs

Grocery store and restaurant projects

Church interventions

Policies

Source: From Schooler et al.,[14] with permission.

or create support for programs in the community organizations participating while allowing for environmental changes supportive of healthy lifestyles.[14] Community interventions targeting only one intervention, however, may be less likely to be successful. The Community Intervention Trial for Smoking Cessation (COMMIT) focused on smoking cessation among 11 matched community pairs but failed to demonstrate differences in smoking prevalence among intervention and control communities.[24] Quit rates in light-to-moderate smokers were affected positively, but there was no effect among heavy smokers.[25] Additional analyses suggest that subpopulations, especially those of lower socioeconomic status, may benefit more from these approaches.[26] A large number of subsequent communitywide programs currently under way will continue to enlarge this experience.[14]

Interventions in schools and youth organizations
Interventions among children attending school offer several advantages to population-based CVD prevention.[27] First, there is good evidence that atherosclerotic disease is well established by the late teenage years, that the risk factors measured in childhood track into adulthood, and that exercise, eating, and smoking behaviors are well established by the early teenage years. Second, school-based programs can involve venues other than the classroom, including school nutrition programs and physical education curricula. Third, school is mandatory, allowing most of the population to be reached. Finally, schoolchildren are an excellent vector for transmitting health messages home to their parents.

Over the past 20 years, a large number of school-based programs to reduce CVD risk have been implemented and evaluated, and 16 have been studied in detail.[27] In general, a variety of theoretical models were employed, with interventions using a wide range of educational techniques, durations and intensities of intervention, and target age groups. A meta-analysis of the studies suggests that interventions targeted at smoking behavior and knowledge about CVD and its risk factors were most effective; interventions to improve blood pressure and obesity were least effective; and diet, blood cholesterol, stress, and physical activity interventions were in-

termediate. Programs with multiple components seemed more effective than single-component interventions.[7] An interesting conclusion was that behavior change may be a more appropriate target for change in children, whose physiologic measures are changing rapidly during growth and development.

Intervention in religious organizations   Religious organizations also offer a number of advantages as sites for primary prevention of CVD. Religious communities often have strong influences on health behavior, and religious organizations offer social support, facilities, volunteers, and networks for communication.[28] Hard-to-reach subpopulations such as specific ethnic and racial groups may be accessed through their religious leaders. Despite this, very few studies have rigorously evaluated communities of faith as a means to reduce CVD risk. In one review, only six well-designed studies could be identified, and most are in progress.[28] At this point, it can best be concluded that religious organizations offer enormous untapped potential for development of effective CVD prevention programs.

Interventions at work sites   Work sites also offer a rich opportunity to influence employee behavior. Increasingly, employers are responsible for the health care costs of their work force, and replacement of skilled workers disabled or deceased from CVD is an added cost. Managed care organizations that have capitated contracts to provide health services to workers have an additional incentive to prevent rather than treat disease. Moreover, work sites can be more than sites to provide health education messages. Environmental interventions such as smoke-free areas and heart-healthy food services can be initiated. The employer can further provide incentives to reduce CVD through reduced health insurance premiums, hiring policies, etc.

A total of 12 well-documented studies of work-site CVD prevention programs have been identified.[29,30] A review of these studies suggests that brief, low-intensity interventions targeted at the entire work force show little evidence of effectiveness, whereas counseling provided to high-risk employees identified within the entire work force has had the best results. As employers and health care providers become increasingly concerned about costs, it is likely that work-site programs will expand as a means of identifying and modifying CVD risk in employees.

Summary

In general, there is cautious optimism that community-based interventions will influence CVD risk at relatively low cost. The continued emphasis on and assessment of the burden of CVD and its implications to health are important first steps. Media might be selected according to audience and the type of message that is to be conveyed. A variety of organizations need to get involved; it is unlikely that the health care system, a single voluntary organization, or even a government body can have substantial impact working alone. The role of regulations and policy to modify the environment has had increasing relevance, particularly with regard to tobacco and nutrition. These strategies can then be applied to schools, religious organizations, work sites, or even whole countries. The results have been mixed and are often difficult to interpret. However, many of the improvements have been widely disseminated as communities search for ways to prevent the CVD epidemic.

Individual Approaches to High-Risk Populations

Health care facilities should be included as important community settings for populationwide CVD risk reduction.[31] Physicians remain among the most credible sources of health information for the population, and the majority of the population has contact with the medical care system at least once a year. Surveys of CVD prevention-related services such as smoking-cessation advice, measurement and treatment of lipid disorders, and physical activity assessment and counseling are often disappointing.[32,33] A variety of factors at the levels of the patient, physician, health care setting, and community/society may interfere with the provision of these services (Table 22–2).[34]

As a first step in rectifying this problem, the American Heart Association has published a consensus panel statement putting forth recommendations for

TABLE 22–2 Barriers to Implementation of Preventive Services

Patient
  Lack of knowledge and motivation
  Lack of access to care
  Cultural factors
  Social factors
Physician
  Problem-based focus
  Feedback on prevention is native or neutral
  Time constraints
  Lack of incentives, including reimbursement
  Lack of training
    Poor knowledge of benefits
    Perceived ineffectiveness
    Lack of skills
  Lack of specialist-generalist communication
  Lack of perceived legitimacy
Health care settings (hospitals, practices, etc.)
  Acute care priority
  Lack of resources and facilities
  Lack of systems for preventive services
  Time and economic constraints
  Poor communication between specialty and primary care providers
  Lack of policies and standards
Community/society
  Lack of policies and standards
  Lack of reimbursement

Source: From Pearson et al.,[34] with permission.

the primary prevention of CVD in individuals (Table 22–3).[35] These guidelines include advice about risk-factor assessment, lifestyle modification, and pharmacologic interventions as well as recommendations regarding individual risk factors such as blood pressure,[36] blood lipids,[37] physical activity,[38] obesity,[39] and smoking.[40] Guidelines that highlight preventive cardiology strategies in women have also been issued.[41]

Individual Risk Assessment

A key recommendation is that CVD risk should be assessed in all patients through careful history, physical examination, and selected laboratory testing. Tobacco, diet, and physical activity should be routinely inquired about; blood pressure, height, weight, and waist/hip

TABLE 22–3   Guide to Primary Prevention of Cardiovascular Diseases

Risk Intervention	Recommendations	
Smoking: *Goal* **complete cessation**	Ask about smoking status as part of routine evaluation. Reinforce nonsmoking status. Strongly encourage patient and family to stop smoking. Provide counseling, nicotine replacement, and formal cessation programs as appropriate.	
Blood pressure control: *Goal* **<140/90 mmHg**	Measure blood pressure in all adults at least every $2\frac{1}{2}$ years. Promote lifestyle modification: weight control, physical activity, moderation in alcohol intake, and moderate sodium restriction. If blood pressure >140/90 mmHg after 3 months of life habit modification or if initial blood pressure >160/100 mmHg: add blood pressure medication, individualize therapy to patient's other requirements and characteristics.	
Cholesterol management: *Primary goal* **LDL <160 mg/dL** **if 0–1 risk factors** **or** **LDL <130 mg/dL** years **if ≥2 risk factors** *Secondary goals* **HDL >35 mg/dL;** **TG <200 mg/dL**	Ask about dietary habits as part of routine evaluation. Measure total and HDL cholesterol in all adults ≥20 years and assess positive and negative risk factors at least every 5 years. For all persons: promote AHA Step I Diet (≤30% fat, <10% saturated fat, <300 mg/day cholesterol), weight control, and physical activity. Measure LDL if total cholesterol ≥240 mg/dL or ≥200 mg/dL with ≥2 risk factors of if HDL <35 mg/dL. If LDL: ≥160 mg/dL with 0–1 risk factors; or ≥130 mg/dL on 2 occasions with ≥2 risk factors; then Start Step II Diet (≤30% fat, <7% saturated fat, <200 mg/dL cholesterol) and weight control. Rule out secondary causes of high LDL (LFTs, TFTs, UA). If LDL: ≥160 mg/dL plus two risk factors; or ≥190 mg/dL; or ≥220 mg/dL in men <35 y; or in premenopausal women; then consider adding drug therapy to diet therapy for LDL levels > those listed above that persist despite Step II diet.	Risk factors: age (men ≥45 years, women ≥55 or postmenopausal), hypertension, diabetes, smoking, HDL <35 mg/dL, family history of CHD in first-degree relatives (in male relatives <55 years, female relatives <65 years) HDL ≥60 mg/dL: Subtract 1 risk factor from the number of positive risk factors.

ratio should be assessed regularly, and serum total and HDL cholesterol levels should be measured in all adults 20 years of age and older. This assessment should not be time-consuming or expensive and is amenable to performance at settings outside of health care facilities, such as work sites, pharmacies, etc. Another key part of the recommendations is the establishment of goals for the various risk factors (Table 22–3). The definition of "desirable levels" serves as a means of identifying and prioritizing behavioral interventions. These levels provide goals for behavioral and pharmacologic intervention.

Another approach is the development of a *global risk score*. The concept here is to factor in the contribution of all of an individual's risk factors to an overall risk of CVD. One benefit of this approach is the identification of those who are at high risk not because of a high level of a single risk factor but rather because of the presence of several moderately elevated risk factors. It is likely that a larger pro-

Risk Intervention	Recommendations			
Cholesterol management (continued):	Suggested drug therapy for high LDL levels (≥160 mg/dL) (drug selection priority modified according to TG level)			
	TG <200 mg/dL	TG 200–400 mg/dL	TG >400 mg/dL	HDL <35 mg/dL: Emphasize weight management and physical activity, avoidance of cigarette smoking. Niacin raises HDL. Consider niacin if patient has ≥2 risk factors and high LDL (except patients with diabetes).
	Statin Resin Niacin	Statin Niacin	Consider combined drug (niacin, therapy fibrates, statin)	
	If LDL goal not achieved, consider combination drug therapy.			
Physical activity: **Goal** **Increase amount of exercise regularly 3–4 times per week for 30 min**	Ask about physical activity status and exercise habits as part of routine evaluation. Encourage 30 minutes of moderate-intensity dynamic exercise 3–4 times per week as well as increased physical activity in daily life habits for persons who are inactive. Encourage regular exercise to improve conditioning and optimize fitness level. Advise medically supervised programs for those with low functional capacity and/or comorbidities. Promote environmental factors conducive to health (e.g., golf courses that permit walking).			
Weight management: **Goal** **Achieve and maintain desirable BMI (21–25 kg/m²)**	Measure patient's weight and height, BMI, and waist-to-hip ratio at each visit as part of routine evaluation. Start weight management and physical activity as appropriate. Desirable BMI range: 21–25 kg/m². BMI of 25 kg/m² corresponds to percentage desirable body weight of 110%; desirable waist-to-hip ratio for men, <0.9; for middle-aged and elderly women, <0.8.			
Estrogens:	Consider estrogen replacement in all postmenopausal women, especially those with multiple CHD risk factors, such as elevated LDL. Individualize recommendation consistent with other health risks.			

Key: TG, triglycerides; LFTs, liver function tests, TFTs, thyroid function tests; UA, uric acid; CHD, coronary heart disease; BMI, body-mass index.

Source: Grundy et al.,[35] with permission.

portion of the population at high risk falls into this latter group and not into that comprising those with a single elevated risk factor.[42] The Framingham Risk Equation has recently been updated.[43] It includes total serum low-density-lipoprotein (LDL) cholesterol, systolic and diastolic blood pressure, age, sex, HDL cholesterol, diabetes, and smoking grouped into categories to which scores are assigned and summed so as to provide estimates of both relative and absolute risk (see Chap. 1, Figs. 1–2 and 1–3). The estimates of relative risk have been generally robust from one population to the next. Estimates of absolute risk likely require additional calibration to take into account the underlying risk of the population being assessed. The Joint European Societies have used this multiple-risk approach to develop figures that allow the visual calculation of a previous absolute risk of developing CHD over the next 10 years based on age, sex, smoking, systolic blood pressure, and total cholesterol level[44] (Fig. 22–7).

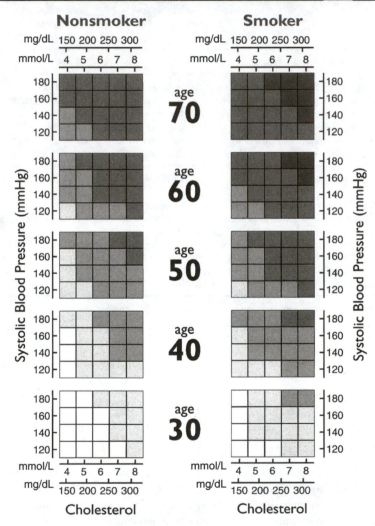

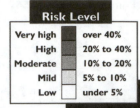

Risk Level

Very high		over 40%
High		20% to 40%
Moderate		10% to 20%
Mild		5% to 10%
Low		under 5%

MEN

Risk of Coronary Heart Disease

Nonsmoker

mg/dL 150 200 250 300
mmol/L 4 5 6 7 8

Systolic Blood Pressure (mmHg)

age **70**
age **60**
age **50**
age **40**
age **30**

mmol/L 4 5 6 7 8
mg/dL 150 200 250 300

Cholesterol

Smoker

mg/dL 150 200 250 300
mmol/L 4 5 6 7 8

Systolic Blood Pressure (mmHg)

mmol/L 4 5 6 7 8
mg/dL 150 200 250 300

Cholesterol

How to use the Coronary Risk Chart for Primary Prevention

The chart is for estimating coronary heart disease (CHD) risk for individuals who have not developed symptomatic CHD or other atherosclerotic disease. Patients with CHD are already at high risk and require intensive lifestyle intervention and, as necessary, drug therapies to achieve risk factor goals.

- **To estimate a person's absolute 10-year risk of a CHD event,** find the table for their gender, smoking status, and age. Within the table, find the cell nearest to their systolic blood pressure (mmHg) and total cholesterol (mmol/L or mg/dL).

- **The effect of lifetime exposure to risk factors** can be seen by following the table upwards. This can be used when advising younger people.

- **High-risk individuals are defined as those whose 10-year CHD risk exceeds 20% or will exceed 20% if projected to age 60.**

A

FIGURE 22–7 Coronary risk charts for men (*A*) and women (*B*). (From Pyrola K et al., with permission.[44])

Risk Level		
Very high		over 40%
High		20% to 40%
Moderate		10% to 20%
Mild		5% to 10%
Low		under 5%

WOMEN
Risk of Coronary Heart Disease

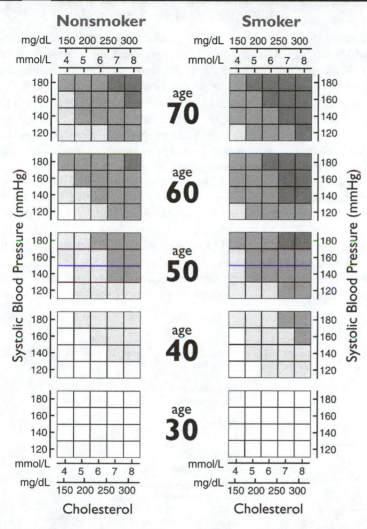

Nonsmoker

Smoker

mg/dL 150 200 250 300

mmol/L 4 5 6 7 8

age **70**

age **60**

age **50**

age **40**

age **30**

Systolic Blood Pressure (mmHg)

Cholesterol

- **CHD risk is higher than indicated** in the chart for those with
  - Familial hyperlipidemia
  - Diabetes: risk is approximately doubled in men and more than doubled in women
  - Those with a family history of premature cardiovascular disease
  - Those with low HDL cholesterol. These tables assume HDL cholesterol to be 1.0 mmol/L (39 mg/dL) in men and 1.1 (43) in women
  - Those with raised triglyceride levels >2.0 mmol/L (>180 mg/dL)
  - As the person approaches the next age category.

- **To find a person's relative risk,** compare their risk category with that for other people of the same age. The absolute risk shown here may not apply to all populations, especially those with a low CHD incidence. Relative risk is likely to apply to most populations.

- **The effect of changing** cholesterol, smoking status, or blood pressure can be read from the chart.

B

It is likely that additional methods for risk assessment will be developed and prove to be cost-effective in the health care setting. In this context, it is useful to differentiate risk factors from risk markers. The term *risk factor* is usually reserved for a characteristic felt to be etiologically related to a disease. The implication is that modification of the factor will prevent the disease's development or progression. Other characteristics may be associated with a disease, but not necessarily in an etiologic fashion. Such characteristics are called *risk markers,* which can be used to identify persons at high risk for the disease in whom aggressive intervention may be worthwhile. A variety of new risk markers have been proposed, including measures of inflammation (e.g., C-reactive protein), prothrombotic diathesis (e.g., fibrinogen), altered endothelial function (e.g., endothelium-dependent brachial reactivity), physiologic evidence of atherosclerosis (e.g., ankle-brachial blood pressure index), or noninvasive evidence of atherosclerosis (carotid artery intima/media thickness ratios, coronary calcification on electron beam computed tomography). Many of these new risk assessment approaches are promising but have not been fully examined in primary prevention settings for efficacy or cost-effectiveness. Well-designed clinical studies,

such as the ongoing National Institutes of Health–sponsored Multiethnic Study of Atherosclerosis (MESA),[45] will further define the role of a number of screening modalities in cardiovascular risk assessment.

Matching the Level of Risk with the Intensity of the Intervention

The use of information about an individual's risk may differ between the patient, the care provider, and the payer for health care services.[46] Traditionally, risk estimation has been used to inform the patient of the importance of changes in risk behaviors or the need for treatment. Increasingly, however, health care providers and payers have used risk stratification to better reserve aggressive (and often expensive) interventions for those at highest risk. Interventions to lower LDL cholesterol serve as a good illustration (Fig. 22–8).[37,47] Clinical trials of HMG-CoA reductase inhibitors have demonstrated efficacy in virtually every stratum of risk, from persons with elevated LDL-cholesterol levels and myocardial infarction to persons without evidence of coronary disease and relatively normal LDL-cholesterol levels. The recent Air Force/Texas Coronary Atherosclero-

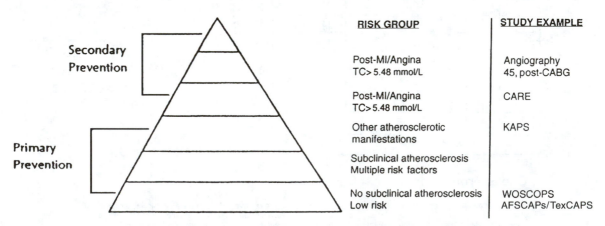

FIGURE 22–8 Pyramid of risk. CARE, cholesterol and recurrent events; KAPS, Kuopio Atherosclerosis Prevention Study; post-CABG, post-coronary artery bypass grafts; 4S, Scandinavian Simvastatin Survival Study; MI, myocardial infarction; TC, total cholesterol; WOSCOPS, West of Scotland Coronary Prevention Study; AFCAPS/TexCAPS, Air Force/Texas Coronary Atherosclerosis Prevention Study. (From Downs JR et al.,[48] with permission.)

sis Prevention Study (AFCAPS/TexCAPS) serves as a good example.[48] In the trial, 85 percent of participants would not have met treatment criteria for the National Cholesterol Education Program,[37] yet there was a statistically significant reduction in coronary endpoints. The primary consideration in the use of these agents then moves to one of cost-effectiveness rather than efficacy. The rationale is to limit expensive interventions to those among whom the expected reduction in the number of expensive cases of vascular disease is great enough to counterbalance the cost of the preventive intervention.[49]

Guidelines for the National Cholesterol Education Program[37] and the Sixth Report of the Joint National Committee on Prevention, Detection, Evaluation, and Treatment of High Blood Pressure (JNC VI)[36] are based on concepts of risk stratification. These guidelines vary the thresholds for initiation of treatment and the goals of therapy depending on the presence of vascular disease and the number of coexisting cardiovascular risk factors, as in the case of LDL-cholesterol levels for initiation and goals of treatment (Table 22–4). The Joint European Societies have taken this one step further and have recommended the use of pharmacologic therapy based on estimation of absolute risk.[44] For example, pharmacologic therapy for LDL-cholesterol levels equal to or greater than 3.0 mmol/L (115 mg/dL) is reserved for those with an absolute risk of coronary disease of greater than 20 percent over the next 10 years.

Strategies to Improve Primary Prevention in Clinical Settings

A large number of studies have examined interventions in health care practice settings to improve the level of preventive interventions.[31] While many of the studies have involved patients with CVD in secondary prevention programs, a large number have involved primary care practices and patients prior to onset of symptomatic disease. Both single-risk-factor interventions and multiple-risk modifications have been studied. Although the secondary prevention studies demonstrated greater impact, a number of lessons have been learned about the implementation of primary prevention in clinical settings. First, education and training programs of health care providers can increase the quantity and quality of preventive services, especially when combined with performance feedback and practice guidelines.[34] Second, an important step is the reorganization of

TABLE 22–4 LDL-Cholesterol Thresholds for Initiation and Goals of Treatment: The National Cholesterol Education Program Adult Treatment Panel Guidelines

Risk Stratum	Low-Density-Lipoprotein Cholesterol (mg/dL)		Treatment Goal
	Initiation of Therapy		
	Diet	Drug	
No coronary disease <2 risk factors*	≥160	≥190	<160
No coronary disease, 2+ risk factors*	≥130	≥160	<130
Coronary or other vascular disease	≥100	≥130	<100

*Risk factors include male ≥45 years or female ≥55 years or premature menopause without estrogen replacement therapy; family history of myocardial infarction in first-degree male relative < 55 years or first-degree female relative < 65 years; current cigarette smoking; hypertension; HDL-C < 35 mg/dL; and diabetes. An HDL-C ≥60 allows one risk factor to be subtracted.

Source: Expert Panel on Detection, Evaluation and Treatment of High Blood Cholesterol in Adults, National Cholesterol Education Program,[37] with permission.

the practice setting to an emphasis on prevention, providing the physician with resources and tools to both speed the process and to improve the quality of the intervention. Third, the practice of reorganization often entails formation of a multidisciplinary team, with some members such as nurses, nutritionists, and counselors, etc., often being more accessible to the patient and more effective than physicians in providing risk-factor counseling and other preventive services. They should be given the training, responsibility, and tools to carry out various aspects of the intervention. Thus, a systems approach to primary prevention may increasingly allow the health care system to play a larger role in population-based primary prevention. Chapter 24 provides further details regarding the organization of preventive cardiology services.

Conclusions

A cornerstone of any approach to reduce the population's burden of CVD must be a primary prevention program aimed at reduction of risk behaviors on a populationwide basis and on the identification, stratification, and selected treatment of high-risk individuals prior to their development of disease. These two approaches should be complementary. The health care system should benefit from population-wide efforts via health education, environmental intervention, or legislation to reduce the burden of deleterious health behaviors. These changes should facilitate risk-factor change in the clinical setting. On the other hand, policymakers, employers, and community leaders look to health care providers to provide advice and leadership. Both the capacity to prevent CVD and the will to implement policies and programs will be necessary to reduce CVD in communities *and* physicians' offices.[11]

References

1. Swan HJC, Gersh BJ, Grayboys TB, Ullyot DJ: Evaluation and management of risk factors for the individual patient (case management). *J Am Coll Cardiol* 1996; 27:1030–1047.

2. Pearson TA, Jamison DT. Trejo-Gutierrez J: Cardiovascular disease. In: Jamison DT, Mosley WH, Measham AR, and Bobadilla JL (eds): *Disease Control Priorities in Developing Countries.* New York, Oxford University Press, 1993: 577–594.

3. Rose G: Sick individuals and sick populations. *Int J Epidemiol* 1989; 14:32–38.

4. Carleton RA, Dwyer J, Findberg L, et al: Report of the Expert Panel on Population Strategies for Blood Cholesterol Reduction. *Circulation* 1991; 83:2154–2232.

5. Blackburn H: Epidemiological basis of a community strategy for the prevention of cardiopulmonary disease. *Ann Epidemiol* 1997; 7(suppl):S8–S13.

6. *The President's Health Security Plan: The Clinton Blueprint.* New York, Times Books, 1993.

7. Stone EJ, Pearson TA, Fortmann SP, McKinley JB: Community-based prevention trials: challenges and directions for public health practice, policy, and research. *Ann Epidemiol* 1997; 7(suppl):S113–S120.

8. Carleton RA, Lasater TM: Population intervention to reduce coronary heart disease incidence. In: Pearson TA, Criqui MH, Luepker RV, et al (eds): *Primer in Preventive Cardiology,* Dallas, American Heart Association, 1994: 285–292.

9. Committee on Research: *Development, and Institutional Strengthening for Control of Cardiovascular Diseases in Developing Countries.* Washington, DC, National Academy Press, 1998.

10. Advisory Board of the International Heart Health Conference: *The Victoria Declaration on Heart Health.* Victoria, British Columbia, Dept. of Health and Welfare, 1992.

11. Pearson TA, Bales VS, Blair L, et al: The Singapore Declaration: Forging the Will for Heart Health in the Next Millennium. *CVD Prevention* 1998; 1:182–199.

12. Flora JA, Saphir MN, Schooler C, Rimal RN: Toward a framework for intervention channels: reach, involvement, and impact. *Ann Epidemiol* 1997; S104–S112.

13. Pearson TA: Population strategy. In: Rifkind BM (ed): *Lowering Cholesterol in High Risk Individuals and Populations.* New York, Marcel Dekker, 1995: 149–166.

14. Schooler C, Farquhar JW, Fortmann SP, Flora JA: Synthesis of findings and issues from community prevention trials. *Ann Epidemiol* 1997; 7(suppl):S54–S68.

15. Shea S, Basch CE: A review of five major community-based cardiovascular disease prevention programs: Part I. Rationale, design, and theoretical framework. *Am J Health Promotion* 1990; 4:203–213.

16. Mittelmark MB, Luepker RV, Jacobs DR, et al: Community-wide prevention of cardiovascular disease: education strategies of the Minnesota Heart Health Program. *Prev Med* 1986; 15:1–17.

17. Maccoby N, Farquhar JW, Wood PD, Alexander J: Reducing the risk of cardiovascular disease: effects of a community-based campaign on knowledge and behavior. *J Community Health* 1977; 3:100–114.

18. Farquhar JW, Wood PD, Breitrose H, et al: Community education for cardiovascular health. *Lancet* 1977; 1:1192–1195.

19. Puska P, Tuomilehto J, Nissinen A, Vartiainen E (eds.): *The North Karelia Project: 20 Year Results and Experiences.* Helsinki: National Public Health Institute, KTL, 1995.

20. Farquhar JW, Fortmann SP, Flora JA, et al: The Stanford Five-City Project: Effect of community-wide education on cardiovascular disease risk factors. *JAMA* 1990; 264:359–365.

21. Luepker RV, Murray DM, Jacobs DR, et al: Community education for cardiovascular disease prevention: risk factors changes in the Minnesota Heart Health Program. *Am J Public Health* 1994; 84:1383–1393.

22. Carleton RA, Lasater TM, Assaf AR, et al: The Pawtucket Heart Health Program: community changes in cardiovascular risk factors and projected disease risk. *Am J Public Health* 1995; 85:777–785.

23. Baranowski T, Lin LS, Wetter DW, et al: Theory as mediating variables: Why aren't community interventions working as desired? *Ann Epidemiol* 1997; 7(suppl):S89–S95.

24. The COMMIT Research Group: Community Intervention Trial for Smoking Cessation (COMMIT): II. Changes in adult cigarette smoking prevalence. *Am J Public Health* 1995; 85:193–200.

25. The COMMIT Research Group: Community Intervention Trial for Smoking Cessation (COMMIT): I. Cohort results from a four-year community intervention. *Am J Public Health* 1995; 85:183–192.

26. Winkleby MA: Accelerating cardiovascular risk factor change in ethnic minority and low socioeconomic groups. *Ann Epidemiol* 1997; 7(suppl):S96–S103.

27. Resnicow K, Robinson TN: School-based cardiovascular disease prevention studies: review and synthesis. *Ann Epidemiol* 1997; S7:S14–S31.

28. Lasater TM, Becker DM, Hill MN, Gans KM: Synthesis of findings and issues from religious-based cardiovascular disease prevention trials. *Ann Epidemiol* 1997; 7(suppl):S46–S53.

29. Jeffery R, Forster J, French S: The Healthy Worker Project: a worksite intervention for weight control and smoking cessation. *Am J Public Health* 1993; 83:395–401.

30. Pelletier K. A review and analysis of the health and cost-effective outcome studies of comprehensive health promotion and disease prevention programs at the worksite: 1993–1995 update. *Am J Health Promotion* 1996; 19:380–388.

31. Ockene JK, McBride PE, Sallis JF, et al: Synthesis of lessons learned from cardiopulmonary preventive interventions in healthcare practice settings. *Ann Epidemiol* 1997; 7(suppl):S32–S45.

32. Kottke TE, Brekke ML, Solberg LI: Making time for preventive services. *Mayo Clin Proc* 1993; 68:785–791.

33. Miller M, Konkel K, Fitzpatrick D, et al: Divergent reporting of coronary risk factors before coronary artery bypass surgery. *Am J Cardiol* 1995; 75:736–737.

34. Pearson TA, McBride PE, Houston-Miller N, Smith SC Jr: Organization of preventive cardiology service. *J Am Coll Cardiol* 1996; 27:1039–1047.

35. Grundy SM, Balady GJ, Criqui MH, et al: Guide to primary prevention of cardiovascular diseases: a statement for healthcare professionals from the task force on risk reduction. *Circulation* 1997; 95:2329–2331.

36. The Sixth Report of the Joint National Committee on Prevention, Detection, Evaluation, and Treatment of High Blood Pressure. *Arch Intern Med* 1997; 157:2413–2446.

37. Expert Panel on Detection, Evaluation, and Treatment of High Blood Cholesterol in Adults, National Cholesterol Education Program: Second Report of the Expert Panel on Detection, Evaluation, and Treatment of High Blood Cholesterol in Adults (Adult Treatment Panel II). *Circulation* 1994; 89:1329–1445.

38. Wenger NK, Foelicher ES, Smith LK, et al: *Cardiac Rehabilitation.* Clinical Practice Guideline no.17. Rockville, MD, Agency for Health Care Policy and Research and the National Heart, Lung, and Blood Institute, 1995.

39. NHLBI Obesity Education Initiative Expert panel in the Identification, Evaluation, and Treatment of Overweight and Obesity in Adults: Clinical guidelines on the identification, evaluation, and treatment of overweight and obesity in adults—the evidence report. *Obesity Res* 1998; 6(suppl.2):51S–210S.

40. Fiore M, Bailey W, Cohen S, et al: *Smoking Cessation: Clinical Practice Guideline No. 18.* Rockville, MD, U.S. Department of Public Health and Human Services, Public Health Service, Agency for Health Care Policy and Research, 1996.

41. Mosca CJ, Grundy JM, Judelson D, et al: A Guide to preventive cardiology in women. AHA/ACC Scientific Statement, Consensus Panel Statement. *Circulation* 1999; 99:2480–2484.

42. Grundy SM, Balady GJ, Criqui MH, et al: Primary prevention of coronary heart disease: Guidance from Framingham. A statement for healthcare professionals for the AHA Task Force on Risk Reduction. *Circulation* 1998; 97:1876–1887.

43. Wilson PWF, D'Agostino RB, Levy D, et al: Prediction of coronary heart disease using risk factor categories. *Circulation* 1998; 97:1837–1847.

44. Pyorala K, De Backer G, Graham I, et al: Prevention of coronary heart disease in clinical practice: recommendations of the Second Joint Task Force of European and Other Societies on Coronary Prevention. *Eur Heart J* 1998; 19:1434–1503.

45. National Heart, Lung, and Blood Institute National Institutes of Health: NHLBI-HC-98-XX. *Subclinical Cardiovascular Disease Study.* Request for proposals. Washington, DC, NHLBI/NIH, 1998.

46. Califf RM, Armstrong PW, Carver JR, et al: 27th Bethesda Conference: matching the intensity of risk management with the hazard for coronary disease events. Task Force 5: Stratification of patients into high, medium, and low risk subgroups for purposes of risk factor management. *J Am Coll Cardiol* 1996; 27:1007–1019.

47. Werner RM, Pearson TA: LDL-cholesterol: A risk factor for coronary artery disease—from epidemiology to clinical trials. *Can J Cardiol* 1998; 14(suppl B): 3B–10B.

48. Downs JR, Clearfield M, Weis S, et al: Primary prevention of acute coronary events with lovastatin in men and women with average cholesterol levels: results of AF-CAPS/TexCAPS: Air Force/Texas Coronary Atherosclerosis Prevention Study. *JAMA* 1998; 279:1615–1622.

49. Goldman L, Garber AM, Grover SA, Hlatky MA: 27th Bethesda Conference: matching the intensity of risk factor management with the hazard for coronary disease events. Task Force 6: Cost effectiveness of assessment and management of risk factors. *J Am Coll Cardiol* 1996; 27: 1020–1030.

CHAPTER 23

Secondary Prevention

Robert D. Brook
Philip Greenland

econdary prevention of cardiovascular disease (CVD) comprises medical interventions and behaviors of patients that aim to reduce complications, recurrent cardiac events, and underlying CVD progression. Cardiovascular event rates in CVD patients are approximately five to seven times higher than event rates in previously healthy individuals.[1,2] Owing to the high absolute risk of clinical events in patients with established CVD, secondary prevention is both important and potentially highly efficient.

Risk-factor modification is the primary route by which secondary prevention is accomplished. Major national organizations such as the American Heart Association[3] and the American College of Cardiology[2] have advocated risk-factor modification as the cornerstone of optimal medical care in patients with CVD. Similar emphasis on secondary prevention has been a focus of clinical recommendations outside of the United States as well.[4] This chapter reviews approaches toward risk assessment in persons with preexisting coronary heart disease (CHD) as well as evidence and recommendations regarding the risk factors for which intervention is of proven, probable, or possible benefit.

Cardiovascular Risk Assessment in Persons with Preexisting Coronary Artery Disease

Risk stratification of patients with CHD involves considering the following five categories of patients:

(1) those with stable CHD, (2) those with unstable angina, (3) patients with acute myocardial infarction, (4) those who have undergone coronary artery bypass surgery, and (5) patients who have had percutaneous coronary intervention. All have diseased arteries susceptible to plaque fissuring and subsequent thrombosis. Figure 23–1 shows that the patient hospitalized with myocardial infarction or unstable angina is at particularly high risk during the initial month following hospitalization, during which the myocardium is subject to sudden electrical instability or the disrupted plaque may undergo rethrombosis. Figure 23–2 shows that the risk after bypass grafting is highest during the first year, when there is an increased risk of graft occlusion.[2,5]

In evaluating the patient with preexisting coronary artery disease for future risk of cardiovascular events, the value of the medical history, physical examination, 12-lead electrocardiogram, and appropriate laboratory tests needs to be recognized. The Framingham Heart Study has assembled algorithms for determining the 2-year risk of CHD events, stroke, or cerebrovascular disease death in women (Table 23–1) and men (Table 23–2) with existing CHD. These tables may be useful for initial risk stratification, but they should be considered only approximate guides to risk assessment. Clinical presentation, including angina or the chest-pain type, as well as comorbidities also figure into the determination of prognosis (Table 23–3). Other risk markers, such as fibrinogen, or more detailed information about symptoms, coronary anatomy, left ventricular function, or results from stress testing

FIGURE 23–1 Risk of future cardiac events as a function of time since the event or procedure. (From Smith et al.,[5] with permission.) *Key:* MI, myocardial infarction.

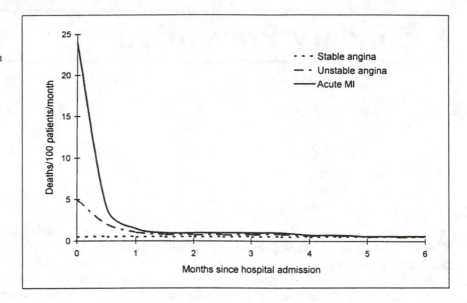

FIGURE 23–2 Risk of occlusion due to thrombosis or mechanical obstruction as a function of time from coronary artery bypass surgery. (From Smith et al.,[5] with permission.)

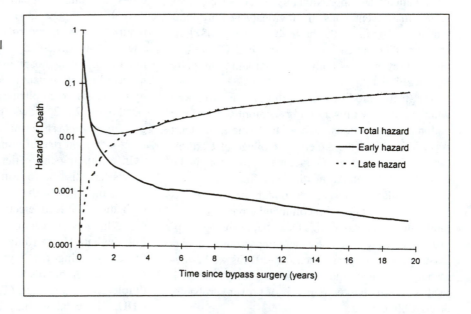

can provide important additional information for risk assessment.

The major CHD risk factors also remain important predictors of long-term prognosis in persons with CHD. Over an average of nearly 10 years of follow-up, systolic blood pressure, total cholesterol, and diabetes remained important predictors for the risk of reinfarction or coronary heart disease death among subjects who sustained a previous myocardial infarction in the Framingham Heart Study.[6]

TABLE 23–1 Risk of Coronary Artery Disease Event, Stroke, or Cerebrovascular Disease Death in Women with Existing Coronary Artery Disease

Age, years	Points	Total-C, mg/dL	Points by HDL-C, mg/dL									SBP (mmHg)	Points
			25	30	35	40	45	50	60	70	80		
35	0	160	4	3	3	2	2	1	1	0	0	100	0
40	1	170	4	3	3	2	2	2	1	1	0	110	0
45	2	180	4	3	3	2	2	2	1	1	0	120	1
50	3	190	4	4	3	3	2	2	1	1	1	130	1
55	4	200	4	4	3	3	2	2	2	1	1	140	2
60	5	210	4	4	3	3	3	2	2	1	1	150	2
65	6	220	5	4	4	3	3	2	2	1	1	160	2
70	7	230	5	4	4	3	3	3	2	2	1	170	3
75	7	240	5	4	4	3	3	3	2	2	1	180	3
		250	5	4	4	4	3	3	2	2	1	190	3
		260	5	5	4	4	3	3	2	2	1	200	3
		270	5	5	4	4	3	3	2	2	2	210	4
Other	Points	280	5	5	4	4	3	3	3	2	2	220	4
Diabetes	3	290	5	5	4	4	4	3	3	2	2	230	4
Smoking	3	300	6	5	4	4	4	3	3	2	2	240	4
												250	4

Average 2-year Risk in Women with CVD

Total Points	2-year Probability, percent	Age, years	Probability, percent
0	0	35–39	<1
2	1	40–44	<1
4	1	45–49	<1
6	1	50–54	4
8	2	55–59	6
10	4	60–64	8
12	6	65–69	12
14	10	70–74	12
16	15		
18	23		
20	35		
22	51		
24	68		
26	85		

Key: HDL-C, high-density-lipoprotein cholesterol; SBP, systolic blood pressure; CVD, cardiovascular disease.

Source: From Califf et al.,[2] with permission.

TABLE 23–2 Risk of Coronary Artery Disease Event, Stroke, or Cerebrovascular Disease Death in Men with Existing Coronary Artery Disease

Age, years	Points	Total-C, mg/dL	Points by HDL-C, mg/dL									SBP (mmHg)	Points
			25	30	35	40	45	50	60	70	80		
35	0	160	6	5	4	4	3	2	1	1	0	100	0
40	1	170	6	5	5	4	3	3	2	1	0	110	1
45	1	180	7	6	5	4	4	3	2	1	1	120	1
50	2	190	7	6	5	4	4	3	2	2	1	130	2
55	2	200	7	6	5	5	4	4	3	2	1	140	2
60	3	210	7	6	6	5	4	4	3	2	1	150	3
65	3	220	8	7	6	5	5	4	3	2	2	160	3
70	4	230	8	7	6	5	5	4	3	3	2	170	4
75	4	240	8	7	6	6	5	4	4	3	2	180	4
		250	8	7	6	6	5	5	4	3	2	190	4
		260	8	7	7	6	5	5	4	3	2	200	5
		270	9	8	7	6	6	5	4	3	3	210	5
Other	Points	280	9	8	7	6	6	5	4	4	3	220	5
Diabetes	1	290	9	8	7	7	6	5	4	4	3	230	6
		300	9	8	7	7	6	6	5	4	3	240	6
												250	6

Average 2-year Risk in Men with CVD

Total Points	2-year Probability, percent	Age, years	Probability, percent
0	2	35–39	<1
2	2	40–44	8
4	3	45–49	10
6	5	50–54	11
8	7	55–59	12
10	10	60–64	12
12	14	65–69	14
14	20	70–74	14
16	28		
18	37		
20	49		
22	63		
24	77		

Key: HDL-C, high-density-lipoprotein cholesterol; SBP, systolic blood pressure; CVD, cardiovascular disease.
Source: From Califf et al.,[2] with permission.

TABLE 23–3   Risk of Mortality at 1 Year: Clinical History Variables

1. Find points for each risk factor:

Age, years	Points	Angina, pain type	Points	Comorbid Factor	Points*
20	0	Nonanginal pain	3	CVD	20
30	13	Atypical angina	25	PVD	23
40	25	Typical angina		Diabetes	20
50	38	Stable	41	Prior MI	17
60	50	Progressive	46	Hypertension	8
70	62	Unstable	51	Mitral regurgitation	
80	75			Mild	19
90	88			Severe	38
100	100				

2. Sum points for all risk factors:

 ____Age____ + ____pain score____ + ____comorbidity____ = ____point total____

3. Look up risk corresponding to point total:

Total Points	Probability of 1-year Death	Total Points	Probability of 1-year Death
84	1%	184	20%
106	2%	199	30%
120	3%	211	40%
136	5%	220	50%
160	10%	229	60%

*Zero points for each "no."

Key: CVD, cerebrovascular disease; MI, myocardial infarction; PVD, peripheral vascular disease.

Source: From Califf et al.,[2] with permission.

Risk-Factor Modifications of Proven or Likely Benefit in Patients with Cardiovascular Disease

The value of specific risk interventions among patients with coronary or other vascular disease is well recognized. The American Heart Association[3] consensus panel statement for preventing heart attack and death in patients with coronary disease provides specific recommendations and goals for risk reduction (Table 23–4). The evidence and rationale for the major recommendations for modifiable risk factors are described below.

Cholesterol as a Risk Factor and Evidence from Secondary Prevention Trials

Serum cholesterol level is a well-established major risk factor for CVD outcomes in otherwise healthy people.[7,8] Cholesterol levels are associated with increased rates of initial coronary events or death in large population studies such as the Framingham

TABLE 23–4 Guide to Comprehensive Risk Reduction for Patients with Coronary and Other Vascular Disease

Risk Intervention	Recommendations			
Smoking: <u>Goal</u> complete cessation	Strongly encourage patient and family to stop smoking. Provide counseling, nicotine replacement, and formal cessation programs as appropriate.			

Lipid management:
  <u>Primary goal,</u>
  LDL <100 mg/dL
  <u>Secondary goals,</u>
  HDL >35 mg/dL;
  TG <200 mg/dL
	Start AHA Step 2 Diet in all patients: ≤30% fat, <7% saturated fat, <200 mg/day cholesterol.
	Assess fasting lipid profile. In post-MI patients, lipid profile may take 4 to 6 weeks to stabilize.
	  Add drug therapy according to the following guide:			

	LDL <100 mg/dL	LDL 100 to 130 mg/dL	LDL >130 mg/dL	HDL <35 mg/dL
	No drug therapy	Consider adding drug therapy to diet, as follows:	Add drug therapy to diet, as follows:	Emphasize weight management and physical activity. Advise smoking cessation. If needed to achieve LDL goals, consider niacin, statin, fibrates.
		Suggested drug therapy		
		TG <200 mg/dL Statin Resin Niacin	TG 200 to 400 mg/dL Statin Niacin	TG >400L mg/dL Consider combined drug therapy (niacin, fibrates, statin)	
	If LDL goal not achieved, consider combination drug therapy.			

Physical activity:
  <u>Minimum goal</u>
  30 min 3 to 4
  times per week
	Assess risk, preferably with exercise test, to guide prescription.
	Encourage minimum of 30 to 60 min of moderate-intensity activity three or four times weekly (walking, jogging, cycling, or other aerobic activity) supplemented by an increase in daily lifestyle activities (e.g., walking breaks at work, using stairs, gardening, household work). Maximum benefit 5 to 6 h a week.
	Advise medically supervised programs for moderate- to high-risk patients.			

Weight management	Start intensive diet and appropriate physical intervention, as outlined above, in patients >120% of ideal weight for height. Particularly emphasize need for weight loss in patients with hypertension, elevated triglycerides, or elevated glucose levels.			
Antiplatelet agents/ anticoagulants	Start aspirin 80 to 325 mg/day if not contraindicated. Manage warfarin to International Normalized Ratio = 2 to 3.5 post-MI patients not able to take aspirin.			
ACE inhibitors post-MI	Start early post-MI in stable high-risk patients (anterior MI, previous MI, Killip class II [S_3 gallop, rales, radiographic CHF]). Continue indefinitely for all with LV dysfunction (ejection fraction ≤40%) or symptoms of failure. Use as needed to manage blood pressure or symptoms in all other patients.			
Beta blockers	Start in high-risk post-MI patients (arrhythmia, LV dysfunction, inducible ischemia) at 5 to 28 days. Continue 6 months minimum. Observe usual contraindications. Use as needed to manage angina, rhythm, or blood pressure in all other patients.			

(continued)

Estrogens	Consider estrogen replacement in all postmenopausal women. Individualize recommendation consistent with other health risks.
Blood pressure control:	Initiate lifestyle modification—weight control, physical activity, alcohol moderation, and moderate sodium restriction—in all patients with blood pressure >140 mmHg systolic or 90 mmHg diastolic.
Goal ≤140/90 mmHg	Add blood pressure medication, individualized to other patient requirements and characteristics (i.e., age, race, need for drugs with specific benefits) **if** blood pressure is not less than 140 mmHg systolic or 90 mmHg diastolic in 3 months **or** if *initial* blood pressure is >160 mmHg systolic or 100 mmHg diastolic.

Key: LDL, low-density lipoprotein; HDL, high-density lipoprotein; CHF, congestive heart failure; ACE, angiotensin-converting enzyme; MI, myocardial infarction; TG, triglycerides; LV, left ventricular.

Source: American Heart Association,[3] with permission.

Heart Study[7] as well as in large primary prevention trials such as the Lipid Research Clinics Primary Prevention Trial[8] and the Multiple Risk Factor Intervention Trial.[9]

The prognostic value of serum cholesterol levels in patients with established CVD has also been demonstrated. In a population-based observational study in survivors of myocardial infarction (MI), Framingham Heart Study data showed the importance of cholesterol levels for predicting recurrent infarction and total mortality.[10] Survivors of MI with cholesterol levels of 275 mg/dL or greater compared with MI survivors in the reference range of less than 200 mg/dL were found to have a relative risk of 2.8 for recurrent MI. This association held true for men and women as well as for the elderly.[10] Similarly, in the Lipid Research Clinics Prevalence study, men with a cholesterol level of 240 mg/dL or greater had a three to four times higher risk of death due to CVD as compared with men whose cholesterol levels were less than 200 mg/dL. Relative risks were also elevated for high low-density-lipoprotein cholesterol (LDL-C) and for low high-density-lipoprotein cholesterol (HDL-C) (hazard ratios each about 6.0).[11] A review of the relatively small-scale studies conducted prior to 1990 stressed the causal importance of cholesterol levels of reinfarction in observational studies as well as in controlled clinical trials.[1]

In the 1990s, secondary prevention trials demonstrated further the important role of blood lipids in patients with preexisting CHD. For example, in an analysis of the Scandinavian Simvastatin Survival

Study, a positive relation was found between several lipid measures (with the exception of apolipoprotein A-I) and the subsequent risk of major cardiovascular events. Non-HDL-C, triglycerides, and total cholesterol/HDL-C ratio were most highly correlated with recurrent coronary events.[12]

During and prior to the 1980s, secondary prevention trials such as the Coronary Drug Project sought to determine the effect of cholesterol reduction in patients with CVD.[13] Most of the early trials demonstrated modest reductions in cardiovascular events, but no benefits on total mortality. In the 1990s, with the use of hydroxymethylglutaryl coenzyme A (HMG-CoA) reductase inhibitors, the benefit of cholesterol reduction has become more definitive, particularly in patients with established CVD.

In 1994, the Scandinavian Simvastatin Survival Study (4S) trial (14) was published, showing a total mortality benefit associated with cholesterol reduction in patients with CVD. Over a trial duration of 5.4 years, 4444 patients aged 35 to 70 years old with a history of angina or MI were randomized to receive placebo plus diet versus simvastatin plus diet. The study included men and women, diabetics, and patients with peripheral vascular disease. In 4S, prerandomization cholesterol levels were high (5.5 to 8.0 mmol/L, or approximately 212 to 308 mg/dL); thus, only a portion of the highest-risk coronary patients were included. The simvastatin group had a highly significant reduction in total mortality (the primary trial endpoint) with a relative risk of 0.70

(95 percent CI = 0.58 to 0.85). In the simvastatin group, 182 patients died (8 percent), as compared with 256 (12 percent) in the placebo group, with no significant difference in non-CVD mortality. Most of the total mortality benefit was accounted for by a marked reduction in coronary deaths. There were 189 coronary deaths in the placebo group as compared with 111 in the simvastatin group, a relative risk of 0.58 (95 percent CI = 0.46 to 0.73). The secondary endpoint, any major coronary event, was also significantly reduced in the simvastatin group, with a relative risk of 0.66 (95 percent CI = 0.59 to 0.75). Rates of coronary revascularization were also reduced in the simvastatin group. Subgroup analyses showed that both women and the elderly (age >59 years) benefited from simvastatin therapy. Diabetics also benefited from simvastatin therapy as much as and possibly even more than nondiabetics. All main trial endpoints were reduced in diabetic patients treated with simvastatin.[15] Evidence of clinical benefit seemed to begin at about 1 year after randomization.

The Cholesterol and Recurrent Events (CARE) trial studied the effect of cholesterol reduction on secondary prevention of CVD in patients with more modestly elevated cholesterol levels than in the 4S trial.[16] In CARE, 4159 men and women with a mean cholesterol level of 209 mg/dL were randomized to treatment assignments of pravastatin plus diet versus placebo plus diet. Eligible patients were 21 to 75 years old with a history of a MI. Asymptomatic patients with left ventricular ejection fraction as low as 25 percent were included. The combined primary endpoint in CARE was a fatal coronary event or a nonfatal MI. In the pravastatin group, 212 patients (10.2 percent) as compared with 274 (13.2 percent) in the placebo group had a primary event, a 24 percent risk reduction (95 percent CI = 9 to 36 percent). A significant reduction in the need for revascularization procedures also occurred in the pravastatin group, and there was a similar but not statistically significant 23 percent reduction ($p = .10$) in death from coronary disease in the pravastatin group. The reduction in total mortality in the pravastatin group of 9 percent also was not statistically significant. Both younger and older people and men as well as women benefited from pravastatin, as did pa-

tients with either a normal or low ejection fraction. Stroke event rates were also reduced significantly in the pravastatin group (31 percent relative reduction). In CARE patients with an initial LDL-C concentration below 125 mg/dL, there was no benefit of further cholesterol reduction by pravastatin.

The LIPID trial[17] also evaluated an HMG-CoA reductase inhibitor in patients with CVD. The LIPID (Long-Term Intervention with Pravastatin in Ischemic Disease) study was stopped prior to planned completion date because of a significant reduction in trial endpoints in the pravastatin group. The trial was designed to determine whether cholesterol reduction with pravastatin reduces CHD mortality in patients with previous MI or unstable angina and cholesterol levels between 155 and 271 mg/dL. Over 9000 patients, men and women, 31 to 75 years old, were enrolled and randomized to a pravastatin plus diet regimen or to placebo plus diet. CHD events were significantly reduced in the pravastatin group: a 29 percent lower rate of MI, a 24 percent lower rate of coronary artery bypass grafting (CABG), 18 percent lower rate of percutaneous transluminal angioplasty (PTCA), and an 11 percent lower rate of unstable angina pectoris. CHD mortality was lower by 24 percent in the pravastatin group with 19 CHD deaths prevented per 1000 treated patients over 6 years.[18] This study adds further evidence to support the value of cholesterol reduction by statins in secondary prevention.

Cholesterol lowering with HMG-CoA reductase inhibitors has produced other clinically relevant results in addition to effects on coronary events and mortality. In a follow-up analysis of 4S, simvastatin group patients also had a reduced use of hospital services.[19] Thirty-four percent fewer hospital days ($p = .0001$) over the course of the trial in the simvastatin group resulted in a 31 percent reduction in associated costs. Admissions for heart failure were also reduced in the simvastatin group. The placebo group had a total of 334 days in hospital for heart failure compared with 194 for the simvastatin group, suggesting that the course of heart failure may have been beneficially affected by the use of a cholesterol-lowering agent.

In an ancillary analysis of the 4S trial,[20] new or worsening symptoms of claudication were reported to be reduced by 38 percent in the simvastatin group. Additionally, the risk of developing a new carotid bruit or the worsening of an existing bruit was less in the simvastatin group, with a relative risk of 0.52 (95 percent CI = 0.32 to 0.85). If additional data can confirm these subgroup analyses, HMG-CoA reductase inhibitors could become standard and proven therapy for patients with peripheral vascular disease and hypercholesterolemia.

Stroke incidence has also been reduced with cholesterol-lowering agents, in particular by HMG-CoA reductase inhibitors in coronary patients. Established risk factors for stroke are age, hypertension, diabetes, and cigarette smoking.[21] In observational studies, the relation between cholesterol levels and stroke has been inconsistent. The incidence of thromboembolic stroke has been higher with higher cholesterol levels in some observational studies,[22] but other studies have found no association between cholesterol level and stroke.[23] However, a metanalysis of 28 cholesterol-lowering trials found a significant risk reduction for stroke with the use of HMG-CoA reductase inhibitors.[24] In hypercholesterolemic patients, the treatment group had a risk ratio of 0.76 (95 percent CI = 0.62 to 0.92). Of the eight trials that used HMG-CoA reductase inhibitors, seven were secondary prevention trials in patients with CVD. The benefit of cholesterol-lowering with other cholesterol-lowering agents, perhaps related to the less powerful effect of those medications, was not demonstrated. Thus, in patients with known CVD and elevated cholesterol, HMG-CoA reductase inhibitors appear also to be an effective means for the prevention of strokes. Among recent secondary prevention trials, the CARE study[16] reported a 19 percent reduction (95 percent CI = 0 to 34 percent) in stroke incidence, and in the LIPID study,[17] a 31 percent reduction (95 percent CI = 3 to 52 percent) in stroke incidence was reported.

Mechanisms of Benefit from Lipid Lowering

Clinical event reductions in both the 4S and CARE trials have been greater than that expected by the small amount of atherosclerosis regression produced in angiography trials.[2] Mechanisms other than regression in the size of atherosclerotic lesions are likely to be involved in the improved clinical endpoints seen in these trials. Plaque stabilization is one commonly proposed mechanism. According to this concept, fibrous plaques can be rendered more "stable" and less likely to initiate thrombosis after cracking or fissuring.[25]

It has also been demonstrated that hypercholesterolemia impairs the normal function of vascular endothelium.[26] Several trials have demonstrated a favorable effect of lipid reduction on endothelial function, including two trials[27,28] that compared lovastatin versus placebo in hypercholesterolemic patients. Initial coronary angiograms were repeated after several months of therapy (in one trial in 5.5 months and the second trial after 1 year). The first trial[27] also used the antioxidant probucol in addition to lovastatin. Endothelial function was determined by intracoronary injections of acetylcholine with measurements of the change in coronary lumen diameter. All patients had significant endothelial dysfunction at the start of the trial, manifest by paradoxical vasoconstriction in response to acetylcholine (ACh) injections. After the follow-up period, both treatment groups demonstrated improvement, and there was significantly less vasoconstriction seen in both the lovastatin alone and the lovastatin-plus-probucol groups in response to ACh. These data suggest that endothelial dysfunction can be relatively rapidly improved by lipid modification, and this mechanism may explain rapid clinical benefits seen in HMG-CoA reductase inhibitor trials.[27–29]

Silent myocardial ischemia may also be attenuated by cholesterol reduction. A trial involving 40 patients with known coronary disease, high serum cholesterol levels, and a history of ST-segment depressions on ambulatory electrocardiographic (ECG) monitoring was undertaken to test the benefit of lovastatin therapy on myocardial ischemia.[30] At baseline, an average of four episodes of ischemia per 48 h were recorded in patients randomized to lovastatin or to placebo. Follow-up ambulatory ECG monitoring was performed 4 to 6 months later. During the two monitoring sessions, there were no patient reports of angina; therefore, all ECG ST-segment ischemic changes were "silent" ischemic episodes. There was no significant change in the number of ST-depression episodes recorded in the control group. However, in the lovastatin group, in 13 of 20 patients, there was complete resolution of all ST-segment depressions (compared to 2 out of 20 in the control group). In the placebo group, the total number of minutes of ischemic changes on ECG was unchanged at a median 52 min per 48 h, while the lovastatin group had a median duration of 0 min per 48 h. In a multivariate model, treatment group assignment was the most significant predictor of a reduction in the amount of measured ischemia. This study demonstrates the potential for rapid reduction in myocardial ischemia via cholesterol-lowering therapy. Thus, secondary preventive benefits may be related to various mechanisms including plaque stabilization, ischemia reduction, and atherosclerosis regression or delayed progression.

Lipid Management Guidelines

The National Cholesterol Education Program (NCEP) has published guidelines for cholesterol-lowering therapy.[31] Goals are based on levels of LDL-C, the lipoprotein most strongly associated with atherosclerotic disease. Target levels of therapy are based on the risk of cardiovascular events. Increased risk, as assessed by a higher number of risk factors, mandates a lower LDL-C target goal. Patients at the highest risk level are those with established CVD. It follows that all patients undergoing cholesterol reduction for secondary prevention of CVD fall into this most aggressive LDL-C–lowering category. The recommended target LDL-C is 100 mg/dL or lower in this group of patients.

Several studies have addressed the question of an ideal LDL-C level in secondary prevention. The Post–Coronary Artery Bypass Graft Trial studied 1351 patients with a previous history of coronary bypass surgery.[32] Baseline LDL-C levels ranged from 130 to 175 mg/dL, and all study participants were randomized to receive lovastatin. Patients were assigned to either an "aggressive" treatment range

(goal 60 to 85 mg/dL) or to a "moderate" treatment range (130 to 140 mg/dL). The main endpoint was angiographic evidence of graft atherosclerosis after an average follow-up of 4.3 years. In the "aggressive limb," 27 percent of grafts had atherosclerotic progression as compared with 39 percent in the "moderate treatment" group ($p < .001$). There was also a 29 percent lower rate of revascularizations in the aggressive LDL-C group ($p = .03$). The trial found no difference in clinical outcomes, but it had not been designed to test this difference. The authors concluded that the lower levels of LDL-C achieved in the aggressive limb (actual levels of 93 to 97 mg/dL) as compared with the moderate limb (actual levels of 132 to 136 mg/dL) resulted in less progression of atherosclerosis. This study provides preliminary evidence favoring more aggressive cholesterol lowering than has been recommended to date by the NCEP.

Substudies of the 4S and CARE trials also examined the issue of optimal LDL-C for secondary prevention.[12,33] The 4S subanalysis found that the beneficial effect in the simvastatin group was associated mainly with magnitude of the reduction in LDL-C, as there was a curvilinear graded reduction in coronary events correlating with cholesterol reduction. Each 1 percent lowering of total cholesterol resulted in a 1.9 percent reduction in coronary events ($p = .00005$). The incremental benefit became progressively smaller as the cholesterol reduction increased further. However, no threshold was found below which additional cholesterol lowering was of no further benefit.

In a CARE substudy, different conclusions were reached, but substantive differences between the parent trials may explain the different results.[33] CARE patients started the trial with lower baseline cholesterol levels than those in 4S. In the CARE substudy, there was a progressive reduction in events to an LDL-C level of 125 mg/dL. Beyond this level, no benefit from further cholesterol reduction was achieved. Despite these conflicting data, most experts contend that an optimal LDL-C in secondary prevention is less than or equal to 100 mg/dL, which should be attained provided that cost, tolerability, and safety concerns are met.

Hypertension as a Risk Factor in Secondary Prevention

Both systolic and diastolic blood pressures have continuous, graded, strong, independent, and etiologically significant relationships to the development of cardiovascular disease.[34] Systolic blood pressure may be of even greater importance than diastolic pressure.[35] In patients with established cardiovascular disease, hypertension continues to confer an increased risk for the progression of disease and for the recurrence of adverse events.

In the past, the prognostic role of high blood pressure (BP) following a myocardial infarction was uncertain, possibly due to analytic problems. Confusion may have arisen because in initially hypertensive patients, a drop in blood pressure can cause apparent normalization of BP associated with postevent LV dysfunction. In such patients, post-MI BP level may not correlate with subsequent prognosis. An analysis of Framingham Heart Study data clarified the importance of hypertension in this situation.[36] When patients who experienced a decline in blood pressure after a myocardial infarction were excluded, hypertension persisting after MI was clearly associated with increased mortality and overall cardiovascular risk. Specifically, in patients whose blood pressure continued to be elevated (>160/95 mmHg), the 5-year mortality risk ratio was nearly 2.0 ($p < .05$) as compared with normotensive patients.

The Sixth Report of the Joint National Committee on Prevention, Detection, Evaluation, and Treatment of High Blood Pressure (JNC VI) published updated guidelines for the treatment of hypertension.[37] Included in this consensus statement is the recommended treatment of patients with established CVD. Compelling indications are given for beta-blocker use after a Q-wave MI and for angiotensin converting enzyme inhibitor (ACEI) use in patients with a compromised left ventricular function. ACEIs are also advised in diabetic patients with renal disease involvement, including microalbuminuria.

Mechanisms of Risk from Hypertension

Hypertension results in cardiovascular damage via multiple mechanisms. Maladaptive remodeling of the arterial wall media and intima, as well as endothelial cell dysfunction and altered vasodilator response, worsen overall function of the vasculature in hypertensive patients.[38,39] Hypertrophy of the left ventricle, often as a result of hypertension (and even small increases in mass below usual definitions of hypertrophy), is independently associated with a higher cardiovascular mortality.[40,41] Finally, a complex metabolic picture of insulin resistance, hyperinsulinemia, dyslipidemia, central obesity, and hypercoaguability is often associated with hypertension, and these may contribute to a magnified cardiovascular risk.[42]

Evidence from Secondary Prevention Trials

A plethora of primary prevention trials have demonstrated reduction of CVD accruing from antihypertensive treatment. On the other hand, antihypertensive trials in secondary prevention are sparse. The Hypertension Detection and Follow-up Program (HDFP) compared two treatment assignments to determine the effectiveness of aggressive antihypertension therapy. One group was prescribed a stepped-care approach to treatment, as contrasted with a routine (usual) care group identified from the general population. The overall primary endpoint was a lower total mortality in the stepped-care group. A subgroup analysis was performed in HDFP subjects who had evidence of CVD at the outset of the trial.[43] Patients with baseline CVD included those with evidence of previous MI, left ventricular hypertrophy, major end-organ damage, or any probable preexisting clinical heart disease. All CVD patient subgroups in stepped care benefited in risk reduction when contrasted to patients in the referred care group. For example, 1018 (9.3 percent) patients in the trial had evidence of a previous MI. As had been found in patients without evidence of a prior MI, those with prior MI also had a 20 percent reduction in 5-year death rates in the stepped-care group as compared to the usual-care group. A similar pattern held true for most other subgroups, including patients with evidence of any existing heart disease. Therefore, this subgroup analysis suggests that hypertension treatment is beneficial in patients with established CVD.

Other trials using specific antihypertensive medications suggest the importance of blood pressure treatment in secondary prevention. Beta blockers have been used for years as cardioprotective agents in patients with MI. Immediate beta-blockade shortly after onset of ischemia has proven effective in reducing in-hospital mortality.[44] Additionally, long-term use of beta blockers improves prognosis after MI over many years of follow-up. An overview of beta-blocker trials by Yusuf et al. assessed the effectiveness of their long-term prophylactic use post-MI.[44] Aggregate results show that long-term beta-blocker therapy reduces total mortality by approximately 20 percent with a pooled relative risk of death of 0.77 (CI = 0.70 to 0.85: $p < .00001$). Nonfatal reinfarction and sudden death are also reduced by about 25 and 30 percent, respectively. Overall, data on beta blockers suggest that the most effective beta blockers are those without intrinsic sympathomimetic activity, and the greatest risk reductions can be expected within the first year following MI. Because beta blockers lower blood pressure, it has been difficult to separate the BP lowering effects of beta blockers from the myriad other mechanisms of vascular protection that these agents also provide (antiarrhythmia, decreased ventricular wall tension, weak antiplatelet activity, or antianginal effects). Despite considerable evidence of the short- and long-term benefits of beta blockade after MI, many patients do not receive them.[45] The elderly, nonwhites, and patients with low ejection fractions appear especially unlikely to receive beta blockers post-MI. Evidence indicates that these high-risk subgroups also benefit from beta blockade, and physicians should be encouraged to employ this therapy in most patients[45] regardless of BP level, although ACEIs are generally recommended as initial therapy for those with heart failure or decreased left ventricular ejection fraction.[37]

ACEIs are a class of antihypertensives of special interest with regard to the prevention of CVD. As a group, these agents possess properties that potentially make them uniquely effective in secondary prevention. Recent clinical trials in congestive heart failure (CHF) patients using ACEIs provide hints as to this special role in CVD prevention. The Survival and Ventricular Enlargement (SAVE) trial[46] and the Studies of Left Ventricular Dysfunction (SOLVD) trial[47] both demonstrated the mortality benefit ACEIs confer in patients with reduced left ventricular function. In the SOLVD trial,[48] the ACEI enalapril significantly reduced MI, unstable angina, and the rate of cardiac mortality in patients with a low left ventricular ejection fraction as compared with the placebo-treated group. Within a follow-up period averaging 40 months, 362 patients in the placebo group suffered MI versus 288 in the enalapril group (risk reduction 23 percent; 95 percent CI = 11 to 34 percent; $p < .001$). Systolic blood pressure was 6 mmHg lower and diastolic pressures were 4 mmHg less in the enalapril group. In multivariate analysis, blood pressure reduction in the enalapril group did not appear to account fully for the total reduction in risk of MI. The SOLVD authors also cited metanalysis data suggesting that a 5 to 6-mmHg lowering of blood pressure is associated with only about a 14 percent reduction in CHD risk.[35] Therefore, enalapril seemed to provide additional cardiovascular protection than would be predicted from BP lowering alone. This finding may be explained by the higher absolute risk of cardiovascular events in the SOLVD trial group (a trial of patients with established disease) as compared with the metanalysis patients (mostly primary prevention). However, it is also possible that properties of the ACEI enalapril itself may have accounted for the greater risk reduction as compared with diuretics and beta blockers used in comparison trials. Clinical trials are currently under way to address the cardioprotective effects of ACEIs further.

Calcium-channel-blocker (CCB) use and CVD is a complex issue that is discussed here only briefly. Several relatively early clinical trials raised concern about precipitation of ischemic events by CCBs in patients with established CHD, particularly with use of high doses of short-acting agents.[49–52] However, the use of longer-acting agents less likely to stimulate reflex-increased sympathetic tone has suggested more encouraging results, but not in typical secondary prevention (post-MI) patients.[53,54] To date, only one secondary prevention trial[55] using the long-acting CCB verapamil has demonstrated a positive outcome. In DAVIT-II (the Danish Verapamil Infarction Trial II), verapamil-treated patients had a reduction in reinfarction. In a prespecified subgroup without heart failure, verapamil-treated patients had reduced overall mortality. In spite of the DAVIT-II data, it is generally held that CCBs are not advisable during or after acute MI. Clarification of this complex problem awaits the conclusion of several ongoing clinical trials.

Mechanisms of Benefit from Controlling Hypertension

Like hyperlipidemia, hypertension is associated with endothelial dysfunction, and the possibility that antihypertensive agents might minimize or reverse endothelial dysfunction has been studied. The TREND (Trial on Reversing Endothelial Dysfunction) study used the ACEI quinipril in normotensive patients with established CHD.[54] Angiograms monitored the diameter of the coronary arteries in response to acetylcholine. Treatment with quinipril improved the baseline endothelial dysfunction. Reversal of endothelial dysfunction in patients with established atherosclerosis may be a mechanism by which ACEIs can be effective in secondary prevention.

In patients with essential hypertension, remodeling of resistance vessel structure may play a role in CVD. There is a decreased lumen diameter and an increase in the ratio of wall thickness to lumen diameter. This process, known as *eutrophic remodeling,* may contribute to adverse outcomes in hypertensive patients.[56]

Traditional blood pressure medications (e.g., beta blockers) have not proven to affect this process. ACEI therapy, on the other hand, appears to reverse this problem.[57,58] Both cilazapril and perindopril caused a significant increase in lumen diameter and a reduction of media-to-lumen ratio. This additional positive effect of ACEIs may prove clinically relevant in future clinical trials.

Left ventricular hypertrophy (LVH) is associated with increased cardiovascular mortality,[40,41] and hypertension is a common precursor of LVH. BP control itself, particularly with ACEI therapy, has repeatedly been associated with reduction in LVH.[59] A retrospective analysis of Framingham Heart Study[60]

participants was conducted comparing clinical outcome in people with ECG criteria for LVH. Individuals who had a serial decline in ECG voltage in addition to BP reduction were at a lower risk for the development of cardiovascular complications (men: adjusted odds ratio, 0.46; 95 percent CI = 0.26 to 0.84); women: adjusted odds ratio, 0.56; 95 percent CI = 0.30 to 1.04). This analysis suggests that BP control plus LVH reduction may provide an even more powerful means of secondary prevention of CVD than blood pressure reduction alone.

Many questions in hypertension treatment remain unanswered. One of the key questions, optimal level of BP reduction, was recently addressed in the largest hypertension trial to date. The Hypertension Optimal Treatment (HOT) trial included 3080 patients with coronary heart disease.[61] The lowest incidence of major cardiovascular events occurred at a mean achieved diastolic BP of 82.6 mmHg. Only for MI was there a trend ($p = .05$) for lower event rates at lower target BPs (a nonsignificant 25 percent event reduction in the target group ≤85 mmHg and a 28 percent reduction in the target group ≤80 mmHg, as compared with the target group ≤90 mmHg). No effect on stroke incidence was observed. Of interest, the first-line antihypertension agent used in all patients was the long-acting CCB felodipine. The HOT study provided the first evidence from a randomized controlled trial that reduction in diastolic BP below the usual target value of <90 mmHg is both safe and beneficial in patients with or without coronary heart disease.

Hemostasis as a Risk Factor and Antiplatelet Therapy

Thrombosis and coagulation contribute to the occurrence of acute cardiovascular events as well as to atherosclerosis itself. Measurements of fibrinogen,[62] platelet activity and platelet counts,[63] and tissue plasminogen activator levels[64] have been associated with increases in CVD risk. Trials to date have not focused on manipulation of single elements in the cascade but rather on therapy that affects the entire process of hemostasis.

In a metanalysis performed by the Anti-platelet Trialists' Collaboration, therapy with antiplatelet agents in the secondary prevention of CVD was shown to be effective.[65] Multiple subgroups of patients were analyzed, including a "high-risk" group of patients with established CVD. The use of antiplatelet agents in this subgroup resulted in a 27 percent reduction in all vascular events, a 32 percent reduction in nonfatal MI, a 31 percent reduction in nonfatal stroke, and a 17 percent reduction in total mortality. There was no evidence that a higher dose of either aspirin or other antiplatelet agents were more effective than medium-strength aspirin alone (75 to 325 mg/day).

Anticoagulation with warfarin after a MI may also be beneficial in secondary prevention as seen in early trials.[66] Recently, the Coumadin Aspirin Reinfarction Study (CARS) trial investigated whether the combination of low-dose aspirin plus fixed low-dose warfarin would prove more effective than either agent alone in patients with CVD.[67] The trial was stopped prematurely when interim results revealed no additional benefit from the combination compared with aspirin alone. Low-dose aspirin therapy alone (160 mg/day) proved to be as effective as a combination regimen in preventing reinfarction, nonfatal stroke, and cardiovascular death.

Ticlopidine inhibits the formation of arterial thrombi, prolongs bleeding time, and normalizes shortened platelet survival. In the Canadian American Ticlopidine Study (CATS),[68] it was shown in stroke patients to reduce cardiovascular events by 30 percent; in the Ticlopidine Aspirin Stroke Study (TASS),[69] ticlopidine showed a slight advantage over aspirin in preventing death from any cause or nonfatal stroke.

Clopidogrel is a new drug that blocks platelet activation in a manner similar to ticlodipine but with fewer adverse effects. In a recent study (CAPRIE), clopidogrel was compared with aspirin in the secondary prevention of vascular events.[70] There was a significant 8.7 percent relative risk reduction compared with aspirin in the clopidogrel group for the combined occurrence of stroke, MI, or vascular death. Side-effect profiles were similar between the two treatment groups. Although the trial illustrates the superiority of clopidogrel to aspirin, the much lower cost of aspirin and the relatively small additional benefit attributable to clopidogrel are likely to result in no change in current recommendations of standard aspirin therapy.

Management Guidelines for Antiplatelet Therapy

The use of lifelong aspirin therapy by all patients with established CVD is widely recommended in secondary prevention protocols.[2,3] Although the "ideal dose" is uncertain, doses in the range of 81 to 325 mg/day appear to provide benefit with a lower risk of bleeding than higher doses. Other antiplatelet agents or warfarin are currently recommended only if patients cannot tolerate aspirin. Clopidogrel is an effective and safe alternative to aspirin in the aspirin-intolerant patient. Warfarin may also be a valuable substitute for aspirin in the post-MI patient with LV dysfunction who is also at risk for LV thrombosis and arterial embolization.

Cigarette Smoking

Cigarette smoking worsens CVD by several mechanisms. Angiographic studies have revealed that smoking is associated with the progression of atherosclerosis. Smoking induces an increase in fibrinogen levels, increases platelet activity, and increases blood viscosity. Vascular tone is enhanced and endothelial dysfunction occurs. HDL-C levels are lowered, while more LDL-C is oxidized. BP, heart rate, and sympathetic tone are also increased in response to cigarette smoking.[71]

There are no randomized controlled trials in the secondary prevention of CVD using smoking cessation. However, observational evidence overwhelmingly supports the need for smoking cessation in secondary prevention. One such analysis was performed in patients from the Coronary Artery Surgery Study (CASS) with angiographically documented atherosclerosis.[72] In the total CASS cohort, patients who continued to smoke had a statistically higher adjusted relative risk of death than did patients who quit (RR = 1.7, 95 percent CI = 1.4 to 2.0; $p < .001$). The relative risk of MI was also higher in those who continued to smoke (RR = 1.5, 95 percent CI = 1.2

to 1.7; $p = .001$). Subgroup analyses in CASS showed that elderly patients and women benefited from smoking cessation, as did younger people and men. Also, patients at all levels of coronary risk (assessed by risk scores) benefited from smoking cessation. The CASS data confirmed results of earlier studies that smoking cessation reduces both cardiovascular events and total mortality in all groups of patients with established CVD.[73] Smoking cessation should be included in recommendations to all patients, especially those with documented vascular disease.

Dietary Therapy and Exercise: Management and Recommendations

Dietary therapies have been studied in patients with existing CVD. The overall benefit from reduction in dietary fat intake is less striking in clinical trials than it is for lipid lowering trials using HMG-CoA reductase inhibitors. Several trials have, however, shown a positive impact of dietary modifications.[74–76] In the most striking study,[74] after an average of 17 months, a "Mediterranean-type" alpha-linolenic acid–rich diet produced a 76 percent reduction in mortality after MI. The dietary modification group also had a relative risk of 0.27 (95 percent CI = 0.12 to 0.59; $p = .001$) for the combination of nonfatal MI and cardiac death in comparison with the "usual-diet" group. Of note, average serum cholesterol values were similar in both diet groups in this trial, leading to the hypothesis that the diet-modification group benefited via mechanisms other than lipid lowering. In two other trials, one using a fish-enriched diet[75] and the other using an American Heart Association Step 2 Diet[76] in patients with established CVD, both special diet groups showed improved cardiovascular outcomes compared to usual diets. Trials using dietary modification have also demonstrated slowing of the atherosclerotic process as measured by serial angiograms.[77,78] The Lifestyle Heart Trial studied the combination of a very low fat diet (about 10 percent of calories from fat), moderate exercise, yoga, and stress management,[78] while the Heidelberg Regression Trial studied exercise therapy in addition to dietary therapy.[79] Aggregate data from these trials support the recommendation of a low-fat, low-cholesterol diet in patients with CVD.

Exercise and cardiac rehabilitation in post-MI patients have also been demonstrated to reduce recurrent cardiovascular events. Two metanalyses conducted in the late 1980s concluded that in patients with CHD, exercise rehabilitation programs reduce overall and cardiac mortality by 20 to 25 percent.[80,81] Exercise rehabilitation programs also result in considerable improvements in cardiac symptoms and other measures of quality of life.[82–84] Thus, a program of exercise rehabilitation is a well-justified component of the secondary prevention schema.[2,3,82]

Risk-Factor Modifications of Probable or Possible Benefit

Diabetes Mellitus

Diabetes conveys an increased risk of cardiovascular events and mortality in patients with CVD.[6] No secondary prevention trial has been completed specifically in regard to diabetes control and cardiovascular endpoints. Information on reduction of macrovascular events in a large primary prevention trial appears promising and may apply to patients with established disease.[85] In addition, a recently completed large primary prevention trial in 3867 newly diagnosed type II diabetics revealed a borderline significant ($p = .052$) reduction in occurrence of first MI related to intensive blood glucose control.[86] It remains possible but still unproven that control of blood glucose to relatively normal levels (avoiding hypoglycemia) will result in less macrovascular disease and fewer adverse events in diabetics with CVD.

Subgroup analyses in diabetics suggest highly beneficial effects of lipid lowering or achievement of ideal blood pressure. Among diabetics with pre-existing CHD enrolled in the Scandinavian Simvastatin Survival Study (4S) study, a 55 percent lower risk ($p < .002$) of major coronary events was observed among those receiving simvastatin versus placebo.[87] Recently, the Hypertension Optimal Treatment (HOT) Study showed a 51 percent reduction in major cardiovascular event among those diabetics assigned to a diastolic blood pressure target level below 80 mmHg as compared with a level below 90 mmHg (p value for trend = .005).[61] Although this study was done primarily in those free of preexisting CHD, it is not unreasonable to expect these benefits to occur in secondary prevention as well.

The need for a large-scale clinical trial testing the efficacy of intensive glycemic control by different agents (e.g., those influencing versus not influencing insulin resistance), as well as lipid and blood pressure control on reducing the risk of macrovascular disease, has been recently recognized by the National Institutes of Health.

Hormone Replacement Therapy

Over 30 observational studies have demonstrated a decreased cardiac risk in healthy women taking hormone replacement therapy (HRT),[88] particularly conjugated equine estrogens, including the large Nurses' Health Study.[89] Five of the observational studies included women with coronary artery disease. Risk reduction in total mortality ranged from 10 to 30 percent.[88] A few trials, in particular the PEPI trial, have assessed possible mechanisms of estrogenic benefit.[90] Benefits of estrogen treatment include positive modifications of lipid and lipoprotein values, including lipoprotein (a), reduction in coagulation risk and fibrinogen levels, improved vascular reactivity, and normalized endothelial function.[90,91] Recently, raloxifene (a selective estrogen-receptor modulator) has been shown to share a portion of the cardioprotective properties of conjugated equine estrogens, but the magnitude of the beneficial effect has been less than that with standard estrogen regimens.[92] The potential value of hormone replacement therapy for secondary prevention has received attention in various guidelines,[2,3] but clinical trial data were entirely lacking until 1998.

The Heart and Estrogen/Progestin Replacement Study (HERS) results represent the first data from a large randomized clinical trial on the effect of HRT in women with preexisting heart disease.[93] The HERS trial found that in 4 years of follow-up in postmenopausal women with a uterus, the use of estrogen (as conjugated equine estrogen) and progestin (as continuous daily medroxyprogesterone acetate) did not prevent further heart attacks or death from CHD. The lack of overall effect of this HRT regimen occurred despite positive effects of the treatment on LDL-C, HDL-C, and other cardiovascular risk traits. The HRT regimen used in HERS also increased the risk of venous thrombosis and pulmonary embolism by about threefold compared with placebo.[94] Clearly, the HERS results were surprising in light of the many previous observational studies that had suggested a protective effect of postmenopausal estrogen use in CVD. When the overall results were examined by year of treatment, the investigators discovered a trend toward higher risk of events such as MI during the first year of therapy, but this negative trend was reversed during the third and fourth years of HRT therapy. A possible explanation for these findings might be an increase in thrombotic events early after starting HRT, which is eventually overcome by favorable influences on atherogenesis. Despite these possible differing effects early and late in treatment, the HERS data put a damper on the rush to employ HRT in secondary prevention. HERS did not study other estrogen preparations or other progestins, and there was no estrogen-only arm in hysterectomized women. Clinical judgment is still required in dealing with CHD patients who do not resemble those studied in HERS. Judgment as to the appropriateness of HRT should be withheld for a few years following the coronary event.

HDL-C and Triglycerides

Low HDL-C has been repeatedly associated with an increased cardiovascular risk. Isolated low HDL-C levels in patients with normal total cholesterol levels and established CVD is a predictor of subsequent mortality and adverse vascular events.[95] In one study, isolated low HDL-C conveyed an increased relative risk of adverse cardiovascular events of 2.0 (95 percent CI = 1.2 to 3.3; p = .01). Other studies have demonstrated that an isolated low HDL-C is a common lipoprotein abnormality in CHD patients, accounting for approximately 25 percent of all lipid abnormalities in such patients.[96,97]

There are only limited data relating to modification of HDL-C in coronary patients. The Lopid Coronary Angiography Trial (LOCAT) used gemfibrozil in patients with coronary artery disease and an isolated low HDL-C and provided preliminary evidence that raising HDL-C may be beneficial.[98] LOCAT found less angiographic progression of atherosclerosis in the gemfibrozil group than in the placebo-treated group. Post hoc analysis attributed most of the treatment effect to the raising of low HDL-C. With a small study size, clinical endpoints were not different between groups. Similar results were found in BECAIT, a double-blind, placebo-controlled intervention trial using bezafibrate versus placebo in 81 patients.[99] The study involved male survivors of MI below 45 years of age at the time of MI. Angiographic endpoints were significantly improved in the bezafibrate-treated patients compared with those who were given placebo. The cumulative coronary event rate was also significantly lower among bezafibrate-treated than among placebo-treated patients (3 versus 11 patients, $p = .002$). These findings occurred in association with favorable changes in total serum cholesterol (-9 percent), very low density lipoprotein cholesterol (-35 percent), serum triglycerides (-31 percent), and plasma fibrinogen (-12 percent). HDL-C was also significantly increased with bezafibrate ($+9$ percent). Thus, BECAIT and LOCAT were highly suggestive of beneficial effects with the use of fibrates in coronary patients.

Two large-scale secondary prevention trials have been underway in coronary patients with low HDL-C. The Veterans Affairs Cooperative HDL Intervention Trial (HIT) showed a 22 percent reduction in the risk of CHD death or nonfatal MI in patients randomized to gemfibrozil or placebo who had evidence of CHD and an HDL-C of below 40 mg/dL and LDL-C below 140 mg/dL.[100] The Israeli Bezafibrate Infarction Prevention Study (BIP)[101] was presented in preliminary form in August 1998. BIP was designed to assess whether bezafibrate could reduce coronary endpoints (fatal and nonfatal MI or sudden death) in patients with previous MI or angina, by elevating low HDL-C and reducing triglycerides. The trial was a double-blind, placebo-controlled study us-

ing 400 mg of bezafibrate daily. Study inclusions were recent MI (6 months to 5 years before entry) and/or angina for prior 2 years, total cholesterol 180 to 250 mg/dL, LDL-C less than or equal to 180 mg/dL, HDL-C less than or equal to 45 mg/dL, and triglycerides less than or equal to 300 mg/dL. Over 15,000 patients were screened, and 3122 were eventually enrolled in BIP. At enrollment, mean HDL-C was about 35 mg/dL in both treatment groups.

Results of BIP showed no overall benefit of bezafibrate in the primary analysis.[102] Adverse effects were low in both the bezafibrate and placebo groups. HDL-C increased by 15 percent and triglycerides decreased by nearly 20 percent in the bezafibrate patients. Subgroup analyses suggested beneficial effects of bezafibrate in patients with marked HDL-C increases (≥ 5.2 mg/dL) and in patients with baseline triglycerides equal to or greater than 200 mg/dL. Overall, BIP results leave the issue of the raising of HDL after MI in an uncertain state.

Other Risk Factors

Homocysteine[103] and oxidative stress[104] have both been implicated in the process of atherosclerosis. Cardiovascular events are higher in patients with elevated homocysteine levels.[103] No clinical secondary prevention data exist to date in regard to homocysteine reduction. Recommendations on when, how, and to what level to lower homocysteine await clinical trials. Many observational studies have analyzed anti-oxidant therapy and possible reduction of adverse cardiovascular events.[104] A randomized controlled secondary prevention trial—the Cambridge Heart Antioxidant Study (CHAOS)—demonstrated a striking 77 percent reduction in nonfatal MIs in patients taking vitamin E as compared with patients taking placebo[105]; however, overall mortality was not reduced by vitamin E in this trial. Trials with vitamin C and beta carotene have shown no CVD benefit.[104] Based on limited observations to date, these other factors are not yet considered proven targets for secondary prevention efforts.

Selected Patient Groups

Elderly

In several trials of risk-factor modification, elderly patients benefited as much as or more than younger patients, even in the presence of established vascular disease. In subgroups of lipid-lowering trials, both the 4S[14] and the CARE[16] studies demonstrated benefit of cholesterol reduction in patients as old as 75 years of age. It is currently not established whether patients older than 75 would also benefit from lipid lowering. In some of the secondary prevention hypertension trials discussed earlier,[44,48] elderly patients had event reductions similar to those in younger patients. The smoking cessation observational data from CASS[72] also suggest that there was no diminution of beneficial effect of smoking cessation with older age. Last, in the metanalysis of antiplatelet agents,[65] elderly high-risk patients (those with established vascular disease) derived as much as or even more benefit from antiplatelet drugs as did younger patients. All this evidence is in support of risk-factor modification as an effective method of secondary prevention of cardiovascular events in elderly patients with established CVD. Because of the absence of definitive clinical trial data in the elderly, clinical judgment in drug utilization is generally advised.

Women

Women with CVD generally appear to benefit from secondary prevention treatments as much as men. Both the 4S[14] and CARE[16] studies included women. As with the elderly, women benefited from cholesterol reduction as much as did men. CARE data suggested that women may have an even greater reduction in major coronary events (46 percent) than do men (20 percent). Therefore, in women known to have CVD, aggressive management of serum cholesterol is as important as it is for men. Hypertension therapy also seems to be of benefit in women. For example, in the analysis of the SAVE trial,[48] the use of an ACEI reduced combined cardiovascular events in women by 35 percent as compared with 19 percent for men. A metanalysis comparing the effects of antihypertensive drug treatment in men and women has been published.[106] Although most of the data were drawn from primary prevention trials, blood pressure treatments did not differ in terms of reduction of relative risk for men and women. Absolute risk reduction was greater in men (reflecting the baseline higher risk in men). Since men and women benefited about equally in antihypertensive trials, it seems reasonable to recommend BP control in both groups for both primary and secondary prevention of CVD. Last, both smoking cessation[72] and antiplatelet agents[65] have produced similar proportional reductions in men and women in metanalyses and large observational studies.

Conclusions

In the patient who has suffered a coronary event, the risk of recurrent events or mortality is greatest within the first month following the event and decreases in a nonlinear fashion thereafter. It is crucial to stratify individuals appropriately as to risk, not only on the basis of functional tests but also on the basis of the physical examination and information as to risk factors obtained during the casual office visit. In the last decade, the efficacy of risk-factor modification for secondary prevention of CHD, particularly lipid and hypertension control and antiplatelet therapy, has been demonstrated. Immediate risk-factor modification is necessary—particularly control of dyslipidemia, hypertension, cigarette smoking, as well as administration of antiplatelet therapy and appropriate dietary modification and physical activity—all of which have proven or are likely to be beneficial. Close monitoring to ensure compliance to prescribed therapy and lifestyle modifications is vital for the secondary prevention of CHD.

References

1. Rossouw JE, Lewis B, Rifkind BM: The value of lowering cholesterol after myocardial infarction. *N Engl J Med* 1990; 323:1112–1119.
2. Califf RM, Armstrong PW, Carver JR, et al: Task Force 5: stratification of patients into high, medium, and low

risk subgroups for purposes of risk factor management. *J Am Coll Cardiol* 1996; 27:1007–1019.

3. Smith SC Jr, Blair SN, Criqui MH, et al: AHA consensus panel statement: preventing heart attack and death in patients with coronary disease. The Secondary Prevention Panel. *J Am Coll Cardiol* 1995; 26:292–294.

4. Pyorala K, De Backer G, Graham I, et al: Prevention of coronary heart disease in clinical practice recommendations of the Task Force of the European Society of Cardiology, European Atherosclerosis Society and European Society of Hypertension. *Atherosclerosis* 1994; 110:121–161.

5. Smith LR, Harrell FE Jr, Rankin JS, et al: Determinants of early versus late cardiac death in patients undergoing coronary artery bypass graft surgery. *Circulation* 1991; 84:(suppl III):III-245–III-253.

6. Wong ND, Cupples LA, Ostfeld AM, et al: Risk factors for long-term coronary prognosis following initial myocardial infarction: the Framingham study. *Am J Epidemiol* 1989; 130:469–480.

7. Anderson KM, Castelli WP, Levy D: Cholesterol and mortality. 30 years of follow-up from the Framingham study. *JAMA* 1987; 257:2176–2180.

8. The Lipid Research Clinics: The Lipid Research Clinics Coronary Primary Prevention Trial results: I. Reduction in incidence of coronary heart disease. *JAMA* 1984; 251:351–364.

9. Martin MJ, Hulley SB, Browner WS, et al: Serum cholesterol, blood pressure, and mortality: implications from a cohort of 361,662 men. *Lancet* 1986; 2:933–966.

10. Wong ND, Wilson PW, Kannel WB: Serum cholesterol as a prognostic factor after myocardial infarction: the Framingham Study. *Ann Intern Med* 1991; 115:687–693.

11. Pekkanen J, Linn S, Heiss G, et al: Ten-year mortality from cardiovascular disease in relation to cholesterol level among men with and without preexisting cardiovascular disease. *N Engl J Med* 1990; 322:1700–1707.

12. Pedersen TR, Olsson AG, Faergeman O, et al: Lipoprotein changes and reduction in the incidence of major coronary heart disease events in the Scandinavian Simvastatin Survival Study (4S). *Circulation* 1998; 97:1453–1460.

13. Canner PL, Halperin M: Implications of findings in the coronary drug project for secondary prevention trials in coronary heart disease: the Coronary Drug Project research group. *Circulation* 1981; 63:1342–1350.

14. The Scandinavian Simvastatin Survival Study Group: Randomised trial of cholesterol lowering in 4444 patients with coronary heart disease: the Scandinavian Simvastatin Survival Study (4S). *Lancet* 1994; 344:1383–1389.

15. Pyorala K, Pedersen TR, Kjekshus J, et al: Cholesterol lowering with simvastatin improves prognosis of diabetic patients with coronary heart disease: a subgroup analysis of the Scandinavian Simvastatin Survival Study (4S). *Diabetes Care* 1997; 20:614–620.

16. Sacks FM, Pfeffer MA, Moye LA, et al: The effect of pravastatin on coronary events after myocardial infarction in patients with average cholesterol levels. Cholesterol and Recurrent Events Trial investigators. *N Engl J Med* 1996; 335:1001–1009.

17. Long-Term Intervention with Pravastatin in Ischemic Disease study group: Design features and baseline characteristics of the LIPID (Long-Term Intervention with Pravastatin in Ischemic Disease) study: a randomized trial in patients with previous acute myocardial infarction and/or unstable angina pectoris. *Am J Cardiol* 1995; 76:474–479.

18. The Long-Term Intervention with Pravastatin in Ischemic Disease (LIPID) study group: Prevention of cardiovascular events and death with pravastatin in patients with coronary heart disease and a broad range of initial cholesterol levels. *N Engl J Med* 1998; 339:1349–1357.

19. Pedersen TR, Kjekshus J, Berg K, et al: Cholesterol lowering and the use of healthcare resources: results of the Scandinavian Simvastatin Survival Study. *Circulation* 1996; 93:1796–1802.

20. Pedersen TR, Kjekshus J, Pyorala K, et al.: Effect of simvastatin on ischemic signs and symptoms in the Scandinavian Simvastatin Survival Study (4S). *Am J Cardiol* 1998; 81:333–335.

21. Tell GS, Crouse JR, Furberg CD: Relation between blood lipids, lipoproteins, and cerebrovascular atherosclerosis: a review. *Stroke* 1988; 19:423–430.

22. Neaton JD, Blackburn H, Jacobs D, et al: Serum cholesterol level and mortality findings for men screened in the Multiple Risk Factor Intervention Trial: Multiple Risk Factor Intervention Trial research group. *Arch Intern Med* 1992; 152:1490–1500.

23. Pekkanen J, Linn S, Heiss G, et al: Ten-year mortality from Cholesterol, diastolic blood pressure, and stroke: 13,000 strokes in 450,000 people in 45 prospective cohorts. Prospective studies collaboration. *Lancet* 1995; 346:1647–1653.

24. Bucher HC, Griffith LE, Guyatt GH: Effect of HMG-CoA reductase inhibitors on stroke: a meta-analysis of randomized, controlled trials. *Ann Intern Med* 1998; 128:89–95.

25. Ross R. The pathogenesis of atherosclerosis: a perspective for the 1990s. *Nature* 1993; 362:801–809.

26. Vita JA, Treasure CB, Nabel EG, et al: Coronary vasomotor response to acetylcholine relates to risk factors for coronary artery disease. *Circulation* 1990; 81:491–497.

27. Anderson TJ, Meredith IT, Yeung AC, et al: The effect of cholesterol-lowering and antioxidant therapy on endothelium-dependent coronary vasomotion. *N Engl J Med* 1995; 332:488–493.

28. Treasure CB, Klein JL, Weintraub WS, et al: Beneficial effects of cholesterol-lowering therapy on the coronary endothelium in patients with coronary artery disease. *N Engl J Med* 1995; 332:481–487.

29. O'Driscoll G, Green D, Taylor RR: Simvastatin, an HMG-coenzyme A reductase inhibitor, improves endothelial function within 1 month. *Circulation* 1997; 95:1126–1131.

30. Andrews TC, Raby K, Barry J, et al: Effect of cholesterol reduction on myocardial ischemia in patients with coronary disease. *Circulation* 1997; 95:324–328.

31. Summary of the second report of the National Cholesterol Education Program (NCEP) Expert Panel on Detection, Evaluation, and Treatment of High Blood Cholesterol in Adults (Adult Treatment Panel II). *JAMA* 1993; 269:3015–3023.

32. The Post Coronary Artery Bypass Graft Trial Investigators: The effect of aggressive lowering of low-density lipoprotein cholesterol levels and low-dose anticoagulation on obstructive changes in saphenous-vein coronary-artery bypass grafts. *N Engl J Med* 1997; 336:153–162.

33. Sacks FM, Moye LA, Davis BR, et al: Relationship between plasma LDL concentrations during treatment with pravastatin and recurrent coronary events in the Cholesterol and Recurrent Events Trial. *Circulation* 1998; 97:1446–1452.

34. Stamler J, Stamler R, Neaton JD: Blood pressure, systolic and diastolic, and cardiovascular risks: U.S. population data. *Arch Intern Med* 1993; 153:598–615.

35. MacMahon S, Peto R, Cutler J, et al: Blood pressure, stroke, and coronary heart disease: Part 1, Prolonged differences in blood pressure: prospective observational studies corrected for the regression dilution bias. *Lancet* 1990; 335:765–774.

36. Kannel WB, Sorlie P, Castelli WP, McGee D: Blood pressure and survival after myocardial infarction: the Framingham study. *Am J Cardiol* 1980; 45:326–330.

37. National High Blood Pressure Education Program: The sixth report of the Joint National Committee on Prevention, Detection, Evaluation, and Treatment of High Blood Pressure. *Arch Intern Med* 1997; 157:2413–2446.

38. Chobanian AV: 1989 Corcoran lecture: adaptive and maladaptive responses of the arterial wall to hypertension. *Hypertension* 1990; 15:666–674.

39. Lüscher TF, Noll G: Endothelial function as an end-point in interventional trials: concepts, methods and current data. *J Hypertens* 1996; 14(suppl 2):S111–S121.

40. Levy D, Garrison RJ, Savage DD, et al: Prognostic implications of echocardiographically determined left ventricular mass in the Framingham Heart Study. *N Engl J Med* 1990; 322:1561–1566.

41. Koren MJ, Devereux RB, Casale PN, et al: Relation of left ventricular mass and geometry to morbidity and mortality in uncomplicated essential hypertension. *Ann Intern Med* 1991; 114:345–352.

42. DeFronzo RA, Ferrannini E: Insulin resistance: a multifaceted syndrome responsible for NIDDM, obesity, hypertension, dyslipidemia, and atherosclerotic cardiovascular disease. *Diabetes Care* 1991; 14:173–194.

43. Langford HG, Stamler J, Wassertheil-Smoller S, Prineas RJ: All-cause mortality in the Hypertension Detection and Follow-up Program: findings for the whole cohort and for persons with less severe hypertension, with and without other traits related to risk for mortality. *Prog Cardiovasc Dis* 1986; 29:29–54.

44. Yusuf S, Peto R, Lewis J, et al: Beta blockade during and after myocardial infarction: an overview of the randomized trials. *Prog Cardiovasc Dis* 1985; 27:335–371.

45. Gottlieb SS, McCarter RF, Vogel RA: Effect of beta blockade on mortality among high-risk and low-risk patients after myocardial infarction. *N Engl J Med* 1998; 339:489–497.

46. Pfeffer MA, Braunwald E, Moye LA, et al: Effect of captopril on mortality and morbidity in patients with left ventricular dysfunction after myocardial infarction: results of the survival and ventricular enlargement trial. The SAVE Investigators. *N Engl J Med* 1992; 327:669–677.

47. The SOLVD Investigators: Effect of enalapril on survival in patients with reduced left ventricular ejection fractions and congestive heart failure. *N Engl J Med* 1991; 325:293–302.

48. Yusuf S, Pepine CJ, Garces C, et al: Effect of enalapril on myocardial infarction and unstable angina in patients with low ejection fractions. *Lancet* 1992; 340:1173–1178.

49. Collins R, Peto R, MacMahon S, et al: Blood pressure, stroke, and coronary heart disease: Part 2. Short-term reductions in blood pressure—overview of randomised drug trials in their epidemiological context. *Lancet* 1990; 335:827–838.

50. The Multicenter Diltiazem Postinfarction Trial Research Group: The effect of diltiazem on mortality and reinfarction after myocardial infarction. *N Engl J Med* 1988; 319:385–392.

51. Furberg CD, Psaty BM, Meyer JV: Nifedipine. Dose-related increase in mortality in patients with coronary heart disease. *Circulation* 1995; 92:1326–1331.

52. Goldbourt U, Behar S, Reicher-Reiss H, et al—SPRINT II Study: Early administration of nifedipine in suspected myocardial infarction. *Arch Intern Med* 1993; 153:345–353.

53. Staessen JA, Fagard R, Thijs L, et al: Randomised double-blind comparison of placebo and active treatment for older patients with isolated systolic hypertension: the systolic hypertension in Europe (Syst-Eur) Trial Investigators. *Lancet* 1997; 350:757–764.

54. Mancini GB, Henry GC, Macaya C, et al: Angiotensin-converting enzyme inhibition with quinapril improves endothelial vasomotor dysfunction in patients with coronary artery disease: the TREND (Trial on Reversing Endothelial Dysfunction) Study. *Circulation* 1996; 94:258–265.

55. DAVIT-II Study—Danish Study Group of Verapamil in Myocardial Infarction: The effects of verapamil on mortality and major events after myocardial infarction. *Am J Cardiol* 1990; 66:779–785.

56. Elliot HL: Post hoc analysis: use and dangers in perspective. *J Hypertens* 1996; 14(suppl 2):S21–S25.

57. Schiffrin EL, Deng LY, Larochelle P: Effects of a beta blocker or a converting enzyme inhibitor on resistance arteries in essential hypertension. *Hypertension* 1994; 23:83–91.

58. Thybo NK, Stephens N, Cooper A, et al: Effect of anti-hypertensive treatment on small arteries of patients with previously untreated essential hypertension. *Hypertension* 1995; 25:474–481.

59. Gottdiener JS, Reda DJ, Massie BM, et al: Effect of single-drug therapy on reduction of left ventricular mass in mild to moderate hypertension: comparison of six antihypertensive agents: the Department of Veterans Affairs Cooperative Study Group on Antihypertensive Agents. *Circulation* 1997; 95:2007–2014.

60. Levy D, Salomon M, D'Agostino RB, et al: Prognostic implications of baseline electrocardiographic features and their serial changes in subjects with left ventricular hypertrophy. *Circulation* 1994; 90:1786–1793.

61. Hansson L, Zanchetti A, Carruthers SG, et al: Effects of intensive blood-pressure lowering and low-dose aspirin in patients with hypertension: principal results of the Hypertension Optimal Treatment (HOT) randomised trial. HOT Study Group. *Lancet* 1998; 351:1755–1762.

62. Yang XC, Jing TY, Resnick LM, Phillips GB: Relation of hemostatic risk factors to other risk factors for coronary heart disease and to sex hormones in men. *Arterioscler Thromb* 1993; 13:467–471.

63. Trip MD, Cats VM, van Capelle FJ, Vreeken J: Platelet hyperreactivity and prognosis in survivors of myocardial infarction. *N Engl J Med* 1990; 322:1549–1554.

64. Ridker PM, Vaughan DE, Stampfer MJ, et al: Endogenous tissue-type plasminogen activator and risk of myocardial infarction. *Lancet* 1993; 341:1165–1168.

65. Antiplatelet Trialists' Collaboration Collaborative overview of randomised trials of antiplatelet therapy—I: Prevention of death, myocardial infarction, and stroke by prolonged antiplatelet therapy in various categories of patients. *BMJ* 1994; 308:81–106.

66. Smith P, Arnesen H, Holme I: The effect of warfarin on mortality and reinfarction after myocardial infarction. *N Engl J Med* 1990; 323:147–152.

67. Coumadin Aspirin Reinfarction Study (CARS) investigators: Randomised double-blind trial of fixed low-dose warfarin with aspirin after myocardial infarction. *Lancet* 1997; 350:389–396.

68. Gent M, Blakely JA, Easton JD, et al: The Canadian American Ticlopidine Study (CATS) in thromboembolic stroke. *Lancet* 1989; 1:1215–1220.

69. Hass WK, Easton JD, Adams HP, et al: A randomized trial comparing ticlopidine hydrochloride with aspirin for the presentation of stroke in high-risk patients. *N Engl J Med* 1989; 321:501–507.

70. CAPRIE Steering Committee: A randomised, blinded, trial of clopidogrel versus aspirin in patients at risk of ischaemic events (CAPRIE). *Lancet* 1996; 348:1329–1339.

71. Fuster V, Gotto AM, Libby P, et al: Task Force 1: pathogenesis of coronary disease: the biologic role of risk factors. *J Am Coll Cardiol* 1996; 27:964–976.

72. Hermanson B, Omenn GS, Kronmal RA, Gersh BJ: Beneficial six-year outcome of smoking cessation in older men and women with coronary artery disease: results from the CASS registry. *N Engl J Med* 1988; 319:1365–1369.

73. The Coronary Drug Project Research Group: Cigarette smoking as a risk factor in men with a prior history of myocardial infarction. *J Chronic Dis* 1979; 32:415–425.

74. de Lorgeril M, Renaud S, Mamelle N, et al: Mediterranean alpha-linolenic acid-rich diet in secondary prevention of coronary heart disease. *Lancet* 1994; 343:1454–1459.

75. Burr ML, Fehily AM, Gilbert JF, et al: Effects of changes in fat, fish, and fiber intakes on death and myocardial reinfarction: diet and reinfarction trial (DART). *Lancet* 1989; 2:757–761.

76. Singh RB, Rastogi SS, Verma R, et al: Randomised controlled trial of cardioprotective diet in patients with recent acute myocardial infarction: results of one year follow up. *BMJ* 1992; 304:1015–1019.

77. Effects on coronary artery disease of lipid-lowering diet, or diet plus cholestyramine, in the St Thomas' Atherosclerosis Regression Study (STARS). *Lancet* 1992; 339:563–569.

78. Ornish D, Brown SE, Scherwitz LW, et al: Can lifestyle changes reverse coronary heart disease? the Lifestyle Heart Trial. *Lancet* 1990; 336:129–133.

79. Shuler G, Hambrecht R, Schlierf G, et al: Regular physical exercise and low-fat diet: effects on progression of coronary artery disease. *Circulation* 1992; 86:1–11.

80. O'Connor GT, Buring JE, Yusuf S, et al: An overview of randomized trials of rehabilitation with exercise after myocardial infarction. *Circulation* 1989; 80:234–244.

81. Oldridge NB, Guyatt GH, Fischer ME, Rimm AA: Cardiac rehabilitation after myocardial infarction: combined experience of randomized clinical trials. *JAMA* 1988; 260:945–950.

82. Wenger NK, Froelicher ES, Smith LK, et al: *Cardiac Rehabilitation: Clinical Practice Guideline No. 17.* AHCPR Publication No. 96-0672. Rockville, MD: U.S. Department of Health and Human Services; Public Health Service; Agency for Health Care Policy and Research; and the National Heart, Lung, and Blood Institute, 1995.

83. Balady GJ, Fletcher BJ, Froelicher ES, et al: Cardiac rehabilitation programs: a statement for healthcare professionals from the American Heart Association. *Circulation* 1994; 90:1602–1610.

84. Greenland P, Chu JS: Efficacy of cardiac rehabilitation services—with emphasis on patients after myocardial infarction. *Ann Intern Med* 1988; 109:650–663.

85. Diabetes Control and Complications Trial Group: Effect of intensive diabetes management on macrovascular events and risk factors in the Diabetes Control and Complications trial. *Am J Cardiol* 1995; 75:894–903.

86. UK Prospective Diabetes Study (UKPDS) group: Intensive blood-glucose control with sulphonylureas or insulin compared with conventional treatment and risk of complications in patients with type 2 diabetes (UKPDS 33). *Lancet* 1998; 352:837–853.

87. Pyorala K, Pedersen TR, Kjekshus J, et al: Cholesterol-lowering with simvastatin improves prognosis of diabetic patients with coronary heart disease. *Diabetes Care* 1997; 20:614–620.

88. Stampfer MJ, Colditz GA: Estrogen replacement therapy and coronary heart disease: a quantitative assessment of the epidemiologic evidence. *Prev Med* 1991; 20:47–63.

89. Grodstein F, Stampfer MJ, Colditz GA, et al: Postmenopausal hormone therapy and mortality. *N Engl J Med* 1997; 336:1769–1775.

90. The Writing Group for the PEPI Trial: Effects of estrogen or estrogen/progestin regimens on heart disease risk factors in postmenopausal women: the Postmenopausal Estrogen/Progestin Interventions (PEPI) trial. *JAMA* 1995; 273:199–208.

91. Wild RA, Taylor EL, Knehans A: The gynecologist and the prevention of cardiovascular disease. *Am J Obstet Gynecol* 1995; 172(1 pt 1):1–13.

92. Walsh BW, Kuller LH, Wild RA, et al: Effects of raloxifene on serum lipids and coagulation factors in healthy postmenopausal women. *JAMA* 1998; 279:1445–1451.

93. Hulley S, Grady D, Bush T, et al: Randomized trial of estrogen plus progestin for secondary prevention of coronary heart disease in postmenopausal women: Heart and Estrogen/progestin Replacement Study (HERS) Research Group. *JAMA* 1998; 280:605–613.

94. Grady D, Hulley SB, Furberg C: Venous thromboembolic events associated with hormone replacement therapy (letter). *JAMA* 1997; 278:477.

95. Miller M, Seidler A, Kwiterovich PO, Pearson TA: Long-term predictors of subsequent cardiovascular events with coronary artery disease and "desirable" levels of plasma total cholesterol. *Circulation* 1992; 86:1165–1170.

96. Ginsburg GS, Safran C, Pasternak RC: Frequency of low serum high-density lipoprotein cholesterol levels in hospitalized patients with "desirable" total cholesterol levels. *Am J Cardiol* 1991; 68:187–192.

97. Milani RV, Lavie CJ: Prevalence and effects of nonpharmacologic treatment of "isolated" low-HDL cholesterol in patients with coronary artery disease. *J Cardiopulm Rehab* 1995; 15:439–444.

98. Frick MH, Syvanne M, Nieminen MS, et al: Prevention of the angiographic progression of coronary and vein-graft atherosclerosis by gemfibrozil after coronary bypass surgery in men with low levels of HDL cholesterol: Lopid Coronary Angiography Trial (LOCAT) study group. *Circulation* 1997; 96:2137–2143.

99. Ericsson CG, Hamsten A, Nilsson J, et al: Angiographic assessment of effects of bezafibrate on progression of coronary artery disease in young male postinfarction patients. *Lancet* 1996; 347:849–853.

100. Bloomfield-Rubins H, Robins SJ, Collins D for the Department of Veterans Affairs HIT Study Group: Presentation at the 71st Scientific Sessions, American Heart Association, Dallas, November 1998.

101. Goldbourt U, Behar S, Reicher-Reiss H, et al: Rationale and design of a secondary prevention trial of increasing serum high-density lipoprotein cholesterol and reducing triglycerides in patients with clinically manifest atherosclerotic heart disease (the Bezafibrate Infarction Prevention Trial). *Am J Cardiol* 1993; 71:909–915.

102. Kaplinsky E for the BIP Study Group: *The Bezafibrate Infarction Prevention (BIP) Study Results.* European Society of Cardiology Annual Congress; Vienna, August 24, 1998. Brussels, European Society of Cardiology, 1998:2.

103. Wald NJ, Watt HC, Law MR, et al: Homocysteine and ischemic heart disease: results of a prospective study with implications regarding prevention. *Arch Intern Med* 1998; 158:862–867.

104. Diaz MN, Frei B, Vita JA, Keaney JF Jr: Antioxidants and atherosclerotic heart disease. *N Engl J Med* 1997; 337:408–416.

105. Stephens NG, Parsons A, Schofield PM, et al: Randomised controlled trial of vitamin E in patients with coronary disease: Cambridge Heart Antioxidant Study (CHAOS). *Lancet* 1996; 347:781–786.

106. Gueyffier F, Boutitie F, Boissel JP, et al: Effect of antihypertensive drug treatment on cardiovascular outcomes in women and men: a meta-analysis of individual patient data from randomized, controlled trials. The INDIANA Investigators. *Ann Intern Med* 1997; 126:761–767.

CHAPTER 24

Establishing a Preventive Cardiology Program

Nathan D. Wong
Julius M. Gardin
Henry R. Black

To be effective in reducing the burden due to atherosclerotic coronary heart disease (CHD), both community and academic medical care facilities need to have an appropriate infrastructure for providing preventive cardiology services. Although many health care facilities do have active cardiac rehabilitation programs, effective programs for evaluating and treating high-risk persons without preexisting CHD and for long-term secondary prevention are frequently lacking. Appropriate services for the screening and identification of those at risk and for the management of cardiovascular risk factors are the cornerstones of such a preventive cardiology program. However, a well-rounded program will also provide professional and community education opportunities as well as a research component. Both consensus-based statements for primary[1] and secondary[2] prevention as well as guidelines for the identification and management of major coronary risk factors[3–5] are available. The fact that these are often inadequately implemented in a general practice setting[6–8] provides a basis and rationale for preventive cardiology programs.

In this chapter, we describe the components of preventive cardiology services, as well as the resources needed and challenges faced in developing such office- and clinic-based approaches. In addition, barriers to the implementation of preventive services are discussed, as are the needs for professional and community education, community services, and research. This chapter is intended to provide a general overview and foundation for the development of such a program that will be applicable to many health care settings.

Priorities for Preventive Cardiology Services

No single structure will necessarily satisfy all the needs of a preventive cardiology program. Often, a combination of approaches, integrated into the health care system, may be needed to optimize effectiveness. What is necessary is close cooperation and communication among a wide range of physician and nonphysician health care specialists who have in common the mission to deliver an effective, efficient, and cost-effective service. Screening (or identification of patients at risk), treatment, follow-up, and ongoing professional and patient education are crucial components of an effective program. Components recommended by the Second Joint Task Force of European and Other Societies on Coronary Prevention[9] include (1) lifestyle and cardiovascular risk assessment, (2) behavioral change, (3) education, (4) family-based intervention, (5) risk-factor management, and (6) screening of first-degree relatives.

Prioritization of Patients

Priority for services should be reserved for those with established CHD or other atherosclerotic disease and

TABLE 24–1 Priorities of Coronary Heart Disease Prevention in Clinical Practice

1. Patients with established coronary heart disease (CHD) or other atherosclerotic vascular disease.

2. Asymptomatic subjects with particularly high risk (subjects with severe hypercholesterolemia or other forms of dyslipidemia, diabetes, or hypertension; subjects with a cluster of several risk factors).

3. Close relatives of patients with early-onset CHD or other atherosclerotic vascular disease; asymptomatic subjects with particularly high risk.

4. Other subjects met in connection with ordinary clinical practice who are identified or reported to have one or more CHD risk factors.

Source: Adapted from Swan et al.,[10] with permission.

those who are at high risk of developing such diseases in the future.[9,10] Table 24–1 lists priorities regarding types of patients that should be considered for preventive strategies. In addition to patients with established CHD, priority patients include those with familial hyperlipidemias, a strong family history of premature CHD, diabetes mellitus, other lipid profile abnormalities, hypertension, obesity, and unhealthful lifestyle practices such as a high-fat diet or cigarette smoking.[10] The probability of future events can be high in such individuals, particularly if multiple risk factors are present. By dealing first with those at highest absolute risk, the service will prevent the most events per dollar spent and thus be more justifiable from an economic perspective.

Identification of Patients at Risk

Many key candidates for risk-factor modification are not currently being identified, either because of failure of physicians to request the appropriate tests (e.g., lipid profiles in patients with established CHD, or blood pressure follow-up of those with high normal blood pressure or who are hypertensive) or the inability of health care systems to adequately identify patients needing such tests. The current reimbursement environment provides few if any incentives to follow these individuals aggressively. Partly

because of the failure adequately to identify those with risk factors that warrant treatment, risk-factor management is often lacking, even among patients with preexisting CHD (Table 24–2).[6,11,12] A recent chart audit of nearly 50,000 patients in the United States with CHD showed only 44 percent to have annual diagnostic testing of low-density-lipoprotein cholesterol (LDL-C), and of those tested, only 25 percent reached the target goal of 100 mg/dL or less. Only 39 percent were taking lipid-lowering therapy.[6] Also, a European survey among 4863 patients with CHD showed that 53 percent still had elevated blood pressure and 44 percent had elevated cholesterol. Of those receiving blood pressure- or lipid-lowering drugs, approximately half were not adequately controlled, and only 21 percent reported being advised to have their relatives screened for coronary risk factors.[12]

The components and examples of questionnaires and tools used for cardiovascular risk assessment are discussed in earlier chapters in this book dealing with primary (Chap. 22) and secondary (Chap. 23) prevention, physical activity (Chap. 12), nutrition (Chap. 13), and psychosocial characteristics (Chap. 14). Key algorithms have also been provided in Chap. 1, based on levels of key major risk factors, for determining the probability of experiencing CHD, stroke, or intermittent claudication.

Accurate risk assessment begins with ensuring that the appropriate patients receive the necessary

TABLE 24–2 Estimated Compliance with Secondary Prevention Measures in Patients Surviving Myocardial Infarction

Referral to a cardiac rehabilitation program	<5%
Smoking cessation counseling	20%
Lipid-lowering drug therapy	25%
Beta-blocker therapy	40%
Angiotensin-converting enzyme inhibitor therapy (for reduced left ventricular ejection fraction)	60%
Aspirin	70%

Source: Adapted from Pearson et al.,[11] with permission.

tests. At a minimum, a physician's patient rolls should be reviewed to ensure the performance of certain tests, where clearly indicated (e.g., lipid profiles for all patients with CHD). Although this can be done manually by a member of the physician's office staff, computerized patient-tracking databases can streamline the process. Interrelated databases—e.g., electronic medical records with patient diagnoses, laboratory data, and pharmacy prescriptions—are rapidly becoming a standard for larger health care organizations. Computer identification of abnormal cholesterol values is more likely to lead to preventive or follow-up treatment,[13] as are reminder checklists attached to outpatient records,[14] or computer or nurse-generated preventive care reminders.[15,16] Others have also shown a significant increase in physician compliance with treatment guidelines prompted by a structured message pasted on patients' charts sum-

marizing their risk and the appropriate guideline recommendations.[17]

Quality of Care and Performance Monitoring

Quality-assurance programs should include risk-factor management as a key indicator of quality of care and performance monitoring. A list of 10 key measures (Table 24–3)[12] has been proposed as a starting point, which may be modified as new risk factors, and the efficacy of interventions designed to decrease or reverse them, become established. Reliable mechanisms to monitor the level to which clinical guidelines, practice standards, and other goals in preventive cardiology are being carried out should be developed and implemented. With the advent of new Health Employer Data Information Set (HEDIS) measures from the National Committee on Quality

TABLE 24–3 Key Measures of Quality of Preventive Care*

1. Smoking status should be documented in all patients with coronary or other vascular disease.

2. Organizations should have a smoking cessation program suitable for the smoking patient and his or her family.

3. All eligible patients hospitalized with coronary or other vascular disease should be offered, as documented in the medical record, physician advice and self-help materials to stop smoking.

4. All patients with coronary or other vascular disease should have a fasting lipoprotein profile documented at the appropriate time within the first 3 months after onset of disease if the patient is deemed appropriate for diet or pharmacologic intervention.

5. All patients with coronary or other vascular disease should be offered, as documented in the medical record, nutritional evaluation and counseling at the time of diagnosis.

6. All patients with coronary or other vascular disease who have an LDL cholesterol level ≥ 130 mg/dL after nutritional therapy should be prescribed, as documented in the record, lipid-lowering pharmacologic therapy if the patient is deemed appropriate for intervention.

7. All patients with coronary or other vascular disease should be assessed and provided with exercise counseling/prescription at the time of diagnosis if the patient is deemed appropriate for intervention.

8. Aspirin therapy should be offered to all patients eligible at the time of diagnosis of coronary or other atherosclerotic disease. If aspirin therapy is contraindicated, the contraindication should be documented in the medical record.

9. All patients with coronary or other vascular disease should have a blood pressure measurement documented at every visit.

10. If the average of three blood pressure measurements is equal to or greater than 140 mmHg systolic or 90 mmHg diastolic, lifestyle and pharmacologic treatment plans should be offered and documented at the time of diagnosis.

*As endorsed by the American Heart Association and American College of Cardiology to be implemented in patients with established cardiovascular disease. Some of these strategies can be used to create performance monitoring measures to assess quality of care.
Source: From Pearson et al.,[11] with permission.

Assurance (NCQA) mandating evidence for LDL-C screening and control (to <130 mg/dL within 1 year after discharge) for patients with established cardiovascular disease and for the rates of control of hypertension, the motivation for developing these systems becomes even stronger.

Preventive care can also be enhanced with varying degrees of success by using computer-based clinical support systems.[18] Monitoring systems can provide data for individual and organizational feedback,[19] as in a "report card" format, facilitating quality assurance efforts to provide performance data and reinforcement of organizational and provider behavior.[11] Such systems should ideally be able to provide physician-specific lists of names and contact information on patients who, for example, have CHD or diabetes (as identified by the appropriate ICD-9-CM codes) and who have not had a lipid profile performed in the last year. For those in whom a recent lipid profile is available, a list of patients can be provided whose LDL-C level is above a specified target level for treatment and where cholesterol-lowering treatment (if any) is listed.

Organizational Structures for Preventive Cardiology Services

A system of preventive cardiology services can be implemented by solo practitioners, small group practices, and hospital-based or other clinics, as well as by large providers, such as managed care or governmental organizations (such as the Department of Veterans Affairs).[10] However, clinical preventive services cannot be effectively implemented unless clinicians accept responsibility for providing and directing them. If physicians have limited time to provide these services, they can design the system, determine the indications for such services, and delegate the implementation to colleagues. However, they must provide staff implementing these services with the necessary direction, resources, and unambiguous support for the concept.[20]

Office-Based Approach

In many cases, risk-factor identification and management will be the responsibility of the primary health care provider, with intervention accomplished one patient at a time.[21] In this model, there may be multiple (perhaps hundreds) primary care physicians within a given health care organization serving as a focal point for prevention efforts for a given panel of patients.

The vast majority of uncomplicated cases of dyslipidemia, hypertension, diabetes, and individuals with other risk factors are currently managed through relatively short office-based visits. During such visits, the physician can be most effective in explaining the clinical significance of the problem and the necessity for the patient to comply with prescribed lifestyle modifications and, when necessary, pharmacologic therapy. Increased efforts in this regard, particularly, are needed, since surveys suggest that after 1 year, up to half of patients stop prescribed preventive therapy, such as cholesterol-lowering drugs or estrogen replacement therapy.[22] Reasons for this lapse in compliance are numerous, but include (1) the failure of the medical care profession to agree on appropriate strategies, (2) the failure of physicians to implement risk-reduction therapies, (3) poor patient adherence to such therapies, (4) patient-presumed adverse reactions to the treatment, and (5) lack of reimbursement for such therapies.[18] For many of these issues, the physician is in the best position to ensure that they do not become barriers to patient compliance. Practice models for incorporating CHD prevention strategies, including educational and counseling components, have been developed.[23]

As the office-based approach provides limited opportunity for adequate patient education, a responsible prevention program entails recommendations (or "prescriptions") to obtain needed education for risk-factor management from other members of the health care team—including nurses, dietitians, exercise specialists, pharmacists, psychologists, and, if necessary, vocational staff (Table 24–4).[9] The management of risk factors is a complex process, involving not only educating patients but also teaching them the skills to change and maintain healthful behaviors and to adhere to prescribed regimens.[11] This may involve establishing appointments or referrals with a dietitian with expertise in cardiovascular nutrition, a

TABLE 24–4   Recommended Resources for Cardiac Prevention and Rehabilitation Programs

Physicians

Cardiologists and other physicians in the hospital and in the community have a central role to play because of their professional relationship with the patient and are ultimately responsible for all aspects of their care. They need to give leadership to the organization of such a service, ensuring that it becomes an integral part of the health care delivery system.

Nurses

Specially trained cardiac nurses can help recruit patients and organize lifestyle assessments, risk-factor screening, and health promotion sessions. Training in models of behavioral change, health promotion, and psychosomatic aspects of disease is essential.

Dietitians

The dietitian provides important management and professional advice for assessment and recommendation of dietary changes that need to be made. Most nurses and doctors have not received any formal training in this area, and if professional dietitian staff are not available, such training needs to be provided on key aspects of nutrition using well-written educational materials.

Exercise Specialists

Exercise evaluation and prescriptions are important for all patients and for those with CHD; supervised exercise is an important component of patient management.

Pharmacists

Pharmacists have an educational role in relation to the use of drugs, their clinical indications, mode of action, side effects, and benefits. Their increasing role in providing general health education necessary for successful risk reduction is also recognized.

Psychologists

Mental health staff—including psychologists, psychiatrists, or other qualified staff—can design necessary programs and inform patients about how to address the psychological consequences of developing CHD, including how to cope with and manage stress. This can have an important impact on the patient's quality of life and improve compliance to achieve other goals in the program, such as weight loss or smoking cessation. Helping patients to understand and manage their emotions and reactions to stress, psychologists can also help to increase their motivation to make and sustain appropriate lifestyle changes as well as to return to a full and active role in the community.

Vocational Support

Adequate assistance may be needed by some patients to help them return to work or find more suitable alternative employment.

Facilities

These should include office space for staff, an area for individual and family lifestyle and risk-factor assessment, a private area for counseling, and an area for group activities, including education and health promotion sessions and supervised physical activity.

Source: Adapted from the Second Joint Task Force of European and Other Societies on Coronary Prevention,[9] with permission.

clinical psychologist, and/or an exercise physiologist as needed.

Protocols should be developed for the type of specialty services each team member will provide, which patients are to receive them, and to what extent and in what format (e.g., initial group sessions followed by individualized counseling sessions to address individual needs and so on). As is often the case, however, the physician may bear the burden of much of this education about risk factors and, if so, should have had the training (or utilize appropriate team members within the office visit) to provide such education. For instance, a 15-min physician office visit may need to be extended to 30 min to provide appropriate dietary advice, and perhaps 40 to 45 min to provide appropriate consultation on physical activity and/or stress management. The constraints on physician time in the managed care era make this unrealistic in many cases, but physicians should spend the time that is needed to provide the best care for patients.

Finally, a key to the success of this model for preventive services lies in the ability to provide—and ensure—that preventive services personnel obtain appropriate training, so that there is some standard (ideally based on nationally recognized and agreed upon guidelines) for the management strategies that are being prescribed. For more complicated risk-factor management needs, referral is recommended to a specialty physician provider—e.g., a cardiologist, endocrinologist, lipid specialist, or hypertension specialist.[4] In addition, the general internist might have an arrangement with an appropriate specialist for periodic review of evaluation and treatment plans.[10]

A schedule should be developed for regular follow-up visits by patients to the primary care physician, with appointments scheduled in advance if possible. At these visits, progress made in controlling risk factors should be reviewed and appointments with the above recommended specialists should be scheduled as necessary. The provider should have a system implemented to remind patients of their visits in order to promote better compliance.

Physician-Directed Specialty Clinic

The hallmark of a preventive cardiology program is often a specialty clinic, such as a "risk reduction" or "prevention and reversal" clinic. Such clinics can be particularly attractive from a marketing standpoint, potentially offering a unique program that appeals to the public. In many regions, these clinics are still relatively uncommon except in certain well-known medical centers and clinics, some of which have been involved in this specialty for more than a decade. Some health care facilities have become aggressive at providing a heart disease prevention and reversal program, with an educational program for the pub-

lic (a "cardiac college") directed toward reducing suffering and death due to heart disease.[24]

A preventive cardiology clinic in the academic setting might have as its focus the management of a particular disorder—such as dyslipidemia or hypertension—by virtue of its physician director having a particular academic expertise. Ideally, however, the clinic should provide services for managing multiple risk factors—including smoking, obesity, and physical inactivity—since most of the patients seen are likely to exhibit multiple risk factors. As diabetes programs normally exist at major hospitals, these specialty programs will normally receive the referrals for many of the diabetic patients.

A preventive cardiology clinic should be prepared to handle more difficult-to-manage cases of dyslipidemia and hypertension as well as problems related to obesity and tobacco use. The initial visit will normally require a comprehensive medical history and physical examination (see Appendix 24–1). Frequently, it will be desirable to conduct a battery of assessment tests—including a blood chemistry and fasting lipid profile, nutritional and exercise inventory, and a behavioral health survey—and have them completed prior to the initial physician visit. These results should be made available to the physician in advance of the patient visit, so that a preliminary review and initial plan (see Appendix 24–1) can be drafted and, if necessary, modified at the initial visit.

A single physician director and, if necessary, other trained physicians with expertise in the major risk-factor therapeutic areas will usually provide medical supervision for the program. In some cases, there will be a research or administrative director responsible for research operations or general management. A nurse or other allied health care provider, such as a clinical pharmacist, will frequently be employed as a clinic manager for the facility, and additional nurses and administrative staff will provide the needed support services (Fig. 24–1).

As in the office-based approach, access is needed to a specialized team of allied health care providers, including dietitians, exercise physiologists, psychologists, and other personnel (Table 24–4, Fig. 24–1).[9] For the specialty clinic, such individuals will ideally be on staff, either part or full time, dedicated to pro-

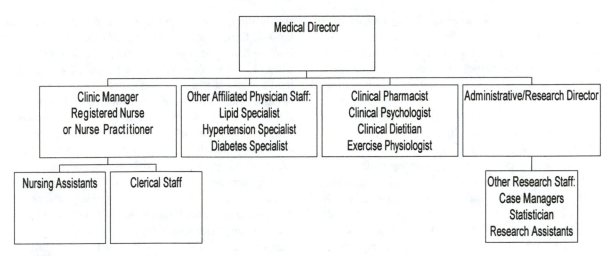

FIGURE 24–1 Schematic diagram of a physician-directed specialty clinic for preventive cardiology services.

viding the highest quality of care for patients seen by the clinic. Patients should normally be able to do "one-stop" preventive care for cardiovascular disease, where most services will be available in a single facility.

Pharmacist and Nurse or Nurse Practitioner Case-Management Approaches

In an increasing number of health care settings, particularly within managed care, the role of the pharmacist or nurse/nurse practitioner has been expanded to provide, with the assistance of a physician supervisor, a wide range of preventive services. One scenario is the operation of a lipid or hypertension clinic using a case-management approach. While such a clinic is usually overseen by a physician, the nurse or pharmacist may be the focal point of care. A pharmacist-coordinated clinic may be appropriate where multiple or complex medication algorithms need to be followed and where the patient can benefit from advice on how to best comply with prescribed medications. A nurse-based case-management system may be most useful for more general risk-factor reduction or lifestyle modification efforts. Ultimately,

available resources will be an important factor in determining the precise administrative structure.

Protocols for pharmacologic management of lipid disorders (and/or hypertension), can be followed closely by the pharmacist in conjunction with the physician, who approves all prescriptions. This type of setting can be successful in managing thousands of patients in a given facility who attend follow-up visits with staff within a pharmacist-based clinic. The pharmacist is well prepared to provide patient education, particularly with respect to information about cardiovascular risk factors and their control, and to ensure compliance with the prescribed medication regimen. One study demonstrated a community pharmacy to be an easily accessible, well accepted, and effective site for cholesterol screenings, with a high degree of follow-up of abnormal results.[25] In many cases, basic lifestyle counseling can also be delivered by a pharmacist.

Case-management systems for risk factor modification, such as those operated by trained nurses, can not only be more efficacious but are often more cost-effective than physician-staffed risk-factor modification approaches. This is true partly because of full-time, dedicated staff often involved and reliance by some systems on phone and mail contact rather than face-to-face visits. Nurses can be hired and trained to devote their time completely to such an activity, whereas physicians must often divide their efforts among numerous responsibilities. Patient satisfaction and convenience are often enhanced by such approaches.

A nurse or nurse practitioner case-management approach has been shown to be effective in the management of hypertension,[26] diabetes,[27] smoking cessation,[28] and hyperlipidemia.[29] Among patients with CHD, a physician-directed, nurse-managed, home-based case-management system for coronary risk-factor modification showed, compared to usual care, a significantly greater confirmed smoking cessation rate (70 versus 53 percent, respectively), better LDL-C control (107 versus 132 mg/dL), and improved functional capacity [9.3 versus 8.4 metabolic units (METs)].[30] A recently published trial of 19 nurse-run general practice clinics involving 1173 patients with CHD showed after 1 year significant improvements in aspirin use, blood pressure control, lipid management, physical activity, and diet modification, but not smoking cessation.[31]

A case-management approach, such as that offered by a dedicated pharmacist or nurse, can improve the efficacy of risk-factor modification because three important objectives are achieved: (1) patients can be encouraged to adhere to drug and diet regimens; (2) patients can be instructed in the self-monitoring of weight, blood pressure, blood glucose, or smoking relapse; and (3) patients can be taught to take appropriate action in response to new or worsening symptoms. Such a system can be integrated into the usual care of patients with the use of existing facilities (hospital or outpatient clinics) and convenient channels of communication (telephone, mail, and even the Internet).[10] Physicians can be kept apprised of patients' progress, and be involved in approving prescriptions and management strategies.

Approach to Preventive Care

The approach to delivering preventive cardiology services begins with the traditional workup by medical history and physical examination, as in a traditional practice. The clinical and laboratory findings should then be summarized and related to a general level of CHD risk, as by using a health appraisal or Framingham-type risk algorithm (such as presented in Chap. 1). The risk level should be linked to the patient's personal behavior and genetic makeup as well as family and social behaviors. Smoking, eating, physical activity, and weight change should be reviewed and possible causes of excess risk discussed. The entire family should be engaged in making healthy lifestyle choices, reducing risk if it is high, and preventing increases in risk at all ages. The patient should be encouraged to set goals and be given guidance on how to reach them. Progress should be reviewed at each visit and there should be a focus on success rather than failure. Whether a patient is at low, medium, or high risk based on the evaluation, positive messages related to preventive strategies should be given.[32]

Barriers to Implementation of Preventive Services

A number of barriers—patient, physician, and external—have been identified that can affect the delivery of, and compliance with, preventive services.

Patient factors may involve lack of knowledge and motivation, lack of access to care, cultural factors, and social factors. Physicians frequently perceive patients as unmotivated or noncompliant, but patients indicate preventive services as a high priority in their health care and frequently cite physicians' failure to order certain tests or communicate results of such tests.[11,20]

Physician barriers to implementing preventive services may include their fundamental focus on and increasing time commitment to acute care—often including noninvasive and invasive procedures. In addition, the pressures of the managed care environment have tended to result in shorter times being allotted to patient visits. Also, while reimbursement for acute interventions is frequently perceived as acceptable, reimbursement remains generally poor for risk-factor interventions[11]—particularly dietary and other ancillary services—a major reason for their not being appropriately utilized. Risk-factor interventions may also be accompanied by patient complaints of side effects. Finally, lack of training or confidence in implementing risk-reduction strategies—such as smoking cessation, dietary counseling, or even treatment with cholesterol-lowering medications—is cited by a substantial proportion of primary care physicians[33] as an important barrier to the delivery of preventive services. Cardiologists do not fare much better in terms of reporting adequate training and confidence in applying preventive strategies. This is not surprising, given that most cardiology programs do not have specialists in treatment of lipid disorders or risk-factor management, resulting in inadequate training in preventive cardiology.[11,34]

Although physicians and other health care providers may be ready and able to provide preventive services, hospitals often create obstacles to their implementation. Often, the focus of care in secondary and tertiary care hospitals is on acute conditions that prompt hospital admission. Furthermore, once the patient is hospitalized, there is frequently limited time to interact with (and educate) the patient because of the pressures for early discharge.[11] In addition, patients are not necessarily in the best condition to discuss nutrition, exercise, or other preventive strategies. However, while they are in the acute care setting, they are often highly impressionable and can be encouraged to make such changes. Unfortunately, there is frequently a lack of infrastructure or resources, including facilities and staffing, to allow health care professionals to focus on risk-factor management. Staff nurses are often trained to deal with acute management issues, and neither physicians nor nurses have undergone formal training in the behavioral aspects of risk-factor modification. Finally, most hospitals do not ensure adequate continuity of care after the hospitalization, making long-term risk-factor modification difficult to ensure.[11]

Educational Programs

Professional

Although postgraduate continuing medical education programs frequently provide courses and symposia directed at cardiovascular risk reduction, few physician training programs (e.g., internal medicine residencies or cardiology fellowships) provide sufficient background in preventive cardiology. Subspecialty training programs should include requirements for adequate instruction on (1) the pathophysiologic roles of risk factors and epidemiologic and clinical trial evidence supporting the efficacy of treatment in reducing the risk of cardiovascular disease, (2) comprehensive assessment of individual risk factors and overall risk, and (3) techniques to modify risk factors using both lifestyle and pharmacologic interventions.[35,36] It is also important that training take place in an academic medical center or institution with a strong commitment to academic training and appropriate certification. Trainees in adult cardiology training programs should have adequate preparation in the biological, physical, and epidemiologic sciences basic to medicine.[36] The American College of Cardiology has proposed content for such a training program at three levels (Table 24–5).[36]

Family practice physicians frequently see patients with major coronary risk factors; they should be able to assess an individual patient's overall risk and provide advice and counseling to reduce that risk. Teaching-consultation clinics have been developed where family practice residents learn from knowledgeable faculty with expertise in preventive cardiology how to assess cardiac risk in the general patient and develop counseling skills to manage that risk.[37]

Once a preventive cardiology clinic is established, mechanisms for integrating participation in the clinic by cardiology fellows and internal medicine residents should be developed. In addition, opportunities should be provided to enhance training of dietetic, exercise physiology, and behavioral medicine interns as members of the preventive cardiology health care team. Patient conferences reviewing specific cases and involving input from all members of the team can be an invaluable educational experience while also enhancing the quality of patient care by obtaining input from multiple disciplines simultaneously.

Community Education

Educational programs on preventing heart disease aimed at the community can potentially provide

TABLE 24–5 Recommended Content for Training in Preventive Cardiovascular Medicine

Level 1

This includes training that should be part of the knowledge base of all clinical cardiologists and includes exposure to the following general and specific areas.

General content areas:

1. Vascular biology of the heart and blood vessels (It is important for future cardiovascular medicine trainees to understand the language of molecular biology as well to continue self-study and critical review of published medical reports.)
2. Clinical epidemiology and biostatistics
3. Principles of clinical trials and outcomes research
4. Principles of clinical pharmacology

Exposure to the following specific content areas is also essential:

1. Diagnosis and treatment of primary and secondary hypertension
2. Diagnosis and treatment of primary and secondary dyslipidemias
3. Diagnosis and treatment of thrombosis and hypercoagulable states
4. Management of smoking cessation and nicotine addiction
5. Cardiac rehabilitation
6. Exercise physiology
7. Nutrition and its effects on the cardiovascular system
8. Psychosocial and behavioral aspects of cardiovascular diseases
9. Diagnosis and treatment of peripheral vascular disease

Training in these areas should be integrated into consultative, inpatient, and outpatient rotations and into didactic components of the core cardiovascular medicine programs. The time allotted should be equivalent to 1 month of full-time training. Alternatively, this goal could be met by 1 month of block time followed by experience in continuity clinics.

Level 2

Level 2 training should achieve a level of expertise for the cardiovascular specialist so that the trainee could serve as an independent consultant to other cardiovascular practitioners in the management of cardiovascular risk factors. This should involve 6 to 12 months of training within the 36 months of a cardiovascular training program and include block time for direct evaluation of patients with advanced atherosclerosis, resistant hypertension or hyperlipidemia, or recurrent thrombosis.

This could involve block time in hypertension and lipid clinics or services or both, coagulation laboratories, peripheral vascular laboratories, clinical and cardiac rehabilitation services, and additional exposure to behavioral medicine, exercise physiology, clinical epidemiology, outcomes research, and vascular biology.

The clinical application of information contributed by newly emerging fields, such as vascular biology and medicine, lends itself to the development of the clinician/scientist and the expert teacher/clinician.

Level 3

Level 3 requires advanced training to qualify as a director of a clinical service or research program or both. Examples include director of a preventive cardiology, hypertension or lipid service; director of a cardiac rehabilitation program; director of a vascular biology laboratory; or a trainee who obtains a Master of Public Health degree in clinical epidemiology, outcomes research, or both.

Training to this level would require at least 1 year of a 36-month program. Alternatively, 2 to 3 years in a vascular biology laboratory or health services outcomes research/clinical epidemiology program would be required to attain expertise in these fields, possibly leading to an advanced degree.

information of interest and relevance to most lay attendees. Participating physicians, dietitians, and other members of the health care team should conduct community outreach seminars on such popular topics as (1) how to optimize cholesterol control, (2) nutritional strategies for preventing heart disease, (3) preventing heart disease in women, and (4) preventing heart disease in the elderly. The public is eager to learn all they can about how to prevent a disease that has likely affected many of their friends if not themselves. They are often anxious, whether in a lecture or small group setting, to obtain informed advice by professionals specializing in the topic on which they are being addressed—information that they frequently are unable to obtain from their limited contact with their primary health care provider.

Often, such talks are an integral part of community education programs offered by senior centers, corporations, local hospitals, and organizations such as the American Heart Association. Physicians and other health care personnel with the appropriate expertise should be encouraged to participate on community education speaker bureaus.

Educational community outreach programs are especially needed for minority and underserved communities. An example is the National Heart Lung and Blood Institute (NHLBI) Latino Community Cardiovascular Disease Prevention and Outreach Initiative, Salud para su Corazon. This heart disease prevention and education campaign addresses language preferences and cultural values by developing educational materials and interventions targeting the Latino community.[38]

Research

An active preventive cardiology program will often be engaged in research—basic, epidemiologic, and/or clinical—investigation aimed at elucidating mechanisms of atherosclerosis development or plaque stabilization, epidemiologic projects studying newer risk factors or subclinical disease assessment, or clinical trials testing the efficacy of newer pharmacologic agents for risk-factor reduction. Such research—particularly projects that have national recognition or those that offer unique treatments or services—can help to establish the program as a center of excellence, enhancing its reputation in the community. Furthermore, patients are often interested (sometimes because of financial need) in participating in ongoing clinical trials, such as those testing newer cholesterol-lowering agents, that provide them with medications, limited risk-factor evaluation, and consultative services to which they may not otherwise have access.

Conclusions

While the provision of preventive services can be challenging in the current health care environment, most providers express a desire to implement such services, and a high proportion of the public expects such services and is willing to pay for them.[10] A team effort to implement preventive cardiology services and a process of continuous quality improvement will promote the delivery of high-quality preventive services.[10] Physicians and other health care providers must reflect on the strengths, limitations, resources, and goals at hand and settle on the systematic practice of preventive cardiology as a routine component of medical care.[32] Physicians and all health care providers must decide themselves to implement the lessons we have learned regarding the value of prevention. We all would prefer to prevent our own heart attack or stroke rather than join a rehabilitation program or relearn how to speak or walk all over again. This message should be emphasized to our patients and colleagues whenever and wherever we can.

APPENDIX 24-1 SAMPLE CLINIC FORMS FOR INITIAL ASSESSMENT, INITIAL PLAN, PHYSICAL EXAMINATION, PERSONAL MEDICAL HISTORY, PROGRESS, AND FOLLOW-UP

Initial Assessment

Date of Services _____

Referral: ☐ self   ☐ send copy to Dr. _____

Summary: _____ year old (Cauc Hisp Black Oriental Am. Indian) M / F   for (evaluation   treatment) of

_____

_____

_____

_____

_____

_____

_____

_____

_____

_____

_____

#1   **Hyperlipidemia Dx:** Heterozygous / Homozygous Familial Hypercholesterolemia (FH)   definite / probable
Familial Defective Apo B (apo B_{3500} or FDB) polygenic   Other IIa _____

Familial Combined Hyperlipidemia (FCHL) type IIb   type III   type IV   LPL deficiency   type I/V   low HDL   high
Lp(a)   other _____

_____

_____

_____

Molecular Defect(s) (if known): _____

Contributing cause(s): overweight   inactivity   smoking   diabetes   menopause   estrogen   hypothyroidism

hepatic disease   renal disease   alcohol   other _____

_____

_____

Risk for pancreatitis (trig):   ☐ minimal (<1000 mg/dL)   ☐ moderate (1000-2000 mg/dL)   ☐ high (>2000 mg/dL)

Current diet: ☐ poor ("typical" American)   ☐ fair (step1)   ☐ good (step 2)   ☐ excellent (step 3)
☐ vegetarian with very low saturated fat _____

_____

_____

Medications (indications / rationale): _____

_____

_____

_____

_____

Additional indicated Rx: control 2° cause   diet   weight loss   exercise   sugar control   added fiber
fish   fish oil   alcohol restriction   modest alcohol OK   estrogen replacement   decrease estrogen
change to estrogen patch   antioxidants (Vit E, Vit C)   vitamin therapy for high homocysteine

_____

_____

_____

#2   Coronary Artery Disease: ☐ none suggested   ☐ possible   ☐ probable   ☐ needs evaluation
☐ definite (prior Dx):   Events (ages): MI _____   CABG _____   PTCA _____
Chest pain: none   nonanginal   old / new   angina (atypical   definite   unstable) _____

_____

Physiology: CHF (mild   moderate   severe)   EF _____%   Arrhythmias _____

Other CAD risk reduction indicated: ☐ ASA   ☐ β blocker   ☐ ACE inhibitor   ☐ Cardiac rehab

_____

#3   Other Cardiovascular Disease: ☐ TIA (age of onset) _____   (most recent) _____
☐ Stroke (ages) _____   [thrombotic / embolic (source) _____ / hemorrhagic]

_____

☐ Peripheral vascular disease _____

_____

☐ Hypertension _____

_____

_____

#4   Other CV Risk Factors: +FHx   smoking   diabetes   overweight   high homocysteine   other

_____

_____

_____

_____

_____

From Cardiovascular Genetics Research. University of Utah, Salt Lake City, UT, with permission.

Initial Plan

Date of Services _____

1. **Diet & Exercise Therapy:** *(in all cases a diet low in saturated fat and cholesterol is strongly encouraged)*
    - ☐ Meet with dietitian   ☐ Diet classes   ☐ Controlled sugar   ☐ Added fiber   ☐ Encourage fish
    - ☐ Fish oil (dose) _____   ☐ Antioxidants (Vit E 400-800 IU qd   Vit C 250-500 mg qd)
    - ☐ Very low fat diet (≤10% calories fat) _____
    - ☐ Vitamin therapy for high homocysteine _____
    - ☐ Weight loss _____
    - ☐ Exercise _____
    - ☐ Other _____
    _____

2. **Lipid Meds:** ☐ Continue current therapy   ☐ Discontinue _____
    - ☐ Add / Change _____
    _____

    - ☐ Information sheet(s) given: statins   resins   niacin   gemfibrozil   antioxidants   high homocysteine   weight loss
    _____

3. **Other Medications:** ☐ ASA _____ mg qd _____
    _____
    _____
    _____

4. **Initial Labs:** <u>Date</u> _____ ☐ Extended lipid panel (circle method: ultracentrifugation / direct LDL)
    - ☐ Coronary risk (total cholesterol, triglycerides, HDL, calculated LDL)   ☐ Lp(a)   ☐ apo E genotype
    - ☐ Liver panel (Alk Phos, ALT, AST, GGT, bilirubin total & direct)   ☐ CK (total)   ☐ T4   ☐ TSH
    - ☐ Chemistry panel (glucose, uric acid, creatinine, BUN, albumin)   ☐ Electrolytes (Na, K, Cl, Bicarb, Ca)
    - ☐ Homocysteine   ☐ Hgb_{A1c} ☐ SPEP   ☐ CBC with auto diff   ☐ urinalysis (blood, protein, sugar)
    _____

    Other Labs: _____ ☐ Extended Lipid Panel (circle method: ultracentrifugation / direct LDL)
    - ☐ Coronary Risk (total cholesterol, triglycerides, HDL, calculated LDL)   ☐ Lp(a)   ☐ apo E genotype
    - ☐ Liver panel (Alk Phos, ALT, AST, GGT, bilirubin total & direct)   ☐ CK (total)   ☐ T4   ☐ TSH
    - ☐ Chemistry panel (glucose, uric acid, creatinine, BUN, albumin)   ☐ Electrolytes (Na, K, Cl, Bicarb, Ca)
    - ☐ Homocysteine   ☐ Hgb_{A1c} ☐ SPEP   ☐ CBC with auto diff   ☐ urinalysis (blood, protein, sugar)
    _____

5. Return to clinic in _____ Consider: _____
    FLC 7/5-98 uucvg   Resident/Fellow _____ Clinic Physician _____

From Cardiovascular Genetics Research. University of Utah, Salt Lake City, UT, with permission.

Initial Physical Exam

Date of Services _____

(See reverse side for additional narrative history)   M.D. Initials _____

☐ *performed*   ☐ *deferred*   *(Underline heading if examined and normal, circle and describe abnormalities)*

Vital signs: Height _____ (in / cm)   Weight _____ (lbs / kg)   BMI _____ (kg/m²)

sitting-BP: R _____ / _____ L _____ / _____ Heart Rate _____ bpm (reg / irreg)

Orthostatics: lying BP _____ / _____ HR _____   standing BP _____ / _____ HR _____

Temp _____ ° C / F Resp _____ Comments: _____

_____

General appearance: overweight (central / diffuse   mild / moderate / morbid)   Cushingoid   acromegaly (pos / def)

_____

Head, neck, lymphatics: thyroid   earlobe crease present   lymph nodes _____

_____

Eyes: arcus (partial / complete)   xanthelasma   lipemia retinalis   definite arteriolar narrowing   wiring (silver / copper)

A-V nicking   hemorrhages   exudates   microaneurysms   neovascularization _____

_____

Chest: crackles   wheezes   rhonchi   expiratory delay   diminished sounds   dullness _____

_____

Cardiovascular: elevated JVP _____   enlarged heart   S1 (increased / decreased)   S2 (paradoxical split / S2>S1 apex)

S3   S4   mid-systolic click   Murmurs: systolic ejection (likely innocent / likely pathological / uncertain)

holosystolic   late systolic   diastolic   Pulses: decreased (R / L carotid   R / L radial   R / L femoral   R / L PT

R / L DP)   Osler's +   bruit (R / L carotid   sys / dia aortic   R / L renal   R / L femoral)   abdominal aneurysm

Doppler: Arm systolic: R _____ L _____   Ankle systolic: R _____ L _____   Ankle/Arm index _____

_____

_____

Abdomen: R / L enlarged kidney   hepatomegaly   splenomegaly   ascites _____

_____

_____

Extremities & neurological: edema   xanthomas   reflexes (unequal   delayed relaxation)   Babinski   Gait   Other

_____

_____

Other findings and comments: _____

_____

FLC 11/5-98 uucvg   Intern/Resident _____ Clinic Physician _____

From Cardiovascular Genetics Research. University of Utah, Salt Lake City, UT, with permission.

Personal Medical History

Name _____

Age _____ Birthdate _____ Date filled out this form _____

Referred by: _____ Address _____

Primary care physician: _____ Address _____

Main reason you are seeking help at this time: _____

_____

_____

Current Medications *(List all medicines and supplements you are currently taking.)*

Medication or supplement name (include aspirin, etc.)	Pill size or dose	Times taken per day	Date started (approximate)	Why started, any problems
Example - Lovastatin	20 m	2	9/89	High cholesterol
_____	_____	_____	_____	_____
_____	_____	_____	_____	_____
_____	_____	_____	_____	_____
_____	_____	_____	_____	_____
_____	_____	_____	_____	_____
_____	_____	_____	_____	_____
_____	_____	_____	_____	_____
_____	_____	_____	_____	_____
_____	_____	_____	_____	_____
_____	_____	_____	_____	_____

Current Medical Problems *(describe any active problems you are currently being seen for)*

_____

_____

_____

_____

_____

_____

Allergies *(also note reaction to each)*

Food: _____

_____

Medications: _____

_____

Other (such as hay fever): _____

_____

Past Medical Problems *(please circle if you have ever been diagnosed with any of the following problems. If none, check "none")*

Head and Eye Problems: None ☐

head injuries   frequent headaches   migraines   glaucoma   cataracts   macular degeneration   serious eye injury
serious eye infection

Other: _____

Ear, Nose and Throat Problems: None ☐

hearing loss   vertigo   chronic sinusitis   nasal polyps frequent nose bleeds   recurrent throat infections

Other: _____

Respiratory Problems: None ☐

asthma   chronic obstructive pulmonary disease (COPD)   emphysema   pulmonary embolism   sleep apnea

Other: _____

Cardiovascular Problems: None ☐

Heart attack(s) (date, age, hospital): _____

_____

_____

_____

Angioplasty or atherectomy (date, age, hospital): _____

_____

_____

_____

Coronary bypass surgery (date, age, hospital): _____

_____

_____

_____

Angina (duration, severity): _____

_____

_____

_____

Most recent angiogram or treadmill (date, results): _____

_____

_____

_____

Arrhythmias, valvular or other heart disease: _____

_____

_____

Stroke or transient ischemic attack (age, hospital): _____

_____

_____

Claudication or aortic aneurysm (age of onset, surgeries):

_____
_____

Venous thrombosis (date or age, hospital): _____
_____
_____

Varicose veins (any surgeries, procedures): _____
_____

Other: _____
_____
_____

Gastrointestinal Problems *(circle):*   None ☐
esophageal spasm esophagitis acid reflux hiatal hernia ulcer (stomach or duodenal) gastritis
liver cirrhosis hepatitis: (type _____) pancreatitis (age _____) irritable bowel diverticulosis diverticulitis colitis
Other: _____

Genitourinary Problems*(circle):*   None ☐
frequent bladder infections urethritis prostatitis
glomerulonephritis nephrotic syndrome kidney stones   vaginitis candida infections renal vascular disease
Other: _____

Nervous System Problems: None ☐
Alzheimer's multiple sclerosis peripheral neuropathy
Other: _____

Blood and Lymph Problems: None ☐
Anemia (low blood count) Clotting disorder lymphoma
Other: _____

Cancer *(give age, therapy, and outcome):*   None ☐
breast lung colon prostate cervix uterus blood melanoma other skin (type)
Other: _____
_____
_____
_____

Endocrine & Metabolic Problems: None ☐
high cholesterol high triglycerides low HDL diabetes low thyroid (hypothyroidism) high thyroid Grave's gout
severe obesity Cushing's pituitary insufficiency
Other: _____

Muscle, Bone, Joint Problems: None ☐
low back pain osteoarthritis rheumatoid arthritis osteoporosis systemic lupus erythematosus
Other: _____

Skin and Hair Problems: None ☐
severe acne psoriasis alopecia severe skin infections

Other: _____

Emotional Problems: None ☐

depression   anxiety   panic attacks   schizophrenia

Other: _____

_____

Surgeries *(list age and type of surgery)*

_____

_____

_____

_____

_____

_____

_____

_____

Risk Factors *(check all that apply)*

Blood Pressure

My last blood pressure check was (date) _____. Results: systolic _____ / diastolic _____

Was this result typical? (Circle) yes / no   If not, what is your usual blood pressure? _____ / _____.

☐   I was never told that my blood pressure was high.

☐   I am currently taking medications for high blood pressure. First started medications age _____.

☐   My blood pressure was borderline/high in the past but is now normal without special treatment.

☐   My blood pressure was borderline/high in the past but is well controlled with diet and/or exercise.

☐   I have been told I have borderline or high blood pressure but it was **never treated**.

☐   My blood pressure increased in **pregnancy** to a degree that my physician(s) was/(were) concerned, or I had **toxemia**.

List any blood pressure medications you have had in the past and why you stopped taking them (side effects, etc):

_____

_____

_____

Diabetes

☐   I have never been told that I have diabetes.

☐   I have had diabetes since (age) _____.

☐   My diabetes is controlled with weight loss and diet.

☐   I take oral medication for my diabetes (yrs _____).

☐   I take insulin for my diabetes (yrs _____).

☐   I check my blood sugar levels at home regularly.

Prior diabetes medications: _____

_____

Exercise

☐ I do not exercise regularly.

☐ I walk for _____ minutes _____ times per week.

☐ I do other moderate exercise (gardening, playing tennis, etc.) 3 or more times each week but do not keep track of my pulse rate.

☐ I engage in vigorous exercise 3 or more times each week which raises my heart rate to a good training level (about 75% of my maximum) for at least 20 minutes without interruption.

☐ I engage in vigorous sports (basketball, racquetball, soccer, other) _____ times each week.

☐ I engage in weight training or resistance exercises.

☐ I am not able to exercise because of pain or limitation (specify):

_____

_____

Tobacco

☐ I have never smoked cigarettes

☐ I smoked cigarettes in the past but have quit:

Number of years since quit: _____

Average packs per day while smoking _____

Total number of years smoked: _____

☐ I currently smoke cigarettes:

Average packs per day: _____

Total number of years smoked: _____

☐ I smoke a pipe. # per day _____ for _____ yrs

☐ I smoke cigars. # per day _____ for _____ yrs

☐ I use snuff or chew tobacco.

Alcohol

☐ I never drink alcoholic beverages (skip to the next section)

☐ I have less than one drink per week (skip to the next section)

☐ I have one or more drinks per week (list amounts):

_____ cans of beer

_____ glasses of wine

_____ shots of whiskey, vodka, rum, etc.

☐ I have felt a need to cut down on my drinking.

☐ I have sometimes felt annoyed by criticism about my drinking.

☐ I have felt guilty at times about drinking.

☐ I sometimes have a morning "eye-opener."

Serum Cholesterol History *(Please call your physician's office for past results if you do not have them.)*

Date	Weight	Total Cholesterol	Serum Trigl	HDL Chol	LDL Chol	Treatment for cholesterol at the time of other test results, comments
_____	_____	_____	_____	_____	_____	_____
_____	_____	_____	_____	_____	_____	_____

_____	_____	_____	_____	_____	_____	_____	_____
_____	_____	_____	_____	_____	_____	_____	_____
_____	_____	_____	_____	_____	_____	_____	_____
_____	_____	_____	_____	_____	_____	_____	_____
_____	_____	_____	_____	_____	_____	_____	_____

List below any cholesterol or triglyceride lowering drugs you have tried or that were prescribed for you in the past (including niacin and fish oil) and any adverse effects you may have experienced while using them:

_____

_____

_____

Caffeine Intake *list cups or cans per day of:*

caffeinated coffee: _____   decaffeinated coffee: _____

regular tea: _____   caffeinated soda pop: _____

Sleep

Usual number of hours of sleep: _____

Heavy snoring? Y / N   Sleep apnea? Y / N

Other sleep problems: _____

Vaccinations *(list approximate year of most recent)*

Tetanus and diphtheria _____

Pneumovax (pneumococcal vaccine) _____

Flu _____   Hepatitis B _____

Measles _____   Mumps _____   Rubella _____

Social History

Circle: Single   Married   Divorced   Spouse deceased

Number in household (include self) _____

Number of close friends or relatives near you: _____

Are you active in a religious or social group? Y / N

Years of education (12 = high school grad.) _____

Occupation: _____

Occupational Exposures *(circle):*   None ☐

loud noise   paints   solvents   dyes   mineral dust   organic dust (hay, flour, etc.)

Other: _____

Seat belts worn in the car: always   sometimes   never

For Women

Age when period first started _____

Number of live births _____ Miscarriages _____

Age at first pregnancy _____ Complications? Y / N

_____

Passed <u>menopause</u>? Y / N Age at menopause _____

Bleeding problems/spotting? Y / N _____

_____

<u>Hysterectomy</u>? (Age) _____ Ovaries removed? Y / N

Birth control pills ever? Y / N Years since used _____

Last breast exam _____ Mammogram _____

Any problems noted? _____

Last PAP smear _____ Normal? Y / N

<u>Estrogen replacement therapy</u>: Age started _____

Age stopped _____ Problems? : _____

_____

From Cardiovascular Genetics Research. University of Utah, Salt Lake City, UT, with permission.

Progress Note

Date of Services_____

Referral: ☐ self ☐ send copy to Dr. _____

HISTORICAL (include current diet compliance):- _____

_____

_____

_____

_____

_____

_____

_____

_____

_____

Medications, Dose	Compliance (%)	Side Effects, Other Problems, Changes, Comments
	( )	
	( )	
	( )	
	( )	
	( )	
	( )	
	( )	
	( )	

Exercise Level/Tolerance: _____

_____

Other CV Risk Factors: smoking hypertension diabetes overweight high homocysteine _____

_____

_____

_____

Cardiovascular Symptoms/Events/Procedures Update: _____

_____

_____

☐ definite CHD (ages): MI _____ CABG _____ PTCA _____ Other _____

☐ CVD (ages): stroke: _____ TIA_____ ☐ PVD _____

From Cardiovascular Genetics Research. University of Utah, Salt Lake City, UT, with permission.

OBSERVATIONS: Height _____in   Weight _____lbs   BP_____

_____

Physical Exam: ☐ deferred   ☐ performed   Findings (include xanthoma changes): _____

_____

_____

Labs: Date_____   Chol _____   Trig _____   HDL _____   LDL (calc / meas) _____
meas VLDL _____   meas VLDL / Trig _____   Estimated β-VLDL Chol _____   Apo E _____
Lp(a) _____   Homocysteine _____   Glucose_____   T4 _____   TSH _____
Abnormal LFT's / Renal / Uric Acid/Other Labs: _____

_____

ASSESSMENT

#1   Hyperlipidemia: Dx & contributing cause(s): _____

_____

Risk for pancreatitis (trig): ☐minimal (<1000 mg/dL)   ☐moderate (1000-2000 mg/dL)   ☐ high (>2000 mg/dL)
Diet assessment: ☐ poor ("typical" American)   ☐ fair (step1)   ☐ good (step 2)   ☐ excellent (step 3+)
Medications (indications / rationale): _____

_____

_____

_____

Additional indicated Rx: control 2° cause   diet   weight loss   exercise   sugar control   added fiber
fish   fish oil   alcohol restriction   modest alcohol OK   estrogen replacement   decrease estrogen
change to estrogen patch   antioxidants (Vit E, Vit C)   vitamin therapy for high homocysteine

_____

_____

#2   Coronary Artery Disease: ☐ none suggested   ☐ possible   ☐ probable   ☐ definite (prior Dx)
Chest pain: none   nonanginal   old / new angina (atypical   definite   unstable)   ☐ needs evaluation
Other CAD risk reduction indicated: ☐ ASA   ☐ β blocker   ☐ ACE inhibitor   ☐ Cardiac rehab

_____

_____

_____

_____

_____

_____

_____

_____

_____

_____

From Cardiovascular Genetics Research. University of Utah, Salt Lake City, UT, with permission.

Follow-up Plan

Date of Services _____

1. Diet & Exercise Therapy: *(in all cases a diet low in saturated fat and cholesterol is strongly encouraged)*

   ☐ Meet with dietitian   ☐ Diet classes   ☐ Controlled sugar   ☐ Added fiber   ☐ Encourage fish

   ☐ Fish oil (dose) _____   ☐ Antioxidants (Vit E 400-800 IU qd   Vit C 250-500 mg qd)

   ☐ Very low fat diet (≤10% calories fat) _____

   ☐ Vitamin therapy for high homocysteine _____

   ☐ Weight loss _____

   ☐ Exercise _____

   ☐ Other _____

   _____

2. Lipid Meds: ☐ Continue current therapy   ☐ Discontinue _____

   ☐ Add / Change _____

   _____

   _____

   ☐ Information sheet(s) given: statins resins niacin gemfibrozil anti-oxidants high homocysteine weight loss

   _____

3. Other Medications: ☐ ASA _____ mg qd _____

   _____

   _____

   _____

4. Next Labs: Date _____   ☐ Extended lipid panel (circle method: ultracentrifugation / direct LDL)

   ☐ Coronary risk (total cholesterol, triglycerides, HDL, calculated LDL)   ☐ Lp(a)   ☐ apo E genotype

   ☐ Liver panel (Alk Phos, ALT, AST, GGT, bilirubin total & direct)   ☐ CK (total)   ☐ T4   ☐ TSH

   ☐ Chemistry panel (glucose, uric acid, creatinine, BUN, albumin)   ☐ Electrolytes (Na, K, Cl, Bicarb, Ca)

   ☐ Homocysteine   ☐ Hgb_{A1c} ☐ SPEP   ☐ CBC with auto diff   ☐ urinalysis (blood, protein, sugar)

   _____

   Other Labs: _____   ☐ Extended lipid panel (circle method: ultracentrifugation / direct LDL)

   ☐ Coronary Risk (total cholesterol, triglycerides, HDL, calculated LDL)   ☐ Lp(a)   ☐ apo E genotype

   ☐ Liver panel (Alk Phos, ALT, AST, GGT, bilirubin total & direct)   ☐ CK (total)   ☐ T4   ☐ TSH

   ☐ Chemistry panel (glucose, uric acid, creatinine, BUN, albumin)   ☐ Electrolytes (Na, K, Cl, Bicarb, Ca)

   ☐ Homocysteine   ☐ Hgb_{A1c} ☐ SPEP   ☐ CBC with auto diff   ☐ urinalysis (blood, protein, sugar)

   _____

5. Return to clinic in _____   Consider: _____

   _____

   Resident/Fellow _____   Clinic Physician _____

From Cardiovascular Genetics Research. University of Utah, Salt Lake City, UT, with permission.

References

1. Grundy SM, Balady GJ, Criqui MH, et al: Guide to primary prevention of cardiovascular diseases. A statement for health care professionals from the task force on risk reduction. *Circulation* 1997; 95:2329–2331.

2. Smith SC, Blair SN, Criqui MH, et al: Preventing heart attack and death in patients with coronary disease. *Circulation* 1995; 92:2–4.

3. Adult Treatment Panel: Summary of the Second Report of the National Cholesterol Education Program (NCEP) Expert Panel on Detection, Evaluation, and Treatment of High Blood Cholesterol in Adults. *JAMA* 1993; 269:3015–3023.

4. The Sixth Report of the Joint National Committee on Detection, Evaluation and Treatment of High Blood Pressure (JNC-VI). *Arch Intern Med* 1997; 157:2413–2446.

5. National Institutes of Health, National Heart, Lung, and Blood Institute: *Clinical Guidelines on the Identification, Evaluation, and Treatment of Overweight and Obesity in Adults: The Evidence Report.* Washington, DC, U.S. Department of Health and Human Services, 1998.

6. Sueta CA, Chowdhury M, Boccuzzi SJ, et al: Analysis of the degree of undertreatment of hyperlipidemia and congestive heart failure secondary to coronary artery disease. *Am J Cardiol* 1999; 83:1303–1307.

7. Burt VL, Cutler JA, Higgins M, et al: Trends in the prevalence, awareness, treatment, and control of hypertension in the adult U.S. population: data from the health examination surveys, 1960 to 1991. *Hypertension* 1995; 26:60–69.

8. Abrams J: Reporting of coronary risk factors. *Am J Cardiol* 1995; 75:716–717.

9. Joint Task Force of European and Other Societies on Coronary Prevention. Prevention of coronary heart disease in clinical practice. *Eur Heart J* 1998; 19:1434–1503.

10. Swan HJC, Gersh BJ, Graboys TB, Ullyot DJ (Task Force 7): 27th Bethesda Conference: matching the intensity of risk factor management with the hazard for coronary disease events: Task Force 7: evaluation and management of risk factors for the individual patient (case management). *J Am Coll Cardiol* 1996; 27:1030–1039.

11. Pearson TA, McBride PE, Miller NH, Smith SC (Task Force 8). 27th Bethesda Conference: matching the intensity of risk factor management with the hazard for coronary disease events: Task Force 8: organization of a preventive cardiology service. *J Am Coll Cardiol* 1996; 27:1039–1047.

12. EUROASPIRE: A European Society of Cardiology survey of secondary prevention of coronary heart disease: principal results. EUROASPIRE Study Group. European Action on Secondary Prevention through Intervention to Reduce Events. *Eur Heart J* 1997; 10:1569–1582.

13. Reed RG, Jenkins PL, Pearson TA: Laboratory's manner of reporting serum cholesterol affects clinical care. *Clin Chem* 1994; 40:847–848.

14. Williams BJ: Efficacy of a checklist to promote a preventive medicine approach. *J Tenn Med Assoc* 1981; 74:489–491.

15. McDonald CJ: Protocol-based computer reminders, the quality of care and the nonperfectibility of man. *N Engl J Med* 1976; 295:1351–1355.

16. Davidson RA, Fletcher SW, Retchin S, Duh S: A nurse-initiated reminder system for the periodic health examination. Implementation and evaluation. *Arch Intern Med* 1984; 144:2167–2170.

17. Weingarten SR, Riedinger MS, Conner L, et al: Practice guidelines and reminders to reduce duration of hospital stay for patients with chest pain: an interventional trial. *Ann Intern Med* 1994; 120:257–263.

18. Johnston ME, Langton KB, Haynes RB, Mathieu A: Effects of computer-based clinical decision support systems on clinician performance and patient outcome: a critical appraisal of research. *Ann Intern Med* 1994; 120:135–142.

19. Vuori HV: *Public Health in Europe, 1982.* Copenhagen: World Health Organization, 1982.

20. Kottke TE, Brekke ML, Solberg LI: Making time for preventive services. *Mayo Clin Proc* 1993; 68:785–791.

21. Smith SC: The challenge of risk reducing therapy for cardiovascular disease. *Am Fam Physician* 1997; 55:491–500.

22. Smith SC: The need for broad preventive therapies in the new millenium: a challenge to change. Lecture delivered June 5, 1999 at Reducing Cardiovascular Risk in the New Millennium: One Heart at a Time, Leesburg, VA (personal communication).

23. Makrides L, Veinot PL, Richard J, Allen MJ: Primary care physicians and coronary heart disease prevention: a practice model. *Patient Educ Counsel* 1997; 32:207–217.

24. Reddell JR: Expansion of an existing program for the prevention and reversal of heart disease. *J Cardiovas Mgt* 1997; 8:33–35.

25. Madejski RM, Madejski TJ: Cholesterol screening in a community pharmacy. *J Am Pharm Assoc* 1996; NS36:243–248.

26. Reichgott MJ, Pearson S, Hill MN: The nurse practitioner's role in complex patient management: hypertension. *J Natl Med Assoc* 1983; 75:1197–1204.

27. Weinberger M, Kirkman MS, Samsa GP, et al: A nurse-coordinated intervention for primary care patients with non-insulin-dependent diabetes mellitus: impact on glycemic control and health-related quality of life. *J Gen Intern Med* 1995; 10:59–66.

28. Taylor CB, Houston-Miller N, Killen JD, DeBusk RF: Smoking cessation after acute myocardial infarction: effects of a nurse-managed intervention. *Ann Intern Med* 1990; 113:118–123.

29. Blair TP, Bryant FJ, Bocuzzi S: Treatment of hypercholesterolemia by a clinical nurse using a stepped-care protocol in a nonvolunteer population. *Arch Intern Med* 1988; 148:1046–1048.

30. DeBusk RF, Miller NH, Superko HR, et al: A case-management system for coronary risk factor modification after acute myocardial infarction. *Ann Intern Med* 1994; 120:721–729.

31. Campbell NC, Ritchie LD, Thain J, et al: Secondary prevention in coronary heart disease: a randomised trial of nurse led clinics in primary care. *Heart* 1998; 80:447–452.

32. Kottke TE, Blackburn H, Brekke ML, Solberg LI: The systematic practice of preventive cardiology. *Am J Cardiol* 1987; 59:690–694.

33. Shea S, Gemson DH, Mossel P: Management of high blood cholesterol by primary care physicians: diffusion of the National Cholesterol Education Program Adult Treatment Panel guidelines. *J Gen Intern Med* 1990; 5:327–334.

34. Roberts WC: Getting cardiologists interested in lipids. *Am J Cardiol* 1993; 72:744–745.

35. 25th Bethesda Conference: Future personnel needs for cardiovascular health care, Nov. 15–16, 1993. *J Am Coll Cardiol* 1994; 24:275–328.

36. Sullivan JM, Frohlich ED, Lewis RP, Pasternak RC: Guidelines for Training in Adult Cardiovascular Medicine. Core Cardiology Training Symposium (COCATS). Task Force 10: training in preventive cardiovascular medicine. *J Am Coll Cardiol* 1995; 25:33–34.

37. Cable TA, Delaney MJ: Teaching preventive cardiology: the consultation clinic. *Am J Prev Med* 1996; 12:161–164.

38. Moreno C, Alvarado M, Balcazar H, et al: Heart disease education and prevention program targeting immigrant Latinos: using focus group responses to develop effective interventions. *J Commun Health* 1997; 22:435–450.

Index

ISBN 0-07-071856-3

90000

9 780070 718562